AN INTRODUCTION TO THE
US HEALTH CARE INDUSTRY

AN INTRODUCTION TO THE US HEALTH CARE INDUSTRY

BALANCING CARE, COST, AND ACCESS

DAVID S. GUZICK, MD, PHD

Johns Hopkins University Press

Baltimore

Johns Hopkins University Press
2715 North Charles Street
Baltimore, Maryland 21218-4363
www.press.jhu.edu

Library of Congress Cataloging-in-Publication Data

Names: Guzick, David, author.
Title: An introduction to the US health care industry : balancing care, cost, and
    access / David S. Guzick, MD, PhD.
Description: Baltimore : Johns Hopkins University Press, [2020] | Includes
    bibliographical references and index.
Identifiers: LCCN 2019052376 | ISBN 9781421438825 (hardcover ; alk. paper) |
    ISBN 9781421438658 (paperback ; alk. paper) | ISBN 9781421438665 (ebook)
Subjects: MESH: Health Care Sector—economics | Delivery of Health Care |
    Quality of Health Care | United States
Classification: LCC RA410.53 | NLM W 74 AA1 | DDC 338.4/73621—dc23
LC record available at https://lccn.loc.gov/2019052376

A catalog record for this book is available from the British Library.

*Special discounts are available for bulk purchases of this book. For more information, please
contact Special Sales at specialsales@press.jhu.edu.*

Johns Hopkins University Press uses environmentally friendly book materials, including
recycled text paper that is composed of at least 30 percent post-consumer waste, whenever
possible.

CONTENTS

PREFACE

Although the United States spends much more on health care than other nations, its population is in poorer health. Why is this? And what can be done about it? This book attempts to answer these two questions.

In comparison with 10 other high-income nations, per capita health care expenditures in the United States are almost twice as high, yet the US has the lowest life expectancy at birth, the highest rates of infant and neonatal mortality, and the most inequitable access to physicians when adjusted for need.[1]

These health outcomes are for the US population as a whole. The rich, however, are in much better health than the poor. At age 40, men and women at the highest level of income have life expectancies that are 14.6 and 10.1 years greater, respectively, than men and women at the lowest income level.[2]

What can one conclude from these data and the varied experience that Americans have with its "system" of health care? One might say that, in comparison with other countries with high per capita incomes:

"The United States has the best medical care for some but not for others."

or

"The United States has the best health care system for some but not for others."

or

"The United States has the best medical care *and* the best system for some but not for others."

All of these statements are largely true. I am in the fortunate last group, having experienced the best of our nation's medical care *and* health care system. In July 2017, I was diagnosed with an advanced-stage cancer. I received state-of-the-art (and, so far, curative) treatment. I had access to a wonderful facility and an extraordinary health care team at the University of Florida—where each patient receives care that is technically advanced while being highly personalized, attentive, and convenient. And although the fees for my treatment as paid by my employer's self-insurance plan were expensive, my personal "out-of-pocket" cost, including my deductible and coinsurance payments, was less than 10 percent of the total fees paid.

Others are less fortunate. Many in our nation have less access to the best contemporary treatment and much higher out-of-pocket costs.

In an August 6, 2010, *New York Times* op-ed piece, the highly respected health economist Uwe Reinhardt (1937–2017) began with an excerpt from a 2010 television talk show in which the host, William Shatner, has an exchange with Rush Limbaugh:[3]

> Shatner: "Here's my premise and you agree with it or not. If you have money, you are going to get health care. If you don't have money, it's more difficult."
>
> Limbaugh: "If you have money, you're going to get a house on the beach. If you don't have money, you're going to live in a bungalow somewhere."
>
> Shatner: "Right, but we're talking about health care."
>
> Limbaugh: "What's the difference?"
>
> Shatner: "The difference is we're talking about health care, not a house or a bungalow."
>
> Limbaugh: "No, no. You're assuming that there is some morally superior aspect to health care than there is to a house."

For more than a century, our nation has been struggling to find the right way to balance care, cost, and access in a manner that is consistent with our values. Specifically, we have struggled to balance several widely held, but conflicting, values and beliefs:

1. Individuals with significant illness (e.g., genetic disease, work injury, accidental trauma, life-threatening cancer, heart disease, neurologic conditions, or other significant illness) should be provided with high-quality, compassionate medical care.

2. In a market-based economy, there will be a large and acceptable variation in the financial capability of individuals to consume a variety of goods and services, including health care.
3. Public expenditures should be limited to avoid large governmental deficit and debt; that is, we should avoid the enormous public expense (and potentially inefficient private expense) of providing free (or almost free) access to medical care for all individuals and all types of illness.

As our century-long struggle to resolve these conflicting values failed to strike a balance between care, cost, and access, a large, complex, and internationally unique collection of entities with many moving parts evolved to create what can be called the "United States health care industry." While I used the more conventional term, "health care system" at the beginning of this preface, in the United States we really have more of an industry than a "system" because the latter would imply an organized, purposeful structure forming a unified whole. Rather, we have an industry of health care comprising a confederation of stakeholders.

This industry is now responsible for almost one in five dollars that circulate in our economy. But it is not in balance. The balance is tipped decidedly toward cost and spending without commensurate results regarding care and access. The goal of this book is to analyze the economic underpinnings, history, and current functioning of the US health care industry and to suggest ways in which we can strike a better balance among care, cost, and access.

ACKNOWLEDGMENTS

Over many decades, I was privileged to practice medicine and work as a researcher, educator, and administrator. More recently, as I experienced illness and medical care as a patient, the idea of a book about health care took shape in my mind. Translating these fuzzy thoughts into writing turned out to be quite another matter. As my rendition of the economic underpinnings, history, and current functioning of the US health care industry began to unfold, I realized I needed help. I reached out to individuals with expertise in a wide variety of disciplines. I am indebted to the following people who gave so generously of their time to answer my questions, clarify my writing, and provide their insights.

Carmen Allegra, William Friedman, Andrew Guzick, Daniel Ho, David Nelson, and William Slayton made edits and/or provided language for the examples of medical progress in chapter 1. Mark Flannery and Richard Romano clarified my presentation of economic principles. Discussions with David Cutler, Joseph Dielman, Alan Garber, Joseph Newhouse, Louise Sheiner, and Jonathan Skinner improved my understanding of results reported in the health economics literature, which hopefully translated into a clear presentation of those topics. Discussions with the following individuals about specific aspects of the US health care industry were extremely helpful: Bill Robinson and Paul Lipori (finance); Steve Ondra and Jill Sumfest (health insurance); Elliot Sussman (Medicare Advantage); Kari Cassel and Gigi Lipori (information technology and electronic health records); Elizabeth McGylnn (evidence-based practice); Robert Navarro (pharmaceutical supply chain); Desmond Schatz (insulin pricing); Haesuk Park and Doug Owens (cost-benefit and cost-effectiveness analysis); Mike Perri and Tom Pearson (social and behavioral determinants); Ray Dorsey (environmental determinants); Robert Califf (drugs and devices); and Marvin

Dewar, Ed Jimenez, and Jill Sumfest (hospitals and physicians). Abe East-man ensured that references were in accordance with the *Chicago Manual of Style* and Tamara Freeman converted data on historical National Institutes of Health funding into graphic form.

A number of individuals served as readers for one or more chapters and provided valuable edits: Hunter Beebe, Kari Cassel, Mark Flannery, Randy Jenkins, Ed Jimenez, David Lambert, Gigi Lipori, Chip Mainous, Steve Ondra, James Roberts, Richard Romano, Eric Rosenberg, Scott Rivkees, Elizabeth Rusczyk, Desmond Schatz, John Smulian, and Jill Sumfest. I am indebted to James Roberts for taking major responsibility for the chapter on health law.

Steve Ondra filled in historical details pertaining to the Affordable Care Act. He also provided informed insight and contributed language to my presentation of health policy, both content and process.

All of the tables and figures were created by Laura Huntley. Her skill in these endeavors was matched by her sophistication in translating my conceptual points in the best way.

On a daily basis, I bounced ideas off my wife, Donna Giles, and she bounced them back. Sometimes an idea was appropriately retired; for those that made some sense, she helped me sharpen these thoughts and put them in the right place. She also served as preliminary copy editor on all chapters.

Any opinion expressed in this book is my own, and I am responsible for any errors of commission or omission, notwithstanding all of the assistance listed above.

AN INTRODUCTION TO THE US HEALTH CARE INDUSTRY

SETTING THE STAGE
HEALTH AND HEALTH CARE
OVER THE PAST CENTURY

People are living much longer than did their parents and grandparents. In 1965, when President Lyndon B. Johnson signed into law legislation that amended the Social Security Act to establish Medicare and Medicaid, life expectancy at birth for males and females in the United States was 66.8 years and 73.8 years, respectively.[1] By 2017 life expectancy at birth for males and females had increased to 76.1 years and 81.1 years, respectively.[2] Thus, in the past 50 years, life expectancy has increased by almost a decade for males and 7.3 years for females.

When we track back another 50 years, life expectancy at birth in 1915 for males and females was 52.5 years and 56.8 years, respectively.[3] Thus, the *previous* half-century from 1915 to 1965 showed a more dramatic jump in life expectancy at birth—14.3 years for males and 17 years for females—than the most recent half-century (figure 1.1), despite the latter being an era of extraordinary biomedical discoveries that were translated into effective treatments for a broad range of diseases.

Much of this paradox can be explained by public health initiatives in the first part of the twentieth century that preferentially benefited young people. At the turn of that century, the three leading causes of death were microbial: pneumonia, tuberculosis, and diarrhea/enteritis.[4] Heart disease, which accounted for 32 percent of deaths by the end of the twentieth century, was the fourth leading cause of death in 1900 at only 8 percent. Cancer, responsible for 23 percent of deaths by the century's end, caused only 4 percent of deaths in 1900. Improvement in life expectancy during the first half of the twentieth century was largely due to initiatives that reduced infectious diseases, including major public health initiatives such as sewage disposal projects; chlorination and other water treatments; food safety; immunization against major killers such as typhoid, diphtheria, tetanus, influenza,

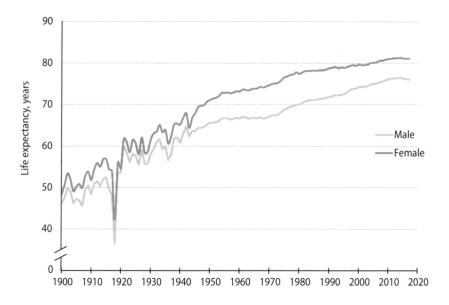

Figure 1.1. Life expectancy at birth, 1900–2017. Arias, Heron, and Xu, "United States Life Tables, 2014"[1]; Murphy et al., *Mortality in the United States, 2017.*[2]

poliomyelitis, and smallpox; and the introduction of antibiotics. These public health advances also affected adults: the expected years of life remaining at age 40 in the first half of the twentieth century increased from 27.3 years to 30.8 years for males and from 29.1 years to 35.1 years for females (figure 1.2).

Of particular note in the curve for life expectancy in figure 1.1 is the influenza pandemic of 1918, which affected about 500 million people worldwide (about a third of the world's population at that time) and had a very high mortality rate, even among previously healthy young people. Worldwide, about 50 million people died, one million of whom were Americans, producing a dramatic reduction in US life expectancy of about 12 years from 1917 to 1918. The isolation of the influenza virus in 1933 led to the development of vaccines that have successfully mitigated the impact of influenza epidemics by taking account of changes in the antigenic composition of the influenza virus.

Having dramatically reduced mortality due to bacteria and viruses during the first half of the century, attention then turned to emerging causes of morbidity, mortality, and disability, including heart disease, cancer, neurologic disorders, genetic conditions, and others. This transition in the United States parallels a shift in global mortality and disease patterns that Abdel Omran has described as a proposition in the theory of epidemiologic

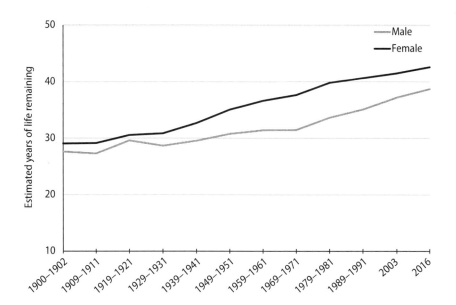

Figure 1.2. Life expectancy at age 40, according to death-registration time periods. Arias, Heron, and Xu, "United States Life Tables, 2014."[1]

transition: "During the transition, a long-term shift occurs in mortality and disease patterns whereby pandemics of infection are gradually displaced by degenerative and man-made diseases as the chief form of morbidity and primary cause of death."[5] To address these man-made diseases, the second half of the twentieth century became an era of accelerating breakthroughs in biomedical science and medical technology, as well as one of improved appreciation of the behavioral causes of acquired disease.

Overall, whether measured from birth or at age 40, the US population has gained about 7 to 9 years of life expectancy in the past 50–60 years. (As an unfortunate commentary on more recent trends in life expectancy, there has been an overall decline in life expectancy since 2014 due mainly to midlife deaths from drug overdoses, alcohol abuse, and suicides.)[6] Much of the gains in life expectancy since the mid-twentieth century can be attributed to progress in medical diagnosis and treatment, and in our understanding of health-making (prevention and wellness) behaviors. Later in this chapter, I summarize some examples of these advances, which have improved life expectancy and quality of life. But along with this progress in science and medicine has evolved a health care industry in the United States that is costly, complex, and inequitable.

Regarding cost, there wasn't much in the way of effective medical treatment on which to spend much money back in 1965 at the time that Medicare and Medicaid were enacted. Per capita national health care expenditure in 1965 was a mere $146.[7] But when government funding of Medicare and Medicaid began in 1965, increases in expenditures also began: third-party payments for health care, inclusive of Medicare, increased from 35 percent of total outlays in 1950 to 56 percent by 1967.[8]

The per capita national health care expenditure of $146 in 1965 ballooned to $10,739 in 2017, a 7,255 percent increase (figure 1.3). For comparison, the consumer price index increased only one tenth as fast during this time period, and the medical care price index increased about one fifth as fast.[9] The rapid growth in health care spending from midcentury until the 1990s was due to increases in both the price and utilization of medical care. The growth in utilization was due to the rising prevalence of major chronic diseases and the emergence of a variety of medical advances to treat them, as well as the advent of employer-sponsored health insurance, Medicare, and Medicaid. Since the 1990s most of the growth in health care spending has been due to price increases.

As a concrete way to set the stage for an examination of the roots of the US health care industry and its current functioning, let's review some examples of the extraordinary breakthroughs that have occurred in medical

Figure 1.3. National health expenditures, per capita, 1960–2017. "NHE Summary including share of GDP, CY 1960–2017" (data spreadsheet), National Health Expenditures Data, Centers for Medicare and Medicaid Services, accessed March 8, 2019, https://www.cms.gov/Research-Statistics-Data-and-Systems/Statistics-Trends-and-Reports/National-HealthExpendData/NationalHealthAccountsHistorical.html.

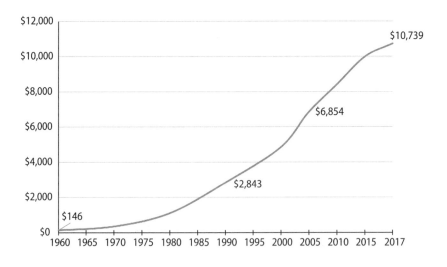

care over the past half-century. As the saying goes, "the plural of anecdote is not data," but these examples will provide a pertinent backdrop to an analysis of the US health care industry. Recognizing that medical innovations have come at significant financial cost, we still embrace them because they extend and improve our lives. But we do so while keeping in mind that as a nation we must strike a balance: while we want to make such innovations available to all those who could benefit, we also recognize that not all illnesses are equally harmful, not all treatments are equally efficacious, and not all illness-treatment combinations are equally costly relative to their benefit.

Medical Breakthroughs of the Past Half-Century

For clinicians of recent generations—in virtually every field of medicine, dentistry, and other health professions—the knowledge and technology with which we care for patients have advanced in fundamental ways that were unimaginable during our training. These major steps forward have been associated with vastly improved patient outcomes but in some cases have been accompanied by unintended consequences, especially involving markedly increasing costs of health care services and associated inequities in access. The remainder of this chapter describes examples of advances in medical and surgical care and contrasts these with the continuing challenges of access and cost.

Let's start with my own field of gynecology and reproductive endocrinology. The impact of oral contraceptives on the social and economic fabric of modern society, first approved for use by the Food and Drug Administration (FDA) in 1960, was powerful. Three additional examples of advances in this field are treatment of tubal ectopic pregnancy, development of in vitro fertilization, and the early detection and prevention of cervical cancer.

Ectopic Pregnancy

A tubal ectopic pregnancy occurs when a fertilized egg, on its way from the end of the fallopian tube to the uterus, gets stuck in the tube and implants there. About 2 in 100 pregnancies are ectopic. Locations for ectopic pregnancy other than the fallopian tube can occur, but tubal ectopic pregnancy is by far the most common. Having implanted in the lining of the fallopian tube, the pregnancy begins to grow but obviously can't expand much; after a relatively brief period of time the fallopian tube ruptures, leading to profuse bleeding into the pelvic portion of the abdominal cavity.

In the early 1900s, the mortality rate from ectopic pregnancy was 80–90 percent unless it was diagnosed early enough to be surgically treated by excising the tube, which in those days was a major surgical procedure carrying significant risk of morbidity and mortality. A quote from the 1913 edition of a well-known textbook of gynecology states, "Today ectopic pregnancy treatment is exclusively surgical. Every extra-uterine pregnancy when diagnosed should be operated on. . . . Expectant treatment gives 86% of death, and operation 85% of cures."[10]

In the late 1970s and early 1980s, ectopic pregnancy was still generally not diagnosed until it was a surgical emergency. This was because pregnancy tests that could be performed in real time in emergency rooms were not very sensitive for human chorionic gonadotropin (hCG), the hormone of pregnancy. These tests did not turn positive until about five to six weeks from the last menstrual period, which was about when the circulating concentration of hCG exceeded 1,500 mIU/ml. (Currently, an over-the-counter urine pregnancy test turns positive at a concentration as low as 6 mIU/ml, which is 95 percent accurate for pregnancy detection on the day of a missed menstrual period.)[11] Moreover, ectopic pregnancies produce hCG less efficiently than intrauterine pregnancies, so positive hCG levels would be even more difficult to detect in early ectopic pregnancy.

Therefore, up until the early 1980s, when a woman with a tubal ectopic pregnancy had lower abdominal pain at five to six weeks since her last menstrual period, the urine pregnancy test was often negative. Ultrasound was in its infancy and of little help. The only way to diagnose the ectopic pregnancy was if it had already ruptured. In such cases, patients had severe lower abdominal pain and were lightheaded due to low blood pressure from internal bleeding. Accumulating blood in the basin of the pelvis could be readily aspirated through a needle passed through the back of the vaginal canal. The diagnosis of tubal ectopic pregnancy was now made but the situation had become a surgical emergency due to intra-abdominal bleeding requiring a surgical incision through the abdominal wall, resection of the fallopian tube, and often blood transfusion.

During the 1980s and 1990s, tests for hCG became much more sensitive, and the advent of high-resolution transvaginal ultrasound meant that an intrauterine gestational sac could be seen very early in the pregnancy. The *absence* of an intrauterine gestational sac, in combination with an hCG concentration above the level at which the sac *should* be seen, means that there is an ectopic pregnancy by exclusion. With the diagnosis made early, open abdominal surgery is not needed and the ectopic pregnancy can now be removed from the tube using a laparoscopic approach with very small incisions; or better yet, in many cases of early ectopic pregnancy, it can be treated with medication, avoiding surgery altogether. Thus, over the last century tubal pregnancy transitioned from a condition with a high mortality rate to one that could be treated effectively with surgery (albeit often on an emergency basis) to one that can now be diagnosed early with laboratory testing and imaging technology and frequently treated with medication rather than surgery.

In Vitro Fertilization (IVF)

In the foreword to *In Vitro Fertilization Comes to America*,[12] which the pioneering reproductive surgeon and IVF innovator Howard W. Jones Jr., MD, published when he was 104 years young, Dr. Jones reprinted the Robert Frost poem "The Road Not Taken." It ends with the lines

Two roads diverged in a wood, and I—
I took the one less traveled by,
And that has made all the difference.

Taking the road less traveled is the story of IVF in a nutshell, and it is also a strategy that pertains to many of the other scientific and medical discoveries that I summarize below. The idea of IVF was introduced as science fiction by Aldous Huxley in his 1932 novel *Brave New World*, but it became reality when IVF pregnancies were established in rabbits in 1959. It wasn't until 1978, however, that the first human baby, Louise Brown, was born through IVF after what was reported to be over 100 failed attempts in other infertile patients.[13] The team responsible for this achievement was Patrick Steptoe, a British gynecologist who learned laparoscopy as a fellow under Dr. Jones and subsequently developed a laparoscopic method for egg retrieval, and Robert Edwards, a reproductive biologist based at the University of Cambridge who developed culture media for the fertilization of oocytes and early embryo development. Talk about persistence. Can you imagine counseling the 100th couple about undergoing an experimental procedure that hadn't worked in the previous 99 couples? Drs. Steptoe and Edwards were blazing a new path and were determined to be successful.

Since then, the field of IVF has exploded scientifically and technologically, such that there were 68,908 live births (resulting in 78,052 live infants) in the United States from IVF in 2017.[14] IVF is now responsible for about 1.7 percent of all infants born in the United States. In 2010, Dr. Edwards received the Nobel Prize in Physiology or Medicine for this achievement. (Dr. Steptoe died in 1988 and therefore was not eligible to receive the prize.)

In 1981, the husband-wife team of gynecologists Howard and Georgeanna Segar Jones and embryologist Lucinda Veeck established the first successful IVF pregnancy in the United States: Elizabeth Jordan Carr was born on December 28, 1981. While live birth rates in the early 1980s were in the range of 10 percent per IVF attempt, the excitement in the field, nationally and internationally, led to a series of exciting scientific and clinical innovations that have increased success rates dramatically.

As an interesting historical note—and a commentary on changing perspectives regarding age—in 1979 Dr. Howard Jones retired from his position as professor at the Johns Hopkins College of Medicine. He had been at Hopkins since 1931 as a medical student, resident, and faculty member, but he had reached (what had been at that time) Hopkins's mandatory retirement age of 70. What did he and his wife (also a noted Hopkins medical faculty member) do upon "retirement"? They visited their friend and former fellow Patrick Steptoe in England, learned IVF, brought it to the new Eastern Virginia Medical School, and ran the most successful IVF program in the United States for the next decade.

Early Detection and Prevention of Cervical Cancer

In the first half of the twentieth century, cervical cancer was a major cause of death among women in the United States, with a mortality rate of over 10 per 100,000 per year. Since then, screening with Pap smears reduced mortality significantly. The Pap smear involves taking a sample of cells from the uterine cervix with a wooden spatula or brush and examining them under a microscope to detect cellular abnormalities that are precursors of cancer. If precancerous cells are seen, a biopsy can be taken to confirm that a problem exists and simple treatments can be employed to destroy the abnormal cells and prevent invasive cancer. Cervical cancer mortality declined from 10.7 deaths per 100,000 women in 1946 to 2.3 per 100,000 in 2015, a decline of 79 percent (figure 1.4).

Epidemiologic evidence had long suggested that cervical cancer was caused by a sexually transmitted agent, but it was not fully understood until the 1980s that virtually all cases of cervical cancer are caused by specific types of human papillomaviruses (HPVs). Among the fifteen or so HPV types that are carcinogenic, two that are particularly "high-risk," HPV-16 and HPV-18, cause 70 percent of cervical cancers. High-risk HPV types can be identified by DNA testing, which has resulted in an updating of screening recommendations.[15] If both the Pap smear and high-risk HPV DNA are negative, for example, the screening interval can be extended to three or more years.

In the 1990s a vaccine was developed against the cancer-causing human papillomavirus. This vaccine now promises to almost eradicate the disease, at least in developed countries. The story of scientific discovery behind the development of the vaccine against HPV is, like many of the other medical advances described below, a sterling example of translational research. I was fortunate to be dean of the medical school at the University of Rochester that developed the virus-like particle responsible for eliciting the immunologic response that is the basis for the vaccine's efficacy. Several other scientists around the world contributed additional technologies to the vaccine; that said, the story of the Rochester group is noteworthy as a wonder-

Figure 1.4. Age-adjusted cervical cancer mortality rates, United States, 1946–2015. Source for 1946–1975 data: Hershel W. Lawson, *Cancer of the Cervix: An Overview* (Atlanta, GA: Centers for Disease Control and Prevention, June 2006), https://www.cdc.gov/cliac/docs/addenda/cliac0606/AddendumD.pdf. Source for 1975–2015 data: "Cancer Stat Facts: Cervical Cancer," Surveillance, Epidemiology, and End Results Program (SEER), National Cancer Institute, accessed November 20, 2018, https://seer.cancer.gov/statfacts/html/cervix.html.

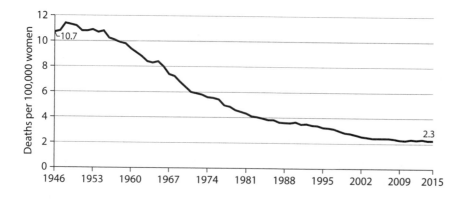

ful example of the sometimes chance combinations of events, people, and experiences that culminate in scientific discovery. (Although, as Louis Pasteur famously said, "Chance favors only the prepared mind.")

Richard Reichman, MD, was director of the Division of Infectious Disease in the Department of Medicine at Rochester, bringing with him three years of training in a National Institues of Health (NIH) virology lab after residency and subsequent NIH-funded virology research as a faculty member. Along the way, he was told by Dr. King Holmes, a founding father of sexually transmitted disease research, to pursue research on papillomaviruses as a line of work that would potentially be of tremendous public health benefit and would build on Dr. Reichman's background in virology. Dr. Reichman followed Dr. Holmes's advice. He quickly realized that he needed an HPV antigen with which to do immunologic studies but did not realize at the time that the search for this antigen would lead to the technological basis for the HPV vaccine. Enter William Bonnez, MD, who, although the first in his family to attend college, was trained in a French medical school that gave him the opportunity to supplement his medical training with work in physics and chemistry. After finishing medical school and his residency in internal medicine, Dr. Bonnez was recruited by Dr. Reichman as a fellow to work on the HPV antigen and a method for measuring its concentration in blood.

Now came the third link in the chain, Robert Rose, also a first-generation college graduate, who was then a technician working with Drs. Reichman and Bonnez. Rose was also a graduate student and needed a PhD thesis. In July 1990, he attended a meeting of the American Society for Virology, where he listened to a talk on the use of the baculovirus system for producing HIV virus–like particles. A light bulb came on in his head—he recognized that this system could be used to generate HPV virus–like particles that could be used not only as an antigen for serodiagnosis but also as a basis for a human vaccine. This became his PhD dissertation. He produced the major HPV capsid protein using the baculovirus system and found that this protein could spontaneously fold into a full capsid, forming a virus-like particle for HPV. These virus-like particles had the same immunologic properties as native HPV viral particles but were not infectious. This work, conducted as Dr. Rose's PhD thesis under Dr. Reichman as mentor, became the immunologic basis for the HPV vaccine.

The first HPV vaccine licensed for use, in 2006, was Gardasil. This was followed by Cervarix. Both vaccines are highly effective against high-risk

HPV types. The vaccines are now approved for the vaccination of males and females from the ages of 9 to 26. A recent study has documented a decline in the incidence of cervical cancer: Comparing four-year intervals before and after introduction of the HPV vaccine, annual incidence rates for cervical cancer in 2011–2014 were 29 percent lower than those in 2003–2006 for women between ages 15 and 24, and 13.0 percent lower among females between ages 25 and 34.[16] There should be an even greater decline in incidence as more individuals are vaccinated against HPV, which should lead to a decline in mortality from cervical cancer downstream.

Treatment of Premature Babies

About 1 in 10 babies in the United States are born preterm, defined as a birth prior to 37 weeks' completed gestation since the mother's last menstrual period. The improved survival of babies born before term gestation is another example of the extraordinary scientific and clinical achievements that have occurred since the middle of the twentieth century.

Premature birth is typically subdivided based on birth gestational age.[17] "Late preterm" infants are those born 34 to less than 37 weeks' gestation; "moderate preterm" infants are those born between 32 and 34 weeks' gestation; "very preterm" infants are those born between 28 and 32 weeks' gestation; and "extremely preterm" infants are those born less than 28 weeks' gestational age. The subgroup of extremely preterm births comprises approximately 6 percent of all preterm births. Overall rates of preterm birth are influenced by race and ethnicity. For example, in 2016 the rate of preterm birth among black women (14 percent) was about 50 percent higher than the rate of preterm birth among white women (9 percent).[18]

Early innovations in neonatal care occurring in the first half of the twentieth century included the development of incubators to foster a favorable environment of heat, humidity, and oxygen for the premature infant; recognition of the importance of handwashing by staff and family members to avoid causing infection of the baby; and laboratory measurements to measure the baby's lung maturity when still in utero. Still, through the 1960s, the probability of survival for extremely preterm infants was very low. Patrick Bouvier Kennedy, son of then President John F. Kennedy and Jackie Bouvier Kennedy, was born at 34 weeks' gestation with respiratory distress syndrome (RDS) and died 39 hours after birth. Since the 1970s, however, a number of advances in maternal-fetal medicine and neonatology have greatly improved the survival of premature babies, including the extremely premature, and reduced the significant long-term morbidity of prematurity. These advances have included

- treatment of maternal infection with antibiotics prior to delivery to prevent significant neonatal infection,
- administration of steroids to pregnant women at risk of premature delivery for prevention of RDS in the baby,
- continuous positive airway pressure mechanical ventilation to achieve targeted oxygen saturation in the premature baby,
- administration of surfactant to premature babies after delivery to take the place of the surfactant their lungs would normally produce, also to prevent RDS, and
- fine-tuned nutritional management of the baby to achieve appropriate growth targets.

These and other measures have improved survival from 59 to 82 percent for babies born at 26 weeks' gestation, and from 11 to 63 percent for babies born at 24 weeks' gestations.[19]

Neonatologists continue to improve the outcomes of premature infants. Many new strategies to minimize injury, preserve growth, and identify interventions (e.g., via antioxidant and anti-inflammatory pathways) are now being evaluated. As in other medical fields, methods to prevent and treat long-term deficits are constantly evolving.

Childhood Acute Lymphoblastic Leukemia

As a triumph of the interplay between biomedical research and cooperative clinical trials, an extraordinary achievement during the past 50 years is the dramatically improved cure rates in children with acute lymphoblastic leukemia (ALL). Fifty years ago this disease was universally fatal; today, greater than 90 percent of children with ALL are cured.

What has driven this incredible advancement? During the earliest years, clinicians and scientists at centers such as Boston Children's Hospital and St. Judes Research Hospital collaborated to understand the biology and unique vulnerabilities of pediatric patients with ALL, using alternating series of chemotherapy to kill surviving leukemia cells that were tolerant of the previous series. This work resulted in the discovery of the blood-brain barrier and prompted direct injection of chemotherapy into the space be-tween the thin layers of tissue that cover the brain and spinal cord (called "intrathecal chemotherapy") to eradicate leukemia that survived in the central nervous system.

The dramatic improvement in cure rate was fueled by the rise of the co-operative clinical trials groups, including the Children's Cancer Group and the Pediatric Oncology Group. Alternative treatment approaches were tested against the standard of care in treatment sites across the country, producing data regarding which approach was better. Iteratively, over the years these efforts improved survival rates in pediatric ALL to the point that nearly all children are being cured, a triumph of biomedical science and clinical research. Innovation continues in this field, with the potential for immunotherapy to narrow the gap of those who do not survive and for new molecular agents that may replace the need for bone marrow transplants in some patients.

Progress in Cancer Treatment

The early detection and prevention of cervical cancer, and the use of che-motherapy to treat childhood acute lymphoblastic leukemia, are two exam-ples of major progress in the fight against cancer. While treatment of some other types of cancers have not shown the same degree of success, signifi-cant progress has occurred for virtually all types of cancer. The five-year survival rate for all cancer sites combined, from 1975 through 2009, shows good progress against the goal set by the US Department of Health and Human Services in their Healthy People 2020 campaign (figure 1.5).

A timeline of progress in the prevention and treatment of cancer can be delineated alongside these upward trends in cancer survival:

- In 1971, the National Cancer Act established national cancer research centers and national cancer control programs. This set the stage for scientific advances in the fundamental understanding of cancer biology along with their translation into better methods for prevent-ing, diagnosing, and treating cancer.
- Adjuvant chemotherapy for breast cancer was introduced in 1974 and hormone-receptor therapy (tamoxifen) was approved by the FDA in 1977. In addition to using tamoxifen as a treatment for breast cancer, the National Cancer Institute subsequently funded a study of breast cancer

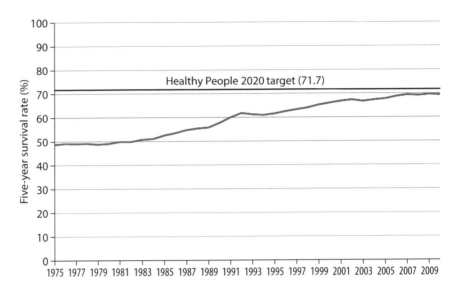

Figure 1.5. Trend line versus Healthy People 2020 target for five-year relative survival for all cancer sites combined, both sexes, age 20 and over, 1975–2009. National Cancer Institute, *Cancer Trends Progress Report* (Bethesda, MD: National Institutes of Health, Department of Health and Human Services, 2018), accessed November 20, 2018, https://progressreport.cancer.gov/sites/default/files/archive/report2018.pdf.

prevention: women who were at high risk for breast cancer (based on age, family history, and other factors) were randomized between tamoxifen and placebo. Six years after its inception, the Breast Cancer Prevention Trial showed a 49 percent reduction in the incidence of invasive breast cancer among participants who took tamoxifen.[20] As a result, investigators released the initial study results about 14 months earlier than expected and notified the 13,388 woman participants of the findings so those women who had been taking a placebo could consider starting tamoxifen therapy after consulting with their personal physicians.

- The critical role of genetics in breast cancer was highlighted in 1979 when the suppressor gene TP53 was discovered as the most commonly mutated gene in human cancer. As a suppressor gene, TP53 helps control cell proliferation and suppresses tumor growth. When it is mutated, it can no longer perform these functions well.
- In 1984, it was discovered that 20–25 percent of breast cancers overexpress a specific gene (HER2/neu). Women with breast cancer who are positive for this gene have more aggressive tumors with a poor prognosis. Because the HER2 protein is a cell surface receptor, it became a

logical target for antibody therapy. At the turn of the twenty-first century, trastuzumab, a monoclonal antibody to HER2, was tested and found to be highly active in patients with HER2 overexpressing metastatic breast cancer. Treatment with standard chemotherapy with or without the antibody showed that use of the antibody resulted in greatly enhanced response rates and survival.[21] The use of trastuzumab was subsequently shown to reduce markedly the risk of recurrence and death of women with operable HER2 overexpressing breast cancer when used as an adjuvant following standard adjuvant chemotherapy.[22]

Since the successes associated with these early clinical trials, a number of additional antibodies, antibody-drug conjugates, and small-molecule kinase inhibitors targeting the HER family of proteins have been developed and found to be highly active in patients with several cancers, including gastric and colon cancers as well as breast cancers that overexpress the HER2 protein.

- In 1994 and 1995, the BRCA1 and BRCA2 tumor suppressor genes were cloned. Germ line mutations of these genes greatly increases the risk of breast and ovarian cancer. As a result, screening is critical for individuals with these mutations. Additionally, cancer cells that harbor these mutations have been found to be particularly sensitive to the chemotherapeutic agents that have been developed to target them.

- A major breakthrough has been the development of "targeted" drug treatments against specific genes or proteins to help stop cancer from growing and spreading. These genes and proteins are found in cancer cells or in cells related to cancer growth, like blood vessel cells. The discovery and application of imatinib for the treatment of patients with chronic myelogenous leukemia (CML) and gastrointestinal stromal tumors by Brian Druker is considered by many to be the "poster child" for the potential utility of targeted therapeutics.

Our molecular understanding of CML dates back to the 1960s and 1970s when investigators in Philadelphia discovered that CML harbors a single genetic defect, namely the translocation of one gene on chromosome 9 to another gene on chromosome 22 resulting in a "fusion protein" that is responsible for the development of CML. It was not until the last decade of the twentieth century, however, that Dr. Druker reasoned that a small molecule inhibitor of the fusion protein may have value for the treatment of patients with CML. Laboratory testing of countless compounds, and tremendous persistence on the part of Dr. Druker, ultimately resulted in the discovery of imatinib, which was extraordinarily potent in inhibiting the activity of the fusion protein. This compound was subsequently tested in patients with CML, which resulted in complete and sustained disappearance of all leukemia cells for almost every treated patient.[23] This startling result was not unlike the use of penicillin for the treatment of bacterial infections some 60 years previously. Subsequently, imatinib was used with tremendous success for the treatment of patients with gastrointestinal stromal tumors,[24] and it remains today the standard to which other targeted therapeutic approaches aspire.

- More recently, immunologic treatments have been developed to treat conditions that previously were intractable, such as metastatic melanoma. Several types of immunotherapy treatments have now been developed and tested in the treatment of advanced melanoma, which heretofore had a median survival time of six months or less. Such treatments include a class of drugs called "checkpoint inhibitors," which work by disrupting the signaling proteins that allow cancer cells to hide from the immune system. The cancer cells are thereby exposed to the body's own T-cells, which can then attack and kill the cancer cells. In metastatic melanoma, a combination of two such immunotherapy drugs resulted in an extraordinary three-year survival rate of 58 percent.[25] Checkpoint inhibitors are now being used in patients with a variety of malignancies.

Hepatitis

The story of hepatitis, an inflammatory liver disease that has been responsible for considerable morbidity and mortality throughout history, is another remarkable example of translational research in action. Worldwide, hepatitis was responsible for 1.34 million deaths in 2015.[26] Starting in the 1960s, recognition that the etiology of the disease was viral in nature led to the discovery of the causative viruses. In the case of hepatitis A and B, identification of the virus culminated in safe and effective vaccines. In the case of hepatitis C, initial, nonspecific antiviral treatments were somewhat successful but had significant side effects and recurrence rates. More recently, direct-acting antiviral (DAA) medications have been developed that achieve cure rates of greater than 95 percent in clinical trials with real-world populations.[27]

Hepatitis is a condition that covers a spectrum of liver infections, caused by different viruses, that result in abdominal pain, lethargy, jaundice, and other symptoms. One form of the disease, transmitted by person-to-person contact or through contaminated food or water, has a short incubation period and results in an acute illness that can often resolve spontaneously, but which can sometimes be severe and result in significant mortality. This disease, which came to be called hepatitis A, was responsible for many of the historical epidemics of hepatitis. The virus responsible for hepatitis A, eventually identified in 1973, was the basis on which safe, effective vaccines were developed and made available in the early 1990s. It is now recommended that all children receive the hepatitis A vaccine at one year of age.

It was recognized historically that many patients with hepatitis seemed to have a different etiology and clinical course than what would be expected with hepatitis A. The hepatitis in these patients seemed to stem either from vaccines that contained serum—leading, for example, to epidemics of jaundice among army personnel during World War II—or from blood transfusions. This form of the disease, called hepatitis B or "serum hepatitis," was more virulent. It had a longer incubation period, was associated with a chronic infection that caused liver scarring or "cirrhosis," had a high mortality rate, and was associated with hepatocellular cancer.

The virus responsible for hepatitis B was discovered in 1965 by Baruch Blumberg, a medical anthropologist and geneticist. Dr. Blumberg went on with his colleague, microbiologist Irving Millman, to develop a blood test for the hepatitis B virus. They also developed the first hepatitis B vaccine in 1969 prepared from heat-inactivated virus. For these achievements, Dr. Blumberg won the Nobel Prize in Physiology or Medicine in 1976. In 1970, a more sensitive assay was developed to detect the presence of minute amounts of the hepatitis B antigen and antibody in blood. Using this assay, blood banks began to screen blood donations, and by 1972 the FDA mandated screening of all blood donations for hepatitis B.

In 1986, a second generation of hepatitis B vaccines were synthetized using DNA recombinant technology. These vaccines are safer than the ones using inactivated virus in that they do not contain blood products and therefore cannot cause hepatitis. It is recommended by the Centers for Disease Control and Prevention (CDC) that all infants should be vaccinated against hepatitis B, receiving their first dose at birth and completing a series of three to four doses by six months of age.

Following FDA-mandated blood bank screening for hepatitis B, the risk of hepatitis B infections from a blood transfusion decreased significantly, but up to 10 percent of blood transfusion recipients still developed post-transfusion hepatitis. Like hepatitis B, this newly identified "non-A, non-B" type of hepatitis could be contracted from infected blood and could result in a chronic liver infection and cirrhosis. However, it differed from hepatitis B in that people with this disease rarely experienced acute symptoms and therefore often developed chronic hepatitis without signs of infection. It wasn't until about 15 years later, in 1989, that the culprit, called hepatitis C virus (or HCV), was discovered by the British biochemist Michael Houghton working with CDC virologists Qui-Lim Choo, George Kuo, and Daniel Bradley.

Chronic HCV infection remains a significant global public health burden, affecting over 70 million persons worldwide, and is associated with substantial morbidity and mortality due to liver cirrhosis and hepatocellular carcinoma.[28] Now, three decades following the discovery of HCV, the development of new treatment options has revolutionized the care of patients with chronic hepatitis C. The first two decades of treatment centered on antiviral, immune modulation therapies (interferon), which resulted in relatively low cure rates and high side-effect profiles. With the discovery of oral direct-acting antivirals in 2014, significant improvements in safety and efficacy have been realized. These newer DAA drugs target various points of the hepatitis C viral replication cycle, resulting in rapid suppression of HCV and cure in as little as eight weeks of oral therapy. Cure rates exceeding 95 percent in all populations have been achieved, also resulting in a significant decrease in both hepatocellular carcinoma and all-cause mortality.[29] In this context, the World Health Organization released in May 2016 a global strategy on viral hepatitis that called for the elimination of HCV infection as a public health threat by 2030, defined by an 80 percent reduction in new HCV infections and a 65 percent reduction in HCV-associated mortality.[30] If successful, these efforts will result in an absolute decrease in annual global HCV-associated deaths from 1.4 million to fewer than half a million.[31]

Thus, in the short time span of 30 years, we have moved from the discovery of the virus causing hepatitis C to the development of curative therapy and the implementation of strategies for global elimination. This series of achievements represents a unique and monumental example of translational science at its best.

Cardiovascular Disease

We now take for granted the knowledge that cigarette smoking and high-fat diets are bad for your heart and blood vessels while regular exercise and lean body mass are good. But until the mid-twentieth century this was not well understood. While heart disease was an uncommon cause of death at the beginning of the twentieth century, by midcentury an increase in atherosclerosis associated with smoking and changes in the American diet made heart disease the most common cause of death. Cardiovascular mortality reached a peak in the 1960s of almost 500 per 100,000 people annually. Death often was the result of a sudden "heart attack" (i.e., infarction of the myocardium, or heart muscle, due to obstruction of a coronary artery).

The dramatic decline in mortality due to cardiovascular disease is another example of how scientific, pharmacologic, surgical, and technological advances have been translated through rigorous clinical research and widespread public education into meaningful reductions in mortality (figure 1.6).

Figure 1.6. Decline in deaths from cardiovascular disease in relation to scientific advances. Acronyms signal sets of randomized clinical trials representing corresponding milestones. From Nabel and Braunwald, "A Tale of Coronary Artery Disease and Myocardial Infarction."[32]

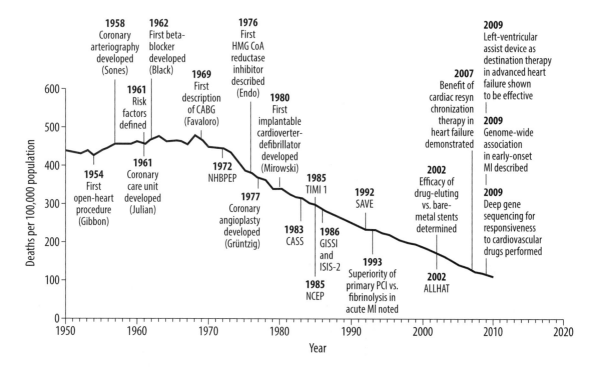

All aspects of cardiovascular disease—prevention, treatment, and improvement in quality of life—have been favorably impacted by these advances.

As conceptualized by two leading cardiologists, Drs. Elizabeth Nabel and Eugene Braunwald, one of the first key steps was the identification of risk factors.[32] This was accomplished through the Framingham Heart Study, a federally funded, longitudinal investigation of risk factors for heart disease among the residents of Framingham, Massachusetts. The study began in 1948 and initial findings were reported in 1961.[33] These early data documented the association between heart disease, hypertension, and high levels of circulating cholesterol. Nabel and Braunwald summarize subsequent events as follows: "With the identification of these coronary risk factors and others that followed, the veil that masked the underlying mechanisms in angina and myocardial infarction was lifted, and the concept that coronary heart disease and its complications could be prevented was introduced. Increasingly large multicenter clinical trials subsequently showed that both primary and secondary prevention was possible when steps were taken to lower blood pressure and serum total cholesterol. Fortunately, drugs to reduce these risk factors safely became available as a result of a series of productive collaborations between industry and academic medicine."[34]

Nabel and Braunwald used acronyms for a series of randomized clinical trials representing these collaborations. The timeline for the introduction of a variety of other technologies was also included, along with associated changes in mortality rates. These include the introduction of coronary angioplasty, implantable defibrillators, coronary catheterization, electrophysiologic interventions such as cardiac resynchronization, treatments for heart failure such as left-ventricular assist devices, and initial forays into "personalized medicine" with gene sequencing to determine the responsiveness to specific cardiovascular drugs.

Added to these advances are more recent data on progress in the treatment of cardiovascular disease, such as the endovascular approach to the treatment of malfunctioning heart valves, discussed next, and innovation in both the surgical and medical treatment of atrial fibrillation.[35]

The future holds promise for further reductions in the occurrence and impact of cardiovascular diseases: for those with existing conditions, there will undoubtedly be new or improved medications, surgical procedures, and other technologies such as wearable devices for monitoring and treatment. Hopefully, however, there will be an enhanced public understanding of the lifestyle and behavioral causes of cardiovascular disease that will lead to fewer instances of these problems developing to begin with.

Treatment of Stroke

Stroke, also known as cerebrovascular accident or "brain attack," is a syndrome caused by a disruption in the flow of blood to part of the brain due to either occlusion of a blood vessel (ischemic stroke, about 85 percent of cases) or rupture of a blood vessel (hemorrhagic stroke, about 15 percent). The interruption in blood flow deprives the brain of nutrients and oxygen, resulting in injury to cells in the affected vascular territory of the brain. When brain cells die, the function of the part of the body parts they control is impaired or lost.

Stroke is a leading cause of death and disability. According to statistics from the CDC, about 800,000 people in the United States have a stroke each year, and stroke kills almost 130,000 Americans each year—or one out of every 20 deaths.[36] On average, one American dies from stroke every four minutes. Among those who have survived a stroke, 20 percent need help walking, 70 percent cannot return to their previous jobs, and 50 percent are unable to return to work. It is the number one cause of adult disability in the United States.

A key turning point in stroke therapy occurred in 1995 with the publication of an NIH-funded randomized trial designed to determine whether clots in blood vessels can be dissolved by treatment with tissue plasminogen activator (t-PA), an enzyme in the body that normally plays an important role in the balance between blood clot formation and dissolution. In this study, t-PA was found to be effective in the treatment of acute stroke,[37] and became the first drug approved by the FDA for this purpose. t-PA is given intravenously to dissolve the clot or clots that are keeping blood from flowing to the brain. It improves the chance of recovery by up to 30 percent when used correctly. But there are two major limitations: the need to begin the treatment within 4.5 hours of the stroke and the risk of intracranial or systemic bleeding.

Since the introduction of t-PA, two other important developments occurred in the evaluation and treatment of stroke. One involves neuroimaging. Advanced imaging with high-resolution computed tomography (CT) scanners provide a window into the real-time physiology of the entire brain. Though time of onset remains a critical determinant in stroke triage and treatment decisions, advanced stroke imaging can show vascular occlusions, compensatory collateral blood flow, and hemodynamic conditions that allows stroke specialists to determine whether salvageable brain tissue remains, irrespective of time of onset.

The other major advance in stroke treatment has been the development of mechanical devices that can remove blood clots within brain arteries (a procedure called "endovascular thrombectomy"). While some of the early mechanical endovascular devices did not show evidence of significant benefit in randomized controlled trials, refinement of the clinical protocols, in conjunction with advances in the engineering of the devices, have resulted in significantly improved patient outcomes.

This journey, taken step by step by experts involved in acute stroke care nationally and internationally, culminated in the 2014 publication of five clinical trials validating endovascular intervention as a clearly superior treatment for patients with blood clots blocking large arteries in the brain. For such patients, endovascular intervention has been defined as the standard of care since 2015, according to American Heart Association / American Stroke Association guidelines. Endovascular treatment often results in poignant and dramatic examples of the "miracles of modern medicine" in real time; a patient with slurred speech or even nonsensical mumbling who is no longer in control of one side of his body can, one day after treatment, develop full strength in his affected arm and leg, walk around his hospital room, and speak with nearly imperceptible hesitation. By day three after treatment, such patients often go home with a level of function that is perceived as normal by family members.

Treatment of Malfunctioning Heart Valves

Like the endovascular neurosurgery described above in the treatment of stroke, there has developed an overall trend in surgery toward "minimally invasive" procedures. These include such things as laparoscopy, robotic surgery, or arthroscopy for a variety of operations that used to be done by making a large incision in the chest, abdomen, or joint. Such approaches mean less morbidity, shorter hospital stays (often "same-day" surgery), and quicker recovery times.

In the cardiovascular field, the placement of stents into coronary arteries via a catheter introduced into a large blood vessel in the groin dates to the 1980s as an alternative to open-heart coronary artery bypass procedures. Instead of major heart surgery, the endovascular catheters could be used to open vessels that are obstructed because of atherosclerosis (build-up of plaque on the inside of an artery). More recently, this technology has been adapted and refined to treat individuals with malfunctioning heart valves due to factors such as infection, rheumatic heart disease, coronary artery disease, or congenital defects.

As the heart muscle contracts and relaxes, the valves that control the entry and exit of blood to the heart and through its chambers sequentially open and close, letting blood flow into the ventricles and atria in a finely tuned manner. Heart valves can develop one of two malfunctions (or both): (1) *regurgitation,* in which the valve does not close completely, causing the blood to flow backward instead of forward through the valve; and (2) *stenosis,* in which the valve opening becomes narrowed or does not form properly, inhibiting the flow of blood out of the ventricle or atria. The heart is forced to pump blood with increased force to move blood through the stiff, stenotic valve. When heart valves fail to open and close properly, the heart's ability to pump blood adequately through the body is hampered, causing heart failure.

There is a long history of surgical innovation and technology in the treatment of heart valve disease. Most of this work has focused on the aortic valve (between the left ventricle and the aorta) and mitral valve (between the left atrium and left ventricle), as these are associated with the highest incidence of disease. Heart valve replacement began in the 1960s with the development of cardiopulmonary bypass, but major open-heart surgery was required. A recent advance has been transcatheter aortic valve replacement (TAVR), which involves delivering a new tissue valve over a catheter into the aortic valve position. TAVR initially was used in patients thought to be too risky for open-heart surgery; clinical trials then showed TAVR was safe for even moderate-risk patients. Clinical trials are now underway to study the efficacy of TAVR in low-risk patients—and soon to come is a preventive clinical trial for patients with severe aortic stenosis before they have any symptoms at all.

Mitral valve repair and replacement also started in the 1960s and has advanced to minimally invasive techniques that allow the mitral valve to be repaired or replaced through a small incision in the right side of the chest. Repairing the patient's own natural valve is always preferred, but rheumatic heart disease often deforms the valve, necessitating replacement. Surgeons and cardiologists have been working for years on a suitable transcatheter replacement for the mitral valve but it has proved much more challenging due to the valve's oval shape and the fact that the mitral valve can sometimes interfere with the aortic valve. In recent years, however, a novel minimally invasive technology has been introduced in which leaky mitral valve flaps can be clipped together under ultrasound-guided imaging to reduce the leak and improve patient symptoms. Clinical trials have shown that younger and healthier patients do better with a mitral valve surgical repair, which is now done through a minimally invasive approach.

Progress in Mental Health

Nearly 19 percent of Americans were estimated to experience a mental health disorder in 2017, and almost 5 percent were considered to have substantial impairment in their ability to function in at least one aspect of their lives.[38] Mental health disorders cause significant functional impairment; the World Health Organization estimates that five of the top twenty diseases causing lost years of life (adjusted for disability level) are mental health disorders, including depressive disorders, anxiety disorders, schizophrenia, and alcohol and substance abuse disorders.[39] The direct medical costs of serious mental illnesses alone are estimated to be about 6 percent of total health care costs, and indirect costs in the form of lost earnings add an estimated $193 billion. This does not include the significant financial burden of clinical and social services or lost earnings for more prevalent, but less severe, mental health disorders.[40]

This impact of mental health disorders has occurred despite the development since the 1950s of numerous psychopharmacologic and behavioral approaches that are effective in relieving the suffering caused by these disorders. Until the 1950s, patients with severe mental illness were primarily confined to asylums notorious for their inhumane conditions. Asylums separated patients from society, and their illness was managed with physical restraints. Sedatives and hypnotics were often used, which masked the underlying disease rather than addressing the underlying causes, whether rooted in biochemistry, neurocircuitry, and/or behavior.

During the 1950s, the major classes of psychotropic drugs were synthesized: antipsychotics, anxiolytics, and several classes of antidepressants.[41] Psychoactive drugs, which have become more targeted in recent decades, treat mental health disorders by affecting neurotransmitters (biomolecules through which neurons communicate) or hormones. While neurotransmitters travel only a short distance to reach their target at the other side of a neuronal synapse, hormones circulate through the bloodstream before reaching target cells anywhere in the body. These methods are connected: the secretion of some hormones, especially those of the pituitary gland, are controlled by neurotransmitters from the brain. Stefan Leucht and his colleagues analyzed 94 meta-analyses comparing the efficacy of drugs that are used to treat medical and mental health conditions (48 drugs in 20 medical diseases and 16 drugs in 8 psychiatric disorders, which ranged from schizophrenia to bipolar disease, depression, and obsessive-compulsive disorder). Using statistical estimates of effect size (e.g., treatment vs. placebo) as the measure of efficacy, these researchers found that while there were some general medical drugs with clearly higher effect sizes than the psychotropic agents, psychoactive drugs were not generally less efficacious than other drugs.[42]

Sigmund Freud introduced psychoanalysis at the turn of the twentieth century. Scientific evaluation of alternative interventions gave rise to behavioral approaches. Since then, a wide array of evidence-based treatments has evolved under the broad umbrella of "cognitive behavioral therapy." These treatments focus on how people can identify thoughts and actions that may maintain problematic behaviors or emotions and how to respond to them in new, adaptive ways. Various forms of cognitive behavioral therapy have garnered substantial empirical support and have been shown to provide clinically significant relief for the majority of people with depressive disorders, eating disorders, anxiety and obsessive-compulsive disorders, post-traumatic stress disorder, substance use and alcohol-related disorders, childhood behavioral disorders, psychotic disorders, and health syndromes related to psychological stress, such as insomnia and chronic pain.

The challenge for the next 50 years will be finding ways to extend and improve the effectiveness of pharmacologic and behavioral approaches by more closely integrating therapy with insights from neuroscience. There are also promising recent advances in treating abnormal neuronal circuitry in mental health conditions such as depression and obsessive-compulsive disorder with deep brain stimulation or transmagnetic stimulation. These approaches will likely also contribute to progress in improving the lives of individuals with a broader spectrum of mental health conditions in the future.

Radiosurgery

Neurosurgery is inherently risky. Even in the most skilled hands, certain groups of patients, like those harboring arteriovenous malformations (abnormal connections between arteries and veins in the brain, present at birth) or tumors at the base of the skull, are at risk of serious complications. Radiosurgery is a term coined by a Swedish neurosurgeon, Lars Leksell, to describe his vision of focusing hundreds of very small beams of radiation through the intact skull to produce a lesion in the brain that could be therapeutic.[43] Although his original intent with this method was to treat movement disorders and pain, his colleagues later used the same technology to treat tumors and vascular malformations, precisely delivering the radiation using a Gamma Knife, first developed in the 1960s and refined since then. Because of cost and complexity, in the 1980s, linear accelerators used for conventional radiation therapy were modified to perform radiosurgery, with excellent outcomes reported in the 1990s.[44] With these technological developments and favorable results, radiosurgery emerged in the 1990s as an alternative to open neurosurgery.

As practiced today, radiosurgery is a one-time outpatient procedure. The day starts with the attachment of a stereotactic head ring while the patient is under local anesthesia. That ring provides the geometric reference point for all imaging and treatment planning. While the reliable immobilization and target localization associated with the head ring initially established it as the gold standard, several frameless radiosurgery systems have also been developed, most of which rely on optical and/or image guidance. After CT scans and magnetic resonance images are entered into a planning computer, a team of neurosurgeons, radiation oncologists, and radiation physicists then employs computer algorithms to simulate the direction of the beams needed to create a high-dose radiation field that precisely conforms to the shape of the lesion in the brain (e.g., a brain tumor). The treatment is delivered, the ring (if used) is removed, and the patient goes home. In many cases, this one-time outpatient treatment is an alternative to open neurosurgery with its associated risks. Thus, radiosurgery has revolutionized treatment of many diseases of the brain. For smaller benign tumors, arteriovenous malformations, and metastatic brain tumors, radiosurgery generally produces equivalent or better results than open neurosurgery, while the risk of complications is much less.

Balancing Care, Cost, and Access

The advances described in the last few pages are examples of how scientific discoveries can be translated into medical care to save, extend, and improve lives. These advances came about as a result of research and innovation in the United States and around the world. While many emerging economies cannot take full advantage of all this medical progress, the United States and other high-income peer nations share in their ability to access these technologies and treatments.

The United States is unique internationally, however, in the structure of our health care industry. Rooted in a strong belief that market forces should shape all aspects of our nation's economy, our health care industry has evolved in response to events that have unfolded over many generations. A backbone of private health insurance and utilization-driven payments has strengthened over time, increasingly including Medicare and Medicaid in addition to employer-sponsored health plans. Along the way, each of the key stakeholders—physicians, hospitals, insurance companies, pharmaceutical companies, device manufacturers, employers, employees, and politicians— have been able to fashion a place in the industry that works well for them.

Thus, the health care industry in the United States functions well for the individual stakeholders, but it has several key flaws in comparison with other high-income countries: uneven quality of care, inequality of access, and relatively poor health outcomes for the overall population despite much higher costs. While the Affordable Care Act has reduced the percentage of Americans who do not have health insurance to a nadir of 9 percent in 2017 (and now rising again), this compares with essentially 0 percent in other peer countries. And while expenditures on health care in the United States are almost twice as high as other high-income nations, whether measured as expenditures per capita or as a share of national income, population-wide health outcomes are generally among the worst.

Put differently, while remarkable advances in medical care have oc- curred in recent decades, the United States has not achieved a good bal- ance of care, cost, and access. While no country has achieved complete equality of access to the highest quality health care at low cost, the balance between care, cost, and access is more out of kilter in the United States than elsewhere. The task of explaining why we are so unbalanced in health care and how to make things better is approached next in four parts: (1) under- lying economic principles and their applicability to health care, (2) histori- cal evolution of the US health care industry, (3) its current functioning, and (4) how to bring care, cost, and access more into balance.

PART I
ECONOMIC UNDERPINNINGS

PERFECT COMPETITION AND ITS APPLICABILITY TO HEALTH CARE SERVICES

Extraordinary advances in biomedical science and their translation into medical practice have prolonged and improved the quality of our lives. These advances, however, have been accompanied by high cost and inequitable access. How can the United States achieve the right balance between care, cost, and access?

In the ongoing national debate concerning health care, there is often a statement that goes something like this: "Increased free-market competition will reduce cost, improve consumer choice, and enhance quality." Free markets for goods and services are at the core of our capitalist economy. Thus, on the face of it, such a statement has significant appeal. But how does it translate to health care? In the next two chapters, we explore the theory of perfect competition and its underlying assumptions as well as consider whether the predicted outcomes of this theory hold up well for health care services.

The Theory of Perfect Competition

Economists have developed theories about how markets work by employing assumptions that reflect a level of perfection in a variety of conditions that may seem abstract and unrealistic. Recognizing this, economists argue that while there may be some departure from the underlying assumptions in real-life application, the analysis at its core is so powerful and robust that the conclusions are fundamentally and directionally correct. Thus, when a new product emerges that large numbers of consumers would like to have, the high demand for that product can yield substantial early profits for the innovator firm; economic theory would predict that this profitability entices more firms to enter the industry, pushing price and profits down in the longer term. Another example is the prediction that more firms will also enter an industry if the market price for a good or service exceeds its marginal cost of production; this process brings price down toward marginal cost across time. Economic theory also predicts that when a new technology emerges that can lower a firm's marginal cost of production, producers will invest in that technology.

These are but three examples of many in which, according to economic theory, the actions of consumers and producers pursuing their own interests automatically lead to market adjustments that benefit the larger society by creating greater efficiency. Indeed, economic theory leads to the conclusion that, if the underlying assumptions of a perfect market (described next) are met and if consumers follow their desires while producers pursue their profits, society's allocation of resources will be efficient in the sense that nobody can be made better off by any reallocation without making someone else worse off.

This conclusion was first derived by the Italian engineer and economist Vilfredo Pareto, published in his 1906 treatise *Manual of Political Economy*.[1] It follows, however, that in cases where the underlying assumptions do not hold, market imperfections are produced and the economy operates in an inefficient manner. Moreover, economic efficiency does not imply equity in the distribution of wealth or in an allocation of resources that optimally reflects societal values.

Economic Efficiency vs. Optimal Social Welfare in Health Care

A fundamental economic principle is that each consumer has preferences about how to allocate his or her income among items of consumption. A consumer may be indifferent between several different allocations: more of X means less of Y and vice versa. Individuals with larger incomes can have more of *both* X and Y than those with smaller incomes, but "Pareto efficiency" is still achieved if each individual achieves a set of preferences that is best for him or her *given* his or her personal budget constraint.

Sometimes, however, economic efficiency in the Pareto sense is inconsistent with societal values. To illustrate this distinction in the health field and the consequent conundrum in balancing care, cost, and access, we will consider two medical conditions—infertility and cancer—about which there are divergent views on where this balance should be struck.

Let's consider two couples with infertility who are deciding whether to pursue treatment with in vitro fertilization (IVF) at a cost of $15,000. IVF is a procedure to help establish pregnancies among infertile couples in whom simpler techniques have not been successful. It involves the following steps: hormonal medication is given to stimulate the development of several eggs in the woman's ovaries instead of the usual one per menstrual cycle; when the eggs are close to ovulating, they are taken from the ovaries through a needle; the eggs are fertilized by sperm in a laboratory culture dish to create embryos; and after early embryo development, one or more embryos are chosen for transfer to the woman's uterus.

In couple A, the woman is 32 years old and has a 50 percent chance of pregnancy with IVF, but this couple has a limited budget and can barely cover their food, rent, utility, and clothing needs. These necessities have preference over IVF, so they choose not to proceed with IVF. In couple B, the woman is 42 years old and has a 20 percent chance of pregnancy with IVF, but their income is much higher than that of couple A. Given the set of choices on how they can spend their money, they choose to pursue IVF, even with the lower chance of pregnancy. Both couples are making rational choices based on their budgets that are consistent with utility maximization and Pareto efficiency.

In a market economy, insurance will naturally arise to cover unpredictable events like infertility and other illnesses. Risk-averse individuals would gladly pay an actuarially fair insurance premium that represents the average medical costs of others like them in order to avoid the large costs that would be associated with a major unexpected illness. If perfect information (a tall assumption) and other conditions were met, health insurance could be provided efficiently in the Pareto sense. But in that case, individuals participating in a market economy with insurance (but without government intervention) would pay the full premium; that is, the cost of the insurance would not be subsidized by their employer or the government. Some individuals would decide that they could not afford such insurance relative to their other needs.

Now consider a 32-year-old woman who is diagnosed with a type of cancer for which her doctors recommend surgery followed by radiation and chemotherapy. Suppose that the market price for each of these three treatments is $30,000. Of the three recommended treatments, surgery is most important; the tumor mass would be removed, and since the cancer has spread to local lymph nodes, these lymph nodes would also be removed.

Based on data in the literature on patients with clinical circumstances similar to that of this patient, her five-year survival with surgery alone is estimated to be 60 percent. Because of the extent of lymph node involvement, radiation therapy is also recommended, which would increase her five-year survival to 80 percent. There is no evidence of spread beyond the lymph nodes, however, and the data in the medical literature are mixed as to how much additional benefit there might be to adding chemotherapy: the patient's oncologist estimates that chemotherapy might add anywhere from 0 to 10 percent to the patient's five-year survival rate.

In a free-market world, insurance could emerge to cover cancer treatment as noted above, but consumers would pay the full premium cost in advance, without knowing whether they will develop a significant medical condition. If the woman who now has cancer had decided not to purchase this insurance because of its cost, her decision about how to proceed will now be influenced by her budget and other personal needs. One free-market scenario might be that she has very limited income but does have equity in her home; she decides to take out a home equity loan to cover the cost of surgery, but she still cannot afford the radiation and chemotherapy. Another scenario might be that she was laid off from her job, has exhausted her unemployment insurance, and simply has no income or savings to pay for any treatment. A third scenario might be that her annual income is low, but she has savings of several hundred thousand dollars from which she could pay for the entire treatment. In reviewing the literature herself and with her doctor, however, she becomes concerned about the chemotherapy's side effects and concludes that the best studies in the literature do not convincingly demonstrate that chemotherapy has any significant benefit. On this basis, she opts for surgery and radiation, but no chemotherapy. A final scenario might be that our patient has the same financial resources as in the third scenario, but based on her personal preferences she is willing to pay an extra $30,000 for the chemotherapy in the hopes of *some* additional benefit, even with the side effects that she knows will occur.

All of these decisions, like those in the IVF example, represent rational choices based on the patient's budget and personal preferences; they are consistent with utility maximization and Pareto efficiency. However, these "optimal" results from free-market competition—for example, that the patient in scenario 1 does not benefit from the improved survival of radiation therapy or that the patient in scenario 2 does not have *any* treatment—are not consistent with prevailing societal values that patients with cancer should have access to effective treatments, regardless of their financial status. Reflecting these values, our health care industry has evolved such that most patients with cancer indeed have access to treatment, either through employer-sponsored insurance or public programs such as Medicare and Medicaid. But the prevailing value that people with cancer should have access to treatment does not pertain to the 10 percent of Americans who remain uninsured; they would face significant hurdles in obtaining treatment, as would many more who are "underinsured" with high-deductible, limited coverage policies.

Additional wrinkles occur when certain treatments are very expensive but add only a small increment to a positive outcome (e.g., improvement by only a few percent in pregnancy rates or in the probability of survival from cancer) and when definitive evidence of treatment efficacy is lacking, as reflected by decision-making in the third and fourth cancer scenarios just described.

As a final consideration, suppose that the 32-year-old woman with cancer described above is in the early stages of what is destined to be an accomplished career as an artist, scientist, novelist, lawyer, architect, software engineer, athlete, economist, chef, corporate innovator, or some other endeavor. And suppose she has an 80–90 percent chance of complete cure from cancer treatment such that she will live a full life. Do her subsequent contributions to the scientific, artistic, and/or cultural fabric of our society, or her material cumulative contributions to the nation's economy as a producer and consumer, including her cumulative tax payments, justify societal coverage of her cancer treatment at age 32, quite apart from the personal decision she might make at a young age given her limited financial resources? Does the answer change if she were a minimal-wage employee in retail sales who would make a much smaller contribution to cumulative gross domestic product and taxes?

These latter questions pertain to the concept of "externalities," which occur when the production or consumption of a specific good impacts third parties who are not directly related to that production or consumption. The existence of an externality implies a difference between the gain or loss of private individuals and the aggregate gain or loss of the society as a whole. Many externalities are negative, such as pollution. A corporation may implement a technology that increases profits but is harmful to the environment. In the case of our cancer patient, however, society may be *positively* impacted for many years in the future by her current treatment. The same considerations might apply to the child born from IVF who may productively contribute to society over a lifetime, both culturally and economically.

Underlying Assumptions of Perfect Competition

With these examples in mind, let us now return to the widely held belief that increased free-market competition in health care will reduce cost, improve consumer choice, and enhance quality. The desire for market solutions to resource allocations in health care has been such a driving force in shaping the US health care system that it is helpful to understand the theory of perfect competition that has guided the tone of much of the debate. For the remainder of this chapter, therefore, I introduce the basic principles of this theory and its tools of analysis, which are then applied in subsequent chapters.

Under the "general equilibrium theory" of economics, a perfect market is defined by several conditions, collectively referred to as perfect competition. The assumptions that underlie perfect competition are as follows:

- There are a large number of buyers and sellers of a homogeneous product.
- All consumers and producers have perfect knowledge of price, quality, and the real value of the good or service (e.g., in health care, this includes medical need and efficacy).
- Buyers are rational and make purchases of goods or services that maximize their "utility," a concept economists use to reflect the overall satisfaction that buyers obtain from consuming a good or service.
- Suppliers make choices that maximize their profits.
- There are no externalities associated with consumption and production. Only the consumer of the product is affected by its consumption and pays for it; and only the supplier of the product obtains revenues and bears production costs.
- There are no barriers to entry. In health care, this would mean no educational or licensing barriers for physicians and other health care providers, and no Certificate of Need requirements for hospitals and other facilities.
- As a corollary of these assumptions, since there are many buyers of a homogeneous product who are rational consumers with perfect

knowledge, and many independent suppliers, supply and demand are independently determined. Consumers and producers are then price takers at the market clearing price.

When these conditions of perfect competition hold, it can be shown (graphically and mathematically) that the market will reach an equilibrium in which the quantity supplied for every product or service equals the quantity demanded at the equilibrium price. Under perfect competition there is no waste: the production of goods and services is efficient, in that it is carried out at the lowest possible unit cost. And consumption is "efficient" as well, in that individuals allocate their consumption of goods and services in a manner associated with their highest level of satisfaction given their personal budgets.

As already noted, the perfect-competition equilibrium has come to be described as "Pareto efficient" (i.e., an allocation of resources in which, given each individual's income and budget constraint, everyone would be at their highest standard of living because it would be impossible to reallocate resources so as to make any one individual better off without making at least one individual worse). As illustrated by our case examples of IVF and cancer treatment, however, economic efficiency does not imply equity in the distribution of wealth or in an allocation of resources that optimally reflects societal values. The patient of limited means with cancer who can afford surgery but not radiation therapy is making an optimal personal decision given her income, but most Americans would consider this a suboptimal result societally and would be willing to contribute to a tax-advantaged, employer-based insurance program that covers radiation treatment. Many (albeit fewer) would be willing to contribute through government taxation to a program that provides such treatment for those who need it medically but who do not have affordable access to any form of health insurance.

Health insurance can theoretically be provided efficiently in a perfectly competitive market, but this requires "perfect information" about risk and valuation by consumers. Moreover, such insurance carries with it the potential that consumption will increase once insured (i.e., referred to as "moral hazard") and the potential that insurers would charge high prices for individuals with preexisting conditions or other reasons to be at risk for health care utilization. As always, the consumption of insurance will be inequitable in relation to income. Those with higher incomes will be more likely to purchase insurance than those with lower incomes.

Historical Roots

The concept that free-market capitalism leads invisibly and automatically to an economically efficient society—one that operates at the maximum possible business productivity and consumer satisfaction as a result of each business owner and consumer pursuing his or her own interests—has its roots in the writings of economists in the eighteenth and nineteenth centuries. Among others, Adam Smith's *An Inquiry into the Nature and Causes of the Wealth of Nations*[2] and Alfred Marshall's *Principles of Economics*[3] were perhaps the most influential.

Adam Smith

Adam Smith (1723–1790) was a Scottish economist whose *Wealth of Nations* is arguably one of the most influential books ever written. Smith advanced a view of societal interactions that was considered radical at the time. He argued that the population as a whole would prosper most if individuals were free to follow their own interests. The pursuit of self-interest would not produce chaos, he posited, but rather order and concord. The dictums of kings and other monarchs—who often supported vested interests by taxing imports, subsidizing exports, and granting protective monopolies, among other executive actions—would lead to a less advanced and robust society than one in which people were free to trade with one another without intervention by the government; in so doing, Smith argued, the nation's resources would be directed by "an invisible hand" to the ends and purposes that people valued most highly.

Interestingly, it was his book on ethics, *The Theory of Moral Sentiments*,[4] and not *Wealth of Nations*, that first launched Adam Smith as a major scholar of his day. It was in this book that the term "invisible hand" was first used: "The rich . . . are led by an invisible hand to make nearly the same distributions of the necessaries of life which would have been made had the earth been divided into equal portions among all of its inhabitants, and thus without intending it, without knowing it, advance the interest of society."[5]

Smith explored his invisible hand idea from several different angles in *Wealth of Nations*. For example, he writes, "It is not from the benevolence of the butcher, the brewer, or the baker, that we expect our dinner, but from their regard to their own interest."[6] And: "Every individual . . . neither intends to promote the public interest, nor knows how much he is promoting it . . . he intends only his own security; and by directing that industry in such a manner as its produce may be of the greatest value, he intends only his own gain, and he is in this, as in many other cases, led by an invisible hand to promote an end which was not part of his intention."[7]

Thus, the endorsement of free markets and the pursuit of self-interest by the man credited with being its most influential and founding thinker is not an endorsement of greed, as is sometimes believed; rather, Smith posits that such self-interest drives the economy in an automatic, invisible fashion toward the greater societal good.

What a powerful idea! All of us who have lived in a capitalist society such as the United States have witnessed the benefits of these fundamental concepts. It is understandable that, to this day, advocates of free-market capitalism refer back to the fundamental tenets of Adam Smith's *Wealth of Nations* when arguing in favor of an industry, including the health care industry, to be left alone to pursue its interests.

It is sometimes the case, however, that the underlying assumptions do not apply, leading to unwelcome results. For example, if (for a variety of reasons) there is only one seller instead of the large number of sellers posited in the first assumption earlier, a monopoly results. In contrast to perfect competition in which market forces from many sellers push price toward the marginal cost of production, thus driving down profit margins, a monopolist can forever set price above marginal cost, thus generating sustained supernormal profits. Consumers must therefore persistently pay a higher price for the monopolist's products than would be the case if there were many other producers. Such a price would lead to inefficiently low consumption of the product. If the high price of a new, improved drug protected by patent were unsubsidized by insurance, for example, some buyers might then choose a cheaper, but inferior treatment, as an alternative.

Adam Smith voiced concern about these issues even as he advanced the core belief that self-interested competition in the free market would tend to benefit society as a whole by keeping prices low while still building in an incentive for a wide variety of goods and services. He railed against the collusive nature of business interests, warning they can conspire to act as a monopoly, fixing the highest price "which can be squeezed out of the buyers."[8]

Thus, the author of the invisible hand understood that departures from the fundamental assumptions underlying free-market competition would lead to suboptimal results. To what extent does health care deviate from these assumptions and what are the implications of such deviations? To answer this question, we shall introduce the work of two other other historically important economists, Antoine Cournot and Alfred Marshall, who also made landmark contributions that continue to be influential to this day.

Antoine Cournot and Alfred Marshall

With the tremendous rate of change in scientific thought that we have experienced in recent years, we may forget that advances occurred much more slowly in previous centuries. Thus, it is perhaps surprising that the invisible hand concept developed by Adam Smith in the mid-to-late eighteenth century was not translated into the now ubiquitous tools of supply and demand until many decades later, in the works of Antoine Cournot and Alfred Marshall.

Although the British economist Marshall popularized the idea that the interaction of supply and demand determines an equilibrium price as part of his 1890 six-volume publication *Principles of Economics*, it was Cournot, a French mathematician, who laid the groundwork for this work in *Researches on the Mathematical Principles of the Theory of Wealth*.[9] In applying the mathematical tools of functions and probability to economic analysis, Cournot was the first to derive supply and demand equations as a function of price and to draw supply and demand curves on a graph.

Marshall drew on the ideas of Adam Smith and Antoine Cournot, extending their concepts in great detail and also using them as foundational principles for many other areas of economic analysis that he developed. Marshall's body of work largely shaped mainstream economic thought for the next half-century, both through his own analysis and that of his students, such as Arthur Pigou and John Maynard Keynes, who themselves became highly influential.

Prior to Marshall, there was tremendous controversy regarding the question: "What determines the value of a commodity?" Classical economists argued that supply (reflecting the cost of production) was the major force behind value. By contrast, other economists believed that demand, based on marginal "utility" (or consumer satisfaction) was the major determining factor. Marshall's analysis, which showed that it was the *interaction* of supply and demand that determined value, proved to be paradigmshifting in its impact. Marshall likened supply and demand to two blades of a pair of scissors but suggested that it was useless to ask which blade does the cutting: "We might as reasonably dispute, whether it is the upper or under blade of a pair of scissors that cuts a piece of paper, as whether value is governed by utility or cost of production. It is true that when one blade is held still, and the cutting is effected by moving the other, we may say with careless brevity that cutting is done by the second; but the statement is not strictly accurate, and is to be excused only so long as it claims to be merely a popular and not a strictly scientific account of what happens."[10]

In making this case, Marshall embedded two ideas in his writing that have stood the test of time. One was shifting from "value" as the center of analysis and replacing it with price; the other was his emphasis on marginal behavior. It is marginal utility that dictates the downward sloping shape of the demand curve, in that the marginal (additional) benefit to the consumer falls as more of a product is consumed. And, as quantity rises, it is the increasing marginal cost of greater production that leads to the upward sloping supply curve. In this sense, price is then determined by the forces of supply and demand at the margin.

Supply and Demand

With this background, let's look at a classic analysis of supply and demand curves and how they interact to determine price using the demand for IVF procedures in a geographic region (figure 2.1). The y-axis is the price of IVF and the x-axis is quantity of IVF procedures in the region. D–D′ is the demand curve, which is downward sloping to reflect the inverse relationship between price and quantity in a geographic region (i.e., at a lower price more

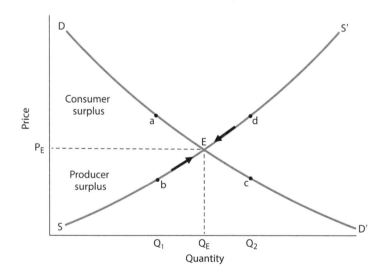

Figure 2.1. Supply and demand for in vitro fertilization: equilibrium price and quantity

infertility patients who are candidates for IVF will purchase the procedure). S–S' is the supply curve, which slopes upward because IVF programs will be willing to perform more procedures as the price rises.

The stage is now set for the analysis of how supply and demand interact to determine price. Marshall's discourse in *Principles of Economics* refers to decisions around bringing "goods to market," but the same principles would apply to bringing "services to market," such as IVF, which requires a team of doctors, embryologists, nurses, and others. Explanatory brackets related to figure 2.1 have been inserted into Marshall's explanation:

> When therefore the amount produced (in a unit of time) is such that the demand price is greater than the supply price [i.e., at quantity Q_1 of IVF procedures, the price at point a is greater than the price at point b], then sellers receive more than is sufficient to make it worth their while to bring goods to market to that amount; and there is at work an active force tending to increase the amount brought forward for sale [i.e., IVF programs will perform more IVF procedures, as shown by the upward arrow along the supply curve]. On the other hand, when the amount produced is such that the demand price is less than the supply price [i.e., at quantity Q_2 of IVF procedures, the price at point c is less than the price at point d], sellers receive less than is sufficient to make it worth their while to bring goods to market on that scale; so that those who were just on the margin of doubt as to whether to go on producing are decided not to do so, and there is an active force at work tending to diminish the amount brought forward for sale [as shown by the downward arrow along the supply curve]. When the demand price is equal to the supply price, the amount produced has no tendency either to be increased or to be diminished; it is in equilibrium [i.e., point E associated with an equilibrium price P_E and quantity Q_E].[11]

Marshall also used equilibrium price to define the concepts of "consumer surplus" and "producer surplus."[12] The former is the difference between the price that buyers actually pay for a good or service—the equilibrium price—and the highest amount they would have paid, while the latter is the difference between the price sellers receive and the lowest price they would have accepted. In figure 2.1 (akin to how Marshall diagrammed it), consumer surplus is the area above the dotted line corresponding to price P_E and below the demand curve, while producer surplus is the area below P_E and above the supply curve. A competitive equilibrium maximizes consumer and producer surplus. Moreover, the "first welfare theorem of economics" (also called the "invisible hand theorem") is that any competive equilibrium is Pareto efficient. However, consumer surplus depends on consumer income; this is the manifestation of the inequities in competitive equilibrium.

Marshall emphasized that under free-market conditions, producers who are responsible for the supply of goods and services do not influence consumer demand. That is, supply and demand curves are independent of one another in producing a market-clearing price at their intersection. He goes on to comment on the dynamics of the process, making analogies to physical phenomena, perhaps in an effort to convey that there are economic "laws" that parallel physical laws:

> When demand and supply are in equilibrium, the amount of the commodity which is being produced in a unit of time may be called the equilibrium-amount, and the price at which it is being sold may be called the equilibrium-price. Such an equilibrium is stable; that is, the price, if displaced a little from it, will tend to return, as a pendulum oscillates about its lowest point; and it will be found to be a characteristic of stable equilibria that in them the demand price is greater than the supply price for amounts just less than the equilibrium amount, and vice versa. . . . When demand and supply are in stable equilibrium, if any accident should move the scale of production from its equilibrium position, there will be instantly brought into play forces tending to push it back to that position; just as, if a stone hanging by a string is displaced from its equilibrium position, the force of gravity will at once tend to bring it back to its equilibrium position.[13]

Although it is attractive to think of the price-setting dynamics of supply and demand as analogous to gravitational forces, deviations from underlying assumptions are much more common in economics than in matters of gravity and other laws of physical science. In the next chapter, we consider the implications of deviations in these assumptions in health care. Before jumping in, though, there is one addition to the analysis of supply and demand that will be helpful.

Again using the supply and demand for in vitro fertilization as an example, as the price of IVF rises there will be a decline in demand for IVF along the demand curve D–D', and an increase in the quantity of procedures that IVF programs will be willing to provide along the supply curve S–S'. However, there are situations in which there may be a *shift in the entire demand and/or supply curves* (figure 2.2).

For example, suppose that IVF pregnancy rates significantly improve due to a new technology. This would shift the market demand curve to the right, for example, from D_1–D_1' to D_2–D_2'. That is, at any given price, more

Figure 2.2. Supply and demand for in vitro fertilization: effects of shifts in supply and demand curves

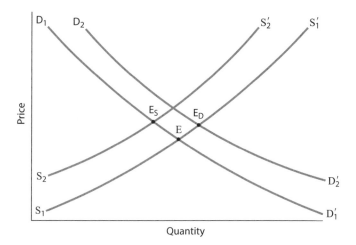

infertility patients would be willing to pay that price and enroll in IVF programs, as their odds of success are higher. Such a shift in the demand curve, if the supply curve remained at S_1–S_1', would imply a shift in the equilibrium price and quantity from E to E_D.

Now suppose that there is an increase in the cost of production for IVF services. The cost of nurses and laboratory personnel may have increased and/or the cost of supplies, for example. If costs rise, fewer procedures can be provided at any given price, so the supply curve shifts inward, or to the left. This would also cause an increase in the equilibrium price, in this case corresponding to point E_S. By contrast, enhanced technology that allows greater productivity of existing staff, or an expansion in the number of IVF programs in the market would lead to the shift in the supply curve outward (not shown) and a reduced equilibrium price.

Of note, advancements in technology that produce better outcomes in health are an example of the "dynamic efficiency" that occurs in the health care industry. Dynamic efficiency occurs over time and is strongly linked to the pace of innovation within a market and improvements in both the range of choice for consumers and the quality of goods or services. This phenomenon is distinguished from the more static allocative and productive efficiency of Pareto. It is sometimes argued that persistent supernormal profits in some health care sectors (e.g., pharmaceuticals) can be justified on the basis of promoting innovation and dynamic efficiency.

All of these principles of supply and demand are used in the next chapter to discuss what happens when there are departures from the underlying assumptions of perfect competition in the market for health care services.

Summary

It is often argued that the introduction of more free-market competition into the market for health care services would lead to reduced costs, improved consumer choice, and better quality. In this chapter I laid the groundwork for a discussion of the market for health care services by reviewing the assumptions underlying the model of perfect competition and providing historical context for the early and still influential economists whose theories of perfect competition as a basis for societal welfare continue to be quite powerful in current policy discussions. Alfred Marshall's description of the dynamics of supply and demand, creating forces that lead automatically to a market-clearing price, was indeed the basis for generations of subsequent economic analyses. All of these began with the same set of perfect competition assumptions, which collectively supported Adam Smith's eighteenth-century vision of the invisible hand.

The basic elements of price-setting mechanisms by supply and demand interactions set the stage for what happens when some of the underlying assumptions of the theory are not met in the health care industry. Given these free-market assumptions, a Pareto-efficient economy would result in which no one could be made better off without making someone else worse off. A Pareto-efficient economy, however, does not necessarily optimize social welfare, as was illlustrated using health care examples.

The overall conclusions of this chapter are that (1) perfect competition is very enticing and powerful in theory, but its functioning depends on a set of underlying assumptions that may not apply to health care; and (2) *if* there were a system in which health care decisions were made in an environment that approximated the free-market competitive model, some of the results may nonetheless be contrary to societal values.

3   IMPERFECTIONS IN THE MARKET FOR HEALTH CARE SERVICES

Stakeholders involved directly or indirectly in the provision of health care (e.g., physicians and other providers, hospitals, insurance companies, pharmaceutical companies, and device manufacturers) are generally quite satisfied that they are contributing to high-quality patient care. Moreover, employers benefit from providing health benefits to employees on a tax-exempt basis and consumers (patients) benefit from receiving such health insurance as part of their employment. And yet, the US health care industry suffers from serious shortcomings in care, cost, and access.

Regarding care, Americans are much less healthy overall than citizens of other countries. For example, among the 35 countries that participate in the Organisation for Economic Co-operation and Development, the United States ranks 32nd in infant mortality[1] (i.e., infant deaths per 1,000 live births), 31st in female life expectancy at age 40, and 27th in male life expectancy at age 40.[2] A series of reports from the National Academy of Medicine have documented substantial deficits in the safety of medical care and disparities in the quality of care.[3] While access to medical services may be readily available for some, tens of millions of Americans have poor access and receive less than exemplary care.

Regarding cost, expenditures on health care per capita in the United States are almost twice as high as other high-income nations, absorbing about 18 percent of the US gross domestic product (GDP). This compares with 7–8 percent of GDP in Ireland and Israel and 9–11 percent of GDP in such other high-income nations as Australia, Austria, Belgium, Canada, Denmark, Finland, Italy, Japan, Norway, Sweden, the Netherlands, and the United Kingdom. The nation with the next highest percent of GDP spent on health care is Switzerland, at 12.3 percent.

Not only do we have poorer health outcomes at higher cost than other high-income nations but also more inequitable access to care. About 10 percent of Americans are uninsured for health care expenses, as compared with universal coverage in virtually all other high GDP-per-capita nations. And many more Americans are underinsured (i.e., they have health insurance policies with limited coverage and high deductibles). Consequently, the extent to which needed health care is forgone due to cost is much greater in the United States than in other high-income nations. For example, 22 percent of consultations are skipped due to cost in the United States, as compared with 12 percent in the Netherlands, 7 percent in Switzerland, and 4 percent in Sweden.[4]

Do the Assumptions of Perfect Competition Hold for Health Care?

Part of the reason the United States has gotten to this state of poorer outcomes, higher cost, and inequitable access is rooted in the nature of health care, which is often inconsistent with the assumptions underlying well-functioning competitive markets:

1. *There are a large number of buyers and sellers of a homogeneous product.*

    Through the first half of the twentieth century, physicians primarily practiced solo or in small groups, hospitals were mainly small or medium-sized individual facilities serving their communities, and patients were billed for services directly by physicians and hospitals. Currently, however, substantial entities are involved in most health care transactions, including government, insurance companies, employers, and large, multisite health systems that employ physicians and other health care providers. Individual consumers rarely interact in the market with individual physicians and hospitals to produce a market price, except for discretionary services that aren't covered by insurance.

    Regarding homogeneity, health care services are clearly heterogeneous in terms of outcomes. Some heart transplant programs have much better patient survival rates than others. Some laser refractive surgery (e.g., LASIK) programs have better patient outcomes and safety profiles than others. Many other examples can be given to support the case that medical services are not homogeneous in their outcomes. And there are other aspects of heterogeneity: some medical offices or hospitals are more convenient in their location; some may provide similar expertise in evaluation and treatment but with greater hospitality and service; the personality of the physician and/or staff may differentiate one practice from another; and differentiation may occur based on reputation or the availability of a particular technology.

2. *All consumers and producers have perfect knowledge of price, quality, and the real value of a good or service (but in health care, real value includes need and efficacy).*

As applied to health care, this assumption is clearly an abstraction—the reader might think it is an absurd abstraction! Economic theorists advanced this assumption about perfect knowledge, which complements their assumption about homogeneous products, with the goal of creating a theory that captures enough reality to be correct in its essence. In the current US health care industry, however, price is opaque and medical knowledge is asymmetric between doctors and patients. Physicians' offices and hospitals do not post prices for all to see. And through their training, clinical experience, and ongoing education, physicians and other providers have a fundamentally different context of knowledge and expertise into which they place information about a patient's history, physical findings, and diagnostic results, even in this era of ubiquitous search engines and artificial intelligence.

3. *Buyers are rational and make purchases of goods or services that maximize "economic utility" (overall satisfaction).*

In many respects, the assumption of consumer rationality and utility maximization holds for health care to the same extent as many other services, but the ability of consumers to remain rational in the face of significant illness, and to make decisions with a goal of maximizing utility in the face of imperfect and incomplete information, is arguably more difficult for health care than for most other services.

4. *Suppliers make choices that maximize their profits.*

This assumption also largely holds for health care to the same extent as it applies to many other services. There are some caveats, however. In making health care recommendations, physicians and other health professionals have a responsibility to serve as their patients' agents, in addition to being mindful of their fees and personal income. Community hospitals and other nonprofit health care institutions have a responsibility to provide community benefit, but they also pursue profit maximization according to the adage "no margin, no mission," attributed to the Daughters of Charity. A similar statement can be made about nonprofit health insurance companies. However, investor-owned hospitals, insurance firms, pharmaceutical companies, device manufacturers, and other for-profit companies in the health care industry have the same return on investment goals as for-profit entities in other sectors of the economy. In practice, while the cultures are quite different between nonprofit and for-profit organizations in health care, the goal to maximize financial margins is functionally quite similar throughout the industry.

5. *There are no externalities associated with consumption and production. Only the consumer of the product is affected by its consumption and pays for it, and only the supplier of the product obtains revenues and bears production costs.*

Some externalities are clearly present in health care. Immunization against communicable disease is one example. Biomedical and clinical research is another. Some externalities are less obvious but important: for example, medical treatments can extend the lives of individuals who then tangibly benefit others by living longer. The intangible benefit to family and friends of an individual receiving successful medical treatment that prolongs his or her life is a profound, but difficult to measure, externality.

6. *There are no barriers to entry (e.g., in health care, no educational or licensing barriers for physicians and other health care providers, and no Certificate of Need requirements for hospitals).*

There are clearly barriers to entry in health care. For the most part, although a departure from the perfect competition model, there are good reasons for such barriers. Patients rely on their health care providers to make the right decisions on their behalf based on deep knowledge and informed clinical experience. Educational and licensing requirements for physicians and other health care providers ensure a requisite level of knowledge and skill to achieve this goal. Most national board certification entities, as well as state licensing authorities and local hospital board privileging systems, require continuing education and recertification, which further ensures that health care providers meet ongoing standards of knowledge and performance throughout their careers. That said, the limited number of residency positions, especially in certain specialties and subspecialties (which continues to this day), has limited the supply of physicians. This shifts the supply curve for physicians to the left, increasing professional fees.

Certificate of Need regulations are currently in place in 36 states and the District of Columbia. Through these certificates, states regulate the number of beds in hospitals and nursing homes and prevent the purchase of more equipment (e.g., magnetic resonance imaging [MRI] machines) than is thought to be necessary. Statutory authority for state agencies to approve such facilities and equipment on the basis of need is contrary to the assumption of free entry under the competitive model.

7. *Independence of supply and demand.*

As a corollary to the first six assumptions, since there is a large number of producers under perfect competition, and large numbers of buyers of a homogeneous product who are rational consumers with perfect knowledge under perfect competition, supply and demand are independently determined. As a result, (a) the market-clearing price is determined by the actions of producers and consumers based on supply and demand forces, (b) consumers are price takers at the market price, and (c) providers do not have the power to influence demand. One could easily argue that the opposite is true for health care. Due to health care coverage by employers and government, the trust that patients place in their doctors, and their imperfect knowledge about medical treatments, the following is more likely true: (a) the price paid to providers is determined not by interaction of supply and demand in the market but by negotiations between a relatively small number of insurers, government agencies, and health systems; (b) the price paid by patients is only a fraction of the negotiated price (i.e., the co-pay); and (c) physicians and other providers can exert a substantial influence on demand.

Implications of Deviations from Perfect Competition Assumptions

Since many of the assumptions of perfect competition do not appear to hold in the field of health care, it logically follows that some of the theoretical implications of the perfect competition model are not likely to hold. But how important are these assumption deviations for health care relative to other industries in the US economy? Are there some features of health care that are more important than others?

Heterogeneous Product

When differentiation of a health care service is present, patients will not be indifferent to the choice of a doctor or hospital as they would under perfect competition with homogeneous services; rather, they will often make active choices for one provider over another according to their preferences. To this extent, monopoly elements are introduced into the market. However, heterogeneity of health care services with respect to location, hospitality and service, perceived quality, and a host of other considerations is shared by most other goods and services in the economy. West Texas Intermediate crude oil and other commodities are essentially homogeneous, but for most consumption items (whether smartphones, clothing, groceries, shampoo, floor tile, or virtually any other good) or services (e.g., auto mechanics, financial advisers, home designers, restaurants, hotels, etc.) there is clearly differentiation such that consumers may have preferences for one seller over another. In this market environment, sellers will be able to exert some level of monopoly influence and price will be higher than under pure perfect competition. This is the main result of the theory of monopolistic competition as described in 1933 by Edward Chamberlin.[5]

Thus, the fact that product and service differentiation exists in health care is not itself a factor that differentiates it from many other products and services. However, for reasons to be discussed, consumers are less likely to shop for medical care at a time of need than they are to shop for other differentiated services.

Fewer Buyers and Sellers

While it may seem like there are large numbers of buyers (patients) and sellers (doctors, hospitals, nursing homes, pharmacists, etc.) in the US health industry, price in our current environment is not set in a free market through the interaction of supply and demand by individual buyers and sellers. Rather, large entities are involved. For most health care prices, organizations such as government (Medicare, Medicaid) or private insurance companies negotiate a fee schedule with large health systems (academic, community, or investor-owned), health maintenance organizations, or other entities that include physicians, hospitals, nursing homes, and pharmacy services. Or, large employers work with actuaries and third-party administrators to create self-insured products in which the prices for health care services and pharmaceuticals are also negotiated. This phenomenon has been an important contributor to prices that are significantly higher for health care services than would be the case under perfect competition or monopolistic competition. As we see in subsequent chapters, the greater per capita expenditures on health care in the United States as compared with other developed countries is largely due to higher prices and greater administrative cost, and less attributable to greater utilization.

Imperfect Knowledge

The question here is whether the assumption of perfect knowledge about health care services—need, quality, efficacy, and price, among other attributes—captures enough reality to be meaningful and pertinent in the actual functioning of the health care industry, or does this assumption depart from reality to such an extent that the theory of perfect competition as applied to health care is no longer correct in its essence.

One thing that physicians (and other providers) quickly appreciate in their training, and repeatedly experience in their subsequent practice, is the strength of the physician-patient relationship and the extent to which physicians are influential in the decision-making process of their patients. While some patients come to a physician having read the entire medical literature on their condition, seek second and third opinions with this knowledge to make decisions on treatment A vs. treatment B, and conduct extensive personal research on which physician and health system should provide that treatment, the vast majority of patients turn to their physicians for their expert advice and simply take it. They *want* to trust their doctor to do the right thing for them. "Whatever you say, Doc," is the recurrent phrase. Most patients don't know much about the underlying pathophysiology of their condition or the evidence in the literature (or lack thereof) in support of the efficacy of the treatment being recommended vs. alternative treatments. They also don't know much about the benefits and risks of active treatment vs. conservative management or the price of treatment. Not only are patients unaware of the price of treatment but many may not care since their insurance company (or government programs) will pay for most of it. Thus, large employers that have offered price transparency to employees have not seen a reduction in health care spending.[6] Typically, whatever knowledge they have is limited and imperfect in comparison to that of the doctor. Even when there is significant out-of-pocket cost, patients will typically follow their doctors' advice. For example, in the case of a diagnostic study that is relatively homogeneous and can be obtained in advance of care such as a lower-limb MRI, a recent study found that patients will generally follow the referral from their physician, even though they could have saved an average of 44 percent of their out-of-pocket costs by price shopping and having the MRI done at a different nearby location.[7]

Nobel laureate Kenneth Arrow summed it up this way in his classic paper entitled "Uncertainty and the Welfare Economics of Medical Care," published in 1963: "Because medical knowledge is so complicated, the information possessed by the physician as to the consequences and possibilities of treatment is necessarily very much greater than that of the patient, or at least so it is believed by both parties. Further, both parties are aware of this informational inequality, and their relation is colored by this knowledge."[8] He referred to this phenomenon as "information asymmetry." Patients want to trust their doctors and will generally follow their advice, but information asymmetry may sometimes leave patients vulnerable to receiving services that are unnecessary or of unproven efficacy and paying more for services than they would have if they had better information on price.

The asymmetry of information that occurs in health care is, in a sense, no different from the asymmetry that can occur with other expert service providers, such as lawyers, financial advisors, electricians, plumbers, wedding consultants, and the like. The implications of information asymmetry pertain most directly to the lack of independent supply and demand curves: if health care providers of all stripes exploit their superior knowledge to create demand (whether for medial or surgical treatments, or for diagnostic studies like MRIs), demand is no longer independent of supply and distortion of both price and quantity is thereby introduced into the market.

Barriers to Entry

Rigorous education and high standards for licensing, board certification, and hospital privileging are important safeguards for quality. Barriers to entry may sometimes compromise the efficient provision of high-quality health care. This can occur when medical societies (whether state, national, or specialty-specific) act as trade organizations protecting its members and restrict the scope of practice of other health professionals (e.g., nurse practitioners, optometrists). Greater provision of services by such individuals on a health care team can allow physicians to focus on patients who present with conditions of higher complexity. While some argue for an end to Certificate of Need requirements for hospitals and other health care entities on the basis of promoting competition, advocates argue that they are necessary to limit supply-induced demand and to prevent the siphoning of insured patients by new hospitals in high-income areas from existing safety-net hospitals.

Consumers Are Not Price Takers at the Market Price and Producers Can Influence Demand

In health care, patients are *not* price takers at the market price, and providers *can* influence demand. The price paid by patients is generally not the full price that providers will be paid by the insurance company or government program but rather the coinsurance payment or "co-pay." And since this co-pay is much less than the full price, it follows from a negatively sloping demand curve that the utilization of health services by patients will be much greater than if they were facing the full price. But since the insurance company or government program pays providers the full price, total expenditures (which equals the full price × higher quantity) are much greater than they would be without insurance. Moreover, when consumers (theoretically) know all there is to know about a service, those who supply that service cannot influence demand. But patients do *not* know all there is to know about a particular medical condition, diagnostic test, imaging study, or treatment. Therefore, the providers of health care, who make recommendations regarding office visits, diagnostic tests, imaging studies, and medical or surgical treatments, can indeed induce demand by influencing a patient's decision to purchase such services, especially when the cost (i.e., co-pay) is low.

Example of Higher Health Care Expenditures Due to Price Subsidies and Increased Demand

Let us return to our in vitro fertilization model as an example of how imperfections in the market can lead to distortions that can dramatically increase total health care expenditures. Fifteen states currently have laws pertaining to health insurance coverage for IVF.[9] Of these, five have mandates that commercial insurers must cover a certain number of IVF attempts or cover IVF up to a financial cap. The remaining 35 states have no laws governing IVF insurance mandates. In those states, IVF is generally not covered by health insurance. Under the assumptions of perfect competition, the price paid by consumers is determined by the intersection of independent supply and demand curves. We will see what that looks like for IVF in states without insurance mandates and then overlay the implications of price subsidies (in states with insurance mandates) and provider-induced demand (figure 3.1).

In graph A, the market demand curve for a state reflects decisions by infertile couples who are candidates for IVF but who may or may not choose to undergo the procedure depending on price. The downward-sloping demand curve D–D' reflects the increasing numbers of couples in the state who would choose to undergo IVF as price declines. The supply curve S–S', which reflects market marginal cost, is the aggregate of the individual cost functions of IVF programs in the state. Competitive equilibrium (E) occurs at price P_C and quantity Q_C. Total expenditures on IVF in the state without an insurance mandate, which are entirely incurred by patients paying for the procedure out of pocket, is shown by the lightly-shaded box and is equal to $P_C \times Q_C$.

Now let's see what happens in a state where the legislature has passed a mandate that insurance companies in the state must cover IVF (graph B). (Most of the state IVF statutes pertaining to mandated insurance coverage were passed in the 1980s and 1990s; Connecticut was the last state to pass such a law in 2005.) Patients will pay a subsidized price (P_S) for IVF services (i.e., the amount of the co-pay). At the subsidized price, the quantity of IVF demanded in the state is Q_S, which exceeds the competitive equilibrium amount of Q_C. But here's the critical issue: at quantity Q_S, the fee paid to the IVF clinics is *not* what the patient pays (P_S); it's what the insurance company pays (P_I). Thus, IVF clinics receive a "producer subsidy" of $P_I - P_S$ for each IVF service. The price and quantity of IVF is now given by the full price that insurers have agreed to pay (P_I) and the increased quantity of IVF procedures (Q_S) demanded by patients at the subsidized price (P_S). Thus, the total statewide expenditure for IVF has now expanded to $P_I \times Q_S$, and the increase in total expenditures is shown by the medium-shaded rectangle.

In addition to the increased utilization and expenditures due to a producer price subsidy, additional expenditures can occur because of induced

Figure 3.1. Supply and demand for in vitro fertilization with and without a state insurance mandate and with induced demand

A. Without insurance mandate

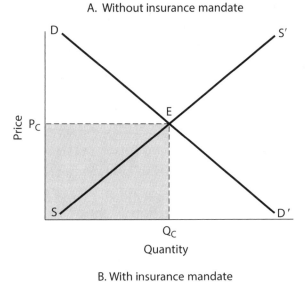

B. With insurance mandate

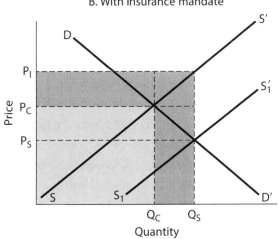

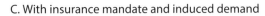

C. With insurance mandate and induced demand

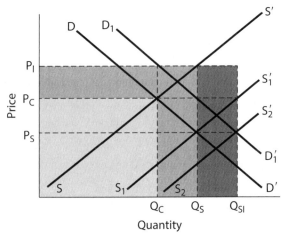

demand (graph C). Induced demand occurs when an infertile couple decides to undergo IVF after their physician recommends it when they wouldn't have done so otherwise. Let D–D' represent a baseline level of demand that is independent of the physician's recommendation, representing perfect competition in which the decisions of consumers are completely independent of the actions of producers. The effect of induced demand is shown by an outward shift of the demand curve to D_1–D_1'.

How do we get to D_1–D_1', a situation in which the statewide quantity of IVF demanded is higher than the baseline amount at every price? Some IVF providers may counsel patients that IVF might be their best treatment option because of a sincere belief that this is the best course of action for them. For other providers, their own financial benefit may be a consideration. In clinical practice, the process is subtle and complex. Consider a couple in which the woman is 33 years old, still well within her normal reproductive years. Twelve months have passed since they decided they wanted to have a baby and discontinued contraception, but no pregnancy has occurred. They technically meet the definition of infertility (12 months of trying without success), but after 12 months this couple by random chance would have about a 10 percent chance of not establishing a pregnancy even if they have absolutely no anatomic or endocrine basis for infertility. This estimate is based on a calculated cumulative probability rate of pregnancy after 12 months among couples who have a probability of pregnancy of 20 percent per month, which is about average. For such couples, the probability of pregnancy during month 13 is the same 20 percent as any other normally fertile couple.

The couple is initially counseled that maybe they should try a little longer, as they are young and might be normally fertile but "unlucky" to this point. But they are also told that if they are anxious about the possibility that something might be wrong, they could undergo an infertility evaluation if they wish, "just to see if there's any specific cause for infertility." They are indeed anxious, and besides, their insurance covers infertility evaluation. A full infertility evaluation is performed and no abnormality is found in either partner. They now have a diagnosis of "unexplained infertility." They are again counseled that maybe they could try a little longer, but they could also try infertility treatment if they wish, as this could help them become pregnant soon rather than waiting and seeing. The couple is worried that something is truly wrong even if the infertility testing was not able to identify a problem. They imagine that maybe the testing is not sensitive or thorough enough. And besides, their insurance covers infertility treatment.

The couple returns to see their physician to discuss possible treatments. Their doctor explains that one option is fertility drugs that increase the number of eggs that are ovulated each month. This approach, however, carries with it a chance of multiple pregnancy, which can be dangerous because of premature birth. IVF is more expensive, but it is covered under their insurance plan. Moreover, the couple is counseled that modern treatments involve only one embryo being transferred to the uterus for implantation, thereby preventing multiple pregnancy. (Any additional embryos can be frozen for future potential use.) Overall, the physician recommends IVF.

In view of all these considerations, the couple chooses to proceed with IVF. All of the couples across the state in this situation who make the decision to undergo IVF contribute to the shifting of the demand curve from D–D' to D_1–D_1'. The quantity demanded under both price subsidies and induced demand is Q_{SI}, and the price paid to IVF clinics remains at P_I, with the fixed-unit subsidy of $P_I - P_S$. Thus, total statewide expenditures on IVF under conditions of an insurance mandate and induced demand is $P_I \times Q_{SI}$, and the increased expenditure due to induced demand is shown by the hatched rectangle. While graph C is just a depiction of tendencies and is not meant to be quantitative (in terms of the sizes of the different shaded boxes), the directionality is clear: total expenditures on IVF are higher than they would be in world of perfect competition, partly due to price subsidies from insurance coverage and partly due to induced demand.

Data are available to support the proposition that insurance mandates for IVF increase utilization. While not recent, a study by Jain, Harlow, and Hornstein[10] compares IVF utilization in states with and without insurance mandates using a straightforward methodology that should hold in any time frame. In this study, rates of IVF utilization in each state for women between the ages of 25 and 45 were calculated using 1998 IVF data as reported to the Center for Disease Control and Prevention and the 2000 US Census. Utilization rates in three states with complete insurance mandates for IVF, and in five states with partial mandates, were compared to the rates in the remaining states without any mandated insurance coverage for IVF. The utilization rate for states with a complete insurance mandate was 3.35 IVF cycles per 1,000 women, as compared to 1.21 for states without coverage. That is, utilization was 2.8 times higher in states with complete insurance mandates than in no-coverage states. Utilization in states with partial coverage, which varied widely in amount, was 1.46.

Summary

Upon analyzing the extent to which perfect competition assumptions hold for health care as well as the implications of deviations from these assumptions, we conclude that the most significant deviation is that consumers of health care do not interact in the market with sellers to create an equilibrium market price. While the price paid to providers is set by negotiation between large entities representing government, insurance companies, and health systems, the price paid by insured consumers is only a fraction of the negotiated price. At this lower price, consumers demand much more health care service than they would if they had to pay the full price. This process leads to high total expenditures on health care, since expenditures are, by definition, the product of the artificially high fixed price paid to providers and the expanded quantity of utilization based on the lower price paid by consumers. This phenomenon is exacerbated by induced demand, which arises from information asymmetry between doctors and patients combined with the trust that patients have in their physicians. Induced demand shifts the demand curve outward, resulting in even greater utilization and expenditure.

4 IMPLICATIONS OF AN IMPERFECT MARKET I
GREATER UTILIZATION DUE TO PRICE SUBSIDIES

Since we have concluded that some of the key assumptions underlying perfect competition do not hold up very well for health care and, as a consequence, total expenditures on health care are higher than they would be under the conditions of a perfect market, where does that leave us? How can we evaluate the impact of market imperfections?

Let's consider in turn

- greater utilization of health care due to the lower (subsidized) price paid by patients (this chapter),
- greater utilization due to induced demand (chapter 5),
- higher price paid to providers due to monopolistic elements and price determination by third-party negotiation (chapter 6), and
- inequality of health care utilization (chapter 7).

Utilization of health care at a price that would be produced by perfect competition (i.e., as a result of market interactions between large numbers of individual health care providers and consumers with perfect knowledge) would be efficient but not necessarily consistent with societal values. This is because, when faced with paying the full price of medical care under perfect competition, consumers of limited financial means making rational decisions about expenditures for food, shelter, and other needs might forego needed medical care. Consumers of moderate means might choose to pay for what they view as essential and (for them) affordable treatment (e.g., dental treatment for a painful tooth, insulin medication for diabetes, repair of a symptomatic hernia), but delay or avoid medical care that is needed but out of financial reach. These potential gaps in access under perfect competition are inconsistent with a value shared by most Americans that people should be able to receive medical care when it is truly needed. To create a bridge between the economic efficiency of competition and our societal values, a complex array of programs in the United States has evolved that entail price subsidies: employer-sponsored insurance plans, government programs such as Medicare and Medicaid, benefits for military veterans and government employees, and others.

While there is some variation in the details of these programs, the subsidy provided is the difference between the full price of care paid to providers and the patient's out-of-pocket payment. Let's first review concepts and data on the impact of price subsidies in the United States on health care utilization before turning to the question of how much subsidy is considered societally acceptable.

Impact of Price Subsidies on Utilization

"Moral hazard" is the name given to negative behavior that can arise from an individual or group being insured and taking on more risk than they would if they were not insured. That is, since people are consuming more of something than they would if they were not insured, it is argued that society's economic welfare is diminished. Economists generally consider the increase in quantity demanded due to price subsidies from insurance as representing moral hazard.

How can we evaluate the effect of such price subsidies—that is, the impact of insurance on the utilization of health care services? One way is to compare utilization in geographic areas with and without insurance. As we learned in the last chapter, for example, utilization of in vitro fertilization is about three times greater in states with mandated insurance coverage for IVF than in states without such a mandate. As another example of the impact of insurance coverage, health care utilization by individuals spikes upward just after they reach Medicare eligibility at age 65 and is associated with a reduction in access disparities.[1]

A more granular approach would be to estimate the increases in quantity (utilization) that occur along the demand curve as price declines; economists call this measure of price sensitivity "price elasticity of demand." As applied to health care, the out-of-pocket price paid by patients declines, for example, when the amount of their co-pay falls. One way to assess price elasticity of demand would be to compare utilization rates by patients who have a variety of insurance policies with different co-pay rates. Thus, for example, utilization of health services by patients with a co-pay of 75 percent could be compared to those with a 50 percent co-pay, 25 percent co-pay, and 10 percent co-pay. (Policies with higher co-pay rates would typically have a lower monthly premium.) A number of such studies have been performed, but they suffer from the potential for adverse selection: that is, patients who sign up for a policy with a 10 percent co-pay are probably those who expect to use more health care than those who sign up for a 75 percent co-pay. To avoid adverse selection, the ideal study would be one in which varying coinsurance rates paid by patients were randomly assigned.

Such a randomized trial was conducted in the 1970s by the RAND Corporation.[2] Although dated, it is not surprising that such randomization has never been repeated, and the RAND project remains the definitive study on the responsiveness of health care utilization to price in the United States. Called the RAND Health Insurance Experiment (RAND-HIE), this study largely avoided adverse selection by randomizing participants to health insurance plans with different coinsurance rates. Between 1974 and 1977, the RAND-HIE study enrolled families who lived in six different rural and urban communities across the nation. Depending upon the insurance plan to which families were randomly assigned, they faced co-pay rates ranging from 0 percent (free) to 95 percent of the health care fees. All plans had an upper limit on out-of-pocket expenses of 5, 10, or 15 percent of family income, up to a maximum of $1,000. Enrollment numbers and study results are shown in table 4.1.

The responsiveness of utilization to price was clear: The likelihood of any use of health care services was 68 percent if participants were respon-

Table 4.1. Results from the RAND Health Insurance Experiment randomized trial

Enrollment			Medical utilization			Dental utilization	
Co-pay	Persons	Person-years	Mean # of visits[a]	Mean # of hospital admissions	Probability of any medical use (%)	Mean # of visits	Probability of any dental use (%)
Free	1,893	6,822	4.6	0.13	86.8	2.5	68.7
25%	1,137	4,065	3.3	0.11	78.8	1.7	53.6
50%	383	1,405	3.0	0.09	77.2	1.8	54.1
90%	1,120	3,729	2.7	0.10	67.7	1.4	47.1

Source: Adapted from Manning et al., "Health Insurance and the Demand for Medical Care."[2]
[a] Visits are face-to-face contacts with MD, osteopath, or other health care provider, exclusive of radiology, anesthesiology, and pathology.

sible for a co-pay equal to almost the full price (up to the deductible limit), but use of services increased step-by-step to 87 percent as the co-pay amount declined to zero. Similar responsiveness of utilization to price can be seen with respect to physicians and dentists. Hospital utilization was lower for families with a co-pay of 25 or 50 percent as compared with 0 percent, beyond which there was no effect of increasing co-pay amounts, since the out-of-pocket deductible for most patients was reached at that point.

Based on the varying utilization among study families in response to the different co-pay rates, the authors of the RAND-HIE study statistically estimated the elasticity of demand for health care services. While there were some differences between ambulatory and hospital care, overall the estimate of price elasticity was about –0.2. This would suggest that a doubling of the co-pay would lead to about a 20 percent reduction in utilization.

Such an increase in co-pay amounts is not hard to imagine. Consider a physician group practice that sees 100 patients per day. If the negotiated fee between an insurance company and a physician practice group is $150 for a doctor visit, but the health plan increases the co-pay from $20 to $40 (a level of increase that has occurred in many health plans of late), this would be seen by patients as a doubling of price, even though the price received by the doctor in both cases is $150 per visit. A price elasticity of 0.2 would imply that patient visits in the group practice would decline, on average, from 100 to 80 per day. This 0.2 estimate is an average of responses across patients, but individual responses will depend on income: a high-income patient will show less of a response to a change in the price of doctor visit from $20 to $40 than a low-income patient. A 2002 review of the literature published as a RAND Monograph Report concluded that the average estimate of price elasticity of demand is –0.17.[3]

More recently, estimates of price elasticity of demand have been obtained in Australia and Japan. The health care system in Australia provides a baseline level of universal health care coverage funded by a 2.0 percent income tax, with a further surcharge for those with high-incomes. However, the system for out-of-pocket payments for physician services in Australia is the inverse of the US system: instead of the negotiated rate being the full amount paid to providers and the co-pay being the fractional amount paid by patients, in Australia the negotiated amount is a floor, above which practitioners are free to charge what they wish. If the physician charges more than this "floor" fee, the patient is required to pay the extra amount, which is known as a "gap" payment. Thus, the presence of gap payments that vary according to differing physician fee schedules provides an excellent natural experiment in which the price elasticity of demand for physician services can be estimated. Jeffery Richardson and Stuart Peacock estimated price elasticity in Australia to be −0.22 on average across different services,[4] a result remarkably similar to that obtained for the United States from the randomized trial in the RAND-HIE study.

Japan has a hybrid government-private health care system. The government pays 70 percent of medical expenses for everyone except for low-income elderly individuals, for whom the Japanese government pays as much as 90 percent. Private health insurance is used to cover the remaining 30 percent—either employer-sponsored or privately purchased. Benefits are the same for everyone and include dental and mental health care. The government contributes a greater subsidy for catastrophic care and for people with disabilities or with specified chronic conditions. Since beginning its national health insurance policy in 1963, the Japanese health insurance system has been comprised of many subsystems, which are operated separately, mainly due to historical events. Across time, these subsystems changed their rules independently. Researchers Yasushi Iwanmoto and Kensaku Kishida were able to identify 19 cases of health insurance reforms that changed the out-of-pocket payment rule for subsets of the population.[5] These "natural experiments" enabled them to estimate price elasticity of demand by finding control populations not affected by the payment changes. From these different natural experiments over 40 years, estimated price elasticity of demand for medical care ranged from 0.1 to 0.3, which is in the same range as estimates obtained by the RAND-HIE study for the United States and by Richardson and Peacock for Australia.

Whether it's called moral hazard or simply the negative slope of a demand curve, it is clear that when the price paid by consumers for health care is lower than the full price paid to providers, consumers will utilize more health care than if they had to pay the full price.

Knowing this, how might one predict health care utilization per capita in the United States, given our varying levels of insurance coverage and government programs, in comparison with other high-income nations, all of which have universal coverage with low or zero co-pays and deductibles? There are competing forces at work:

- *Tendency toward lower utilization.* While the presence of deductibles and co-pays in the United States means that more people have access to health care than they would if they had to pay the full price, *out-of-pocket* expenditures for health care in the United States are still higher than in virtually all other high-income nations. For example, in constant international dollars, out-of-pocket expenditures per capita in the United States is twice as high (or almost twice as high) as they are in Canada, Denmark, France, Germany, Italy, Japan, the Netherlands, Spain, and the United Kingdom.[6] Given an out-of-pocket expense that is higher in the United States, one would predict that health care utilization would be lower. The presence of a large uninsured population, whose use of medical services is below that of insured individuals, would add to the prediction of lower overall utilization in the United States.

- *Tendency toward higher utilization.* The incentive for physicians and hospitals to induce demand, discussed in chapter 5, would lead to greater utilization.

How do these two opposing forces play out? The best data available come from a comprehensive international study reported by Irene Papanicolas and her colleagues.[7] These researchers compared the United States with 10 other high-income countries in which the population prevalence of illness and demographic characteristics are similar. Among these 11 countries, the United States ranked first or second in the per capita utilization of diagnostic modalities and surgical procedures such as MRIs, CT scans, knee replacement, cataract surgery, coronary artery bypass, and coronary angioplasty. This is not surprising since such procedures are among those most sensitive to the potential for physician-induced demand due to asymmetric information and financial incentives.

For outpatient physician consultations, where the presence of US copays and deductibles have a downward impact on utilization, we ranked ninth of the 11 countries studied, averaging about four visits per capita in a given year as compared with an international group mean of about 6.5 visits per capita.

By contrast, we ranked sixth—the middle of the pack—in hospital discharges for common conditions such as pneumonia, chronic obstructive pulmonary disease, mental and behavioral disorders, and heart attack. This is also not surprising: the downward effect of co-pays on utilization is less important for inpatient services than outpatient services, since the cost of hospitalization quickly exceeds the deductible in most insurance plans.

Thus, for hospital discharges, the insurance-based US system (not counting the uninsured) looks a lot more like the universal coverage systems in other countries.

The overall effects of these factors affecting utilization appear to be offsetting empirically. Thus, in the international comparison conducted by Papanicolas and her coauthors, it was concluded that overall health care utilization in the United States was similar to the other countries studied.

Societal Acceptability of Price Subsidies and Increased Utilization

When insurance plans or government programs subsidize the price of medical care, the resulting increased demand means there will be allocative inefficiencies in the Pareto sense. If there were no subsidies, however, rational consumers with limited income would often forego needed medical care in favor of food, shelter, and other necessities. The widespread endorsement of employer-based health insurance and government programs, such as Medicare in the United States, implies that, for programs such as these, greater health care utilization and expenditure associated with subsidized prices are viewed as acceptable trade-offs against allocative inefficiency.

But at what level of health care coverage and price subsidies through insurance and government programs does "acceptable" become "unacceptable"? This question gets to the issue of whether health care should be regarded as a "right." In practice, the United States functions as though health care is "sort of a right" in that about 90 percent of the population have access to health care via private health insurance, government programs such as Medicaid/Medicare, and coverage for military veterans. The stumbling block has always been the uninsured population: people who work for small employers that don't offer employee health insurance, who are self-employed but choose not to purchase individual health insurance, or who are unemployed. For such individuals, apart from "free clinics" and the like, access to health care is mainly through emergency rooms, where by law they must be evaluated and stabilized (chapter 15).

As of this writing, there are 28.5 million individuals who are uninsured in the United States.[8] Faced with the full price of medical care that is usually out of reach, the uninsured often make decisions that other necessities often come first. If they become ill, care is often delayed until the problem becomes acute. In the absence of a regular source of medical care, their main recourse is to go to a hospital emergency room, where they will be evaluated and stabilized but receive high charges for their care. Depending on the hospital, a variable portion of their bill may be written off according to a sliding scale of income, but the remainder will be sought by collection agencies and any lack of payment will follow them in their credit rating.

A challenge for our nation is to determine the level of subsidy for the currently uninsured population that is societally acceptable. Polling data can be informative. In a random sample of 2,410 adults ages 19–64, in a poll conducted in November and December of 2017 by the survey research firm SSRS, 92 percent answered yes to the question, "Do you think all Americans have the right to affordable health care."[9] Endorsement is lower, however, when the question is posed in terms of public financing. For example, in a random sample of 1,019 adults who were surveyed in a poll conducted by the Associated Press-NORC Center for Public Affairs Research, 62 percent said yes to the question, "Is it the responsibility of the federal government to make sure that all Americans have health care coverage?"[10]

The 30 percent difference in the results of these two polls suggests that many people like the idea that all Americans should have access to affordable health care—even that it is a "right"—but are uncomfortable with the implementation of this idea through the federal government. That said, a majority of the population (62 percent) endorses the statement that the federal government should ensure that "all Americans have health care coverage." If the question were asked in terms of coverage for "serious medical conditions" or "medically needed treatment," there would likely be even greater endorsement. But like many issues of public policy, a broad middle ground is not articulated; rather, statements on both sides of the "health care is a right" question state polar positions, such as "health care services should be determined by market forces and ability to pay" vs. "health care should be made available for all without regard to employment or financial resources" (box 4.1).

For the population as a whole, there are few individuals who are totally on one side or the other of this debate. Although polls typically ask questions in a yes/no format about whether health care is a right, or whether the federal government should make sure that everyone should have health care coverage, most people are probably somewhere in the middle, although they might lean strongly in one direction or the other.

Take, for example, a line representing the continuum of medical need and treatment (figure 4.1). At the top end of the line are treatments for serious

Box 4.1. Is health care a right? Pros and cons

PRO

"Quality care shouldn't depend on your financial resources, or the type of job you have, or the medical condition you face. . . . This is the cause of my life. It is a key reason that I defied my illness last summer to speak at the Democratic convention in Denver . . . to make sure, as I said, that we will break the old gridlock and guarantee that every American . . . will have decent, quality health care as a fundamental right and not just a privilege. . . . It goes to the heart of my belief in a just society."

—Edward M. Kennedy, late US Senator, Massachusetts

"At its root, the lack of health care for all in America is fundamentally a moral issue. The United States is the only industrialized nation that does not have some form of universal health care (defined as a basic guarantee of health care to all of its citizens). While other countries have declared health care to be a basic right, the United States treats health care as a privilege, only available to those who can afford it. . . . The Declaration of Independence states there are certain 'inalienable rights,' including life, liberty, and the pursuit of happiness. If Americans believe in an inalienable right to life, how can we tolerate a system that denies people lifesaving medications and treatments?"

—American Medical Student Association

"Our approach to health care is shaped by a simple but fundamental principle: 'Every person has a right to adequate health care. This right flows from the sanctity of human life and the dignity that belongs to all human persons, who are made in the image of God.' Health care is more than a commodity; it is a basic human right, an essential safeguard of human life and dignity. We believe our people's health care should not depend on where they work, how much their parents earn, or where they live. Our constant teaching that each human life must be protected and human dignity promoted leads us to insist that all people have a right to health care."

—The US Conference of Catholic Bishops

CON

"Health care is a service that we all need, but just like food and shelter it is best provided through voluntary and mutually beneficial market exchanges. A careful reading of both the Declaration of Independence and the Constitution will not reveal any intrinsic right to health care, food, or shelter. That's because there isn't any. This 'right' has never existed in America. Rather than increase government spending and control, we need to address the root causes of poor health. This begins with the realization that every American adult is responsible for his or her own health."

—John Mackey, CEO, Whole Foods

"The very idea that health care—or any good provided by others—is a 'right' is a contradiction. The rights enshrined in the Declaration of Independence were to life, liberty, and the pursuit of happiness. Each of these is a right to act, not a right to things. . . . These two concepts of rights—rights as the right to liberty, versus rights as the rights to things—cannot coexist in the same respect at the same time. . . . To reform our health care industry we should challenge the premises that invited government intervention in the first place. The moral premise is that medical care is a right. It is not. There is no 'right' to anything that others must produce, because no one may claim a 'right' to force others to provide it."

—John David Lewis, PhD, late philosopher and political scientist

"With regard to the idea of whether you have a right to health care, you have to realize what that implies. It's not an abstraction. I'm a physician. That means you have a right to come to my house and conscript me. It means you believe in slavery. . . . You're saying you believe in taking and extracting from another person. Our founding documents were very clear about this. You have a right to pursue happiness but there's no guarantee of physical comfort. There's no guarantee of concrete items. In order to give something concrete, you have to take it from someone. So there's an implied threat of force."

—Rand Paul, MD, US Senator, Kentucky

Source: "Pro & Con Quotes: Should All Americans Have the Right (Be Entitled) to Health Care?," ProCon .org, last updated February 23, 2017, https://healthcare.procon.org/should-all-americans-have-the-right -be-entitled-to-health-care-pro-con-quotes.

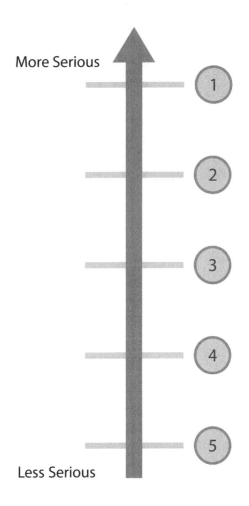

Figure 4.1. Continuum of medical need and potential thresholds for coverage

medical conditions such as sickle cell disease, type 1 diabetes, brain cancer, stroke, lung disease due to workplace asbestos exposure, accidental trauma, and other diseases or injuries that are genetic or randomly acquired in a manner unrelated to lifestyle. At the bottom end are less serious treatments that would be largely viewed as insufficiently essential to justify societal price subsidies, such as plastic surgery for aesthetic purpose or treatments that gain popularity through marketing or social media but without the support of any scientific evidence.

Even those who believe that health care is *not* a right will generally agree that individuals in our society who need treatment for conditions at the top end of the line should receive those treatments. (That is, they would endorse covering conditions above threshold 1.) They understand that individuals born with a genetic disease or who are involved in an accident through no fault of their own are not making a choice as they would, for example, between hamburger or filet mignon for dinner. Health care for such individuals in need *is* different. They might say that for people who don't have insurance, the current emergency room system is an appropriate safety net.

At the other end of the continuum, even those who believe that health care *is* a right will generally agree that some types of health care are discretionary and that if people want to pay for aesthetic plastic surgery or for treatments without scientific evidence of efficacy, they can do so, but such medical care should not be subsidized by public funds or by higher commercial insurance premiums that all employees and employers pay to cover their cost. (That is, they would not endorse the coverage of conditions below threshold 5.)

Thus, people who do and do not believe, in principle, that health care is a right can largely agree in practice that some level of insurance/price subsidy for individuals with conditions at the top end of the continuum should be provided. Where they disagree is how far down the continuum such subsidies should go.

Summary

Greater utilization of needed health care as a result of insurance and associated price subsidies appears to be societally acceptable in the United States because of a broad endorsement of employer-based health insurance and government programs such as Medicare and coverage for veterans. Still, the presence of deductibles and co-pays in the United States, as well as a large number of uninsured Americans, would lead to a prediction of lower utilization in comparison with peer high-income nations. This turns out to be true for physician consultations, which occurs at about three-fifths the rate of the mean of peer nations, but not for imaging studies and surgical procedures that may be subject to induced demand, for which the United States ranks first or second in utilization at a rate that is 50 percent higher than the mean of peer nations.

Opinions about health care programs to cover the uninsured population can become polarized when presented in the context of health care as a right, but there is general endorsement that some level of coverage and price subsidy for needed health care should be provided and financed.

5 IMPLICATIONS OF AN IMPERFECT MARKET II
THE ROLE OF INDUCED DEMAND

Individuals consume greater amounts of health care services not only when the fees they pay are lower than the full amount, as just discussed in chapter 4, but also when demand is "induced" by physicians, hospitals, pharmaceutical companies, or other entities.

Consider the case of rheumatoid arthritis (RA), a condition affecting about 1.5 million individuals in the United States. RA is an autoimmune disease that causes painful, swollen joints as well as morning stiffness. In about 40 percent of cases, other organ systems are involved. The first-line treatment for patients whose symptoms don't respond to exercise and over-the-counter anti-inflammatory drugs is methotrexate, which is available in an inexpensive generic form. For many years, patients with more severe symptoms that did not respond well to methotrexate were given one or two additional drugs, also inexpensive and available as generics. The total price for traditional treatment is about $30–$50 per week.

In recent years, a class of drugs called "biological response modifiers" (usually monoclonal antibodies) have been developed for the treatment of RA. The price paid for such treatments by insurance plans and government programs is in the range of $2,500 to $3,000 per week. For those patients who never received standard therapy and were undergoing treatment for the first time, randomized trials of standard therapy versus a variety of biologicals (or versus a combination that includes biologicals) have shown that the biologicals add no additional benefit or modest benefit, depending on severity and other factors.[1] But individuals with RA who see the television ads for the biologicals may be influenced to visit their rheumatologists and ask about these new drugs. Their rheumatologists might explain that overall there may be a modest benefit and that it seems to work better for some patients than for others, a correct summary. Why not give it a try, especially since the co-pay is low and the pharmaceutical company may have a program that rebates all or part of the co-pay?

The patient tries the new drug and perceives a benefit. Maybe there is a true modest improvement in symptoms, as shown in the clinical trials, or maybe this is a placebo effect (as also occurs in randomized trials). For this modest improvement, would the patient elect to take the drug if she had to pay the full $1,200 or $2,500 per week? Even at the lower co-pay price, knowing that the randomized trials did not consistently show major clinical benefit, would she choose the new drug? Maybe or maybe not, depending on her income and the severity of symptoms. But the average patient is typically not aware of such data; all she knows is what she heard on TV and that her doctor is telling her it might help. Sales for drugs to treat RA totaled $20.3 billion in 2016, which included 55 percent biologicals. Biologicals are projected to increase to about 75 percent by 2025, resulting in projected total sales of $30.4 billion.

Demand can be induced because of imperfect and asymmetric information. Perhaps induced demand for medical care can be traced, as in the RA example here, to direct-to-consumer advertising (more on this in chapter 17) or to other marketing. Because consumers lack ready access to (and/or understanding of) the medical literature, and because they are inclined to trust the recommendations of those they view as experts, demand can also be directly induced by health care providers. While there are many different types of health care professionals, most of the literature focuses on physician-induced demand, which will be used here as shorthand for induced demand by health care providers in general.

Physician-induced demand has been defined in different ways:

- A "physician's alleged ability to shift patients' demand for medical care at a given price, that is, to convince patients to increase their utilization of medical care without lowering the price charged."[2]
- "The amount of demand that exists beyond what would have occurred in a market in which patients are fully informed."[3]
- "Physicians influence patient demand to suit their own interests. They are able to do this because their patients know relatively little about the type or quantity of treatment they need."[4]

While these definitions portray the physician as motivated mainly by profit, a more comprehensive model presents the physician as a "price-taker" at the various prevailing fee schedules from private insurance, Medicare, and Medicaid but also as an agent of the patient. In this type of model, the physician seeks "to maximize the perceived value of health for their patient . . . subject to financial considerations, resource capacity, ethical judgment, and patient demand."[5] The "financial considerations" taken into account by the physicians under this model include not only their own income but the costs faced by patients. Acting not only to advance their own interests but as the patient's agent, this type of physician behavior can result in a quantity of health care services that exceeds the level that would be consumed by the informed patient in the absence of physician advice. Although this has been presented by Skinner as a supply-side effect,[6] the resulting quantity of health care consumed is a point on the consumer's demand curve (which may have shifted outward), so it can also be viewed as a form of induced demand.

While some level of physician-induced demand no doubt occurs, as we shall see there is controversy about the quantitative importance of its contribution to the overall utilization of health care services. Indeed, the phenomenon of physician-induced demand is complex: it involves considerations of ethics, the physician's role as the patient's agent, initiation of provider consultations by patients, and the uncertainty involved in many medical decisions. Before diving into the data on physician-induced demand, let's review these considerations in the context of how consumers make choices about their perceived costs and benefits of consuming health care services.

Patient Decision-Making
A Marginal Cost–Marginal Benefit Model

Ultimately, utilization of health care represents a decision by a patient to access services. This decision lies somewhere on a spectrum ranging from independent analysis of the best information available to following a physician's recommendation without question.

A good place to start this discussion of patient decision-making about health care is with a model of how people generally make consumption decisions, which begins with the consumer demand curve. One idea about why demand curves for individual consumers are negatively sloped (i.e., utilization increases as price declines), which originated with Alfred Marshall as described in chapter 2, is that the marginal "utility" (or benefit) to the consumer declines as more of an item is consumed. That is, each additional unit of consumption is worth less and less as consumption rises. You might be willing to pay quite a bit for that first cup of coffee in the morning at your favorite coffee shop (and endure the time cost of waiting in line!), but at that high price you might only buy one cup. If the price were lower, you might buy a second cup, but would only buy three cups (maybe saving it for later) if the price were lower still.

How might this apply to health care? It is awkward to translate the concept of declining marginal benefit with increasing consumption to health care, since "units" of health care come in different sizes and shapes. In terms of an individual's decision-making about utilization of health care services, it's difficult to conceptualize how this applies to the *number* of MRIs or surgical procedures that an individual might demand at different prices because such decisions tend to be one-zero (i.e., yes-no) at any given price and time.

Thus, while a market demand curve can be constructed for individual yes-no decisions aggregated across the population of a region, creation of such a demand curve for an individual is more tricky. Consider, for example, individuals living in a specific region who have arthritis of the hip that causes a moderate amount of chronic pain and reduced mobility. At each price point for a hip replacement, there will be a specific number of individuals in the region who will decide to undergo surgery (i.e., make the "yes" decision). At very high prices, most people would endure the hip discomfort with anti-inflammatory medication and only a few would make the decision in favor of hip replacement. As price declines, however, more and more people would decide to proceed with hip replacement, producing a negatively sloped *market* demand curve. But for the individual, we have a stair-step *individual* demand curve with two steps: zero hip replacements above a specific price and one hip replacement below that price.

While it may seem artificial, for the purpose of developing a conceptual model of individual demand curves for health care, envision the concept of "units" of health care service in an aggregated fashion. That is, when you add up all health care services together, and imagine a conversion factor such that one surgical procedure equals X amount of medication, Y number of physician visits, and so on, you can envision the idea of a horizontal axis showing an increasing quantity of units of health care as it heads to the right (figure 5.1). Along the negatively sloping demand curve, consumption of more and more health care becomes less and less beneficial (e.g., the fifth physician visit for an episode of illness is less valuable than the first visit).

Figure 5.1. Utilization of health care based on marginal benefits (MB) and marginal cost (MC)

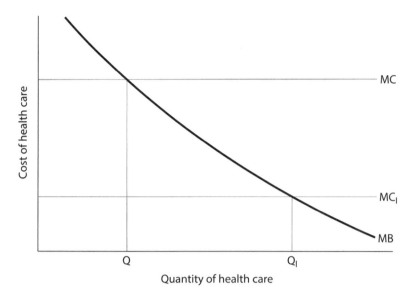

How does an individual determine how much health care he or she will consume? Here's where economists create models with assumptions that may seem abstract and oversimplified in order to make predictions about the *direction* of change: conceptually, individuals consume a marginal unit of health care only if its cost were lower than its benefit. Therefore, the total quantity consumed should be the number of health care units at which marginal cost equals marginal benefit. Let's assume that the price (marginal cost) of a doctor visit, rehab session, or so on is constant, no matter how many are purchased. We also assume that patients have perfect knowledge about the benefits they would receive from the services consumed, about the price, and about other costs such as the value of lost time from work, the risks of any procedures or medications, and so on.

In this scenario, which represents an extension of an analysis originally presented by Victor Fuchs,[7] MC is the fixed marginal cost of consuming successive units of health care for those *without* health insurance, and Q is the quantity of health care consumed where marginal benefit equals margincal cost (MB = MC). For individuals without insurance, if quantity were greater than Q, marginal cost would be greater than marginal benefit and consumers would cut back on utilization. Conversely, if quantity were less than Q, marginal benefit would exceed marginal cost and consumers would expand consumption.

Now consider the situation for those *with* health insurance. MC_I is the cost of consuming units of health care for such individuals, which is the co-pay amount plus the costs of time and other factors. Q_I is the quantity of health care consumed at which $MB = MC_I$. At quantities above or below Q_I, differences between marginal benefit and marginal cost would drive quantity back to Q_I for individuals with insurance.

Given this scenario, what is the "correct" amount of health care consumption, from the standpoint of the individual or society? Is it Q? Is it Q_I? Is it some other quantity? There is no easy answer.

For the individual *without* insurance, perfect information about the benefits of health care services and all pertinent costs would lead to the consumption of Q units of health care, *given his or her level of income and other financial resources*. If the consumer's income were very limited, his or her medical care for chronic illness such as hypertension or diabetes may be subordinate to essential needs such as food and shelter. Moreover, treatment for major illness such as cancer would likely be at a cost that is simply out of reach. While the consumer may be making the best personal decisions given his or her financial circumstances, our society's values may support some level of cost subsidy, whether for the treatment of chronic disease or acute illness.

What about the individual *with* insurance who consumes Q_I units of health care? A modest co-pay because of producer price subsidies will lead to the consumption of Q_I units of health care. This greater utilization due to the price subsidy might be consistent with a re-allocation of society's scarce resources that is in accordance with its values. But if the co-pay were very low (or zero) and the quantity of health care utilized were consequently very high, it might be that the price subsidy provided by employers or government results in such a large amount of health care consumption that it diverts resources away from uses that are more beneficial to society, whether the diverted funds are corporate resources spent on health insurance premiums or taxpayer resources spent on government programs or tax subsidies for employer-sponsored health insurance.

The Role of the Physician as the Patient's Agent

While the MB–MC model might hold for many goods and services in the economy, it is less applicable to health care. Because of the asymmetry of information between patient and physician, and the uncertainty about so many health care decisions due to ambiguous medical data, patients don't typically make independent decisions about health care based on a personal assessment of marginal benefit and marginal cost. Instead, they generally rely on the judgment and advice of their physicians. Even if patients obtain as much information they can from lay publications or the professional literature, individuals who normally feel well informed and "empowered" in consumption decisions will typically defer to their physicians' judgment at a time of illness, especially significant illness.

In this setting, physicians act as the patient's agent in helping them make decisions about whether his or her marginal benefit outweighs marginal cost, or vice versa. In serving as the patient's agent, physicians must balance their estimate of benefits (e.g., the informational value of a proposed diagnostic test, the treatment efficacy of a proposed procedure, etc.) against its cost, which comprises not only the financial expense but the potential harms, including short-term and long-term side effects, and any adverse impact on the patient's work and family life. For patients without insurance who must pay the full price of visits, tests, and procedures, physicians acting *strictly* on behalf of the patient's interests would advise a quantity of health care service at about Q in figure 5.1; for patients with insurance, they would advise a quantity of service at about Q_I. In practice, physicians also act in their own interest;[8] thus, the actual quantity of service recommended represents a balance between their own income and the perceived net benefit to the patient of the treatment provided.

With this background, the phenomenon of induced demand can perhaps be understood more clearly. The word "induced" is not intrinsically pejorative. Physicians can induce demand in a warranted manner when acting as the patient's agent based on data in the medical literature about which the patient may be unaware. In addition, a physician consultation may be initiated by a patient who is anxious about a condition; such patients are typically receptive to recommendations about diagnostic studies and treatments about which he or she might not be aware. A decision to proceed with treatment is "induced," in this scenario, by the patient-initiated decision made jointly with the physician.

Induced demand becomes unwarranted when physicians use their influence to recommend services that a fully informed patient would not choose and/or recommend services despite the provider's belief that the estimated benefits are minimal relative to the patient's financial costs and risk of morbidity. Unwarranted provider-induced demand is reflected in an observed utilization rate that exceeds the quantities Q_I and Q for patients with and without insurance, respectively.

The use of "warranted" and "unwarranted" corresponds to terminology popularized by John Wennberg that grew out of his work on small area variation[9] and is explained further by Skinner: induced demand that is warranted corresponds to "effective care" and induced demand that is unwarranted corresponds to "supply-sensitive treatments with unknown or marginal benefits."[10] Understandably, there is an in-between category that pertains to the large fraction of medical decisions that are made by patients and their physicians when the data are ambiguous.

In balancing benefits and costs when serving as the patient's agent, the physician is guided by the ethical traditions of the medical profession that grew out of early writings, most notably Hippocrates. Unwarranted provider-induced demand would be an example of patient harm, which conflicts with the dictum "Above all, do no harm." Although this phrase is often thought to be part of the Hippocratic Oath that generations of new doctors take when graduating medical school, it actually arises in "Of the Epidemics," which is part of a collection of ancient medical texts called the Hippocratic Corpus. Written in Hippocrates's native Greek around 400 BCE, one translation of the pertinent text, as related by Gary Schwartz, is as follows: "The physician must . . . have two special objects in view with regard to disease, namely, to do good or to do no harm."[11] This is a more nuanced admonition than "Above all, do no harm." The phrase in the original text describes physicians as striking a balance between beneficence and nonmaleficence.

In terms of doing good, the modern-day efficacy of a wide variety of therapies gives physicians an unprecedented arsenal of warranted, highly effective medical and surgical treatments, some of which were summarized in chapter 1. There remains, however, a large number of conditions in which the medical literature has not yet provided definitive evidence of treatment efficacy; in such cases, there are often observational studies to guide decisions that represent best current practice, backed by specialty society guidelines. It is here that the patient makes a decision informed to some extent by his or her own research, but mainly by the physician's explanations about benefits and risks, and the level of uncertainty surrounding the likelihood of these outcomes. Acting as the patient's agent, the physician is following Hippocrates's ethical principles of balancing beneficence and nonmaleficence.

When a doctor recommends a procedure of questionable efficacy despite believing that the costs outweigh the benefits, he or she is violating the dictum of nonmaleficence and is entering the realm of unwarranted induced demand.

But even in cases where available data do not support a treatment, the label of "unwarranted" service, while objectively accurate, does not always reflect the complexities of real-life clinical interactions between human beings. This is because physicians sometimes *believe* that a treatment is efficacious based on their "clinical experience" even if objective data in the literature do not support intervention. Moreover, when patients present to physicians with a clinical problem, practitioners are inclined to "do something" to resolve the problem. Surgeons are inclined to help patients with something that *might* benefit from an operation; non-procedural physicians are inclined to write a prescription when faced with a patient who *might* benefit from a medication.

All of these considerations lead to increased utilization of health care services, partly initiated by patients with low out-of-pocket costs wanting "something" to be done for a perceived medical problem, and partly induced by doctors wanting to help.

These situations can sometimes move one step further, however, in the direction of physician-induced demand that is financially motivated. In such cases, even if a physician does not believe that a procedure will produce significant net benefit for the patient, physicians may nonetheless recommend the procedure to generate a professional fee. This phenomenon can be exacerbated when the physician making a recommendation for medical services (e.g., MRIs or outpatient surgery) has an ownership interest in the facility where they will be obtained.[12] That is, additional income can be generated when groups of specialty physicians who own imaging equipment and/or laboratories and/or outpatient surgical centers refer patients there for CT scans, MRIs, diagnostic tests, or procedures. Despite the clear conflict of interest, as discussed in chapter 15, such a scenario can occur in fields such as orthopedics, ophthalmology, gastroenterology, and radiation oncology. A similar situation arises when specialists such as medical oncologists, neurologists, and rheumatologists financially benefit from treatments using intravenous infusions of expensive pharmaceuticals. In such cases, these specialists benefit not only from professional fees for patient care visits, but from selling them directly to patients and receiving income from the difference between the retail and wholesale price of the drugs.

Empirical Data Regarding Provider-Induced Demand

Evidence to support the presence of provider-induced demand is often based on variations in the rates of medical treatments in different communities and their correlation with the number of providers. Correlation does not equal causation, however, and adjustment for other factors that may explain variation in health care utilization and expenditure, such as patient health status and local physician practice styles and beliefs, must be considered. Sometimes, "natural experiments" can occur in which the role of induced demand or supply-side factors in general can be inferred.

Historical Studies of Geographic Variation

The earliest paper on treatment variation was a 1938 report on tonsillectomy among school children in England and Wales, published in the *Proceedings of the Royal Society of Medicine*.[13] Tonsillectomies in school-age children increased when the School Medical Service in England began paying for the procedure before World War I. In his paper, Glover reported on the dramatic rise in tonsillectomy rates throughout England, but also on differences in tonsillectomy rates across geographic areas that were up to tenfold, without observable differences in the health outcomes of children in the different areas. As an example, Glover provides the following comparison of two counties:

> Let us take the nine years 1928–1936. . . . We will take two rural counties A and B, not far apart and not unlike save in size. During these nine years A, with an average attendance each year of about 2,207 elementary school children, . . . had 1,010 children operated upon. If B, with an average attendance of 8,621 children, had had operations in the same proportion as A, we should "expect" that 3,945 children in B would have been tonsillectomized during this period. But the actual number was 335. Environment and circumstance were not very different, so that it seems 3,610 children, who would have been operated upon had they lived in A, were not operated upon because they lived in B.[14]

During the early 1900s, although advances were occurring in surgical technique, surgical hygiene, and general anesthesia, surgery was still fraught with danger. Glover estimated that eight deaths from tonsillectomy surgery occurred for each death attributable to medical complications associated with tonsillitis. Given this risk, Glover makes the following concluding statement regarding the large numbers of tonsillectomies that were performed in some regions compared to others: "The strange bare facts of incidence seem to support the opinion expressed on other grounds by the

Schools Epidemic Committee of the Medical Research Council that it is a little difficult to believe that among the mass of tonsillectomies performed today, all subjects for operation are selected with true discrimination, and one cannot avoid the conclusion that there is a tendency for the operation to be performed as a routine prophylactic ritual for no particular reason and with no particular result."[15]

In an updated analysis of cross-sectional Vermont data from the late 1960s, Wennberg and Gittelsohn found "surgical signatures" in tonsillectomy rates, ranging from 13 to 151 per 10,000 people in the different regions of Vermont.[16] To this day, tonsillectomy remains one of the most frequently performed operations in children in the United States, and widespread variation persists in the rate at which it is performed in different regions. For example, the rate per 10,000 children was reported by Boss, Marsteller, and Simon to be 125.1 in the South as compared with 28.9 in the West; and 118.4 in medium/small metro areas as compared with 42.1 in large central metropolitan areas.[17]

Given these data, how can we assess the role of physician-induced demand in explaining the variation? Consider the case of a 4-year-old girl whose mother brings her to a pediatric surgeon on the advice of an emergency department physician. The girl had a bout of tonsillitis a year ago, which resolved spontaneously. A month earlier, she had a mild fever and sore throat and was seen by her pediatrician, who cultured her tonsils (negative for a streptococcal infection) and encouraged watchful waiting. This episode ran its course over the next week but two nights earlier the patient again developed similar symptoms, was seen in the emergency room, and was sent to the pediatric surgeon. Her tonsils were moderately enlarged and somewhat pustular, and she complained of significant pain. Over the past year, her sleep has not been affected by enlarged tonsils. Based on the results of randomized trials,[18] watchful waiting for this patient will be associated with slightly more days of sore throat over the next year in comparison with tonsillectomy (23 days vs. 18 days). Although the financial cost to the patient's family is low, due to a small health insurance co-pay, the health system revenues from commercial insurance (fees paid to providers) total about $5,000 taking into account the fees paid to the surgeon and anesthesiologist as well as payments for lab tests and the hospital's outpatient surgery facility fee. (This estimate is based on data from UF Health Shands Hospital, Gainesville, Florida, October 2018. Costs may vary widely from hospital to hospital.) But mom does not like to see her daughter in pain, believes that the surgery will help, is unaware of the randomized trials, and defines cost in terms of her co-pay much more than the overall cost to society. The surgeon recommends tonsillectomy because the last two episodes occurred a month apart and because of the extent of pain experienced by the patient. If mom had information about the expected difference in the number of days of sore throat, and if she had to pay the full price, she might say no to the procedure and see whether her daughter will experience fewer episodes across time; but, it becomes a yes in practice.

Does this represent financially motivated, physician-induced demand? Maybe . . . but maybe not. Perhaps the surgeon's "beliefs," rooted in her training and clinical experience, have not allowed her to accept the results of the randomized trial, or perhaps she is simply unaware of these findings; maybe her training in the same hospital in which she now practices taught her that tonsillectomy is the best way to proceed for such patients and it has become a local standard of care; maybe her personal clinical experience over many years leads her to the genuine belief that there will be more good than harm if she operates. As concluded by Goodman and Challener: "Well-meaning physicians practice locally defined norms of care, without realizing how different their practices are from well-meaning physicians in other communities."[19]

One factor affecting local conditions may be the number of providers—both doctors and hospitals. Some fraction of the variation across communities in per capita rates of surgical procedures, physician visits, lab tests and imaging studies, and hospital admissions may be explainable by variation in the per capita number of doctors and hospitals. A linkage between capacity and utilization was first reported by Shain and Roemer,[20] who demonstrated a correlation between short-term general hospital beds per 1,000 and the number of hospital days used per 1,000 population. In a subsequent paper, the concept that a built bed becomes a filled bed that was paid for became known as Roemer's law.[21] The principle that oversupply of facility resources and specialist physicians (especially combined with third party reimbursement and low co-pays) can lead to induced demand became the major impetus for Certificate of Need legislation to counteract the potential for significant unwarranted physician-induced demand.

Feldstein conceptualized Roemer's law as a phenomenon in which a shift in bed capacity (supply) induces an outward shift in the demand curve for hospitalization.[22] To test this hypothesis, he estimated the response of hospital bed utilization across geographic areas to variation in both price and supply (the number of hospital beds per capita). The estimated elasticity of hospital day utilization with respect to hospital bed supply was 0.53; that is, a doubling in hospital beds per capita was estimated to be associated with a 53 percent increase in days of hospitalization per capita.

In a subsequent study of the relationship between hospital bed supply and utilization among Medicare patients, in which a number of methodologic issues regarding price, in-migration, and other considerations were refined, Ginsburg and Koretz estimated that a doubling in hospital beds per capita would increase hospital utilization among Medicare enrollees by about 40 percent.[23] It should be noted that although the language used to describe such elasticity-of-demand estimates often sounds causal (e.g., a doubling of hospital beds *would lead to* a certain percent increase in the utilization of those beds), these are really cross-sectional associations that may be due to other factors.

Contemporary Cross-Sectional Studies

As documented by the Dartmouth Atlas and a major Institute of Medicine (now National Academy of Medicine) report,[24] there is tremendous geographic variation in health care expenditures. The Dartmouth Atlas, for example, configures geographic areas as hospital referral regions (HRRs) in which patients are thought to receive medical care from similar providers based on visit location and referral patterns. The most recent Dartmouth Atlas map (figure 5.2)—showing mean health care expenditures (2015) per Medicare beneficiary (excluding those participating in health maintanence organizations such as Medicare Advantage, but including both acute and post-acute care) for the nation's 306 HRRs—illustrates that the range of mean Medicare expenditure per beneficiary across HRRs, adjusted for age, sex, race and price, is from $7,134 to $13,109.

What are the possible reasons for the large geographic variation in per-beneficiary health care expenditures? One obvious explanation would be that there is variation across areas in the prevalence of disease. Some of the large variation in medical expenditures seen in figure 5.2, after adjusting for age, race and sex, may reflect "demand-side" factors—different disease patterns of populations in different geographic areas. Differences in area disease patterns may be due to variations in smoking and obesity rates, activity levels, environmental exposures, and other factors. Variation in average patient preferences across communities about the intensity of their care for specific

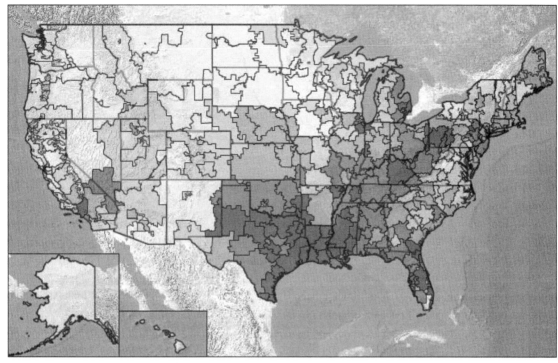

□ No data ▨ $7,134 – <$8,493 (61) ▨ $8,493 – <$9,335 (61) ▨ $9,335 – <$9,935 (61) ▨ $9,935 – <$10,542 (61) ■ $10,542 – <$13,109 (62)

Figure 5.2. Health care expenditures per Medicare enrollee, by hospital referral regions. "Make Your Own Dataset," Dartmouth Atlas Data, Dartmouth Institute for Health Policy Research and Clinical Practice, accessed August 12, 2018, https://atlasdata .dartmouth.edu/long_data/new.

illnesses might also play a role. The effective price of care would also be an important explanatory factor, which would be related to insurance coverage, co-pay amounts, and so on. In figure 5.2, however, insurance coverage is roughly the same (i.e., Medicare), and there is a regional cost adjustment.

Demand-side factors such as disease prevalence, patient lifestyle and behavioral preferences, and price would explain variation in the patient-initiated demand for medical care. But supply-side factors may also be important. Even if disease prevalence, preferences, and price were the same across HRRs, differences in medical care utilization could still vary based on supply-side factors that induce patient demand, which could be motivated by a variety of factors as we have discussed.

Consider the simple correlation between the number of hospital discharges and hospital beds per 1,000 population and hospitals across HRRs (figure 5.3). The strong positive relationship between use and availability pertain

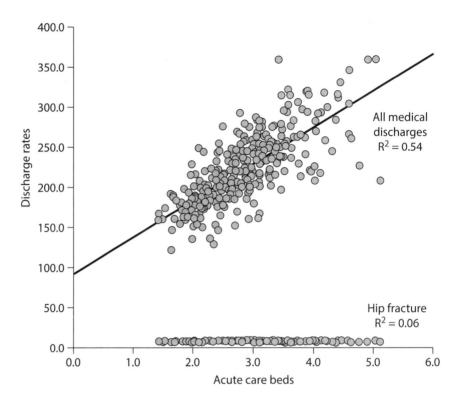

Figure 5.3. Association between hospital beds per 1,000 (1996) and discharges per 1,000 (1995–96) among Medicare enrollees in 306 hospital referral regions. Center for the Evaluative Clinical Sciences, *Supply-Sensitive Care: A Dartmouth Atlas Project Topic Brief* (Lebanon, NH: Dartmouth Atlas Project, January 15, 2007), 2, http://archive.dartmouthatlas.org/downloads/reports/supply_sensitive.pdf.

to all medical admissions, which includes patients whose acuity of medical need for hospital admission (as opposed to outpatient treatment) covers a broad range. It is pertinent that when the data are restricted to a condition that has a high level of medical need for hospital care, such as hip fracture, the number of beds shows no correlation with the number of admissions.

Direct correlations between the supply and utilization of hospital beds have also been found for physician services: for example, in the same 306 HRRs, the correlation between the number of visits per person to cardiologists among Medicare enrollees and the number of cardiologists per 100,000 people (figure 5.4). Similar correlations have been found for other specialties.

As noted with respect to estimates of elasticity of demand for hospital beds, a correlation between two variables like use and supply of cardiology services does not mean that one causes the other. There may be a third

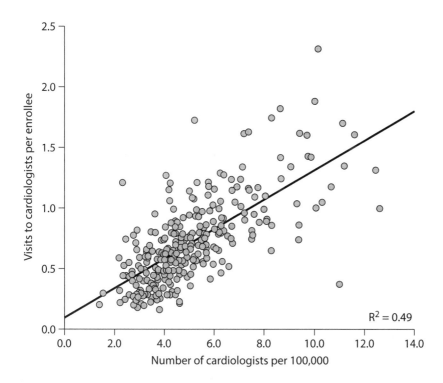

Figure 5.4. Association between cardiologists and visits per person to cardiologists among Medicare enrollees (1996) in 306 hospital referral regions. Center for the Evaluative Clinical Sciences, *Supply-Sensitive Care: A Dartmouth Atlas Project Topic Brief* (Lebanon, NH: Dartmouth Atlas Project, January 15, 2007), 3, http://archive .dartmouthatlas.org/downloads/reports/supply_sensitive.pdf.

factor, such as health status, that is highly correlated with *both* use and supply and therefore accounts for the apparent relationship between the two variables. Perhaps individuals in an area with a greater number of cardiology visits per person have more heart problems, on average, than those in an area with fewer visits. Maybe they live in a community where the residents are more sedentary or have more heart-unhealthy diets. In such a circumstance, the number of cardiologists in this community are greater than other areas because there is more cardiologic disease in that community. Put differently, the correlation between supply and use is not causal but reflective of differences in health status.

Estimates of the extent to which variables such as health status explain the correlation between health care supply and use have been inconsistent, probably because they have been derived from observational data. Since an experimental study (e.g., randomized allocation of different numbers of doctors to different communities) is not feasible, statistical tools must be applied to parse out the "true" effect of supply-side factors in inducing utilization, and to assess the extent to which variations in supply-side factors are represented by differences in the number of physicians, hospitals, and other health care facilities, as well as factors such as differences in physician beliefs and practice styles. Such methods involve statistical adjustment for a variety of factors (e.g., age, race, income, rural/urban, physician/population ratio, patient and physician preferences) that are observed at a moment in time across geographic areas.

Using Medicare Current Beneficiary Surveys from 2000 through 2002 for 6,725 beneficiaries, Zuckerman et al. used standard multivariate regression techniques to analyze Medicare spending variation across HRRs (grouped into five quintiles).[25] Mean spending per beneficiary in their sample (in 2002 USD) was $6,210. Spending in the top-spending quintile of HRRs was $7,183, which was 52 percent higher than the $4,721 expended per beneficiary in the lowest-spending quintile, a difference of $2,462. It was found that demographic and health variables accounted for $902 of the $2,462 difference in per-beneficiary Medicare spending, or 37 percent. Adding income, supplemental insurance and supply of health care resources did not add additional explanatory power to the model.

The National Academy of Medicine (NAM) report already mentioned was a major project that utilized databases from Medicare and commercial health insurance claims (OptumInsight and MarketScan). A variety of small, medium, and large geographic areas were used as units of observation for a variety of cross-sectional analyses and resulted in a representative set of overall findings based on analyses across HRRs (table 5.1).

The NAM results document significant variation in Medicare health care expenditures (adjusted for local prices), with areas at the 90th percentile spending 1.44 times as much as areas at the 10th percentile; the corresponding spending ratios for the OptumInsight and MarketScan commercial health care databases were 1.43 and 1.33, respectively. Consistent with the findings of Zuckerman et al., health status was found to be the major significant explanatory variable: adjusting for health status (using an indicator of health based on hierarchical condition categories) reduced spending variation in all three databases. (In these analyses, health status was measured by hierarchical condition categories, a risk-adjustment method used by the Centers for Medicare and Medicaid Services.) Moreover, it was concluded by the NAM committee members that "after account-

Table 5.1. Ratios of 90th to 10th percentile price-adjusted spending across payers when adjusted for "clusters" of predictors in hospital referral regions

Cluster	Ratio: Medicare	Ratio: Commercial 1 (OptumInsight)	Ratio: Commercial 2 (MarketScan)
Control: _Adjusted for year and partial-year enrollment only_	1.44	1.43	1.33
Cluster 1: _Adjusted for control + age + sex + age-sex interaction_	1.44	1.43	1.26
Cluster 2: _Adjusted for cluster 1 + health status[a]_	1.23	1.37	1.28
Cluster 3: _Adjusted for cluster 1 + race_	1.40	1.43	1.24
Cluster 4: _Adjusted for cluster 1 + income_	1.41	1.40	1.26
Cluster 5: _Adjusted for cluster 1 + race + income + health status_	1.25	1.42	1.27
Cluster 6: _Adjusted for cluster 1 + employer/insurance predictors[b]_	*	1.39	1.30
Cluster 7: _Adjusted for cluster 1 + market-level predictors[c]_	1.44	**	1.26
Cluster 8:[d] _Adjusted for cluster 5 + employer/insurance predictors + market-level predictors_	1.25	**	1.28

Source: Adapted from Institute of Medicine, _Variation in Health Care Spending._[24]

[a] The analysis uses the Center for Medicare and Medicaid Services' 2008 definition of hierarchical condition categories as an indicator of health status.

[b] Employer and insurance predictors include the following variables: benefit generosity, payer/plan type, plan size (OptumInsight only), and data source (MarketScan only).

[c] Market-level predictors include the following variables: hospital competition, uninsured population percentage, supply of medical services, malpractice environmental risk, physician composition, access to care, payer mix, Medicaid penetration, health professional mix, and supplemental Medicare insurance.

[d] Cluster 8 combines all predictors used in clusters 1–7. These include demographic variables, health status, employer and insurance characteristics, and market-level factors. In addition to the specified predictors, this model also includes dummy indicators for institutional status, dual-enrollment status, and supplemental Medicare insurance.

*This regression was conducted using commercial insurance data only, as it was not applicable to the Medicare analysis.

**The methodology used to conduct the OptumInsight market-level analysis differed substantially from that of the other analyses, making the results noncomparable across subcontractors.

ing for differences in age, sex, and health status, geographic variation in spending in both Medicare and commercial insurance is not further explained by other beneficiary demographic factors, insurance plan factors, or market-level characteristics."[26]

Variation in total Medicare spending across geographic areas was found in the NAM study to be mainly due to post-acute services: the share of spending variance explained was estimated to be three times higher for post-acute care than for acute care. Also of note, the NAM study found that variation in expenditures for commercial-pay patients, most of whom were enrolled in employer-based health insurance plans, was mainly due to price markups rather than utilization or input prices. (For Medicare patients, there is essentially no "markup" in price since federal prices for Medicare are preset.)

Finally, an important conclusion from the NAM study was that adjustment for all predictors reduced the ratio of expenditures in high-to-low spending areas only modestly: from 1.44 to 1.25 in the Medicare population, and from 1.33 to 1.27 in the MarketScan population (with little change in the OptumInsight population). Thus, there is still considerable variation in spending that is unaccounted for by the various predictor variables as measured, implying that unknown (or unmeasurable) omitted factors (whether on the demand- or supply-side) may be very salient.

Another important study of variation in Medicare spending was conducted by Louise Sheiner, using state-level data.[27] She argues that although it might be intuitive to control statistically for health and other attributes at the *individual* level, area variation in health spending can best be explained by variation in *area-level* data on health and other characteristics. For example, she points out that "if states all had the same mean levels of health, then individual-level regressions of health spending on health might be helpful in predicting *individual* health spending, but they would not provide any information about *cross-state* variation in spending" (emphasis added).[28] Using this strategy of employing area-level explanatory variables to account for area-level spending, Sheiner's overall conclusion is that health status is the major predictor of health spending.

More specifically, using the prevalence of diabetes in a state as a rough marker of health status, Sheiner documents a strong linear correlation between statewide diabetes rates and Medicare spending on acute care (figure 5.5). When entered into a regression model across states in which acute-care Medicare spending per beneficiary is the dependent variable, diabetes (i.e., the marker for health status) accounts for a substantial share of the variance in spending. Moreover, while per capita income and Medicare price account for 22 percent of variation in spending, adding diabetes prevalence boosts the explanatory power of the model by 50 percentage points to 72 percent. Adding percentage black, percentage uninsured, and age brings the explanatory power of the full model to 81 percent. Sheiner concludes

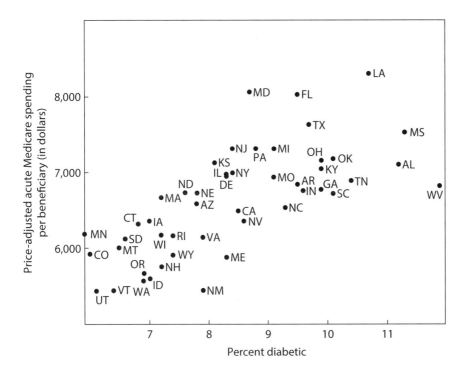

Figure 5.5. Real Medicare spending per beneficiary and diabetes rates, by state, 2008. Sheiner, "Why the Geographic Variation in Health Care Spending Cannot Tell Us Much."[27]

that most of the geographic variation in Medicare spending is explained by differences in state-level health status, in the social and demographic factors that prompt the need for medical care, and in the resources available in the state to financially support such care.

It has been argued that the strength of the estimated effects of health status in some cross-sectional studies may be biased upward because of confounding with medical coding practices. For example, consider two demographically comparable communities that have the same proportion of individuals with osteoarthritis of the knee. If knee arthroscopy is performed at twice the rate in one community than the other, the *apparent* prevalence of osteoarthritis based on the recorded diagnostic codes for knee osteoarthritis will be greater in the community with more knee surgeries, even though the underlying true prevalence is the same. What is really physician-induced demand will be ascribed to differences in the prevalence of disease.

While there will be less confounding when broader measures of health status are used (e.g., in the Sheiner study), it makes sense that there will be some level of bias in using coding-based diagnoses through the hierarchical condition categories (e.g., in the NAM study). At the high end of estimated bias, Song et al. estimated that confounding caused a downward bias of 19 percent in the observed spending differences between the highest and lowest quintiles.[29] In another study that attempted to estimate confounding bias, the researchers used a modified set of hierarchical condition categories in which diagnoses that were thought to be susceptible to diagnosis or coding bias were removed.[30] In this study of 6,000 physicians and 1.5 million Medicare beneficiaries focused on end-of-life care, the estimated bias was estimated at about 8 percent, and the authors concluded that population health explains more than 75–80 percent of the variation in medical spending. Health status can also be measured by self-report, which should not suffer from the confounding bias that occurs when it is measured by the coding of medical claims. When doing so, health status (and demographic variables) has been estimated to account for about 37 percent of the difference in expenditures between high- and low-spending areas.[31]

Quantitative estimates of the importance of health status in accounting for variation in health care spending have been somewhat variable in the cross-sectional studies summarized here as they are observational in nature and potentially confounded by coding practices and a variety of unobserved variables. That said, all of the major studies reviewed above—Zuckerman et al., NAM, and Sheiner—concluded that health status was a major (if not *the* major) contributor to health care expenditures; based on these studies, it would be reasonable to estimate that health status accounts for 25–50 percent of the variation in spending.

Evidence from Natural Experiments

Randomized trials could theoretically tease out the differential effects on health care utilization of health status and physician-induced demand, but these are not feasible. In the absence of randomized trials, there are sometimes "natural experiments" that can provide insight. Two such natural experiments arising from changes in pertinent circumstances over time are (1) an elegant econometric model that exploits information gleaned from Medicare beneficiaries who move from one area to another and (2) an anecdotal example pertaining to the opening and closing of trauma centers in a defined geographic area.

Migration of Medicare Patients

When Medicare beneficiaries move from one area to another, do they continue to have the same rate of medical care utilization and expenditure as before, or does their behavior now reflect the characteristics of their new area? Examining the migration of Medicare patients constitutes a natural experiment that allowed Amy Finkelstein and her colleagues to create a model that separates the role of patient-specific factors such as health status (which travel with them) from factors specific to their new location, such as physicians' incentives and beliefs.[32] For shorthand, patient-specific and place-specific factors are referred to as "demand" and "supply" factors. In terms of the conceptual framework of this chapter, increased utilization of medical care by a Medicare patient in a new area due to his or her new physician having a different set of beliefs and practice styles is a supply factor that leads to a form of induced demand that is operationalized as health care consumption.

The basic idea in the methodology used by Finkelstein and colleagues was as follows: suppose a group of Medicare patients moved from Northern Illinois, an area of low Medicare spending, to Miami, a high-spending area. In the year before their move, the Northern Illinois patients consumed an average of $5,632 on their health care. Assuming that their health status doesn't change when they move to Miami, if they now consumed an average of $15,098 the next year on health care, the mean for Miami, we would infer that the increased spending is due to "place" effects. On the other hand, if they continued to consume an average of $5,632 on health care, we would infer that "place" has no effect and that all health care spending is due to health status.

The actual figure will fall between the two, and the model developed by Finkelstein and her colleagues identifies the relative importance of patient health status and place (i.e., demand and supply). Focusing on utilization rather than expenditure (to avoid the complexity of price variation), they used Medicare claims data for a 20 percent sample of beneficiaries between 1998 and 2008. The HRRs of the Dartmouth Atlas was used as their geographic unit of observation. After applying inclusion and exclusion criteria, their final sample included 2.5 million patients, about one fifth of whom were "movers." Through econometric analysis based on their model of Medicare movers, they inferred that about 47 percent of the difference in utilization between HRRs above and below median utilization is due to patient characteristics, and the remainder is due to place-specific factors.

When the analysis is applied to specific measures of utilization, the results have construct validity in the sense that they reflect the likely degree of patient involvement in decision-making (table 5.2). For utilization decisions that are likely to be made more by a physician than a patient (diagnostic

Table 5.2. Attribution of difference in health care utilization due to patient characteristics and place-specific factors

Percentage (%) share of difference in utilization due to:	Patients	Place
Overall	46.5	53.5
Any emergency room visit	71.4	28.6
Number of preventive care measures	61.1	38.9
Inpatient utilization	24.2	75.8
Number of imaging tests	9.2	90.8
Number of diagnostic tests	14.2	85.8

Source: Adapted from Finkelstein, Getzkow, and Williams, "Sources of Geographic Variation in Health Care," tables 2 and 4.[32]

tests, imaging studies, and inpatient care), a small percent of the utilization difference between areas is attributed to patients (9, 14, and 24 percent, respectively). For utilization decisions that are more patient-driven (preventive care, emergency room visits), a high percent of the utilization difference between areas is attributed to patients (61 and 71 percent, respectively).

Finally, after correcting statistically for the measurement error of health status that varies systematically by area, Finkelstein and her colleagues parsed out the portion of patient effects that are due to health status and other elements of patient demand. They also used survey-based measures that capture physician beliefs about the management of specific patient vignettes to estimate the portion of place effects that are due to physician practice styles based on these beliefs, in addition to estimating effects due to other place-specific variables. Here are some of the highlights of their findings:

- Statistically significant *place-specific effects* (supply-side factors) were associated with HRRs that had more hospital beds per capita, a higher share of physicians who take an aggressive clinical management posture, and a higher share of for-profit hospitals.
- Statistically higher levels of *patient-specific effects* (demand-side factors) were associated with HRRs that had patients who were older, sicker, and had higher levels of income and/or education.
- Patient health status explained between 22 and 37 percent of the utilization difference between HRRs, which is about half of the 47 percent overall that was attributed to patient-specific factors.

Opening and Closing of Trauma Centers

Most states have Certificate of Need statutes that govern the building of facilities like hospitals and trauma centers. Such entities are expensive to create and maintain, and the Certificate of Need process ensures that communities are not "oversupplied" with such facilities that might then become full following Roemer's law and thereby increase overall health care expenditures.

In Jacksonville, Florida, a natural experiment suggestive of supplier-induced demand with respect to trauma centers occurred. Up until 2011, a single hospital (hospital 1) served as the sole regional level 1 trauma center for the northwest portion of Florida. For the years prior to 2011, the baseline volume of trauma patients treated was relatively constant. In November 2011, provisional approval was given to another hospital (hospital 2) to begin a second trauma program in the region, but the program was subsequently closed by the state 16 months later because of various state-defined citations. This situation creates a classic "A-B-A" natural experiment (figure 5.6).

In the 16 months prior to the opening of a second trauma center, from July 2010 to October 2011, there were 5,159 trauma patients treated in the Jacksonville region, all in hospital 1. During the 16-month period of November

Figure 5.6. "A-B-A Experiment" demonstrating supplier-induced trauma cases in Jacksonville, Florida, 2010–2014

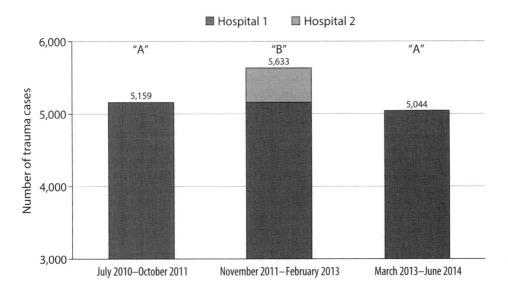

2011 to February 2013, when hospital 2's trauma center was open, hospital 2 treated 1,050 trauma patients. But the trauma volume in hospital 1 was not reduced by 1,050 cases during this period; rather, it treated only 576 fewer trauma cases that year. The total number of trauma cases in the region during the 16-month period in which the second trauma program was open was now 5,633, an increase of 474 cases above baseline. During the 16-month period from March 2013 to June 2014, after hospital 2's trauma program was closed, the volume of trauma cases in the region returned to approximately its baseline number. (Actually, the number of cases fell slightly from baseline, to 5,044.)

Indeed, with the approval of new trauma centers throughout Florida, the phenomenon of apparent supplier-induced demand for trauma care occurred throughout the state. In 2011, provisional approval was granted by Florida to a national, investor-owned hospital corporation to open six new trauma centers throughout the state over three years. Ciesla et al. found that total trauma charges in Florida increased by $1.7 billion between 2010 and 2014, of which $1 billion was due to the new trauma centers.[33] During this period, the general population in the state increased by only 4.7 percent, but the number of cases coded as fulfilling trauma criteria increased by 13 percent and total trauma charges increased by 47 percent.

Often, incremental cases coded as trauma (and therefore eligible for substantial trauma initiation fees and other payments) are older individuals with injuries that would not be coded as trauma were it not for age. Staudenmayer et al. showed that elderly persons referred to trauma centers had the same mortality as those treated in regular, nontrauma emergency departments but had much higher average costs ($35,069 vs. $14,332).[34]

The Role of Physician Beliefs and Clinical Practice Styles

Earlier in this chapter, examples were given of circumstances in which physician beliefs in the face of ambiguous evidence will influence his or her advice and thereby a patient's decision to proceed with treatment. Sometimes differences in practice styles can lead to dramatic results. For example, in a frequently referenced *New Yorker* article about health care costs, Atul Gawande compared two Texas communities: McAllen and El Paso.[35] At that time, Medicare spent $15,000 per McAllen beneficiary, $3,000 more than per capita income. By contrast, Medicare expenditures per beneficiary in El Paso, a community with similar demographics and health status 800 miles up the border, were $7,500. There was no difference between the two areas in available medical technology or in the quality ratings of hospitals. There were large differences between the two communities, however, in the rate at which diagnostic tests, imaging studies, and surgical procedures were performed for patients with the same symptoms. Based on extensive interviews, one of Gawande's conclusions was that a major explanation for the difference between McAllen and El Paso was that the "entrepreneurial" medical environment in McAllen attracted physicians with a style of practice that led to greater utilization and expenditure.

The potential for physician beliefs and practice styles to explain a significant share of geographic "place-based" variation in health care expenditures was explored by Cutler et al. using information gleaned from physician responses to a vignette-based survey.[36] Samples of 999 cardiologists and 1,333 primary care physicians (PCPs) were drawn from the American Medical Association database and the response rates of the two physician groups were 61.5 and 72.5 percent, respectively.

Three patient vignettes were presented, and the physician responses were compared with established evidence-based guidelines that should be well known to the physician groups. Patient A was a patient with a history of angina but who was now stable on current medical therapy, and the other two vignettes were patients who had been treated for heart failure but had few if any reasons for additional intervention. Physicians who "consistently and unambiguously recommended intensive care beyond what would be indicated by current clinical guidelines" were referred to as "cowboys" (which represented 26 percent of cardiologists and 23 percent of PCPs), and those who "consistently recommended palliative care" in the last two patient vignettes were referred to as "comforters" (which represented 27 percent of cardiologists and 44 percent of PCPs). By combining these survey responses with Medicare expenditure and other data in the HRRs in which the physicians were located, the impact of physician practice styles on per capita Medicare expenditures for end-of-life care and myocardial infarction could be estimated. Medicare expenditures were adjusted for price, age, sex, and medical risk at the HRR level. End-of-life expenditures were per-patient spending levels in the last two years of life for a number of fatal illnesses. Acute myocardial infarction (AMI) expenditures were one-year spending levels after admission for an AMI during 2007–2010 for fee-for-service Medicare patients.

Extrapolating from their data analysis using this model, Cutler and his colleagues conclude that if all physicians were comforters who followed clinical guidelines and none was a cowboy, there would be a decline of as much as 35 percent for end-of-life care expenditures and of 12 percent for expenditures on heart disease. Of course, "cowboy" and "comforter" physicians were not experimentally allocated in different proportions to the different communities with utilization tracked prospectively; this was an observational study in which associations were not necessarily causal and might have been due to confounding factors. Nonetheless, it follows from our discussion of induced demand in the context of physicians acting as the patient's agent, and from anecdotal but powerful examples like the ones described by Gawande, that physician preferences and practice styles influence utilization to a significant degree. If about half of the variation in health care utilization by Medicare patients were due to supply factors, then the 12–35 percent of the total variation in utilization attributed by Cutler et al. to "practice style" would account for 24–70 percent of the supply-side half.

Taken together, and recognizing that the results cover a wide range of estimates using a variety of methodologic approaches, we can summarize the factors responsible for the wide variation in health care utilization and spending across geographic areas. In broad terms, it appears that about half of the variation in spending across geographic areas is due to demand (patient) factors, and that about half of this half is due to health status. The remainder of the variation in utilization is due to supply factors (i.e., provider-induced utilization); depending on the nature of the illness for which health care services are being utilized, about 25–70 percent of this supply-side half can be attributed to physician practice styles. This leaves substantial residual, unexplained variation in spending, which might be due to unmeasured variables related to health status, patient or physician preferences, or other pertinent factors. Residual variation might also be due to productivity differences in the delivery of medical care. Such inefficiencies would represent areas of opportunity to achieve better health outcomes at our present level of health care expenditures, or the same health outcomes at lower expenditures, with the savings applied to other parts of the economy.

The Special Case of Induced Demand by the Pharmaceutical Industry

In addition to health providers and hospitals, the pharmaceutical industry can induce demand through marketing. Historically, this had been accomplished mainly through marketing directed at physicians and other health providers, but in recent years there has been substantial growth in direct-to-consumer advertising, a phenomenon that is discussed in detail in chapter 17. An extreme and horrifyingly deadly contemporary example of induced demand for prescription drugs is the promulgation of addiction to opioids. Austin Frakt provides a balanced and cogent discussion of the opioid epidemic, including the role of drug companies, physician groups, the evolution of evidence regarding addiction and its selective dissemination, and historical precedents.[37]

Summary

Patients who are fully informed about the benefits and risks of medical care—based on objective, independent evidence and the value they attach to different outcomes but not affected by physician advice, pharmaceutical marketing or other outside influences—will choose a quantity of medical care consumption where the perceived marginal benefit (improved health) equals marginal cost (including not only price but loss of work time, inconvenience, risk of adverse outcomes, and other tangible and intangible costs). Consumption of health care at the point where marginal benefit equals marginal cost will be greater under a scenario of insurance coverage, since the marginal cost (i.e., "price") is reduced.

Because of imperfect and asymmetric information, real-world patient decision-making will be impacted by physician advice, marketing, and other outside influences. Physicians are trained as part of a profession in which they serve as the patient's agent; thus, physicians try to maximize their patients' health, but they are also mindful of their own income. Using their influence as the patient's agent, physicians sometimes induce medical care utilization beyond the amount associated with the patient's perceived marginal benefit to marginal cost comparison. This influence is often based on evidence-based information regarding the efficacy of a recommended treatment or action. Sometimes, however, it can spring from a practice style that is inconsistent with evidence in the literature. In some cases, physicians can induce utilization because of their own financial interests independent of perceived patient benefit, a phenomenon that can be exacerbated in cases of physician ownership of imaging centers, surgicenters, chemotherapy infusion centers, and the like.

A variety of studies have been performed to tease out the relative contribution of these factors with respect to the consumption of medical care.

Most studies have been cross-sectional analyses of geographic variation in health care expenditures, but some have been longitudinal analyses that exploit natural experiments. Although it would be incorrect to conclude that there is consistency in the findings, a general summary of the current state of knowledge is as follows:

- There is wide variation across geographic areas in health care expenditures for both Medicare and commercial-pay patients, with expenditures in areas at the 90th percentile of spending being 30–50 percent higher than expenditures in areas at the 10th percentile.
- Most of the variation in Medicare spending across geographic areas is due to post-acute services rather than acute-care services.
- Most of the variation in commercial health care spending is due to differences in price markups.
- Based on a natural experiment of "Medicare movers," about half of the variation in medical spending appears to be due to patient (demand-side) characteristics such as health status and demographic characteristics, and the other half to place (supply-side) characteristics, including physician preferences and practice styles. About half of the share of variation attributed to demand factors may be due to health status according to some studies, but others have attributed more importance to health status.
- Studies of supply-side (physician) beliefs and practice styles attribute 12–35 percent of expenditure variation to beliefs that cannot be justified based on patient preferences or evidence of clinical effectiveness.
- There is substantial residual unexplained variation in health care expenditures, which is likely related to unmeasured supply-side or demand-side factors, or to inefficiencies in providing health care.

6 THE ROLE OF PRICE IN HEALTH CARE SPENDING GROWTH

The average utilization of health care in the United States is on par with peer nations due to offsetting factors. Since expenditures equal price multiplied by quantity (E = P × Q), the fact that the average per capita spending on health care in the United States is roughly twice as high as that of peer nations, while utilization is roughly the same, means that the difference in expenditures is accounted for mainly by price.

Put differently, if per capita health care expenditures in country A are twice that of country B, and if the per capita quantity of health care utilized is the same, then the unit price of health care in country A must be twice as high as in country B. This inference is not new. In 2003, Gerard Anderson and his colleagues published a paper in *Health Affairs* entitled "It's the Prices, Stupid: Why the United States Is So Different from Other Countries." Using data from the 30 countries of the Organisation for Economic Co-operation and Development (OECD) in 2000, these researchers found that health care expenditures per capita in the United States were more than twice that of the OECD median ($4,631 vs. $1,983), but on most measures of health care utilization the United States was well below the OECD median. The authors concluded, "Since spending is a product of both the goods and services used and their prices, this implies that much higher prices are paid in the United States than in other countries. . . . It's the prices, stupid."[1]

International data from OECD continue to show such a pattern to this day. Yet, the key role of price in explaining our nation's high expenditures on health care is not fully appreciated; instead, our high spending is often attributed to such things as technology, defensive medicine, physician-induced demand, personal income growth, and other factors. While these factors play a role, there are other data that provide a more comprehensive understanding of the role of price, through both international cross-sectional comparisons and longitudinal analyses within the United States.

One of the authors of the 2003 *Health Affairs* report, Uwe Reinhardt, died in 2017. As a tribute to Professor Reinhardt, the remaining original authors updated their analysis in a 2019 *Health Affairs* paper that came to the same conclusion: "Prices are the primary reason why the US spends more on health care than any other country . . . despite health policy reforms and health systems restructuring . . . that have occurred since the 2003 article's publication."[2]

International Cross-Sectional Comparisons

Based on OECD data from 2016, Irene Papanicolas and her colleagues found that health care expenditures were substantially higher in the United States than peer nations, while utilization rates were on balance approximately the same.[3] This finding led them to conclude, as did Anderson et al. in 2003 and 2019, that the major driver of the expenditure differential between the United States and peer nations is price. In this context, the concept of price is quite broad: it includes not only the specific prices of medical care supplies and other goods such as pharmaceuticals and medical devices but also labor costs (physicians, dentists, nurses, pharmacists, and other health personnel), administrative expenses, and profit.

In the OECD data, "administrative expenses" focus on the transaction costs and associated expenses incurred by insurance companies and/or government. Included in administrative costs as defined by OECD are profit margins of private insurance companies. The administrative costs of hospitals, physicians, and other providers, however, are excluded. Instead, by default, these health care expenditures are embedded in the fees that providers charge to insurance companies and individuals.

Phamaceutical Spending

According to 2016 data reported by Papanicolas, Woskie, and Jha, total pharmaceutical spending per capita in the United States was $1,443, more than twice as high as the mean of $680 for peer nations.[4] (The mean value for the 10 countries other than the United States was calculated by multiplying the mean value for all countries by 11, subtracting the US value from the total, and dividing the resulting figure by 10.) One possible explanation would be that there were proportionately more prescriptions filled per person in the United States. Overall prescribing levels were not provided, but antibiotic prescribing (daily doses per 1,000 population) was 24.0 for the United States, as compared with a mean of 19.8 for the other high-income countries. Thus, taking antibiotic prescribing as a very rough proxy for overall pharmaceutical use, prescribing volume in the United States was 21 percent higher than the other countries, but expenditures were 112 percent higher. Thus, based on this imperfect proxy, most of the difference in pharmaceutical expenditures appears to be attributable to price.

Analysis of four medications that are frequently prescribed internationally for common medical conditions indicates that 2016 prices in the United States are the highest among other peer countries for which data are available (Germany, Canada, France, Japan, and the UK).[5] For three of the four drugs, the US monthly price (after discounts) appears to be more than double that paid in the next highest country:

- Crestor (high cholesterol): US $86 vs. $20–$41 for other countries
- Lantus (diabetes): US $186 vs. $54–$67 for other countries
- Advair (asthma): US $155 vs. $29–$74 for other countries
- Humira (rheumatoid arthritis): US $2,505 vs. $982–$1,749 for other countries

Additional international comparisons of drug prices paid by commercial health plans were compiled by the International Federation of Health Plans (IFHP) for 2015 (table 6.1). Price estimates for pharmaceuticals in the United States are robust, as they represent mean prices derived from data on over

Table 6.1. Comparative 2015 prices (USD) for seven commonly used medications

Drug	United States	United Kingdom	Switzerland	Spain	South Africa
Xarelto (blood clots)	292	126	102	101	48
Humira (rheumatoid arthritis)	2,669	1,362	822	1,253	552
Harvoni (hepatitis C)	32,114	22,554	16,861	18,165	N/A
Truvada (HIV/AIDS)	1,301	689	906	559	N/A
Tecfidera (multiple sclerosis)	5,089	663	1,855	1,399	N/A
Avastin (cancer)	3,930	1,745	1,252	1,534	956
Oxycontin (pain)	265	72	95	36	84

Source: International Federation of Health Plans, *2015 Comparative Price Report: Variation in Medical and Hospital Prices by Country* (London: IFHP), accessed December 29, 2018, https://docplayer.net/48892596 -2015-comparative-price-report-variation-in-medical-and-hospital-prices-by-country.html.

170 million pharmacy claims that reflect prices negotiated and paid to health care providers. Prices listed for the other countries (in US dollars) are not as representative, as they reflect the prices obtained from one private-sector health plan in each country. With those caveats, the price for each of these commonly used drugs is generally two-times to five-times higher in the United States than in the other countries listed. The markedly higher prices paid for pharmaceuticals in the United States are important, since total drug spending here is about 17 percent of total personal health expenditures.

Diagnostic Tests and Hospital-Based Services

The IFHP report also provides comparative prices for a variety of diagnostic tests and hospital-based services and procedures in the United States and six peer countries (table 6.2). Prices reported for the United States are mean values that were derived from over 370 million medical claims, reflecting prices negotiated by commercial health plans and paid to providers. As with pharmaceutical data from IFHP, prices for diagnostic tests and hospital-based procedures in the other countries (in US dollars) may not be as representative, since they are based on data provided by one private-sector health plan in each country. Prices for "hospital/physician" services (such as appendectomy, knee replacement, etc.) reflect the combined hospital and physician fees.

It is clear from this data that prices for virtually all the diagnostic tests and hospital/physician services evaluated are significantly higher in the

Table 6.2. Comparative 2015 prices (USD) for hospital and physician services

Service	United States	United Kingdom	Switzerland	New Zealand	Australia	South Africa	Spain
Hospital cost per day	5,220	. . .	4,781	2,142	765	631	424
Appendectomy	15,930	8,009	6,040	. . .	3,814	1,786	2,003
Normal delivery	10,808	. . .	7,751	. . .	. . .	1,271	1,950
C-section	16,106	. . .	9,965	. . .	7,901	2,192	2,352
Cataract surgery	3,530	3,145	2,114	2,740	3,037	1,186	1,719
Knee replacement	28,184	18,451	20,132	16,508	15,941	7,795	6,687
Hip replacement	29,067	16,335	17,112	15,465	19,484	7,685	6,757
Coronary bypass	78,318	24,059	34,224	32,480	28,888	18,501	14,579
Angioplasty	31,620	7,264	10,066	13,677	11,164	6,510	7,839

Source: International Federation of Health Plans, *2015 Comparative Price Report: Variation in Medical and Hospital Prices by Country* (London: IFHP), accessed December 29, 2018, https://docplayer.net/48892596-2015-comparative-price-report-variation-in-medical-and-hospital -prices-by-country.html.

United States than in the other countries. The only exceptions are angiograms in the United Kingdom and colonoscopies in the United Kingdom and New Zealand, which are somewhat higher than in the United States. For diagnostic tests, prices in the United States are generally twice as high as the mean price in the other countries listed, and for hospital/physician services, prices in the United States are generally two-times to three-times higher.

Administrative Costs

Thus, prices for drugs, diagnostic tests, and hospital/physician services are much higher in the United States than in peer nations. In addition, administrative costs are strikingly higher here. Based on a supplement to Papanicolas, Woskie, and Jha's international comparison of health care spending,[6] the United States spent 8 percent of total health expenditures on administration and governance in 2016, as compared to 2.5 percent for the ten other high-income countries studied (range 1 to 5 percent). This administrative expense is a blend of private insurers and government programs.

As would be expected, those countries with more of an insurance-based approach to their universal coverage (Netherland, Switzerland, Germany) experienced greater administrative expense (i.e., 4 to 5 percent of health expenditures), but they were still below the US level of 8 percent. Ezekiel Emanuel computed per capita costs from these data and found a three- to fivefold higher level of per capita administrative expense in the United States ($752) than in Germany, the Netherlands, and Sweden ($232, $208, and $136, respectively).[7]

It is important to note that the OECD database upon which these analyses are based does *not* include provider-based administrative costs. In the United States, since the vast majority of provider billing is fee-for-service (whether to commercial insurance, Medicare, Medicaid, or other payors), there is enormous cost in the coding, billing, reconciling, and auditing of each and every transaction. This cost falls on hospitals, physicians, and other health care providers who must invest in large numbers of people and costly computerized systems devoted to the electronic medical record, "revenue cycle" activities, and regulatory compliance. A 2010 study of hospital administrative costs by Himmelstein et al. compared the United States with Canada, the Netherlands, England, Scotland, and Wales.[8] They found that the share of gross domestic product (GDP) related to such costs were

1.43 percent in the United States against a mean of 0.59 percent in the other seven countries. Expenditures per capita on hospital administration were $667 in the United States as compared to a mean of $216 (in US dollars) for the other five countries.

Along similar lines, a 2018 study by Tseng et al. estimated physician billing and insurance-related activities in a large medical center (Duke Health) that had adopted electronic medical records.[9] Using detailed time-driven, activity-based costing, but not including the capital cost of the electronic medical records system, they estimated billing costs to be 14.5 percent of professional revenues for primary care visits, 25.2 percent for emergency department visits, 8 percent for medical inpatient admissions, and 3.1 percent for inpatient surgical procedures.

When 8 percent of a premium dollar is used for national insurer and governance overhead, to which is added the administrative cost incurred by providers (physicians and hospitals), it is hard to escape the conclusion that administrative overhead contributes substantially to the higher price of health care in the United States. This topic is explored in more detail in chapter 18.

Longitudinal Studies within the United States

In addition to international comparisons, insights about the role of price in health care expenditures in the United States can be gleaned from longitudinal analyses of the growth in spending. According to the federal National Health Expenditure Accounts, the official source for national health care expenditures, total personal health care spending was $615.3 billion in 1990.[10] Accounting for inflation as measured by the consumer price index, the $615.3 billion would have risen to $1,110 billion by 2016. But actual personal health care expenditures in 2016 were $2,835 billion; thus, in constant dollars, expenditures grew 2.55-fold (from $1.1 trillion to $2.8 trillion) between 1990 and 2016. During this time, the US population grew only 1.26-fold, from 254 million to 322 million.

Since $E = P \times Q$, factors affecting expenditures exert their influence through price and/or quantity. With respect to the "quantity" component of expenditures, increases are potentially comprised of growth in population size; the aging of the population, which would increase utilization per capita; increases in the prevalence of disease; new technologies for the diagnosis or treatment of a disease that replace less effective methods; and a greater number of encounters with the health system per episode of illness.

If quantity (health care utilization) is roughly the same across time for an illness, then since $E = P \times Q$, any increase in expenditure is due to a proportional increase in price. In this context, price is not only the price of supplies, pharmaceuticals, and services, but the intensity of treatment for a specific illness. Across time, a given illness (e.g., prostate cancer) may be treated with more expensive technology (e.g., robotic surgery rather than open surgery) that increases cost compared to traditional surgery. Robotic surgery may reduce length of stay in the hospital, however, which would reduce cost. The "price" is the aggregate cost of treating the prostate cancer (i.e., surgical equipment, hospital services, physicians, drugs, home care, etc.).

Looking to the future, the distinction between the individual prices of different elements of service and the overall price of an episode of illness may become less important, in view of the growing use of payments to providers for the care of a patient during an entire episode of illness, rather than piecemeal payment for each lab test, imaging study, physician visit, medication, procedure, and so on. As discussed in chapter 10, Medicare began such comprehensive payments in the 1980s with the use of diagnosis-related groups, but this approach is now being extended to Medicaid and commercial payers.

Several attempts have been made in recent years to deconstruct the relative contributions of price and quantity in explaining the large increase in US health care expenditures. Roehrig and Rousseau studied the civilian noninstitutionalized population from 1996 to 2006, distributed across 260 medical conditions, using data from the National Health Expenditure Accounts.[11] They adjusted for inflation and population increases to estimate the growth rate in real per capita spending for each medical condition and devised a decomposition of this growth rate into two parts—one part attributable to a change in the "treated prevalence" of the condition, and the other part attributable to the "cost per case" (i.e., a proxy for price). The "treated prevalence" measure does not count all the individuals in a population with a disease; it only counts individuals who are *treated* for their disease. Thus, an individual with diabetes who does not access medical care would not be counted as a treated prevalence case.

Overall, Roehrig and Rousseau found that across all medical conditions, real per capita spending grew at an annual rate of 3.8 percent between 1996 and 2006. During this period the annual growth of real per capita GDP was 2.1 percent. Thus, the annual growth rate for real per capita health expenditures grew faster than per capita GDP by 1.7 percent. Of the 3.8 percent total annual growth in real per capita health care spending, 2.8 percent was attributed to increasing cost per case and 1.0 percent was attributed to increasing treated prevalence of medical conditions.

Dunn, Liebman, and Shapiro of the Federal Reserve Bank of San Francisco used 2003–2007 claims data from a large sample of commercially insured patients using the MarketScan Research Database (Thomson Reuters).[12] Thus, their analysis did not take into account patients treated under Medicaid or Medicare, or in nursing homes. These investigators developed a model that expressed growth in health care expenditures per capita (adjusted for changes in population, geographic location, age, and sex distribution) as being comprised of growth in two factors: treated disease prevalence and expenditure per episode of disease. Expenditure per episode was further divided between service utilization per episode and price. Between 2003 and 2007 there was about a 25 percent increase in overall health care expenditures per capita among commercially insured patients, adjusted for population, age, sex, and geography. About two-fifths of this increase was attributed to increasing treated prevalence of disease and three-fifths was attributed to increasing expenditures per episode. Growth in expenditures per episode was, in turn, attributed entirely to price increases since utilization of services per episode in the aggregate showed no change during the time period under study.

Both of these studies suggest that price was more important than quantity as an explanation for growth in US health care spending. Quantitative inferences from these analyses, however, are constrained by their use of "treated" prevalence rather than the true underlying prevalence rate of disease. In other words, a patient with hypertension is only counted if he or she is *treated* for hypertension. Thus, treated prevalence represents a combination of disease prevalence and health care use. Since some of utilization is incorporated into treated prevalence, the measure of utilization is impacted. And since price is inferred from the ratio of expenditures to utilization, a modified measure of utilization implies a modified measure of price.

To date, the cleanest method for parsing expenditure growth into its price and quantity components was reported by Dieleman et al.[13] These researchers studied the growth in US health care expenditures from 1996 through 2013 using a database from the US Disease Expenditure 2013 Project, which has a number of advantages: it can be scaled to the official estimate of US health spending contained in the National Health Expenditure Accounts; it modeled estimates of spending and volume accurately for 155 health conditions, 38 age and sex groups, and six types of care (ambulatory, inpatient, emergency department, retail pharmacy, and nursing home care); and in assessing price, it distinguished payments from charges. Data on disease prevalence and incidence were extracted from the Global Burden of Disease 2015 study. Prevalence data were used for chronic and other diseases except for cancer and injury; in these cases, incidence data were used because health care for these conditions is associated more with incidence than with prevalence.

Dieleman et al. calculated the growth in spending as an identity equation equal to changes in five factors: population, age and sex distribution, disease prevalence, service utilization, and service price and intensity. This identity equation completely accounts for spending without any residual. For each of the 155 health conditions, this modeling process produced a decomposition of the contribution of each of the five factors to health care expenditure growth. The ability to measure true prevalence of disease (or incidence in the case of cancer and injury), instead of "treated prevalence," allowed these investigators to be able to separate prevalence from utilization more clearly and therefore measure price more accurately. Furthermore, measures of price and quantity were tailored to each of the categories of care. Quantity (utilization) was defined as the number of encounters per prevalent case, where encounters were: (a) doctor visits for ambulatory care, emergency department, or dental care; (b) bed days for hospital and nursing home services; or (c) prescriptions filled for pharmaceuticals. Price was then defined as spending per encounter and thus included not only the pure prices of goods and services, but also intensity of service in terms of technology and other factors.

Between 1996 and 2013, after adjusting for inflation, real annual personal health care expenditures increased by $933.5 billion. The decomposition of the five contributing factors to this growth in annual spending showed that

- population growth and aging accounted for about $400 billion of the expenditure growth,
- disease prevalence/incidence and service utilization made no statistically significant contribution, and
- price (including "intensity of service") was responsible for the residual increase in spending.

Results on inpatient and outpatient services and pharmaceuticals add a refined understanding of these aggregate results:

- A reduction in spending of about $200 billion due to reduced utilization of *inpatient services,* plus an additional reduction of about $20 billion due to reduced prevalence/incidence of disease requiring such services, was more than offset by a $340 billion increase in price.
- Utilization of *ambulatory care and pharmaceuticals* increased during the period under study, but the reduction in bed days per prevalent case (likely due to reduced length of stay and a shift from outpatient to inpatient procedures) acted as an offset such that overall utilization during the period was flat.

Further analyses of specific medical conditions revealed that price increases particularly affected the growth in spending on retail drugs for diabetes, inpatient care for low back and neck pain, and emergency department and inpatient care for falls. Although service utilization had a negligible overall impact on spending growth, it had marked effects on expenditures for specific services: ambulatory care for hypertension and low back and neck pain, and retail pharmacy expenditures for hypertension, hyperlipidemia, and depression.

Longitudinal International Comparisons

In 1996, per capita spending on health care in the United States (in 2010 US dollars) was $4,946, as compared to a mean of $2,688 for 10 peer high-income countries (figure 6.1). By 2016, per capita expenditures rose to $8,932 and $4,647, respectively, for the United States and the other high-income countries (in 2010 US dollars). Thus, the almost 2:1 ratio of spending for health care in the United States as compared with peer nations is longstanding: this ratio was 1.84 in 1996 and 1.92 in 2016. Thus, while health care spending in the other countries was virtually half as much as the United States in 1996, since then spending growth in the other countries has almost kept pace with the United States, as can be seen from the compounded annual growth rates.

Since utilization of health care services has been, in the aggregate, similar between the United States and peer nations in recent decades, based on analyses of 2000 data by Anderson et al. and of 2016 data by Papanicolas, Woskie, and Jha, we are left with the conclusion that the growth in expenditures in the United States over the past two decades, which has been almost mirrored by the growth rate in peer nations, has been primarily due

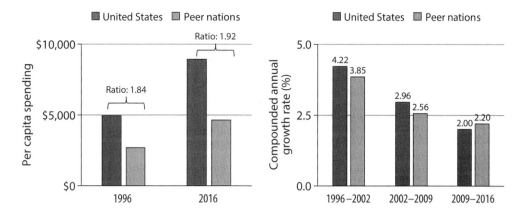

Figure 6.1. International comparisons of health care spending (in 2010 US dollars) and compounded annual growth rates, United States vs. 10 high-income peer nations (Australia, Canada, Denmark, France, Germany, Japan, Netherlands, Sweden, Switzerland, and United Kingdom). "Health Expenditures and Financing," OECD.Stat, Organisation for Economic Co-operation and Development, accessed December 29, 2018, https://stats.oecd.org.

to changes in the price of medical goods and services, above and beyond the growth in general consumer prices.

Summary

Although utilization of certain diagnostic tests, pharmaceuticals, and surgical procedures that are subject to induced demand is greater in the United States than in other high-income countries, overall utilization of other health care services are, on average, comparable. From cross-sectional analyses, the major reason that per capita health care expenditures are currently higher in the United States than other high-income countries is higher US prices, inclusive of administrative services and profits.

Longitudinally, analyses of spending growth in the United States, adjusting for population growth, aging, and disease prevalence, have also concluded that price has been the main driver, not utilization. We conclude that spending growth on health care over the past two decades in the United States has been mainly due to price increases. During this period, spending per capita grew at almost the same rate in peer nations as in the United States, but started from an amount in peer nations that was about one half as high.

7 INEQUALITY OF WEALTH, HEALTH, AND ACCESS TO CARE

Although not shared by all, one prevailing view in the United States is that some of our societal resources should be redistributed to help those in need. This core value is accomplished in part through philanthropy but also though public programs, statutes, and policies. There are many examples in health care:

- Medicare
- Medicaid
- Affordable Care Act, through the health care marketplace exchanges and Medicaid expansion
- Tax policy that exempts health insurance premium payments
- Veterans Benefits Administration health care system
- Statutes such as the Emergency Medical Treatment and Active Labor Act, a 1986 federal law that requires hospital emergency departments to screen every patient who seeks emergency care and to stabilize those with medical emergencies regardless of health insurance status or ability to pay
- Programs such as the Children's Health Insurance Program, which provides low-cost health coverage to children in families that earn too much money to qualify for Medicaid

Such a redistribution of resources is not allocatively "efficient" in the Pareto sense discussed in chapter 2, but it is consistent with prevailing societal values to provide for those in need. There are gaps, however, in the set of insurance and government programs for health care that have evolved over the years, such that about 10 percent of Americans are not currently covered. While this percentage is lower than the 25 percent uninsured prior to Medicare and Medicaid, and the 16 percent uninsured before enactment of the Affordable Care Act,[1] the United States remains unique among other high-income countries in having a sizable minority of individuals who lack coverage for basic health care services.[2] Although access to health care in the United States is more equitable than it would be in a purely competitive market economy, it is less equitable than in all other high-income nations. Thus, for example, 22.3 percent of the US population report that they missed a medical consultation because of cost, as compared to a mean of 9.4 percent for 10 other high-income countries studied.[3]

The goal of more equitable health outcomes was one of the four over-arching objectives of Healthy People 2020, the nation's 10-year list of goals for health promotion and disease prevention that was launched on December 2, 2010. Specifically, the stated objective was "Achieve health equity, eliminate disparities, and improve the health of all groups."[4] Despite the prevailing redistribution of resources in the United States that provides some level of needed medical care across its entire population, and a variety of public and private programs to promote equity in health promotion and disease prevention, substantial variations in health status and health care access remain as a function of income. As a society, although there are wide (and often strongly held) differences of opinion about the degree to which access to health care should be independent of income, over the last century the realities of our political structure, economic system, and stakeholder influence have led to the current state. In many ways, inequalities in health and health care access reflect the same belief systems and cultural influences in the United States that have led to inequality in income and wealth, which is also much greater than that of peer nations.

Inequality in income and wealth is an important context for understanding inequalities in health status and access to care. The link between the two have many impacts, especially on life expectancy. Specifically, data support the relative importance of behavioral factors and health care access in explaining variations in life expectancy.

Inequality in Income and Wealth

While the United States is a multicultural, pluralistic society with a wide variety of views on how income and wealth should ideally be distributed, there is a fundamental belief in the power of free markets to promote overall growth for the greater good, which is widely understood to be intrinsically associated with some degree of inequality in the distribution of income and wealth. It is not surprising, therefore, that over 5,000 individuals participating in a 2005 nationally representative survey (51 percent female, mean age of 44 years) endorsed an ideal distribution of wealth (i.e., assets minus liabilities) that is skewed somewhat toward high-wealth individuals.[5] Survey participants believed that individuals holding wealth in the upper 20 percent of the population should ideally own a little over 30 percent of total wealth. Moreover, survey respondents clearly understood that their *ideal* wealth distribution was more equitable than the actual wealth distribution; on average, they guessed that individuals holding wealth in the upper top 20 percent of the population own about 60 percent of total wealth. In fact, these guesses by survey participants understate the true degree of wealth concentration. At the time of the survey in 2005, individuals holding wealth in the upper 20 percent of the population owned 84 percent of total wealth.

Thus, while a nationally representative sample of Americans believe that an ideal distribution of wealth should not be entirely equal and should be concentrated somewhat at the higher end, and also recognize that actual wealth is probably more skewed than their ideal, the true concentration of wealth is far greater than both their ideal and "guesstimated" levels.

Data computed by Edward Wolff, using Survey of Consumer Finances numbers from the Federal Reserve Board of Washington, show that in 2016, individuals who were in the top 1 percent of income earned 23.5 percent of all income in the nation, and those in the top 1 percent of wealth held 39.6 percent of the nation's wealth (table 7.1). Those in the top 5 percent of income and wealth had 39.7 percent of total income and 66.7 percent of total wealth. By contrast, those in the bottom 40 percent of the population in income had only 9 percent of income and those in the bottom 40 percent of wealth had *no* net assets; in fact, they had net liabilities equal to 0.5 percent of national wealth.

Inequalities in the distribution of income and wealth can be summarized by a statistic called the "Gini coefficient." The Gini coefficient is a useful way of summarizing the degree of inequality in a population and will be used later for international comparisons. It can measure inequality in a variety of variables, although it is typically applied to income and wealth distributions. The Gini coefficient in 2016 for the United States was 0.598 for income and 0.877 for wealth, without adjusting for tax payments and government transfers.

A conceptual understanding of the Gini coefficient can be gleaned from the percentage of total income earned by various proportions of the popu-

Table 7.1. Distribution of income and wealth in the United States, 1962 vs. 2016

Percentage share held by	Income (%)		Net worth (%)	
	1962	2016	1962	2016
Top 1%	8.4	23.5	33.4	39.6
Top 2–5%	11.4	16.2	21.2	27.1
Top 6–10%	10.2	10.2	12.4	12.1
Top 11–20%	16.1	14.1	14.0	11.1
Top 20%	46.0	64.0	81.0	89.9
21–40%	24.0	16.8	13.4	8.8
41–60%	16.6	10.2	5.4	2.4
Bottom 40%	13.4	9.0	0.2	–0.5
Gini coefficient	0.428	0.598	0.803	0.877

Source: Adapted from Edward N. Wolff, "Household Wealth Trends in the United States, 1962 to 2016: Has Middle Class Wealth Recovered?," National Bureau of Economic Research, Working Paper 24085, November 2017, http://www.nber.org/papers/w24085.

lation (figure 7.1). Any point (x,y) on the curves shown (called "Lorenz curves") represents the percentage y of total income in an economy earned by the poorest x percent of the population. The dashed black line represents perfect income equality, with a Gini coefficient of 0. If there were 20 individuals in an economy that generated a total of $1 million income, a Gini coefficient of 0 means that each of the 20 people in the economy earns $50,000. By contrast, the solid dark gray line along the horizontal and vertical axis depicts a Gini coefficient of 1.0, which represents perfect income inequality. This would occur if one person received the entire $1 million of income in the economy while the other 19 individuals received no income. The curved light gray line is the Lorenz curve that reflects the 2016 US income distribution reported in table 7.1. In our 20-person economy with a total income of $1 million, the person with the highest income would have $230,500 in income, while the 8 individuals with the lowest income would together have $90,000 in income. The Gini coefficient is computed as area A divided by area A + B, and is calculated to be 0.598.

Wolff's data also show that the degree of inequality in the distribution of income and wealth became more exaggerated between 1962 and 2016. The share of total income going to the top 1 percent grew from 8.4 percent in 1962 to 23.5 percent in 2016, while the bottom 40 percent experienced a decline in its share of income from 13.4 percent in 1962 to 9.0 percent in 2016. Greater income concentration across time is reflected in the Gini coefficients, which increased from 0.428 in 1962 to 0.598 in 2016. The Gini

Figure 7.1. Lorenz curves corresponding to perfect income equality, perfect income inequality, and the 2016 US income distribution

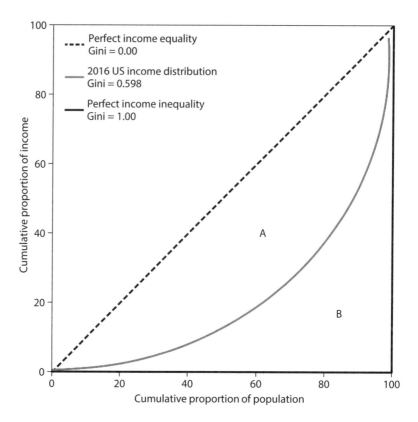

coefficients for the concentration of wealth in the US economy are much greater than that of income and also showed increases in inequality across time: the Gini coefficient for wealth grew from 0.803 in 1962 to 0.877 in 2016.

Like inequality of health care access as analyzed by Papanicolas, Woskie, and Jha, income inequality in the United States is also greater than in other high-income countries (table 7.2). (The Gini coefficients in this table are lower than those in table 7.1 because they are adjusted for taxes and government transfers, but the United States still comes out on top.) Furthermore, the ratio of income earned by the top 20 percent of the population divided by the income of the bottom 20 percent shows the United States as having the highest level of concentration in upper-income strata based on this measure. Interestingly, although Denmark has the most equitable distribution of income among the eleven countries studied, it has a higher GDP per capita than the United States ($53,400 vs. $52,100).

The concentration of financial resources in the United States can be seen in a broader context by comparing trends in the proportion of wealth held by the upper 0.1 percent and bottom 90 percent of the population during the period of 1913 through 2012 (figure 7.2)—drawn from raw data in a pa-

Table 7.2. Comparison of the United States and other high-income countries with respect to measures of income inequality, 2015

Country[a]	Gini coefficient[b]	Top 20% vs. bottom 20%[c]	Gross domestic product per capita ($US)
United States	0.390	8.3	52,100
United Kingdom	0.360	6.1	38,500
Australia	0.337	5.7	45,100
Japan	0.330	6.1	37,500
Canada	0.313	5.2	42,400
Netherlands	0.303	4.6	46,300
Switzerland	0.297	4.6	54,000
France	0.297	4.5	41,000
Germany	0.289	4.4	42,900
Sweden	0.274	4.1	51,600
Denmark	0.256	3.6	53,400

[a] The ten countries chosen for comparison with the United States and their respective gross domestic products come from Papanicolas, Woskie, and Jha, "Health Care Spending."

[b] Gini coefficient for income after taxes and transfers, adjusted for household size. *Source:* "Compare Your Country: Income Distribution and Poverty, Gini Coefficient," Organisation for Economic Co-operation and Development (OECD), accessed February 3, 2020, https://www1.compareyourcountry.org/inequality/en/0/313/datatable, www.oecd.org/social/inequality.htm.

[c] Average income of top 20 percent of income scale as a multiple of average income of bottom 20 percent of income scale. Income after taxes and transfers, adjusted for household size. *Source:* "Compare Your Country: Income Distribution and Poverty, Top 20% vs. Bottom 20%," Organisation for Economic Co-operation and Development (OECD), accessed February 3, 2020, https://www1.compareyourcountry.org/inequality/en/0/315/datatable, www.oecd.org/social/inequality.htm.

per by Emmanuel Saez and Gabriel Zucman, which provides an extraordinarily rich and detailed analysis of wealth concentration using family tax returns as the unit of observation. The wealthiest 0.1 percent of families in the United States (160,000 tax units in 2012) has been increasing its share of wealth since the 1980s and now holds about the same share of wealth—about 22 percent—as the bottom 90 percent (144,600,000 tax units in 2012). Of note, Saez and Zucman found that wealth was 10 times more concentrated than income in 2012. It is also interesting to observe that a similar, but more compressed, pattern of changes in wealth concentration occurred in the 1920s. The relative rise in wealth by the top 0.1 percent in the 1920s dramatically came undone with the financial collapse of the Great Depression, following which there was almost half a century during which the bottom 90 percent gained ground in wealth on a relative basis.

To explain the surge in wealth concentration by the top 0.1 percent in recent decades, Saez and Zucman show that income inequality has a snowballing effect: higher rates of saving at top incomes push up wealth

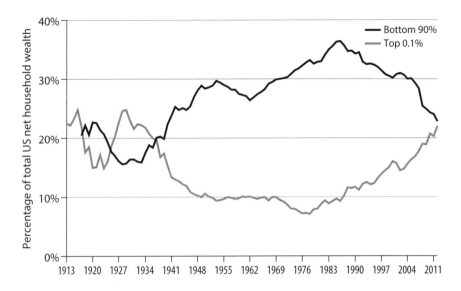

Figure 7.2. Wealth composition, top 0.1 percent and bottom 90 percent. Emmanuel Saez and Gabriel Zucman, "Wealth Inequality in the United States since 1913: Evidence from Capitalized Income Tax Returns," NBER Working Paper No. 20625, National Bureau of Economic Research, Cambridge, MA, October 2014, http://www.nber.org/papers/w20625.

concentration, which in turn leads to a greater concentration of income from capital investments, which then contributes to further increases in their share of income and wealth. By contrast, the lower 90 percent of the population were adversely impacted by a growth in debt in recent decades—mortgages, consumer credit, and student loans—all of which are liabilities that subtract from assets, leading to a fall in savings and wealth.

Inequality in Health and Health Care Access

Income and health are linked. High income essentially serves as a proxy for better education and information access, less toxic environments, healthier behaviors, and a greater capacity to obtain medical care when needed. Thus, it is not surprising that high income is associated with better health, nor that widening differences in health status in the United States are occurring in sync with our widening distribution of income and wealth.

Life Expectancy

Health status in a population can be measured in several ways, but an important aggregate measure is life expectancy, which reflects cumulative health status across the life cycle. The United States ranks last in life expectancy at birth and at age 40, for both males and females (table 7.3) when compared to the 10 high-income countries studied by Papanicolas, Woskie, and Jha.

The general association between income and mortality can be found in European studies going back to the early nineteenth century[6] and continues to this day. A detailed contemporary analysis of this association in the United States is documented by Chetty et al. in a study based on 1.4 billion person-years of tax-return observations between 1999 and 2014.[7] These researchers found that longevity in the United States increases with income throughout the entire range of incomes, and life expectancy for Americans in the upper quartile of income exceeds mean life expectancy in the other high-income countries. Race- and ethnicity-adjusted life expectancy for males and females in the upper quartile of income at age 40 is about 87.5 years and 89.2 years, respectively (figure 7.3), well above the mean life expectancy of high-income countries listed in table 7.3. As would be expected, income and life expectancy are correlated in these other countries as well; evidence from Norway suggests that most of the overall lower life expectancy in the United States is due to lower life expectancy in the lower and middle parts of the income distribution.[8]

As a more telling commentary on the association between income and mortality in the United States, Chetty et al. found that men in the upper quartile of income (mean of $256,000) can expect to live about 10.5 years

Table 7.3. Life expectancy at age 40 and at birth in high-income countries, 2016[a]

Country	At age 40		At birth	
	Female	Male	Female	Male
Japan	87.8	82.0	87.1	81.0
France	86.4	80.6	85.5	79.2
Switzerland	86.3	82.7	85.6	81.7
Australia	85.4	81.8	84.6	80.4
Canada	84.9	81.3	83.9	79.8
Sweden	84.8	81.7	84.1	80.6
Germany	84.2	79.7	83.5	78.6
Netherlands	84.0	81.0	83.2	80.0
United Kingdom	83.9	80.7	83.0	79.4
Denmark	83.5	80.1	82.8	79.0
United States	82.6	78.7	81.1	76.1

Source: "Life Expectancy," OECD.Stat, Organisation for Economic Co-operation and Development, accessed November 13, 2018, https://stats.oecd.org.
  [a] Data are for 2015 for Canada and France.

Figure 7.3. Changes in race- and ethnicity-adjusted life expectancy by income group, 2001–2014. Chetty et al., "Association between Income and Life Expectancy."[7]

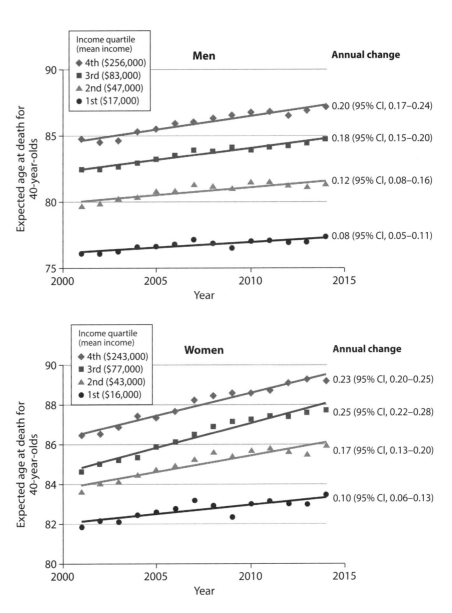

longer than men in the bottom income quartile (mean of $17,000). Similarly, women in the upper quartile of income can expect to live about 6 years longer than women in the bottom income quartile. It is also apparent that, like the widening gaps in income and wealth across time, differences in life expectancy between high- and low-income groups in the United States are also growing. Between 2000 and 2014, the annual rate of increase in life expectancy for men at age 40 in the upper quartile of income was 0.20 years, more than twice the rate of increase for men (0.08) in the bottom quartile. Similarly, life expectancy among upper income women increased at a rate of 0.23 years, more than twice the rate of increase among low-income women (0.10).

Using US counties as the unit of observation, Dwyer-Lindgren et al. analyzed data on inequality in life expectancy from 1980 to 2014.[9] They found enormous variation in life expectancy at birth among US counties in 2014, with a 6.2-year gap between counties in the 10th and 90th percentiles of counties, a 10.7-year gap between the 1st and 99th percentile, and a 20.1-year gap between the lowest and highest life expectancy among all counties. Focusing on inequality in specific age groups, and using the ratio of mortality rates in the 99th to the 1st percentile counties as a measure of relative inequality among counties, a widening of inequality in age-specific mortality was found between 1980 and 2014. This was especially marked for individuals who were between the ages of 5 and 25: the ratio of mortality in the 99th to 1st percentile was already high for this age group, at about 2.8 in 1980, but it climbed to 3.8 in 2014. For individuals 65 to 85 years old, the corresponding mortality ratio showed a smaller but still remarkable increase, growing from about 1.35 to 1.75.

Other Measures of Health Status

While premature mortality is perhaps the ultimate expression of poor health, there are many antecedent measures that impact our day-to-day lives. Those who make healthy dietary choices, engage in regular exercise, don't smoke cigarettes, and follow recommendations on dental hygiene, immunization schedules, and screening tests, will live healthier lives day-to-day by avoiding illness. For individuals who already have a chronic medical condition, their compliance with medication schedules, diagnostic monitoring, and behavioral and other strategies will mitigate the progress of their underlying condition and prevent relapses. Cumulatively, however, if members of the US population make relatively poor dietary choices, don't exercise, smoke cigarettes, engage in other high-risk behaviors, avoid prevention and screening programs, and have poor compliance with recommendations for the management of chronic illness, this will lead to premature mortality and reduced life expectancy. Since the United States has the lowest life expectancy overall among other high-income countries, it isn't surprising that we also show poor outcomes on these antecedent health domains.

These issues were squarely addressed in a report entitled *US Health in International Perspective: Shorter Lives, Poorer Health*, written by a panel of scientists convened by the National Research Council and the Institute of Medicine (now the National Academy of Medicine).[10] The authors of this compendium monograph, which we will call the NRC/NAM study, examined the performance of the United States on nine health domains in comparison with 16 high-income "peer" countries: Australia, Austria, Canada, Denmark, Finland, France, Germany, Italy, Japan, Norway, Portugal, Spain, Sweden, Switzerland, the Netherlands, and the United Kingdom. The summary statement of their findings can be found on pages 2 and 3 of the 400-plus-page report:

1. **Adverse birth outcomes**: For decades, the United States has experienced the highest infant mortality rate of high-income countries and also ranks poorly on other birth outcomes, such as low birth weight. American children are less likely to live to age 5 than children in other high-income countries.

2. **Injuries and homicides**: Deaths from motor vehicle crashes, non-transportation-related injuries, and violence occur at much higher rates in the United States than in other countries and are a leading cause of death in children, adolescents, and young adults. Since the 1950s, U.S. adolescents and young adults have died at higher rates from traffic accidents and homicide than their counterparts in other countries.

3. **Adolescent pregnancy and sexually transmitted infections**: Since the 1990s, among high-income countries, U.S. adolescents have had the highest rate of pregnancies and are more likely to acquire sexually transmitted infections.

4. **HIV and AIDS**: The United States has the second highest prevalence of HIV infection among the 17 peer countries and the highest incidence of AIDS.

5. **Drug-related mortality**: Americans lose more years of life to alcohol and other drugs than people in peer countries, even when deaths from drunk driving are excluded.

6. **Obesity and diabetes**: For decades, the United States has had the highest obesity rate among high-income countries. High prevalence rates for obesity are seen in U.S. children and in every age group thereafter. From age 20 onward, U.S. adults have among the highest prevalence rates of diabetes (and high plasma glucose levels) among peer countries.

7. **Heart disease**: The U.S. death rate from ischemic heart disease is the second highest among the 17 peer countries. Americans reach age 50 with a less favorable cardiovascular risk profile than their peers in Europe, and adults over age 50 are more likely to develop and die from cardiovascular disease than are older adults in other high-income countries.

8. **Chronic lung disease**: Lung disease is more prevalent and associated with higher mortality in the United States than in the United Kingdom and other European countries.
9. **Disability**: Older U.S. adults report a higher prevalence of arthritis and activity limitations than their counterparts in the United Kingdom, other European countries, and Japan.

These findings are based on data gleaned from a variety of sources. For example, health indicators for specific age groups were identified and computed for each of the 17 countries studied (table 7.4). Of the 17 countries, the United States ranked last in the composite ranking for health indicators in *each* of the age groups studied.

The reasons why the United States trails its peers in these health indicators can be analyzed across the life cycle. For the first two age groups (0–4 years and 5–19 years) there is a set of interconnected problems: the teen pregnancy rate in the United States in 2016 was three times higher than the median rate of the other 16 countries studied (21 births per 1,000 women ages 15–19 in the United States vs. 7 births per 1,000 for the other countries) (figure 7.4a). The high teen pregnancy rate leads to greater prematurity and consequently to greater neonatal and infant mortality (figure 7.4b).

Table 7.4. Composite health indicators by age group and rank of the United States among 17 peer countries[a]

Age group (years)	Health indicators	Composite ranking
0–4	Still births; low birth rate; perinatal, neonatal, and infant mortality; days of life lost, males and females	17
5–19	Overweight, boys and girls; dental caries; HIV, boys and girls; adolescent births; adolescent suicides; days of life lost, males and females	17
20–34	BMI, males and females; diabetes, males and females; blood pressure, males and females; cholesterol, males and females; maternal mortality; days of life lost, males and females	17
35–49	BMI, males and females; diabetes, males and females; blood pressure, males and females; cholesterol, males and females; days of life lost, males and females	17

Source: Adapted from National Research Council and Institute of Medicine, *US Health in International Perspective*.[10]
[a] Australia, Austria, Canada, Denmark, Finland, France, Germany, Italy, Japan, the Netherlands, Norway, Portugal, Spain, Sweden, Switzerland, the United Kingdom, and the United States

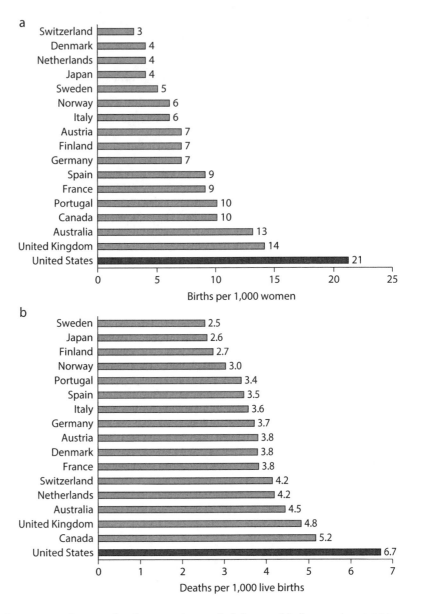

Figure 7.4a. International comparisons of adolescent birth rates (per 1,000 women, ages 15–19, 2016) "Adolescent fertility rate (births per 1,000 women ages 15-19)," United Nations Population Division, World Population Prospects, The World Bank, accessed November 13, 2018, https://data.worldbank.org/indicator/SP.ADO.TFRT.

Figure 7.4b. International comparisons of infant mortality rates, 2005–2009.
National Research Council and Institute of Medicine, *US Health in International Perspective.*[10]

Health indicators for the latter two age groups (20–34 years and 35–49 years) relate to the antecedents of chronic disease and their onset and progress. Obesity, inactivity, and high cholesterol levels among US young adults are associated with the development of diabetes and cardiovascular disease later in life. When Americans turn age 50, they enter their later years in poorer health than their counterparts in peer nations and therefore are more likely to be subject to the ravages of chronic diseases and their attendant morbidity and mortality. For example, the NRC/NAM study found that 18.2 percent of American males between the ages of 50 and 54 had cardiovascular risk in the high or very high level, as compared with 13.6 percent of males in peer countries. The corresponding risk for American females was 10.7 percent, as compared with 4.5 percent in peer nations.

Access to Health Care

Let's return to the statement of William Shatner in his 2010 television exchange with Rush Limbaugh: "Here's my premise and you agree with it or not. If you have money, you are going to get health care. If you don't have money, it's more difficult."[11]

At age 65, Americans have access to Medicare, but for younger adults, Shatner's assessment is largely correct: access to health care for adults under age 65 is variable and dependent on income and insurance coverage. Half of uninsured adults in the United States reported that they had no usual source of care in 2016, as compared with 12 percent who had Medicaid or employer-based or other private insurance.[12] Moreover, 20 percent of uninsured adults reported that they went without care in the past year because of cost, as compared with 8 percent with Medicaid or other public coverage and 3 percent with private coverage.

Similar relationships are seen in international comparisons done by Karen Davis and Jeromie Ballreich.[13] Among Americans across all types of coverage, 28 percent reported in 2013 that they had a medical problem in the past year but did not visit a doctor because of cost, as compared with a mean of 7.7 percent among 10 peer high-income countries. Moreover, 21 percent of Americans did not get a recommended test, treatment or follow-up because of cost, and 22 percent did not fill a prescription or skipped doses because of cost, as compared with means of 6.4 percent and 7.4 percent, respectively, in peer countries. Thirty-nine percent of low-income Americans had a medical problem but did not visit a doctor; 31 percent did not get a recommended test, treatment, or follow-up; and 30 percent did not fill a prescription or skipped doses. This compared with 11, 9, and 11 percent, respectively, for low-income individuals in peer countries.

Medicaid provides access for low-income individuals, mainly focused on children, parents of children, pregnant women, and the disabled. While Medicaid improves access to care overall, specialist care, as already noted, is often difficult to obtain because professional fees paid to specialists by Medicaid are low and they are free to turn away Medicaid patients.

Commercial insurance plans, whether employer-based or individually purchased, have substantially increased cost sharing with patients in recent years.[14] It follows from our earlier discussion of negatively sloped demand curves that when consumers have a greater out-of-pocket cost for health care, they will cut back on utilization. This may be a good thing from the standpoint of reducing expenditures, but not if the reduction in utilization comes at the cost of deferring or curtailing needed medical care. Moreover, people with the worst health are the ones who are most likely to reduce their medical care.[15]

How Can We Explain Our Nation's Poor Health?

In comparison with other high-income countries, the United States ranks last in life expectancy (table 7.2) and last in the nine antecedent health domains studied by the NRC/NAM panel. Since we are unique among these peer countries in not having some form of baseline universal health care, it is understandable that a connection is often made between the lack of universal health care in the United States and our poor health outcomes. While health is no doubt impacted by barriers to health care access in certain segments of the US population, the etiology of our nation's poor health is more complex and rooted in fundamental economic and social considerations.

Explanations across the Life Cycle

Adverse health outcomes in the first five domains studied by the NRC/NAM panel—birth outcomes, injuries and homicides, adolescent pregnancy and sexually transmitted infections, HIV and AIDS, and drug-related mortality—disproportionately affect younger Americans. About two-thirds of the difference in life expectancy at birth for males between the United States and peer countries, and about one-third of the difference for females, is attributable to mortality before age 50.[16] However, most of the adverse health outcomes in these domains, which cumulatively have led to our nation's low probability of surviving to age 50 as compared with peer countries, are not related to health care access.

Consider, for example, the connection between contraception, teen pregnancy, premature birth, and infant mortality. Although one might guess that the higher rate of teen pregnancies in the United States as compared with peer nations is a problem of access to contraception, contraceptive use has improved in recent years and has led to a decline in rates of adolescent pregnancy in the United States.[17] A more fundamental explanation for why the adolescent pregnancy rate remains dramatically higher than in peer nations may be rooted in the greater inequality of our income distribution than other nations, which may lead to a perceived and actual lack of economic opportunity among those at the bottom of the economic ladder.[18]

Once pregnant, adolescents have full access to prenatal and obstetrical care since they qualify for Medicaid. But even with prenatal care, teen pregnancy is associated with a higher risk of preterm birth. In the United States, the proportion of live births that are preterm among adolescents is in the range of 15 to 20 percent, as compared to a baseline of 10 to 12 percent for births to mothers in their 20s and 30s.[19] In the United Kingdom, despite its universal coverage under the National Health Service, a similar increase in the prematurity rate is observed among teenage mothers.[20] The greater rate of preterm birth in the United States leads inexorably to higher rates of neonatal and infant mortality. And unfortunately for preterm birth survivors, there is often greater morbidity throughout life: medical illness as well as adverse academic and social outcomes.[21]

The other health domains studied by the NRC/NAM panel for young adults—injuries and homicides, HIV and AIDS, and drug-related mortality—all pertain to high-risk behaviors that are also more related to social and economic factors than to health care access.

For older adults, the prevalence of obesity and inactivity, and the onset and progression of chronic disease and disability in a population, reflect the balance of preventive measures, early detection and intervention, and vigilant management by both patient and doctor. Where this balance is struck depends on the cumulative behaviors of individuals vs. impact of health care services in the form of counseling and medical treatment. Regarding the role of individual behaviors, just as with younger adults, these are influenced by their social and economic context. For example, US counties with poverty rates of greater than 35 percent have obesity rates that are 145 percent greater than wealthier counties.[22]

Also telling is a 10-year follow-up of more than 12,000 individuals between the ages of 45 and 64 living in a broad cross-section of urban and rural areas in North Carolina, Mississippi, Minnesota, and Maryland, who participated in the Atherosclorosis Risk in Communities Study. Individuals with low socioeconomic status (measured by income and education) were 50 percent more likely to develop heart disease after controlling cardiovascular risk factors such as smoking, high blood pressure, inactivity, and high cholesterol.[23] And in Canada, with universal access to health care, after accounting for risk factors such as high blood pressure, smoking, inactivity, and male gender, individuals with household incomes less than $30,000 had a 70 percent higher prevalence of heart disease.[24]

The Role of Behavioral Factors

In view of these considerations, it is not surprising that both of the major studies of life expectancy discussed earlier found that the main explanation for variations in life expectancy across geographic areas relate more to health behaviors such as smoking, obesity, and exercise, and less to access health care access. The study by Chetty et al. used commuting zones as their unit of observation, which are 741 geographic aggregations of counties based on commuting patterns that completely partition the country.[25] Using cross-sectional analyses of individuals in the bottom and top income quartiles, they found that life expectancy for both groups was negatively correlated with rates of smoking and obesity and positively correlated with exercise and education. For individuals in the bottom quartile, there was no significant correlation between life expectancy and measures of health care access except for a negative correlation with local area hospital mortality. The authors conclude that "any theory for differences in life expectancy across areas must explain differences in health behaviors."[26] These relationships (table 7.5) are correlational and therefore represent associations that are not necessarily causal. Furthermore, multivariate analyses were not performed to try to estimate the independent effect of behavioral and access variables on life expectancy.

Using counties as their unit of observation in cross-sectional analyses, Dwyer-Lindgren et al. performed multivariate studies of the impact on life expectancy of socioeconomic and racial factors, as well as behavioral/met-

Table 7.5. Correlations between life expectancy in the bottom and top income quartiles and local area characteristics

Local area characteristics	Correlation (95% confidence interval) with life expectancy			
	Bottom quartile		Top quartile	
Health behaviors				
Currently smokes	−0.69	(−0.86 to −0.52)	−0.33	(−0.51 to −0.15)
Obesity	−0.47	(−0.67 to −0.26)	−0.29	(−0.46 to −0.12)
Exercise rate	0.32	(0.11 to 0.52)	0.49	(0.35 to 0.58)
Access to health care				
Percent uninsured	0.10	(−0.19 to 0.38)	−0.44	(−0.55 to −0.33)
Medicare dollars per enrollee	−0.09	(−0.28 to 0.10)	−0.50	(−0.62 to −0.37)
30-day hospital mortality index	−0.31	(−0.46 to −0.15)	−0.19	(−0.39 to 0.00)
Index for preventive care	0.05	(−0.19 to 0.29)	0.55	(0.44 to 0.67)

Source: Adapted from Chetty et al., "Association between Income and Life Expectancy."[7]

abolic and health care access variables. When the estimated effect of any given variable took into account an adjustment for the other factors, behavioral and metabolic risk factors emerged as the strongest predictor of life expectancy by far.[27] These included obesity, inactivity, smoking, hypertension, and diabetes. Access to health care was significantly associated with life expectancy, but with a relatively low effect size. The explanatory power of the model that included all categories of variables, including access, was no better than the model that just included the behavioral and metabolic factors. The coefficient of determination (or R^2), a measure of the variance in life expectancy accounted for by explanatory factors, was 0.74 in both models. Like the study by Chetty et al., these findings suggest that the major explanation for geographic variation in life expectancy is variation in the behavioral antecedents of mortality.

The broad conclusion is that behavioral factors seem to make a greater contributor to life expectancy than health care access. This does not change, however, the real-world challenges faced on an individual basis by the 10 percent of Americans who are currently uninsured. It doesn't change, for example, the catch-22 of a person with epilepsy who does not have full-time employment with health coverage due to the epilepsy, which leads to difficulty in accessing medication and, consequently, repeated major seizures for which the emergency room is the only available place to turn. Nor does it change the experience of the young couple, self-employed in a start-up web design business, who choose not to purchase health insurance and must file bankruptcy due to medical bills for the treatment of unexpected cancer. Nor does it change the challenges faced by the individual with hepatitis C whose insurance plan does not cover the new curative medications or the individual with renal failure who receives years of dialysis (covered) instead of the kidney transplant (not covered) that would greatly enhance quality of life. The increasingly common problem of a juvenile-onset, insulin-dependent diabetic who reduces the prescribed dosage of insulin because of rapidly increasing insulin costs—and suffering severe health consequences—is also not a reflection of behavioral factors. To improve the nation's health, the underlying behavioral determinants of health as well as inequalities in health care access must both be addressed.

Summary

The distributions of income and wealth in the United States have become increasingly unequal since the 1980s, such that the top 1 percent earns 23 percent of total income and holds 40 percent of total wealth. This degree of income and wealth inequality is greater than that of peer high-income nations. At the same time, the United States ranks last in health status for the population overall, including life expectancy and antecedent measures of health status. Those in high-income groups in the United States, however, have life expectancies that exceed the mean of all peer nations studied.

Despite the redistribution of resources in the United States to help those in medical need through an array of insurance products, government programs, and philanthropy, a substantially higher percentage of the US population has poor access to health care as compared to peer nations. Behavioral factors, which begin in childhood and adolescence and accumulate through the life cycle, appear to be much more important in explaining poor health outcomes for the US population as a whole than variations in health care access. Moreover, specific instances of how barriers in access adversely impact the lives of uninsured and underinsured cannot be captured by aggregate cross-sectional data and remain inadequately addressed by the current US health care industry.

PART II

HISTORICAL EVOLUTION

8 ORIGINS AND STRUCTURAL UNDERPINNINGS OF THE US HEALTH CARE INDUSTRY

A comparison of health care expenditures in the United States and peer high-income nations can be summarized by a marked divergence in spending growth through 1990 and much less divergence since then (figure 8.1). In the United States in 1970, per capita health care expenditures were $1,453, compared with a mean of $1,164 in peer nations, a ratio of 1.25. Thus, a 25 percent differential in per capita expenditures was already present by 1970. Between 1970 and 1990, however, the ratio of US to peer-nation expenditures grew to 1.76. Since 1990, this ratio has plateaued somewhat, although it continues to gradually increase.

This pattern can be traced to the evolution of structural differences between our health care industry and the health systems of other nations, which are characterized by universal coverage with either a single government payer or highly regulated private insurance with individual mandates and subsidies. Higher spending on health care in the United States and lower rates of coverage are rooted in the historical evolution of health insurance and government-funded health care programs. This chapter begins a history of the US health care industry by describing the origins of health insurance and the emergence of key stakeholders in the United States through 1940. It was during this initial period that the structural features of our health system were shaped.

Conceptual Underpinnings of Health Insurance

It is both natural and intuitive that insurance for health care would develop in a free-market economy. Following Kenneth Arrow's original analysis, let's begin with the assumption that most people are risk averse.[1] What does this mean? As one example, if we were faced with a distribution of incomes having

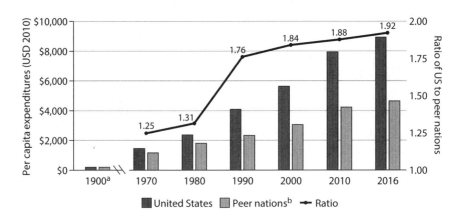

Figure 8.1. Per capita expenditures on health care, United States vs. mean of ten other high-income nations, 1900 to 2016. "Health Spending," OECD Data, Organisation for Economic Co-operation and Development, accessed September 1, 2018, https://data.oecd.org/healthres/health-spending.htm. [a] In 1900 there was little expenditure on health care in the US vs. in peer nations. Data shown for illustrative purposes. [b] Other high-income nations, based on Papanicolas, Woskie, and Jha (see chap. 7, note 2), are Australia, Canada, Denmark, France, Germany, Japan, the Netherlands, Sweden, Switzerland, and the United Kingdom.

a mean of Y dollars from which our actual income would be randomly selected, versus a *certain* income of Y dollars, the assumption of risk aversion would imply that we would choose the certain income.

A similar idea obtains with health insurance since the distribution of medical costs in the course of a year is generally unknown. That is, total medical costs may be relatively small if only minor illnesses occur, but there is always the potential that there will be a very serious illness or accident that would be costly in medical expenses, and also in the loss of work-related income. Suppose the mean of this distribution of medical costs is X dollars. If an insurance company offered a health care policy with an actuarially fair annual premium of X dollars that indemnified individuals against all medical costs, the rational, risk-averse consumer (i.e., gamblers excluded) would gladly pay the premium to avoid the potential for an unpredictable but huge medical bill.

We will see that insurance coverage for medical expenses in the United States did not evolve based on this economic theory. Rather, as in other economic and social arenas, the insurance industry we now have in place reflects a century of history based on deep national ideology combined with the actions of pertinent stakeholders—doctors, hospitals, insurance companies, employers, unions, pharmaceutical companies and device manufacturers, politicians, regulators, and others—advocating for and acting in their own interests.

In the abstraction of a perfect-competition environment, health care prices would be set in a frictionless marketplace by the interaction of 325 million American consumers with 1 million actively licensed physicians, 3 million nurses, 300,000 pharmacists, many other health professionals, 5,500 hospitals with 900,000 staffed beds, and other health care entities. Consumers would have perfect information about their prevention and wellness needs, their illnesses, their need for diagnosis and treatment, and the prices of those services. Physicians and hospitals would enter and exit the market freely based on market forces. Employers, unions, politicians, regulators, and patient advocacy groups would not be involved. And manufacturers of drugs and devices would be part of the supply chain of doctors and hospitals, in their own perfect-competition environment of many buyers and sellers with perfect information on quality and price as well as free entry and exit. Actuarially fair health insurance policies would be available in the market for those consumers who wished to purchase them.

The above scenario is, of course, fanciful. But it makes the point that we are far from a perfect-competition market in health care, and it serves as an idealized counterpoint to the health care industry we now experience, which has evolved as the composite result of diverse interest groups exerting their influence over time. Each interest group has been represented by an industry organization that has lobbied on its behalf (e.g., American Medical Association, American Hospital Association, America's Health Insurance Plans, Pharmaceutical Research and Manufacturers of America, etc.). As stakeholder groups advocated for the interests of their members, there emerged winners and losers. These advocacy efforts were conducted within the crucible of a political process, out of which arose political outcomes, not Pareto-efficient solutions forged in the free market.

Given this history, we now have a relatively stable confederation of structural elements that has served most of the stakeholders well enough to create tremendous support for the status quo and resistance to fundamental change.

- *Doctors* have achieved elevated status in society with comfortable and secure incomes. While currently active physicians trained in previous generations may lament a loss in autonomy, they are practicing in a scientific and technologic age in which they can do more to treat their patients effectively than ever before. Applications for admission to medical school continue to rise and those in training are generally quite appreciative of their opportunities.

- *Hospitals* and health systems have developed powerful financial models in which they have become economic engines for the towns and cities in which they are located, often serving as the area's largest employer. Nonprofit community hospitals have become even stronger local pillars by investing some of their financial margins in capital improvements and providing philanthropy and community service; similar traits characterize university-based or affiliated hospitals, which also support research and education; and investor-owned hospitals provide strong returns to shareholders while serving their communities' health care needs and tax base.

- *Health insurance companies* have also become important economic forces, locally and nationally. They earn substantial profits and have built large reserves; cover two-thirds of Americans under the age of 65; provide health insurance directly but also serve as third-party administrators for self-insurance programs of both public entities and private corporations; and have developed a vast digital infrastructure to support a highly diverse set of provider reimbursement scenarios that cannot be readily replaced.

- *Employers, labor unions, and employees* all benefit from the fact that the value of the health insurance premiums paid for by employers on behalf of employees are not taxable to the employees. This provides union members and other employees access to health insurance plans that, without the tax benefit, would be either more restrictive or constrain wages.

- *Drug companies and device manufacturers* sell their products in an environment that has strong patent protection and limited or no price negotiation by the largest buyers (e.g., Medicare).

- *Consumers* who are covered by health insurance or government programs generally have access to high-quality and affordable health care.

- *Businesses, politicians,* and others who are fearful of universal health care, for ideological and/or financial reasons, are reassured that such a system is unlikely to materialize. This is because our patchwork "system" of private health insurance, bolstered by government programs that provide coverage for children, the elderly and the disabled, along with statutes that ensure emergency room care and a safety net of federal and state funding for the uninsured, has been sufficiently broad-based to fend off any initiatives for universal health care.

So what's not to like? No doubt, these stakeholders will always express concerns and advocate for their interests. Doctors would like more autonomy, more time with patients, less time with electronic medical records, and higher fees. Hospital administrators would like better and broader-based reimbursement along with less regulatory oversight and reporting requirements. Insurers would like to pay out fewer medical claims and have more flexibility in designing benefits. Employers would like lower insurance premiums and greater access to excellent care for their employees. Employees would prefer benefit designs that provide the greatest choice of providers at the lowest out-of-pocket expense. Drug companies and device manufacturers would like broader and longer patents, speedier and less costly paths to FDA approvals, and more protection against price negotiations. Beneficiaries of public programs would like more efficient access, broader coverage, wider choice of providers, and minimal out-of-pocket expense.

Despite these concerns, the interests of all of these stakeholders are sufficiently well addressed in the present health care industry that there is limited broad-based passion to redirect resources toward the minority of people whose needs are poorly taken into account and who have a limited economic and political voice: the uninsured and the underinsured. In addition to inequities in access, the evolution of the US health care industry has produced high prices. But the price of health care does not appear to be a *core* problem for most stakeholders relative to the benefits that they receive from the current system. It has not yet been sufficiently problematic to trigger strong and successful advocacy for fundamental change. Everyone would like lower prices, but we will see that the high price for health care services in the United States is rooted in structural elements that began to take hold a century ago and are now hardwired.[2]

Late Nineteenth Century and Early Twentieth Century

Prior to the twentieth century, people had little reason to insure themselves against medical costs. For one thing, few treatments were effective and many were suspect. For another, the cost of whatever medical care may have been utilized was not a major concern for most households. According to an historical report by the Bureau of Labor Statistics, average annual family income in the United States in 1901 was $750, of which $40 dollars (about 5 percent) was spent on health care.[3]

In those years, hospitals served mainly as sick houses for the poor and for patients with contagious diseases. Doctors saw patients in their homes and did their best to evaluate and treat them with medical history, physical exams, and the supplies in their "little black bags." They were paid with cash or on a barter basis. Competing with a variety of other "healers," the profession of medicine had only modest stature. The folk saying that dates back to the fifteenth century, inscribed on the statue of Dr. Edward Livingston Trudeau at Saranac Lake, New York, applies aptly to that era: *"To cure sometimes, to relieve often and to comfort always."*

As the twentieth century began, two major developments favorably affected the trajectory of medical practice: advances in biomedical science, especially in bacteriology and anesthesiology, and the development of a more uniform approach to science-based medical education, culminating in the paradigm-shifting study of medical education reported by Abraham Flexner,[4] who began this work in 1904 under the aegis of the Carnegie Foundation.

Emergence of Biomedical Science

The revolutionary "germ theory" studies of Louis Pasteur in France and Robert Koch in Germany led to the identification of various infectious agents during this period, including the causative organisms of syphilis, typhus, pneumonia, tuberculosis, cholera, anthrax, and malaria. Diphtheria antitoxin and rabies vaccines were developed in the late 1800s. The first chemotherapeutic drug, Salvarsan, was introduced in the 1910s as an effective treatment of syphilis.

The use of ether for surgery in the mid-nineteenth century was the first major American breakthrough in medicine. This agent, plus chloroform (introduced a year later in Scotland), transformed the potential capabilities of surgeons. However, the longer exposure of open wounds to a nonsterile environment increased the likelihood of post-operative infection and life-ending sepsis. Bed linens, lab coats, and other surgical garb were not washed. Surgeons did not routinely wash their hands before operating. Surgical instruments, which would often be used serially on several patients, were typically only cleaned (but not sterilized) when they were put away for storage. The importance of handwashing, championed by the Hungarian physician Ignaz Semmelweis in the mid-nineteenth century, reduced infection rates, but it wasn't until 1896 that surgical gloves were first introduced by the chief of surgery at the Johns Hopkins Hospital, and later still before a fully sterile environment became the norm in operating rooms. By reviewing a large number of historical photographs, Adams et al. determined that although gowns were consistently worn by surgeons by 1901, caps were not consistently worn until 1930, and masks and gloves not used on a regular basis until 1937.[5]

Surgical activity surged during this time, supported by developments such as the introduction of x-rays in 1895, discovery of blood types in 1901 (which gave rise to blood transfusions in 1914), the introduction of the electrocardiograph in 1903, and the use of novocaine as a local anesthetic in 1905. Tonsillectomies became routine (perhaps to a fault), and there were many firsts in surgery on different organ systems, including neurologic, orthopedic, gynecologic, pituitary, and abdominal surgery. Hospitals were beginning to be viewed as a place where effective treatments could be provided.

Patients were responsible for paying hospital and physician fees, but most families during this time period were more concerned about the loss of income due to illness or injury than the medical expense of illness treatment. Consequently, many households, benevolent societies, and unions were more focused on protecting income through mechanisms like today's disability insurance rather than on protection against medical expense. For example, the 179 US fraternal societies paid out $97 million in benefits in 1917, but only 1 percent were for medical expenses.[6]

Medical Education Reform

In parallel with the scientific progress of the early twentieth century, the 1910 report by Flexner was a critical turning point in the history of the medical profession in the United States. At that time, there were 155 medical schools in North America, many of which were small, for-profit trade schools that were owned by one or more physicians. Admission requirements, curricula, and requirements for graduation varied greatly, instruction was often provided by part-time local doctors who themselves had variable education and training, and there was minimal regulation by state licensure. A degree was often awarded after two years of medical school, often without any prior university preparation. According to Starr,

Sharp contrasts characterized medicine by 1900. The changes in progress at Harvard, Johns Hopkins, and other universities were counterpointed by the continuing growth of commercial medical colleges. . . . [T]he ports of entry into medicine were still wide open, and the unwelcome passed through in great numbers. At proprietary schools and some of the weaker medical departments of universities, the ranks of the profession were being recruited from workingmen and lower-middle classes, to the dismay of professional leaders, who thought such riff-raff jeopardized efforts to raise the doctor's status in society. From the viewpoint of established physicians, the commercial schools were undesirable on at least two counts: for the added competition they were creating and for the low image of the physician that their graduates fostered.[7]

Flexner advocated an educational model then embodied by the university-based medical schools in Europe, which demanded more scientific preparation before entry to medical school and a longer period of study that combined scientific and clinical instruction by full-time faculty. Some of Flexner's key recommendations (box 8.1) reference the Johns Hopkins School of Medicine as the best American example of this approach. And the report had a dramatic impact on medical training (box 8.2).

Setting a high bar for the minimal requirements to practice medicine has obvious benefits from the standpoint of the quality of care that we now take for granted. Any given patient undergoing surgery today in a US hospital, for example, is reassured that his or her anesthesiologist and surgeon have the requisite scientific knowledge and clinical training to be state-licensed, hospital-credentialed, and specialty national-board certified to perform this procedure safely. However, such licensing, credentialing, and certification requirements conflict with the "free entry of suppliers" assumption of perfect competition discussed in chapter 2. Thus, in the first half of the twentieth century, restriction of entry into the medical profession, along with its growing stature as a learned profession rooted in science, led to monopolistic elements, higher fees, and the collective ability of physicians to exert political influence regarding the emergence of health insurance.

First Efforts at a National Paradigm for Health Insurance

The American Association of Labor Legislation (AALL) initiated the first campaign for health insurance in the United States at the 1905 annual meeting of the American Economic Association.[8] By 1915, the AALL's coun-

Box 8.1. Key recommendations of Flexner report

A significant reduction in the number of medical schools and medical students

Requiring more scientific preparation (preferably at least two years of university education) as a prerequisite for medical school

Establishing a four-year medical curriculum divided equally between basic science and clinical training

Incorporating medical schools into universities so that basic science research and education could create a positive feedback loop

Strengthening state licensing requirements and oversight

Source: Flexner, *Medical Education in the United States and* Canada.[4]

Box 8.2. Impacts of the Flexner report on medical training

- More than half of all American medical schools merged or were closed in the 25 years following the report.
- Of the 66 surviving medical degree–granting institutions in 1935, 57 were part of a university.
- Essentially all state medical boards adopted Flexner's recommendations across time, which motivated much of the merger activity and closures and increased the uniformity of curricula.
- The acceleration of medical discoveries and the resulting translation to effective patient care, along with the dramatic changes in medical education and licensure requirements, led to the perception that physicians were part of a learned profession rather than a trade.

Source: Mark D. Hiatt and Christopher G. Stockton, "The Impact of the Flexner Report on the Fate of Medical Schools in North America after 1909," *Journal of American Physicians and Surgeons* 8, no. 2 (2003): 37–40.

---

cil, including recognized national leaders such as Louis Brandeis and Woodrow Wilson, drafted a model state bill for health insurance, versions of which were introduced by 16 states through 1920. Included in most of the state bills were several common provisions (box 8.3).

Although these bills were initially supported at the national level by the American Medical Association (AMA), there was fierce opposition by state medical societies. For example, Anderson quotes a New York physician: "Nowhere has the swinish greed of the debasing propaganda of state socialism been more brazenly exposed than in this merciless attempt to steal the livelihood of the most unselfish profession in the world."[9]

Physician opposition was joined by the American Federation of Labor (AFL), the private insurance industry and business groups opposing the AALL proposal. The AFL was concerned that an insurance system involving government contributions would weaken unions by usurping their role in providing medical benefits. Insurance companies, which depended on insurance policies for working-class families that paid death benefits and covered funeral expenses, opposed the state bills as upending the backbone of their businesses. And some business groups argued that if any public action were taken, employee productivity and health would benefit more from public health measures than from sickness benefits.

Thus, an alliance of organized representatives of physicians, employees, insurance companies, and businesses, along with the beginning of World War I in 1917, ended the first attempt at health insurance in the United States. But the process of working through these state bills, and of solidifying advocacy/lobbying positions by the key stakeholders, foreshadowed what was to come.

1920s and 1930s

Progress in Biomedical Science and Clinical Tranlation

Throughout the 1920s, new drugs and vaccines were developed following lines of research that began in the previous decade. Progress slowed somewhat during the 1930s because of the Great Depression, but significant advances were nonetheless made:

- French researchers perfected a tuberculosis vaccine, bacille Calmette-Guerin, that saved the lives of 98 percent of the infants treated in tuberculosis households.
- The purification of insulin from pancreatic extracts led to the first effective treatment of diabetes, a watershed time that subsequently led to transformation in the prognosis for diabetic patients from "dismal" to "almost normal."
- The clinical meanings of the various deflections that make up normal and abnormal electrical patterns of the heart were better understood using more refined electrocardiography machines.
- Brain waves that were captured in early prototypes of an electroencephalogram were first used to detect brain tumors or injuries.
- George N. Papanicolaou invented the "Pap smear," which used exfoliated cells of the cervix to detect cellular abnormalities that might be forerunners of cancer.
- In 1937, the first link between cigarette smoking and lung cancer was reported, and the first blood bank was established at Cook County Hospital in Chicago.
- Sulfa drugs became the first of the antibacterial wonder drugs, saving thousands of lives from bacterial infections.
- The antibacterial action of the fungus Penicillium notatum was discovered in 1928 and its ability to kill infectious bacteria was demonstrated in 1939; this led to commercial production of penicillin in the early 1940s and its synthesis and mass production in the early 1950s. Penicillin proved to be the drug discovery that saved lives like no other to that point, especially during World War II.

Proposals Regarding Health Insurance

As the benefits of improved diagnosis and treatment became increasingly apparent, there was greater utilization of physician and hospital services in the 1920s. Accordingly, there was an increase in the cost of medical services as a fraction of household income. Also by this time, mandated health insurance had begun to take place in a number of European countries: in 1883, Germany required that workers be covered by the sickness funds maintained by labor unions and various trades. Many other nations followed suit with similar national systems: Austria (1888), Hungary (1891), Serbia (1910), Britain (1911), Russia (1912), and the Netherlands (1913).[10] Because of increasing cost and the existence of European models, the question of coverage for medical illness in the United States arose again. Resurrecting the debates surrounding the AALL proposals, health insurance—whether public, private, or both—became more actively discussed.

In 1927, the Committee on the Costs of Medical Care (CCMC) was established with private funding from six major foundations: the Carnegie Corporation, the Josiah Macy Jr. Foundation, the Milbank Memorial Fund, the Russell Sage Foundation, the Twentieth Century Fund, and the Julius Rosenwald Fund.[11] Chaired by Ray Wilbur, president of Stanford University and former president of the AMA, the committee comprised 42 members (including 17 private practice physicians) and 75 staff. The CCMC published 27 field studies between 1928 and 1932, and a final report in 1932.

The vast amount of data compiled in these reports cannot be easily summarized, but some of the most salient findings, extracted from a longer list summarized in an Institute of Medicine study,[12] were:

- Per capita medical expenses averaged about 4 percent of national income in 1930 (about $25 to $30 per person), but one third of total spending was due to illnesses of 3.5 percent of the population.
- Medical care spending was divided mainly between physicians (30 percent), hospitals (24 percent), medications (18 percent), and dentists (12 percent).
- Unions, lodges, and commercial insurance companies focused on disability insurance and not on medical expenses.
- About 150 multispecialty medical groups were developing strategies for coordinating patient care among different providers and health care settings in a cost-effective manner, which many mem-

bers of the committee viewed as innovative and an important future direction.

The final CCMC report contained both majority and minority reports representing points of view that echo to this day in health care policy discussions (box 8.4). The majority recommended against compulsory insurance as too costly for taxpayers and employers (with some dissent on this

---

Box 8.4. Summary of the majority and minority reports of the Committee on the Costs of Medical Care, 1932

MAJORITY REPORT

- Costs of medical care should be placed on a voluntary group payment basis through the use of insurance, taxation, or both.
- Medical service provided on an individual fee-for-service basis should be available for those who prefer this present method.
- Medical service, both preventive and therapeutic, should be furnished largely by organized groups of physicians, dentists, nurses, pharmacists, and other associated personnel.
- Groups should be organized, preferably around a hospital, to provide complete office and hospital care.
- Organizations should encourage high standards and a personal relationship between patient and physician and should not compete with each other.

MINORITY REPORT

- State or county medical societies should establish and control voluntary nonprofit medical care plans, which should be separate from disability insurance payments and which should not compete with each other.
- Plan enrollees should have free choice of physicians and should pay directly for the care they can afford.
- Plans should maintain the confidentiality of the patient-doctor relationship.
- Participation in plans should be open to all medical society members willing to meet plan conditions, and plans should include all or most medical society members.
- Public care for the indigent should be strengthened and should be assisted (but not paid for) by the medical plan.

Source: Institute of Medicine Committee, *Employment and Health Benefits*, chapter 2, "Origins and Evolution of Employment-Based Health Benefits," table 2-3.[2]

point from progressive committee members), allowed for fee-for-service care for people who preferred this method of payment, and celebrated high standards of care and the doctor-patient relationship. While these recommendations were acceptable to most members of the CCMC, other majority recommendations incited a fervent, hostile response from eight private practitioners plus a representative of the Catholic hospitals, who wrote the minority report. They were particularly concerned about the proposal that medical services should be placed on a voluntary group payment basis through the use of insurance, taxation, or both; that medical care should be provided largely by organized groups of health care teams; and the notion that these medical groups should provide integrated ambulatory and hospital care. The minority report referred to group practice as "the technique of big business . . . mass production," recommended that "government competition in the practice of medicine be discontinued," and suggested that "government care of the indigent be expanded with the ultimate object of relieving the medical profession of this burden."[13]

The majority report also sparked the ire of the AMA. For example, Anderson quotes the editor of the *Journal of the American Medical Association* (JAMA) as stating in a 1932 editorial: "The alignment is clear—on the one side the forces representing the great foundations, public health officialdom, social theory, even socialism and communism, inciting to revolution; on the other side, the organized medical profession of this country urging an orderly evolution guided by controlled experimentation."[14]

And Chapin quotes another JAMA editorial from December 10, 1932: "Let the big businessmen who would reorganize medical practice and the efficiency engineers who would make doctors the cogs of their governmental machines, give a little of their horse power brains to a realization of the fact that Americans prefer to be human beings."[15]

The AMA, representing the interests of its physician members who were largely practicing independent, fee-for-service medicine, saw the proposed initiatives for group practice and the introduction of private insurance and taxation as the forerunners to corporate domination of medical practice followed by government control. Interestingly, both the majority and minority reports of the CCMC agreed that voluntary medical insurance plans should not be administered by private insurance carriers. Many members of the CCMC committee were concerned that administration by health insurance companies would increase administrative cost and forfeit physician involvement in setting medical policy. To this point, as reported by Anderson, one of the CCMC studies of European health insurance concluded that "a comparative study of many insurance systems seems to justify the conclusion that the evils of insurance decrease in proportion to the degree that responsibilities with accompanying powers and duties are entrusted to the medical profession."[16]

Hospital Insurance

Among the different experiments in medical care and health insurance reviewed by the many CCMC reports was one on insurance for hospital care. This idea was not viewed by the committee as addressing the key goals of integrated medical practice and preventive care, and it was not believed to be capable of covering most high-cost illnesses. During this time period, however, quite apart from CCMC recommendations, a structure for hospital health insurance began to take shape in response to economic uncertainty associated with the Depression. Average hospital receipts per person in the nation's voluntary hospitals declined from $236 to $59 one year after the 1929 crash.[17] Two prominent economists at the time, Michael Davis and C. Rufus Rorem, warned that hospitals could not survive if they continued to depend on patients having the resources to pay for all of their bills, and they advocated for prepayment plans to cover populations through insurance.[18]

Attempts at hospital insurance began with individual, single-hospital plans, in which a hospital agreed to provide care to specific groups for a prepaid amount per person. The earliest example was Baylor University Hospital in Dallas, which started such a plan in late 1929. Dr. Justin Ford Kimball, who was a Baylor hospital administrator, noticed that there was a disproportionate number of schoolteachers who had unpaid bills. He addressed this problem by organizing a plan in which teachers could be covered for a three-week hospital stay in a semi-private room by prepaying as little as 50 cents a month. The first group health plan was launched when 1,250 Dallas-area teachers enrolled at once. In creating this plan, Dr. Kimball was credited with launching the prototype model that served as the basis for Blue Cross. Similar single-hospital plans sprang up in Iowa and Illinois.

As an alternative to the single-hospital plans, community-wide plans emerged that served a broader population. The first of these plans was in Sacramento, California, where, in July 1932, employed persons in that community were offered hospital service contracts by a consortium of community hospitals. In February 1933, the American Hospital Association (AHA) approved this form of community-based hospital insurance as a "practicable solution" to the problem of creating an affordable service for hospital expenses, which by their nature are unpredictable in occurrence and highly variable in cost.[19] It was recommended that these plans cover only hospital charges, so as not to compete with physicians. Importantly, the AHA advocated for these community plans *instead of,* not in addition to, the single-hospital plans. The community plans would offer consumers "free choice" of hospitals, but at the same time it should be noted that this thwarted potential competition among hospitals and imprinted the community plans with elements of monopolistic pricing.

In 1934, the Blue Cross name and symbol were developed by E. A. van Steenwyk, executive secretary of Blue Cross of Minnesota, who pioneered the St. Paul, Minnesota, community-based plan. This symbol soon was affixed to hospital insurance plans in other parts of the country. By 1935, there were 36 Blue Cross plans in the United States, with a total enrollment of 1.4 million.[20]

While the Blue Cross plans were beginning to take hold, private insurance companies were reluctant to jump into the hospital insurance business. Insurance companies to that point issued policies grounded in the concept of limited liability, which was counter to the idea of a "service contract" in which expenses for virtually all medical problems, big and small, were covered. Service contracts were viewed as blank checks for patients and hospitals that did not limit the plans' liabilities, and would encourage utilization because of moral hazard (i.e., a negatively sloping demand curve, as discussed in Chapter 4). As the success of Blue Cross plans became evident, however, in 1934 some commercial carriers, "half-dragged and half-lured," began offering coverage to groups for hospital expenses on an indemnity basis.[21] These indemnity plans typically paid a set amount for hospital expenses, with the patient responsible for the balance.

Between the final CCMC report in 1932 and passage of the Social Security Act (SSA) in 1935, signed by President Franklin D. Roosevelt, there were three years to enact some version of the CCMC recommendations or incorporate them into the SSA. Neither occurred. The SSA focused on pension and unemployment benefits paid from workers' payroll taxes, with some provisions for maternal and child health services and for the disabled. Given the overwhelming economic hardships and other crises facing government in association with the Great Depression, combined with vehement opposition by organized medicine to financing medical services by private insurance or taxation, the SSA was passed with no provisions for health insurance, although a follow-on Committee to Coordinate Health and Welfare Activities was created by the Roosevelt administration to explore future potential reforms. Also factoring into the decision not to include health insurance in the SSA was an estimate that it would double the amount of required payroll taxes.[22]

Although the CCMC recommendations were not implemented, another piece of legislation passed in 1935, the National Labor Relations Act, was to have profound effects on the evolution of health insurance because it required company management to negotiate employment benefits with unions, including health insurance benefits.

In the late 1930s, the structure of health insurance for hospitals and doctors continued to take shape. On the hospital side, the single-hospital plans grew less rapidly than the community-wide plans, partly because the single-hospital plans appeared to be less attractive to consumers and partly because they were actively discouraged by the AHA. Commercial plans were still in their infancy and quite small in comparison with the Blue Cross plans. In 1937, the AHA received a grant from the Julius Rosenwald Fund to set up a committee to foster community-based insurance efforts. As summarized by Starr, a set of principles were delineated, including

- specification of territories for the various Blue Cross plans so that they wouldn't compete with one another,
- oversight by state insurance departments, and
- commitment to offer service benefits rather than indemnity benefits, thus distinguishing themselves from the commercial insurance plans.[23]

Physician Insurance

Blue Shield plans got their start in the late 1930s. These were physician insurance policies that ran in parallel to Blue Cross. The Blue Shield system grew out of "medical society plans" that were started by physicians. In general, the AMA preferred that any insurance plans for physicians be indemnity-based; that is, the doctor would receive his or her stated fee from the patient, who would then be reimbursed a set amount. But national AMA leaders tolerated some degree of prepaid programs by their medical societies because "they needed to display the strength of voluntary insurance to thwart government reform proposals."[24]

Blue Cross, for their part, was interested in a partnership with the doctors but wanted to have some influence over the medical society health plans to limit their liability if they were to offer bundled hospital-doctor plans. Such bundling would help Blue Cross in two ways: responding effectively to the burgeoning demand for health insurance by employers and other groups and allowing them to compete with the commercial insurance companies by offering comprehensive coverage across hospital and physician services. Chapin describes the roles of the AMA and Blue Cross in the developmental story of Blue Shield as resembling "that of a child pulled between two parents in a custody battle."[25]

American Medical Association Approval of Health Insurance

Ultimately, although the AMA, Blue Cross, and Blue Shield viewed each other warily every step of the way, they accommodated the basic interests of their three constituencies by separating insurance for hospital and physician services. In this process, these organizations hoped that by providing a private mechanism for health insurance, the perceived need for compulsory health insurance would be reduced. The AMA, in particular, needed to express some measure of support for the general concept of health insurance. This was to address an emerging plan from the federal Committee to Coordinate Health and Welfare Activities, which contained a plank for state-financed compulsory medical insurance. Because of concern that such a plank was gaining support, the AMA met with the committee in July 1938 and forged a compromise in which they agreed with all of the committee's recommendations so long as they dropped their advocacy for compulsory health insurance. AMA leaders realized that they could not be successful in fighting a two-front battle against the growing popularity of health insurance in the market and government-financed health insurance; thus, they decided to express support for private health insurance. At an emergency meeting of the AMA's House of Delegates in 1938, they "approved" private health insurance in the hopes that growth of the private plans would render government programs redundant.[26]

To preserve their core underlying principles, the AMA attached important stipulations to their approval of health insurance. In particular, they insisted that the third-party insurance plans should contract with individual doctors on a fee-for-service indemnity basis. Like the AHA's opposition to single-hospital plans, the AMA opposed prepaid group practice plans. In both cases, competition would be created for their individual hospital and physician members. In the case of physicians, the prepaid group practice plans would be competing against the individual, fee-for-service physician. The AMA also feared that proliferation of doctor groups would lead not only to the prepaid plans but then to the corporatization of medicine and, ultimately, to government insurance.

Impact of Physician Fee and Hospital Rate Models on Price

The fee-for-service system advocated by the AMA at that time involved physicians setting a fee, patients paying the full amount, and a set indemnity payment being sent to the patient by the insurer, which might or might not cover the fee. This system of patient reimbursement was layered onto a common practice by physicians to charge patients on a sliding scale based on ability to pay. (Of note, while a sliding scale of fees may appropriately be viewed as an expression of altruism by physicians, economists would point out that it also represents the behavior of a price-discriminating monopolist, in which the physician is not faced with a single market-clearing price, but rather can charge the highest price possible for each patient.) Together, indemnity payments plus a sliding fee scale led to higher prices due to the effects of subsidized pricing as discussed in chapter 4. To explain this phenomenon, suppose the price for an office visit by a patient with a sore throat during this era was $5 before health insurance, based on the sliding scale of fees. If the same patient presented with an indemnity policy that would pay her $4 for this visit, the physician might increase the visit price to $7, knowing that the patient would have a net payment of $3 ($7 – $4), which is still a lower cost to the patient than before she had insurance. Creating a new sliding scale of fees that incorporates this upcharge at each point on the scale increased the overall cost of health care for that population of patients, simply by the introduction of indemnity insurance.

The structural increase in fee schedules created by indemnity payments formed a baseline of higher fees when, in later years, physicians were paid directly by insurance companies rather than patients. These fee schedules were typically based on what was deemed the physician's "usual, customary, and reasonable fees."

The origins of a similar phenomenon for hospitals also occurred in the late 1930s. Although health insurance was not included in the SSA, some specific programs for special groups were funded. The federal Emergency

Maternity and Infant Care Program developed the first nationwide payment system based on the "actual per diem cost of operating the hospital."[27] Hospitals would then add a fixed percentage to create a financial margin that would pay for needed capital costs. For hospitals, this became known in later years as "cost plus" reimbursement. Each item needed for a patient's care (IV bags, surgical supply sets, medications, etc.) were charged separately, documented, and reimbursed. Under such a scenario, hospital administrators had little incentive to be maximally efficient in hospital operations, knowing that all documented costs that could be defended as legitimate would be reimbursed, and a supplement would be added for capital needs.

Beginning in this era, insurance companies memorialized the higher prices of physicians and hospitals through the premium setting process. The costs of all physician and hospital services in the previous year were calculated, an increment was added based on revised fee schedules negotiated with physicians and hospitals, and an additional amount was added for administrative expenses and a financial margin for capital needs or for cash reserves needed to meet insurance regulatory requirements. This total amount was divided by the number of subscribers and a per capita "community-based" insurance premium was calculated.

Although the last few paragraphs represent a bit of extrapolation to later years, by 1940 the basic structure of health care financing had taken shape, rooted in a health insurance industry that accommodated the interests of the key stakeholders—physicians, hospitals, insurance companies, employers, and unions/employees. Moreover, the evolving health insurance industry had already embedded schedules of physician and hospital prices that, in a circular self-reinforcing way, were higher *because* of the presence of insurance.

Summary

Structural differences between the United States and peer nations in health care began to take shape in the early part of the twentieth century but became more firmly rooted by 1940. This was an important historical period in which the framework for US health care industry was created.

The unpredictability of illness and injury, combined with a risk-averse preference of most consumers, would lead naturally to some form of insurance coverage for health care in a market economy. In the early part of the twentieth century, however, due to the lack of efficacious medical treatments, insurance coverage focused mainly on protection against the loss of income due to illness or injury, and much less on the expense of treatment. The emergence of effective treatment for some infectious diseases, along with fundamental changes in medical education and licensure requirements brought about by the Flexner report, led to physicians being perceived as part of a learned profession rather than a trade, and to a restriction in entry to the medical profession. Greater stature and limited supply allowed organized medicine to exert greater influence in the marketplace. An alliance of the American Medical Association and the organized representatives of employees, insurance companies, and business ended the first significant attempt at state-supported health insurance, as advocated by the American Association of Labor Legislation in the period from 1915 to 1920.

In the 1920s and 1930s, progress in biomedical science led to more efficacious medical and surgical treatments, and thus greater utilization of physician and hospital services. Accordingly, the cost of medical care became a consideration for families, and the question of whether there should be some sort of insurance coverage for medical illness, whether public, private, or both, became more actively debated in the United States. This debate occurred against a backdrop of many European countries adopting different forms of government-supported health insurance. The Committee on the Costs of Medical Care (CCMC), funded by six major foundations, published 27 white papers between 1928 and 1932. Its final majority report in 1932 advocated for the costs of medical care to be placed on a voluntary group payment basis through the use of insurance, taxation, or both, and that medical services should be integrated by organized groups of health care teams who would provide both ambulatory and hospital care.

None of the CCMC recommendations were enacted because of fierce opposition by organized medicine. During this period, however, single-hospital and community-based hospital insurance plans developed, which formed the basis of the Blue Cross system of hospital plans. Although reluctant initially, commercial insurance carriers also entered the market. On the physician side, Blue Shield got its start in the late 1930s. While opposed to any form of insurance at first, the AMA ultimately approved private health insurance in 1938, both in recognition of the reality of the marketplace and as a foil against compulsory, publicly funded insurance. Increasing levels of health insurance, combined with payments to physicians based on usual and customary fees and to hospitals based on cost-plus reimbursement, led to higher structural prices for health care that became embedded in the industry.

9 THE US HEALTH CARE INDUSTRY TAKES SHAPE
THE 1940s THROUGH 1965

Entering the 1940s, various elements came together to shape the US health care industry. These included

- advances in biomedical research;
- translation of research discoveries to the bedside via new diagnostic methods, medications, and procedures;
- increased demand for medical care due to the efficacy of the new treatments;
- attracting the best and brightest to a career in medicine;
- establishment of fee-for-service as the primary mode of payment for health care services;
- continued development of health insurance to distribute and smooth the overall cost of care among individuals in large population groups; and
- expansion of hospital facilities.

As these elements became more solidified, so did the higher pricing structure of physicians (usual, customary, and reasonable fees) and hospitals (cost-based pricing), utilizing the health insurance backbone. From 1940 through the inception of Medicare and Medicaid in 1965, the health care industry that had emerged in the 1920s and 1930s attracted a growing and more interwoven group of stakeholders—doctors, hospitals, employers, unions, and pharmaceutical companies.

Medical Progress and Creation of the National Institutes of Health

Growth in confidence about the efficacy of medical treatments occurred in tandem with increasing recognition of the value of science. The 1940s and 1950s were years of progress in a wide variety of medical and surgical arenas (boxes 9.1 and 9.2, respectively), bolstered by the creation of the National Institutes of Health (NIH). Many of the medical and surgical advances during these decades were strongly influenced by World War II. These medical discoveries and clinical applications paved the way for the truly extraordinary progress that has occurred since then, some of which was summarized in chapter 1.

A key development during this period was the public funding of research through the NIH, which was to become the basis for the ascendency of American biomedical science internationally. Through the early 1940s, medical research was primarily funded by private sources, usually foundations, pharmaceutical companies, or universities. The Rockefeller Institute

---

Box 9.1. Selected medical advances in the 1940s

1940	Influenza: isolation of the influenza B virus
1942	Caudal anesthesia, a type of epidural, was first used on women in labor
1943	TB treatment: streptomycin was first isolated in 1943 and used as an effective treatment for tuberculosis by 1946; isoniazid was developed in 1952 for tuberculosis treatment and is still used to this day
1944	Quinine and chloroquine (1947) synthesized to treat malaria, from which large numbers of American troops in the South Pacific were dying
1946	Fluorinated water: a 15-year experiment began that would establish the dental benefits of adding fluoride to drinking water
1949	The first bone marrow transplant was performed in a mouse, paving the way for this life-saving procedure to treat leukemia and other conditions
1949	The polio virus was grown in human tissue cultures in 1949, making it possible to develop the polio vaccine in the 1950s
1949	The first permanent intraocular lens was successfully used to correct cataracts

---

Box 9.2. Selected medical advances in the 1950s

1950	Smoking and lung cancer linkage: five case-control studies were published associating smoking with lung cancer; by 1954, this association was confirmed more definitively with several prospective cohort studies of British physicians, US veterans, and other groups
1952	Prosthetic heart valves: first implantation of an acrylic ball valve prosthesis into the descending aorta of a 30-year-old woman to correct aortic insufficiency
1953	DNA: James Watson and Francis Crick published the double helix structure of DNA
1953	Heart-lung machine: invented and first used for cardiopulmonary bypass to support the first successful human open-heart surgery
1954	Kidney transplant: first successful transplant, using an identical twin donor
Late 1950s	Cardiac pacing: the first battery-operated wearable pacemaker and the first totally implantable pacemaker
1960	Oral contraceptives: first approved by the FDA after development and testing in the 1950s

for Medical Research was the most richly endowed foundation, with a budget that was manyfold larger than total federal expenditures for medical research. The need to solve biomedical problems related to World War II, however, prompted 450 federal contracts with universities and an additional 150 contracts with research institutes and other organizations.[1]

Breakthroughs in bacteriology and the development of antibiotics saved the lives of tens of thousands of soldiers. Moreover, although German models of science and graduate education were extremely influential in the early twentieth century, a key turning point regarding research occurred during World War II. In stark contrast to the Nazis, who centralized and politicized research while purging universities of scientists, a highly successful system of decentralized biomedical research evolved in the United States, in which a variety of independent institutions were funded on a competitive basis. In parallel, signal achievements in other areas of science related to the war, most notably the development of nuclear weapons, created a desire by American political leaders and its citizenry to expand public investment in science using a decentralized approach.

The National Institute of Health, which began as a single, all encompassing institute, was created in 1930. It began with two buildings and a small budget but began to grow as a significant force in the 1940s. Important events during this period included the private donation of land in Bethesda, Maryland; the legislative basis for NIH's postwar programs through the 1944 Public Health Service Act; renaming of NIH to become the National Institutes of Health (i.e., plural) by incorporating the National Heart Institute and the National Cancer Institute; creation of the National Institute of Dental Research and the National Institute of Mental Health; and a significant increase in the NIH budget. Its federal funding grew from $707,000 in 1940 to $52.7 million in 1950, $399.4 million in 1960, and $959.2 million in 1965.[2]

The organization of NIH as a consortium of institutes directed at specific categories of disease, rather than a single institute for medical research, stemmed from the dramatic fund-raising success of foundations focused on specific diseases, like the March of Dimes. In 1952, more children died of polio than of any other infectious disease. With its assertion that research was winning the battle against polio, the March of Dimes consistently raised more money than any other health campaign. The triumph of the Salk vaccine, proven in double-blind randomized trials in which neither the doctors nor their patients (or the patients' parents) knew whether the injections were vaccine or placebo, heralded an extraordinary breakthrough in clinical medicine and public health. Moreover, it generated great appreciation in the public for both basic and clinical research, and the scientific method in general. A biographer of Jonas Salk put it this way: "Not less than 100 million Americans had a proprietary interest in the vaccine, having financed it with contributions to the March of Dimes. . . . Accordingly, the announcement that the Salk vaccine had been effective against paralytic poliomyelitis made April 12, 1955, a day of uniquely proud jubilation for the American people. It also was a great day in the history of medical science and a great day for the world."[3] Americans surmised that if polio could be prevented, then cancer, heart disease, and other illnesses could be conquered as well. Investing in research made sense.

Hospital Expansion

As progress in medical and surgical treatments unfolded, and as hospital insurance made these treatments more affordable, demand for hospital services grew dramatically. In November 1945, only two months after the official end of World War II, President Harry S. Truman conveyed to Congress five priorities to improve the nation's health. The first and least controversial of these called for constructing hospitals.

In 1946, Congress passed the Hospital Survey and Construction Act (known as the Hill-Burton Act after its Senate sponsors), which gave hospitals, nursing homes, and other health facilities grants and loans for construction and modernization. In return, they agreed to provide a "reasonable volume" of services to persons unable to pay for 20 years after receiving funding. Facilities receiving funding also could not discriminate on the basis of race or national origin. Of note, "separate but equal" facilities were allowed until this provision of the act was overturned by a federal court in 1963. And in contrast to the present political environment in the United States, it is also interesting to note that one month after enactment of the Hill-Burton Act, President Truman (a Democrat) appointed Senator Harold Burton (a Republican) to the Supreme Court. Senator Burton, a namesake of the Hill-Burton Act, was unanimously approved by the entire Senate the same day he was appointed without committee hearings. He joined the Supreme Court the very next day.

States and localities were required to match the federal grant or loan, so that the federal portion would only account for one third of the total cost. The Hill-Burton Act led to a boom in hospital construction. Although industry experts suggested a ceiling of 4.5 hospital beds per 1,000 population, far above the ratio in any state, this ceiling soon became a target. A need was expressed by the hospital industry and local communities to fill any gap between existing ratios and the 4.5 maximum. Between 1947 and 1971, 30 percent of all hospital projects received a contribution from Hill-Burton, at a federal cost of $3.7 billion, which drew matching state and local funds of $9.1 billion.[4] In 1975, Hill-Burton was rolled into bigger legislation known as the Public Health Service Act. By the turn of the 21st century, about 6,800 facilities in 4,000 communities had in some part been financed by the law. These included not only hospitals and clinics, but also rehabilitation centers and nursing homes.

The formula for allocating funds among states favored low-income states, which led to more hospitals being built in the 40 percent of counties without a hospital when the program was conceived in 1945. Within states, however, the matching requirement and a provision that localities provide evidence of financial viability meant that the funds were disproportionately allocated to middle-class communities. For example, de Vise notes that over 25 years of Hill-Burton funding, none was provided to an inner-city hospital in Chicago, while over 20 hospitals in the Chicago suburbs were built or expanded with Hill-Burton support.[5]

Health Insurance Becomes Solidified as the Backbone of the US Health Care Industry

Blue Cross and Blue Shield were the first insurers to enter the health insurance market. Because they were nonprofit entities, they were required to charge the same premium to all members of a community, whether they were healthy or sick (i.e., community rating). They avoided the problem of adverse selection by focusing on large employee groups who would generally be younger and healthier, and who were not individually seeking health insurance. Medical risk was actuarially assessed throughout the employee group and a common premium for all employees was charged to cover the aggregate expectation for medical claims across all employees, which were paid on a fee-for-service basis. This strategy proved to be successful; by the mid-1940s, Blue Cross and Blue Shield were insuring 19 million members nationally.[6]

Commercial Insurance

The success of the Blues attracted the attention of commercial insurers, who then entered the market. Commercial insurers were initially reluctant to do so, mainly because of a concern about adverse selection. Initially, they tiptoed into health-related policies by focusing on lost income due to illness, giving rise to disability insurance for working Americans in the middle class. Beginning as a "frill on the accident form,"[7] but gathering steam beginning in the mid-1940s, commercial carriers began to pursue this line of business. The concern of commercial carriers about adverse selection was ultimately mitigated by two considerations: (1) the success of the Blues in avoiding adverse selection by focusing on employer groups, and (2) since they were for-profit entities, they did not have to abide by community rating.

Commercial insurers differentiated themselves from the Blues by offering coverage for hospitalization insurance (as opposed to "health" insurance), by paying a set amount for each type of hospitalization, and initially covering only surgical fees (as opposed to all physician fees). Adverse selection was addressed by charging higher insurance premiums to some

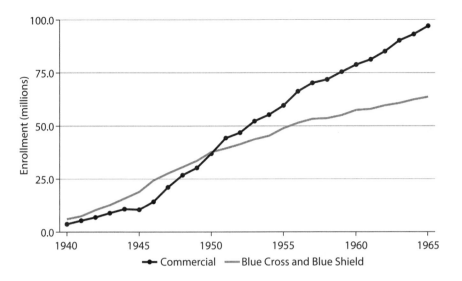

Figure 9.1. Growth of Blue Cross, Blue Shield, and Commercial Insurance, 1940–1966. Reed, "Private Health Insurance Coverage,"[6] and Health Insurance Institute, *Source Book of Health Insurance Data.*[8]

groups than others, based on age and medical history. This is known as "experience" rating, rather than the "community rating" system then employed by Blue Cross and Blue Shield.

Overall, health insurance grew rapidly between 1940 and 1965. In 1940, 9.1 percent of the population had some form of private health insurance, whether individually or as part of a group plan through their employer. The percent insured increased to 50.6 percent by 1950 and to 72.5 percent by 1965.[8] The growth of commercial health insurance grew along with Blue Cross and Blue Shield. By 1950 the total number of people covered by commercial plans reached the number covered by Blue Cross and Blue Shield (about 37 million for each), and by 1955 commercial plan enrollment eclipsed the Blues (59.6 million vs. 48.9 million) (figure 9.1). Through 1965, there was enrollee growth in both the Blues and commercial plans, but the commercial plans became relatively more successful; by 1965, there were 97 million enrollees nationally in commercial plans, as compared with 63.7 million in Blues plans.

Convergence of Commercial and Blues Plans through Acceptance of Both Community and Experience Rating

The Blue plans had their roots in local, community-wide membership. They started with little competition and were therefore able to provide voluntary insurance across a large population at a uniform premium rate. Ultimately, however, they had to adapt to the market, which was driven by commercial plans that used experience rating. The experience-rated indemnity plans gave employers (and individuals) lower-priced premiums for healthy, low-risk workers and were more flexible in their range of benefits and costs.

It's not hard to project where this would have led if the Blue plans did not adapt. Beginning in the 1950s and 1960s, and currently playing out to its logical conclusion, there has been a convergence. For a while, the commercial carriers picked off the low-risk employee groups, leading to a much greater proportion of high-risk groups for the Blue plans, causing substantial losses. Understandably, the Blue plans began to introduce experience-rated products.

Michael Morrisey quotes William McNary, former CEO of Blue Cross of Michigan, as saying, "We fought tooth and nail. To the last gasp. But then you get to the point where the unions are pulling out because they know damn well their experience is better. We would have lost the telephone company. We would have lost the gas company. We would have lost—we did lose—the state employees, 30,000 of them, because we were not experience rating."[9]

Role of Unions in Furthering Convergence of Hospital and Physician Plans

It is estimated that nearly 70 percent of union strikes in the early 1950s were due to health and welfare issues.[10] By the second half of the 1950s, Chapin concludes that "unions were crafting a new gold standard in health insurance: they convinced employers to purchase last-dollar, commercial major medical policies [for doctors] to layer atop first-dollar, nonprofit service plans [for hospitals]."[11] This was the best of both worlds for employees in that they would be covered for any hospitalization flat out without worrying about fee-for-service hospital charges and would be covered for the physician fees (typically also including diagnostic tests and radiology studies) in the "major medical" part of the plan. The tax benefit to employers obscured the full cost of coverage (leading to the increased demand due to price subsidies discussed in chapter 4) and reduced the impulse to ask the unions to consider the possibility of less coverage for lower premium prices. Only 12 percent of Blue Cross subscribers benefitted from employer contributions in 1950, but this grew rapidly; by 1954, employers paid the full cost of health insurance for 62 percent of union members.[12]

Prepaid Group Practice Plans as Forerunners of Health Maintenance Organizations

Below the radar of the huge national expansion in the health insurance plans of the Blues and commercial carriers were a few prepaid group plans that gained size and prominence in selected geographic areas. The impetus for these plans was different in each case. Presented here to round out a description of the mid-century environment, these prepaid plans served as important models for health maintenance organizations, accountable care organizations, and other alternative payment mechanisms that continue to evolve today.

Kaiser Permanente (KP) arose from health care that was provided to construction, shipyard, and steel mill workers for the Kaiser industrial companies, which began in the late 1930s at the height of the Great Depression. Sidney Garfield, MD, a physician treating sick and injured workers who were building the Colorado River Aqueduct Project, borrowed money to build a small hospital, but insurance companies did not pay his bills in a timely manner. As well, he treated all the injured workers regardless of whether they had any health insurance. According to the KP website, "Harold Hatch, an engineer-turned-insurance-agent . . . suggested that the insurance companies pay Dr. Garfield a fixed amount per day, per covered worker, up front. . . . Thus, 'prepayment' was born."[13] This prepayment system was a forerunner to what would be described as "capitation" in today's parlance, which is usually expressed as a fixed payment "per member per month" (PMPM) that is paid to a health plan or health system by an employer or government program.

After this project wound down, Dr. Garfield was asked by Henry J. Kaiser, whose company was building the Grand Coulee Dam, to provide health care to 6,500 workers using a similar financing mechanism. He renovated an existing hospital and recruited a team of physicians to work in a prepaid group practice to serve these workers. With America's entry into World War II, the Kaiser Shipyards in Richmond, California; Portland, Oregon; and Vancouver, Washington, became extremely busy building Liberty ships, aircraft carriers, and related equipment. Mr. Kaiser asked Dr. Garfield to extend his prepaid health care system to 30,000 workers. Although the number of workers covered by this plan was significantly reduced after the war, what Kaiser called the "Permanente Health Plan" was opened to the public in 1945. Currently, KP cares for 12.2 million members in eight states and the District of Columbia.[14]

The Group Health Cooperative of Puget Sound (later named "Group Health") was initially organized in Seattle at the end of World War II by a variety of unions and local supply and food cooperatives. Due to a decline in the local economy at that time, the cooperative was able to buy a prepaid group practice from its physician owners and also a 60-bed hospital. The ability to deliver a full range of care, including hospitalization, protected the cooperative against retaliatory medical society practices that were common at that time. One of the original physicians recalled the critical importance of cooperative ownership of their clinic and hospital: "In the face of firm opposition by the King County Medical Society, which kept our physicians out of the Society, out of the hospitals, and out of post-graduate training courses, our staff would most certainly have had no hospital in which to admit members of the Cooperative."[15] Group Health eventually enrolled upward of 600,000 members in Washington and Idaho. In 2015, it was acquired by Kaiser Permanente.

In 1937, the Group Health Association of New York (which evolved into Group Health Incorporated, or GHI) was established as a small prepaid group practice to provide medical care for New York's working families. This new health care model—built around a network of participating providers—was a precursor to today's preferred provider organizations.

In 1943, New York City Mayor Fiorello LaGuardia learned from the Municipal Credit Union that indebtedness caused by illness was the major source of financial stress experienced by city employees. From a fractious process in which physicians favored a fee-for-service indemnity plan while progressives favored compulsory health insurance, Mayor LaGuardia decided to proceed with an approach based on prepaid group practice. In 1946, 22 medical group practices that included 400 physicians were organized under the Health Insurance Plan (HIP) to provide health care to city workers. New York State law allowed HIP to provide only medical services and not cover hospitalization, so subscribers had to take out a separate policy with Blue Cross for hospital care. Employees who chose the HIP–Blue Cross health insurance benefit paid half of the premium, with the other half paid by the city. By the mid-1950s, HIP was caring for almost a half million city workers.

In order to expand its presence in the upstate New York market, GHI established the GHI Health Maintenance Organization as an incorporated entity in New York State in May 1999. In 2006, GHI and HIP merged to form EmblemHealth, which is now one of the largest nonprofit health plans in the United States with 3.1 million members.

Initially, there were retaliatory efforts against prepaid plans by fee-for-service physicians and organized medicine. In 1959, however, the American Medical Association (AMA) decided to abandon their endorsement of reprisals. There were several considerations: the risk of antitrust prosecution; prepaid plans at that time were limited to a few geographic areas and were small in comparison with commercial insurance and the Blues; and the AMA's finding that there was no evidence of lay interference with medical decision-making.[16]

Private Health Insurance Becomes Solidified as an Alternative to National Health Insurance

The confluence of several factors—more efficacious medical and surgical treatments; an employer tax benefit for health benefits; the growing role of unions that bargained (with statutory support) for generous coverage of hospital and physician care; and a supportive political environment—led to the creation of a health care industry that worked for most stakeholders. Omitted, however, was coverage for retired workers and unemployed individuals who could not afford health insurance. The needs of these groups would be addressed in 1965 by Medicare and Medicaid (chapter 10). Meanwhile, the evolving health care industry worked for enough stakeholders that it protected against three major efforts that were made during the 1940s to enact a comprehensive national program:

1. Incorporating health insurance as part of Social Security (Wagner-Murray-Dingell bill of 1943).
2. A request of Congress by President Truman in 1945 to pass a national program of health insurance.
3. A proposal in 1947 by the financier Bernard Baruch for a national system of voluntary health insurance for high-income Americans and compulsory insurance under Social Security for low-income individuals.

Due to the evolving success of the private health insurance industry and aggressive, well-funded lobbying and marketing efforts against these proposals by the AMA, which characterized them as steps toward "socialized medicine," none of these bills was enacted. During this period, however, establishment of a private health-insurance backbone for fee-for-service payments was solidified.

Growth in Expenditures on Health Care

Between 1940 and 1965, national expenditures on personal health care increased sevenfold (figure 9.2); there were five main reasons for this rapid growth:

1. *Success of health insurance:* The popularity of health insurance grew as a means of protecting against the rising overall cost of medical care, but especially against the prospect of prohibitive expense from one serious episode of illness or injury. The availability of health insurance with full prices paid to providers but subsidized out-of-pocket costs for patients led to greater utilization *and* higher prices.
2. *Union negotiations for health benefits:* In 1948, the National Labor Relations Board ruled in favor of United Steelworkers in a case that established the legal obligation of employers in unionized firms to negotiate over health and welfare benefits.[17] Between 1948 and 1954, the number of workers covered by negotiated health plans increased from 2.7 million to 12 million workers and their families.[18] This set the stage for an era of unions negotiating for health benefits. In

Figure 9.2. Per capita annual total expenditures on health care in the United States, including direct payments from patients as well as private and governmental third parties. Robert M. Gibson, Daniel R. Waldo, and Katharine R. Levit, "National Health Expenditures, 1982," *Health Care Finance Review* 5, no. 1 (1983): 1–31, PMID:10310273.

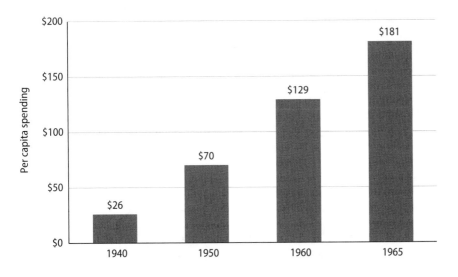

March 2017, the Bureau of Labor Statistics reported that 94 percent of union workers had access to employer-provided health insurance.[19]

3. *Tax policy:* The early success of health insurance, bolstered by union negotiation for health benefits, was significantly enhanced by tax rulings regarding employer-sponsored health insurance. Because of the upward pressure on prices and wages caused by the increased demand for production by war-related industries, and by fewer men available for work due to military service, President Roosevelt imposed wage and price controls through the National War Labor Board. The Labor Board determined, however, that employer-provided health insurance and pensions were not to be considered wages and were therefore excluded from the freeze. This decision enabled employers to offer their employees more expansive insurance plans while still deducting the increased expenses, thereby giving them a tactic to better compete for scarce labor. In 1943, the Internal Revenue Service issued a ruling that the value of employer-provided health insurance was not taxable to employees. While contradictory rulings arose in subsequent years, the Treasury Department under President Dwight D. Eisenhower's administration convinced Congress to enact the Internal Revenue Act of 1954, which exempted the value of employer-sponsored health insurance premiums from federal income taxation.

4. *Medical progress:* Just as the demand curve shifts outward when a given technology becomes more successful, as in our example of in vitro fertilization in chapter 2, the introduction of new, efficacious medications and surgical treatments during this period increased the demand for health care.

5. *Hospital expansion:* The growth in hospital construction, subsidized by the federal government, increased the supply of beds, which raises the issue of Roemer's law and induced demand (chapter 6). Whether the increased supply was in response to demand or its cause, the net result was increased hospital utilization and expenditures.

Summary

The period of 1940–1965 was characterized by further entrenchment of a health care industry built around a health insurance backbone and interwoven with key stakeholders. Growth in private health insurance occurred in tandem with increasing recognition of the value of science and an acceleration of progress in a wide variety of clinical arenas. To support the scientific basis for medical practice and further advances, the National Institutes of Health was formed; across time, its funding was boosted substantially.

Along with the growth in private health insurance was the development of some early prototypes of prepaid group plans. The overall health insurance infrastructure was further solidified by the emergence and growth of employer-based coverage, stimulated by the introduction of tax-exempt insurance premiums and union negotiation for health benefits. Growth in employer-based health insurance codified a higher price structure for physicians and hospitals. Public funds to subsidize the construction or expansion of hospital facilities dramatically increased the availability of hospital services, potentially contributing to increased utilization. The influence of the various stakeholders—doctors, hospitals, insurance companies, employers, and unions—strengthened as the overall size and scope of health care services expanded. Thus, during this period the foundational elements of the US health care industry were put into place: private health insurance that pays full fee-for-service prices to providers; low out-of-pocket costs for those who are covered through their employers, who pay premiums that are not taxable to employees; and a patchwork of public health care funding for the poor.

10 MEDICARE

During the half-century leading up to enactment of Medicare and Medicaid in 1965, a constellation of increasingly entrenched stakeholders gave shape to a burgeoning US health industry. These stakeholders—health insurers, doctors, hospitals, employers, unions, drug companies, medical device manufacturers, and others—pursued their own interests, mindful that periodic partnerships could advance their cause. During this period, private health insurance evolved to provide a common infrastructure through which the network of stakeholders advanced their goals. Just prior to the enactment of Medicare and Medicaid, 75 percent of adults under age 65 had hospital insurance coverage, as did 56 percent of those age 65 and over.[1] Most people with health insurance accessed it through their employers. Some who worked for firms that did not offer health insurance purchased individual health insurance policies, as did some who were self-employed or retired.

In sum, the system was working reasonably well for a large fraction of the population. Left out, however, were individuals who could not access employer-based health benefits and could not afford to purchase individual coverage. This sizable group included almost half of retirees over age 65, about a quarter of adults under age 65, and their children. Enter Medicare and Medicaid, which largely filled the gap for retirees over age 65 and partly filled the gap for the poor, including children. Medicare and Medicaid were passed in 1965 as amendments to the Social Security Act of 1935. In this chapter we will provide historical context and discuss the evolution of Medicare to the present. Chapter 11 will focus on Medicaid.

Historical Context

It will come as no surprise that the enactment of Medicare and Medicaid was the result of a contentious political process.[2] We have seen in previous chapters that attempts at universal health insurance in previous decades were unsuccessful because of opposition by the American Medical Association (AMA) and other stakeholders. The outcries were usually expressed in terms of "socialized medicine" or "government intrusion into private medical affairs." There was also concern over cost.

In 1957, Rhode Island congressman Aime Forand, who had quit school after seventh grade to take care of his ailing father, created a bill with California congressman Cecil King that focused on hospital coverage for older adults under Social Security. Predictably, the AMA mounted a major campaign against the bill as a threat to the doctor-patient relationship. But by concentrating on the health problems of the aged, Forand and King struck a chord with the public and changed the terms of the debate.

In the late 1950s and early 1960s, there was growing clamor among senior citizens for help with the increasing expense of health care. Commercial health insurance, which used experience rating, charged higher premiums to older individuals because of their increased health risks. The Blue Cross and Blue Shield plans, facing stiff competition from commercial insurance, began to shift from community rating to experience-based premiums as well, which were often unaffordable to seniors. Members of Congress were swarmed by older constituents; while there had always been general interest in previous proposals on universal health care, the idea of coverage specifically for the aged drew a groundswell of grassroots support from seniors.

"Medicare," although originally named as a medical care program for families of soldiers serving in the military, was now the term applied to health care proposals for older adults. One legislative proposal included the idea that workers would pay into a Medicare insurance fund for benefits that they would subsequently receive in retirement. President John F. Kennedy ran his 1960 presidential campaign against Richard Nixon expressing strong support for Medicare and reiterated his support on many occasions once elected. In a 1962 speech, he addressed opposition by the AMA, emphasizing physicians' freedom of choice under Medicare and its provisions about physician billing "arrangements" into which the government did not intrude (box 10.1). Nonetheless, Medicare was short of the needed votes in

Box 10.1. Speech by President John F. Kennedy, Madison Square Garden, May 20, 1962

"The point of the matter is that the AMA is doing very well in its efforts to stop this bill. And the doctors of New Jersey and every other State may be opposed to it, but I know that not a single doctor—if this bill is passed—is going to refuse to treat any patient. No one would become a doctor just as a business enterprise. It's a long, laborious discipline. We need more of them. We want their help—and gradually we're getting it. The problem, however, is more complicated because they do not comprehend what we are trying to do. We do not cover doctors' bills here. We do not affect the freedom of choice. You can go to any doctor you want. The doctor and you work out your arrangements with him. We talk about his hospital bill. And that's an entirely different matter. And I hope that one by one the doctors of the United States will take the extraordinary step of not merely reading the journals and the publications of the AMA, because I do not recognize the bill when I hear those descriptions. . . . The fact of the matter is that what we are now talking about doing, most of the countries of Europe did years ago. The British did it 30 years ago. We are behind every country, pretty nearly, in Europe, in this matter of medical care for our citizens."

Source: David Von Pein, "JFK's Speech Health Care Speech from Madison Square Garden (May 20, 1962)," David Von Pein's JFK Channel, August 27, 2013, YouTube video, https://www.youtube.com/watch?v=VXUJErr_vfo.

the Congress until the Democratic sweep in 1964, when Democrats obtained 295 seats in the House and 68 in the Senate.

Medicare and Medicaid were signed into law by President Lyndon B. Johnson in 1965 as amendments to the Social Security Act—titles XVIII and XIX, respectively. Key provisions were the handiwork of Arkansas representative Wilbur Mills, the fiscally conservative Democratic chairman of the House Ways and Means Committee who had resisted earlier efforts at Medicare by refusing to allow a vote in his committee. Recognizing that Medicare was now inevitable given the new political configuration of Congress, he worked to create a bill that would contain costs as much as possible while addressing the desires of the various interest groups. Mills ultimately fashioned what some observers at the time called a "three-layer cake": one layer (Medicare, Part A) was a plan for a *compulsory* hospital insurance program under Social Security, echoing the Forand/King bills of the 1950s; a second layer (Medicare, Part B), was a revised Republican program of *vol-*

untary insurance to cover physicians' services, partly paid by government and partly by enrollees; and the third layer, Medicaid, expanded assistance to the states for medical care for the poor, with significant latitude given to the states for implementation. (Where pertinent, some aspects of Medicaid will be discussed in this chapter in conjunction with Medicare.)

Included in Title XVIII were statutory elements that embedded the basic elements of the US health industry that had been forged to that point.

Rules of Payment for Hospitals

The Medicare legislation adopted the Blue Cross practice of paying hospitals based on their costs. Moreover, rules for calculating costs were extremely favorable to the hospital industry. Even for hospitals that were nonprofit entities, Medicare paid for depreciation and on an accelerated basis. This included Hill-Burton assets (chapter 8), which already contained federal subsidies. At its inception, Medicare reimbursed hospitals on a "cost-plus" basis. The "plus" amounts were termed "return on capital" (ROC) payments: Specifically, nonprofits received an additional 2 percent of costs, and for-profits received an additional 1.5 percent.[3] For-profit hospitals also received a "return on equity" (ROE) payment of 2 percent of equity.[4] In 1969, the ROC payment was replaced by a "nursing" differential, which was 8.5 percent of nursing salary costs.[5] These differential payments were equivalent to about one half to three quarters of the ROC payments. By 1989, both ROE and nursing differential payments were phased out as prospective hospital reimbursement (explained later) was phased in. Thus, cost-plus reimbursement including depreciation was carried forward for the first 25 years of the Medicare program, essentially creating a reimbursement floor when subsequent payment methodologies were introduced.

Rules of Payment for Physicians

Language in the 1965 Medicare bill established the criteria of "usual, customary, and reasonable" (UCR) as the basis for physicians' charges under Medicare. Inserted by Wilbur Mills at the request of the AMA, it became a boon for physicians. In 1992, because of increasing costs due to physician reimbursement at UCR rates, UCR was replaced by a "resource-based relative valued scale" (RBRVS), using a schema developed over a period of years by researchers at Harvard University. Each type of medical, surgical, and diagnostic procedure or service, codified as a Current Procedural Terminology (CPT) code, is assigned a number of relative value units (RVUs) based on the estimated amount of time, skill, and intensity required. This is multiplied by a conversion factor (adjusted for geographic location) to produce a price for that service. Over time, the RBRVS system was adopted by most private insurers. A major consequence of this system has been to incentivize the use of procedures that yield a larger number of RVUs per time unit than office visits. It has also consequently led to a medical workforce in which procedure-based specialties are more attractive to physicians in training than primary care and other office-based specialties.

Use of Fiscal Intermediaries

In order to obtain the support of doctors, hospitals, and insurance companies, the statutory language of Title XVIII established a buffer between providers of health care and the federal government using the existing insurance infrastructure. Hospitals, nursing homes, and home health agencies were reimbursed under Part A through a third party instead of the Social Security Administration. Most providers chose Blue Cross as their intermediary, which provided reimbursement and auditing services. Similarly, private insurers (usually Blue Shield) were chosen as "carriers" to reimburse physicians and other health professionals. In both Part A and Part B, the federal government paid providers through the intermediaries, thus (at least initially) virtually surrendering control of the program and its costs to the providers and insurance industry—an infrastructure that had already evolved to suit the interests of those very providers and insurers.

Taken together in historical context, Medicare reinforced the basic structure of the US health industry that had taken shape in the first half of the twentieth century, as described in chapters 8 and 9: health insurance at subsidized prices for those who are covered through their employer or Medicare, contrasted with a spotty system of public funding (which would now include Medicaid) for the poor. The balance of care, cost, and access in the United States as compared to other high-income nations, which was already somewhat out of kilter by 1965 (chapter 8), was about to evolve into an era in which international disparities would widen. While medical care in the United States would benefit from extraordinary progress in the prevention, diagnosis, and treatment of disease in the second half of the twentieth century (chapter 1), such health care services would be provided in an economic and political environment destined to produce high costs and persistent, significant gaps in access.

The Impact of Health Insurance, Medicare, and Medicaid on Personal Health Care Expenditures since 1965

The growth in health care expenditures (first discussed in chapter 1, figure 1.4) can now be reexplored in the context of the identified forces at work. When comparing 1960 (five years before Medicare and Medicaid), 1970 (five years after Medicare and Medicaid), and each decade through 2010, with the figures for 2018 also provided, the increase in expenditures is striking (table 10.1).

Various factors contributing to this rise have been considered in some detail:

- People born in the mid-twentieth century generally no longer died at a young age from bacterial and viral diseases. Living longer meant an increase in the prevalence of illnesses such as heart disease, cerebrovascular disease, diabetes, and other chronic conditions that occur later in life.
- Progress in biomedical science and clinical research led to effective medical and surgical treatments for these diseases. Overall utilization

Table 10.1. National personal health consumption expenditures, 1960–2018, by source ($ billions)

	1960	1970	1980	1990	2000	2010	2018
Total	24.7	67.0	235.5	674.1	1,285.8	2,450.5	3475.0
Out-of-pocket	12.9	25.0	58.1	137.9	198.9	300.2	375.6
Private health insurance	5.8	15.5	69.2	233.9	458.0	858.5	1243.0
Medicare		7.7	37.4	110.2	224.8	519.8	750.2
Medicaid							
Federal		2.8	14.5	42.6	116.8	266.5	370.9
State		2.5	11.5	31.1	83.5	130.9	228.5
Other[a]	6.0	13.6	44.7	118.5	203.8	374.6	508.8

Source: "National Health Expenditure Data," Historical, NHE Tables (zip file), Table03 (Excel data sheet), Centers for Medicare and Medicaid Services, accessed January 26, 2020, https://www.cms.gov/Research-Statistics-Data-and-Systems/Statistics-Trends-and-Reports/NationalHealthExpendData/NationalHealthAccountsHistorical.

[a]Includes Veterans Affairs, Department of Defense, Children's Health Insurance Program, worksite health care, Indian Health Services, workman's comp, maternal and child health, school health, Substance Abuse and Mental Health Services Administration, and other federal, state, and local programs.

of medical care grew because of the combination of increased disease prevalence and the availability of effective treatments.

- Layered onto the increased utilization was the evolving US health insurance industry. Buoyed by tax-advantaged, employer-based health plans and by Medicare, the combination of producer price subsidies and patient co-pays translated into full-price payments to hospitals, physician, and drug companies. Price *and* quantity both expanded, consistent with the predictions of economic analysis (chapter 3).

- In addition to the increased demand from price subsidies, there was some level of induced diagnostic, procedural, and pharmaceutical demand—more for some diagnoses than for others—that would also percolate through the insurance system at full-price payments.

- Finally, in addition to private insurance and Medicare, the expenditure data in table 10.1 reflects a commitment through Medicaid to a significant level of public funding for the care of people with low-incomes.

These factors evolved in a self-reinforcing manner and collectively contributed to the dramatic increase in health care expenditures over the years. The expenditure increases since the enactment of Medicare and Medicaid also reflect the dynamics of two eras (chapter 6). Spending growth on health care that occurred up until the 1990s was due to increases in both price and utilization; but since the 1990s, spending has grown mainly because of price increases (which includes administrative overhead, profits, and service intensity).

An interesting and perhaps surprising phenomenon resulting from the uniquely American set of circumstances reflected here is that the *out-of-pocket* (OOP) expenses for individuals, on average, have been held (relatively) in check. Specifically, health care paid out of pocket by individuals in the post-Medicare era had a fivefold *decline as a percent of family income* between 1960 and 2016 and only a twofold increase in real dollar spending. Considering this phenomenon in more detail, per capita spending during this period grew from $133 annually to $9,860, a 74-fold increase (table 10.2). The impact of this dramatic expansion in spending was blunted, however, by distributing the burden of the expense to employers, Medicare, and Medicaid (figure 10.1). As a result, per capita *out-of-pocket* spending declined from 52 percent of total health care spending in 1960 to 11 percent in 2016.

Table 10.2. Out-of-pocket health consumption expenditures per capita, 1960–2016

	1960	1970	1980	1990	2000	2010	2016
Per capita expenditures ($)	133	319	1,022	2,657	4,560	7,950	9,860
Percentage out-of-pocket (%)	52	39	25	20	16	12	11
Out-of-pocket amount (nominal $)	69	118	255	531	730	954	1,085
Out-of-pocket, adjusted for inflation ($)[a]	69	90	192	304	401	508	559

Source: "National Health Expenditure Data," Historical, NHE Tables (zip file), Table03 (Excel data sheet), Centers for Medicare and Medicaid Services, accessed January 26, 2020, https://www.cms.gov/Research -Statistics-Data-and-Systems/Statistics-Trends-and-Reports/NationalHealthExpendData/NationalHealthAc countsHistorical.

[a] Calculated from USInflationCalculator.com, accessed October 4, 2018.

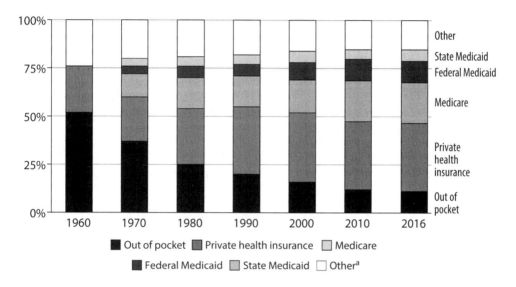

Figure 10.1. Percentage distribution of national personal health consumption expenditures, by source. "National Health Expenditure Data," Historical, NHE Tables (zip file), Table03 (Excel data sheet), Centers for Medicare and Medicaid Services, accessed January 26, 2020, https://www.cms.gov/Research-Statistics-Data-and-Systems/Statistics -Trends-and-Reports/NationalHealthExpendData/NationalHealthAccountsHistorical. [a] Includes Veterans Affairs, Department of Defense, Children's Health Insurance Program, worksite health care, Indian Health Services, workman's comp, maternal and child health, school health, Substance Abuse and Mental Health Services Administration, and other federal, state, and local programs.

The dollar amount of OOP expenditures on health care by individuals can be calculated by multiplying per capita spending by the percent paid out of pocket (table 10.2). Between 1960 and 2016, although *total* per capita spending on health care increased from $133 to $9,860, *out-of-pocket* per capita spending increased from only $69 to $1,085. This was because, as noted earlier, various insurance mechanisms and government programs covered an increasing share of per capita spending. Taking inflation into account as measured by the Consumer Price Index, $69 in 1960 would have the same purchasing power as $559 in 2016. This compares to the *actual* 2016 OOP per capita expenditure of $1,085. Put another way, 2016 OOP expenditures were $134 in 1960 dollars. It is remarkable that the average American's OOP expense for medical care during the post-Medicare era—with all of the enormous and expensive advances in technology and treatments that have occurred—is less than twice the inflation-adjusted equivalent of the $69 that was paid in 1960! That said, these are *average* OOP figures; individuals with high-deductible insurance policies (chapter 12) will have significant OOP expenses if they develop serious illness.

Essential Features of Medicare

Medicare began with coverage for hospitals and medical providers under Parts A and B respectively, in which payments are made on a cost-plus or fee-for-service basis. Across time, two more parts were added (table 10.3). Part C was created with the passage of the Balanced Budget Act of 1997, allowing Medicare enrollees to receive their benefits through capitated insurance plans. While there had been some demonstration projects along these lines dating back to the early 1980s, it was in 1997 that capitated plans were made available to all enrollees. In the Medicare Modernization Act of 2003, most of these plans were rebranded as "Medicare Advantage," which is how we will refer to the Part C plans. Medicare Part D, also made possible with passage of the 2003 Medicare Modernization Act, went into effect on January 1, 2006. It covers outpatient prescription drugs through the various plans that contract with Medicare. The term "traditional Medicare" refers to Parts A, B, and D. Eligibility is shown in figure 10.2. Trends in enrollment for traditional Medicare and Medicare Advantage are shown in figure 10.3.

The different "Parts" of Medicare are administered by private companies, usually insurance firms, under contract with CMS. Some Part C plans are administered (CMS uses the word "sponsored") by health maintenance organizations (HMOs) or similar entities. The Hospital Insurance Trust Fund, which pays Part A expenses, accrues from worker payroll taxes. Part B and D expenses are financed by a separate "Supplementary Insurance Trust Fund," but in contrast to the insurance-style trust fund of Part A,

Table 10.3. Medicare coverage, provisions, deductibles, and financing

	Coverage	Monthly premiums	Deductible/coinsurance	Financing
Part A (1965)	Inpatient hospital Nursing homes (Some) home health visits Hospice care	Usually none[a]	$1,408 + $0–$704 coinsurance per hospital day[a]	2.9% payroll tax, split 50/50 between employer and employee[e]
Part B (1965)	Physician visits Outpatient services Preventive services (Some) home health visits	$144–$491 depending on income[b]	$183 + 20% coinsurance per service[b]	Premiums and general fund revenues
Part C (1997)	Medicare Advantage (MA) plans, including health maintenance organizations and preferred provider organizations; receive all Part A & B benefits and (typically) Part D	$0–$200 depending on plan[c]	Variable, but maximum out-of-pocket spending is $6,700[c]	Uses trust funds from A and B/D
Part D (2003)	Outpatient prescription drugs through private plans, including stand-alone prescription drug plans and MA drug plans		Maximum deductible is $405[d]	Premiums and general fund revenues

[a] *Source:* "Medicare Costs at a Glance," Medicare.gov, accessed January 19, 2020, https://www.medicare.gov/your-medicare-costs/medicare-costs-at-a-glance.

[b] *Source:* "Part B Costs," Medicare,gov, accessed January 19, 2020, https://www.medicare.gov/your-medicare-costs/part-b-costs.

[c] *Source:* "What Are Medicare Part C Costs?," Medicare Matters, National Council on Aging, accessed January 19, 2020, https://www.mymedicarematters.org/costs/part-c.

[d] *Source:* "Yearly Deductible for Drug Plans," Medicare.gov, accessed January 19, 2020, https://www.medicare.gov/drug-coverage-part-d/costs-for-medicare-drug-coverage/yearly-deductible-for-drug-plans.

[e] As of 2013, this payroll tax increased to 3.8% for individuals earning over $250,000 (or over $350,000 for married couples filing jointly).

these expenses are covered on a pay-as-you-go basis—partly by beneficiary premiums but largely by government general revenue. Part C expenses are paid by a combination of the two trust funds, approximately in proportion to their use of Part A, B, and D services.

Hospitals were initially paid for charges pertaining to each individual item of service on a cost-plus basis, as noted above, but this led to

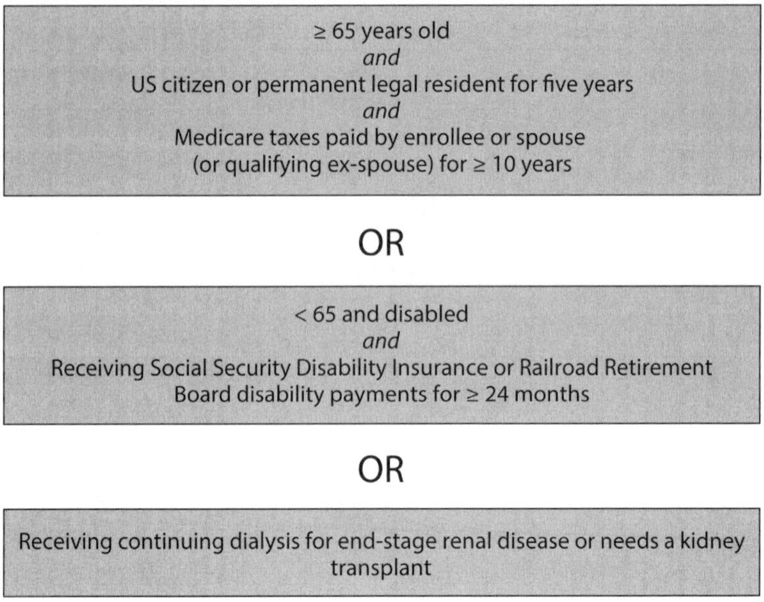

Figure 10.2.
Eligibility for
Medicare

> ≥ 65 years old
> *and*
> US citizen or permanent legal resident for five years
> *and*
> Medicare taxes paid by enrollee or spouse
> (or qualifying ex-spouse) for ≥ 10 years

OR

> < 65 and disabled
> *and*
> Receiving Social Security Disability Insurance or Railroad Retirement
> Board disability payments for ≥ 24 months

OR

> Receiving continuing dialysis for end-stage renal disease or needs a kidney
> transplant

overutilization of many hospital service and supply items. Consequently, an Inpatient Prospective Payment System (IPPS) was developed in which each type of hospital admission is categorized according to a Medicare Severity Diagnosis Related Group (MS-DRG). The DRG classification system, developed at Yale, originally classified hospitalized patients into one of 467 groups based on diagnosis, procedures, sex, comorbidities, and other factors. The basic idea is that patients within each group are clinically similar and are expected to use a similar level of hospital resources.

The first large-scale application of DRGs was in the late 1970s in New Jersey, where the state's Department of Health used DRGs to reimburse a fixed DRG-specific amount for each patient treated in that DRG category, regardless of length of stay and the amount of hospital services or supplies used. In 1983, Congress amended the Social Security Act to include a national DRG-based hospital prospective payment system for all Medicare patients. Physician fees continue to be paid by Medicare according to codes for specific types of office visits, ambulatory procedures, and in-hospital surgery.

This payment methodology is currently evolving toward a system that adjusts payments on the basis of a variety of quality and cost measures. Specifically, the Medicare Access and CHIP Reauthorization Act of 2015

(MACRA), together with accountable care organizations (which had historical roots in prior programs but were codified in the 2010 Affordable Care Act), are both attempting to remodel the payment system for health care services by encouraging coordination/integration between hospitals and physicians, and by modifying the fee-for-service system to include incentives and penalties around reporting, cost, and quality of care. Results have been mixed to date but this is a rapidly evolving area of health care financing and delivery.

Growth of Medicare Expenditures in Relation to Market Imperfections

Medicare evolved as a fee-for-service system for physicians and hospitals with all of the implications of market imperfections in health care discussed in chapters 3–6. In Original Medicare, the prices paid by Medicare for provider and hospital services, as well as drugs, medical equipment and other health care needs, are set by Medicare on the basis of usual and customary fees, cost-based reimbursement, or similar arrangements. The prices paid out of pocket by Medicare beneficiaries, however, are determined by their coinsurance payments, which are much lower—typically 20 percent of the preset price for physician visits and other outpatient services. Thus, the provider price subsidy paid by Medicare is about 80 percent.

The use of preset prices defined by Medicare as provider/manufacturer payments, combined with increased demand due to subsidized prices to patients, results in greater levels of price *and* quantity than would occur in a nonsubsidized market. (In the case of Medicare Advantage, price would be negotiated between the plan and provider.) Indeed, since expenditures equal price multiplied by quantity ($E = P \times Q$), total expenditures are multiplicatively higher than they would be in a nonsubsidized market. Moreover, because of information asymmetry between doctors and patients, there is the potential for induced demand, again exacerbated by subsidized prices, which pushes demand curves outward and contributes to even greater total expenditures. These phenomena, which have been observed in real time since the mid-twentieth century, are consistent with the predictions of the economic analysis of chapter 3. Growth in the population that is 65 years of age or older—due to demographic trends and progress in medical care that

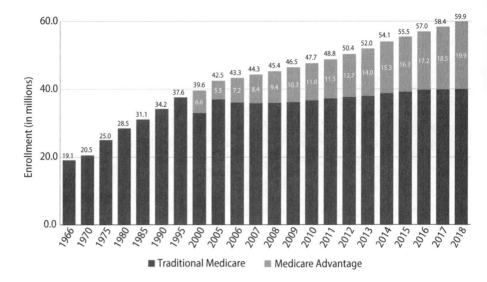

■ Traditional Medicare   ■ Medicare Advantage

Figure 10.3, *opposite.* Medicare and Medicare Advantage enrollment, 1966–2018. Adapted from "Hospital Insurance and/or Supplemental Medical Insurance Program for Total, Fee-for-Service and Managed Care Enrollees," Historical Enrollment Data (zip file), CMS Program Statistics, Centers for Medicare and Medicaid Services, last modified November 25, 2019, accessed March 26, 2019, https://www.cms.gov/Research -Statistics-Data-and-Systems/Statistics-Trends-and-Reports/CMSProgramStatistics /index.html.

prolongs lives—contributes further to substantial growth in total Medicare expenditures.

The nuances of this phenomenon can be understood by considering the expenditures on a specific procedure, service, or drug price and then the aggregate amounts of these expenditures taken together. Consider, for example, hospital expenditures on spine surgery (SS) for low back pain over a given time period, such as a year:

$$E_{SS} = P_{SS} \times Q_{SS}$$

E_{SS} equals annual national hospital expenditures on spine surgery for low back pain, P_{SS} equals the price for spine surgery, and Q_{SS} equals the annual quantity of spines surgeries performed. The price of a DRG-specific spine surgery is set by CMS, but the quantity of spine surgeries performed nationally is determined by several factors:

- Total population size *greater than or equal to* 65 years of age (POP)

- Fraction of the population with back pain $\left(\dfrac{POP_{BP}}{POP} \right)$

- Fraction of the population with back pain undergoing spine surgery

$$\left(\frac{POP_{SS}}{POP_{BP}} \right)$$

- Number of such surgeries per person undergoing spine surgery $\left(\frac{Q_{SS}}{POP_{SS}} \right)$

That is,

$$Q_{SS} = POP\left(\frac{POP_{BP}}{POP} \right)\left(\frac{POP_{SS}}{POP_{BP}} \right)\left(\frac{Q_{SS}}{POP_{SS}} \right)$$

Substituting this equation for Q_{SS} into the original equation for expenditures yields the following equation for national expenditures on spine surgery:

$$E_{SS} = P_{SS} \times POP\left(\frac{POP_{BP}}{POP} \right)\left(\frac{POP_{SS}}{POP_{BP}} \right)\left(\frac{Q_{SS}}{POP_{SS}} \right)$$

Suppose you are the Medicare administrator whose goal is to provide funding for the best care at the lowest cost. Let's look at each of the terms that determine total expenditures on spine surgery. For this exercise, presume that the above equation refers to hospital expenditures for a specific type of spine-surgery DRG. There is nothing you can do about P_{SS}, the hospital charge for the DRG-specific spine-surgery admission that is preset by CMS. Also, there is nothing you can do about the population 65 years of age and older, POP, which is growing. Now consider the prevalence of back pain (i.e., the fraction of the population 65 years of age and older who have this symptom, $\frac{POP_{BP}}{POP}$). In addition to age, key risk factors for low back pain include obesity and the lack of regular exercise involving the back and abdominal muscles. As obesity and inactivity increase in the US population, so does the prevalence of low back pain. You can try to influence colleagues in other agencies to develop prevention programs involving diet and exercise, but in your role as Medicare administrator you will have to take an increasing prevalence of low back pain as a given. You are then left with two critical variables: the fraction of patients with back pain undergoing spine surgery $\left(\frac{POP_{SS}}{POP_{BP}} \right)$ and the number of such procedures per person undergoing surgery $\left(\frac{Q_{SS}}{POP_{SS}} \right)$. The fraction of patients with back pain who undergo spine surgery is potentially subject to significant physician-induced demand. Chart documentation may be one tool at your disposal to determine medical necessity in individual cases, but this is a blunt instrument since a cottage industry of coding consultants has evolved to help hospitals and physicians accomplish chart documentation and payment coding that would pass muster under a Medicare audit. Finally, there is the matter of the number of surgical procedures per surgical patient. Repeat surgical procedures would hopefully be infrequent in the case of spine surgery, and your ability to constrain this number would also be governed by the sophistication of chart documentation. This issue of procedure numbers per patient (or per-patient number of visits, imaging studies, medications, etc.) applies to many other health care services.

For spine surgery, in addition to the equation for hospital expenditures there is a separate equation for expenditures on spine surgeons and anesthesiologists as well as potentially for rehab centers and other cost centers. (Bundled payments are ignored for purposes of this exercise.) Of course, spine surgery is but one example of a wide variety of surgical procedures. Moreover, the same issues apply to medical conditions. Imagine, for example, the same set of decisions for a new method of administering insulin to diabetics, one that is approved by Medicare based on safety and efficacy studies reviewed by the FDA but is only minimally more effective clinically than the current gold standard while being much more costly. The overall Medicare population is growing and the fraction of the population with diabetes is also increasing due to obesity. The fraction of the diabetic population who will be prescribed the new drug is dependent on pharmaceutical company physician marketing and direct-to-consumer advertising, patient preferences, and the degree to which the physician not only acts as the patient's agent but also takes societal cost into account. This scenario plays out across the entire array of medical conditions being evaluated and treated in Medicare patients every day across the nation.

Given these considerations, it is not surprising that the data bear out a steep increase in Medicare expenditures that commenced soon after its enactment into law. Returning to table 10.1, Medicare expenditures were $7.7 billion in 1970, grew 4.5-fold in the 1970s to reach $37.5 billion, and have continued to grow substantially. In 2016, Medicare expenditures were $672.1 billion, representing a compounded annual growth rate of 10.2 percent from its starting position of $7.7 billion in 1970. In 2017, the average expenditure per Medicare beneficiary nationally was $13,185: $5,160 for Part A expenses, $5,915 for Part B, and $2,110 for Part D.[6]

Creation of Part C (Medicare Advantage)

In an effort to reduce cost and improve the quality of care, Part C of Medicare (Medicare Advantage) was created by Congress in 1997. The goals of improved quality and reduced cost were to be accomplished by emphasizing primary care, prevention, and a reduction in avoidable hospitalizations and procedures.

Original Medicare plus Part D is often referred to as "fee-for-service Medicare" or "FFS Medicare." By contrast, Part C works on the basis of a capitated payment. Under Part C, sponsors receive a capitated payment (fixed amount per member per month), adjusted by the risk profile of members. From these revenues the sponsor pays hospitals, physicians, and other providers for services rendered, based on a fee schedule negotiated with them. Thus, while Part C is capitated at the plan level, it is still (in most but not all cases) fee for service at the hospital/provider level.

A Part C (Medicare Advantage) beneficiary must first sign up for both Part A and Part B of Medicare. From the standpoint of the Medicare enrollee, a benefit of Medicare Advantage (MA) is that it sets a limit to annual out-of-pocket spending, while no such limit exists in FFS Medicare. They may also receive additional benefits from the MA sponsor that is not covered in Original Medicare, and "zero premium" plans are also offered. Beneficiaries are free to disenroll from MA each year and return to FFS Medicare. Disadvantages include, for many plans, a restricted choice of physicians and hospitals. It remains difficult for consumers to access network directories to find out whether specific physicians are included, and a 2017 survey of about 400 MA plans found that, on average, a little less than half of area physicians were included in their networks.[7] The typical requirement that a primary care physician serves as a gatekeeper for specialist care may also be viewed as a disadvantage by some beneficiaries. Many of the Part C plans integrate drug coverage in a manner that is similar to the stand-alone Part D prescription drug benefit plan. CMS makes additional capitation payments to the MA plans for these prescription drug benefits.

Congress instituted the Medicare Advantage program in pursuit of two laudable goals: (1) to expand the choices of beneficiaries to include private plans that might provide more coordinated and comprehensive care than provided through traditional Medicare, and (2) to take advantage of presumed efficiencies in managed care that would save Medicare money.[8] Due to the financial advantages to beneficiaries and extensive marketing, Medicare Advantage programs have grown dramatically. Starting at zero in 1997, it has grown to 18.5 million in 2018, which represented 32 percent of Medicare beneficiaries. It is anticipated that MA enrollment will grow to over 30 million enrollees by 2027, increasing the percentage of beneficiaries covered by MA to 41 percent of the Medicare population.[9]

What evidence is available about the impact of MA plans on quality and cost? Regarding cost, there were some early pitfalls. For example, it was reported in 2009 that CMS spent 14 percent more on Medicare Advantage beneficiaries per person than on "like beneficiaries" under Original Medicare.[10] A major part of the problem appeared to be rooted in the payment methodology that CMS uses to pay Medicare Advantage sponsors. Specifically, CMS uses a "benchmark-and-bidding system"[11] in which Medicare establishes a maximum-amount "benchmark" for each county based on its data on traditional Medicare spending per beneficiary in that county. Each sponsor submits a bid that includes the costs of providing medical care as well as its administrative expenses and profits; Medicare pays the sponsor the lower of its bid or the corresponding county benchmark. If a sponsor submits a bid below the benchmark, it receives a bonus "rebate" payment that is used to provide enrollees with additional benefits.

In the early years of Medicare Advantage, benchmarks averaged 118 percent of traditional Medicare spending per beneficiary. Moreover, costs to CMS for Medicare Advantage plans were closely tied to the benchmark level.[12] Analyzing CMS costs across MA plans in different areas, Zuckerman and his collaborators found that every dollar increase in the benchmark was associated with an additional 32 cents in plan costs and an additional 52 cents in rebates.[13] Not surprisingly, Medicare Advantage plans were found to be more plentiful in high-benchmark areas. In Florida, for example, there was a high density of MA plans in South Florida but few plans in North Central or North Florida. Also not surprising, Zuckerman and his colleagues found that insurers with greater market power were able to set higher prices. Under the Affordable Care Act, significant changes were made to the Medicare Advantage program benchmarks: they fell, on average, from 118 percent of traditional Medicare spending per beneficiary in 2009 to 106 percent by 2017.[14]

When a sponsor receives 106 percent of the funds that would be expended by Medicare on "like beneficiaries" in a county, Medicare Advantage can be extremely attractive to health insurance companies and other sponsors (e.g., HMOs). First, for the reasons described earlier related to market imperfections, FFS Medicare leads to high levels of price and utilization that could potentially be reduced with managed oversight in a capitated model. For example, sponsors could pursue a narrow network of hospitals and physicians who would agree to lower prices in return for exclusive access to a defined patient population. Sponsors can also restrict network providers on the basis of practice style profiles that would minimize induced demand, or they could institute a primary care gatekeeper who could potentially reduce the utilization of specialist physicians, procedures, and hi-tech diagnostic procedures and other services. Further, emergency room visits, hospitalizations, and procedures could be reviewed for their appropriateness; based on this review, a fraction of medical claims by providers could be denied.

Thus, there are a variety of approaches that MA sponsors could utilize to reduce both price and utilization. By receiving 106 percent of what CMS would expect to pay under traditional Medicare as revenues, and spending less in the form of medical payments due to reduced price and utilization, the MA sponsor would keep the difference as profit (net of administrative expenses). Furthermore, CMS provides additional avenues by which profit margins of MA sponsors could widen. For example, CMS provides medical risk assessments of the patients in the MA plan; plans with "sicker" patients receive a higher capitated payment. That makes sense, but it also invites "coding gamesmanship" in which consultants to the MA sponsors can advise them how to document and code the medical records of their patients to ensure the highest risk assessment and payment possible. Another example is that additional payments from CMS are provided to the MA sponsor for patients requiring more intensive medical (and sometimes social) attention: dual-eligible beneficiaries (i.e., those eligible for both Medicaid and Medicare—often with disabilities or severe mental health problems) and special needs patients (i.e., those who have one or more of a long list of chronic medical conditions such as diabetes or congestive heart disease). And finally, CMS has created a "star" system for evaluating the quality of care and overall performance of MA sponsors and provides more federal revenue to sponsors having four- or five-star ratings, allowing them to have lower premiums and/or to provide supplemental benefits. There is also the opportunity for five-star sponsors to enroll patients year-round as opposed to just during the open enrollment period. (Sponsors with low star rankings have a reduction in payment, or may be eliminated.)

Under current law, sponsors must spend at least 85 percent of their total capitated payments on medical expenses, leaving up to 15 percent for profit and administrative expenses. The amount of profit relative to administrative expense can be enhanced, however, by counting some types of administrative expense (e.g., case management) as a "medical expense" rather than an administrative expense. Moreover, some large insurance companies have established wholly owned subsidiaries to perform administrative expenses and bill the parent insurance company for these expenses with a built-in profit margin. In this way, the entire face value of the invoice from the wholly owned subsidiary counts toward the 15 percent allowable administrative expense, yet the built-in profit from this administrative activity adds to the main profit margin generated by the capitated payments.

It is therefore no wonder that there has been increased interest in Medicare Advantage among major insurers (table 10.4). It is also telling that there has recently been growing interest among venture capital firms. In October 2018, for example, a new company created to enter the MA market called Devoted Health was valued at $1.8 billion after having raised $300 million in fresh capital, but before even a single insurance policy had been sold.[15] It was also reported that Bright Health raised $240 million from a number of venture capital firms, and Oscar Health raised $375 million from Alphabet to expand into Medicare Advantage.[16]

One concern regarding the overall MA program was a report from the US Government Accountability Office (GAO) indicating that disenrollment by MA beneficiaries in many plans is influenced by health status.[17] The GAO analyzed 252 contracts with MA sponsors in 2014 that met enrollee number and other study criteria and focused on the 126 contracts with disenrollment rates that were above the median rate of 10.6 percent. Of these, 35 contracts were found to have "health-biased disenrollment." That is, beneficiaries in poor health were substantially more likely (on average, 47 percent more likely) in these 35 plans to disenroll in comparison with plan beneficiaries in better health. Beneficiaries tended to leave these plans for reasons related to preferred providers and access to care. The GAO states that "such disparities in contract disenrollment by health status may indi-

Table 10.4. Medicare Advantage enrollees by firm, 2017

United Health	5.1M
Humana	3.5M
Blue Cross Blue Shield (not Anthem)	2.7M
Kaiser Permanente	1.6M
Aetna	1.6M
Well Care Health	0.6M
Cigna	0.4M
All other insurers	4.9M
Total MA enrollees	20.4M

Source: Gretchen Jacobson, Anthony Damico, and Tricia Neuman, *A Dozen Facts about Medicare Advantage* (Menlo Park, CA: Kaiser Family Foundation, November 2018), https://www.kff.org/medicare/issue -brief/a-dozen-facts-about-medicare-advantage.

cate that the needs of beneficiaries, particularly those in poor health, may not be adequately met."[18] The GAO recommended that CMS strengthen its oversight of MA sponsors and contracts.

Regarding quality, a study of ambulatory care from 2003 through 2009 found that beneficiaries in Medicare HMOs were consistently more likely than those in traditional Medicare to receive appropriate breast cancer screening, diabetes care, and cholesterol testing for cardiovascular disease.[19] These early results suggested "that the positive effects of more-integrated delivery systems on the quality of ambulatory care in Medicare HMOs may outweigh the potential incentives to restrict care under capitated payments."[20] A review of studies in the literature on MA vs. traditional Medicare between 2010 and 2014, however, reported mixed results.[21] MA seemed to do better on measures of preventive services and unnecessary hospital admissions but worse on some measures of quality and access.

Recently, a detailed comparison of FFS and MA plans with respect to cost and quality was conducted by Avalere Health, a Washington, DC–based consulting firm.[22] Large, nationally representative samples of the two Medicare populations enrolled for the full year in 2015 were compared (table 10.5). These samples, which were comparable demographically to national enrollment data, included 1.8 million Medicare Advantage beneficiaries and 1.4 million FFS Medicare beneficiaries. Since more than half of the Medicare population have four or more chronic conditions, Avalere Health selected beneficiaries with one or more of the three most prevalent chronic conditions in the Medicare population: hypertension, hyperlipidemia, and

Table 10.5. Comparison of Medicare Advantage and traditional (fee-for-service) Medicare, 2015

	Medicare Advantage	Fee for service
Number in sample	1,813,937	13,753
Medical history (%)		
Severe mental illness	8.5	5.4
Racial/ethnic minority	30.9	15.2
Disability as original reason for enrollment	35.9	22.0
Prevention (%)		
Access to preventive health services	99.4	98.9
LDL testing	77.8	74.0
Hemoglobin A1c testing	90.1	92.0
Breast cancer screening	76.3	67.3
Use and spending		
Hospitalizations/1,000	249	324
ER visits/1,000	511	759
Cost per beneficiary ($)	9,400	9,367
Cost per dual-eligible beneficiary ($)	11,159	13,398

Source: Mendelson, Teigland, and Creighton, *Medicare Advantage Achieves Cost-Effective Care and Better Outcomes.*[22]

diabetes. This design was chosen to provide a potential window into how the FFS and MA plans compare overall in terms of their impact on quality of life and Medicare spending.

Before discussing the Avalere findings in detail, there are two important caveats. First, in analyzing the data we must recognize that patients were not randomized between MA and traditional Medicare. Therefore, there may be selection bias. Second, although Avalere Health's findings are presented at face value as independent and objective, it must be recognized that their study was funded by Better Medicare Alliance, an advocacy group for Medicare Advantage.

Given these caveats, Avalere Health found that among Medicare beneficiaries with chronic medical conditions, MA beneficiaries had the following characteristics in comparison with their FFS counterparts:

1. A higher proportion of beneficiaries in the MA plans have clinical and social risk factors known to affect health outcomes and cost. These include a higher proportion of beneficiaries who enrolled in Medicare

due to disabilities, a higher proportion of racial/ethnic minorities, and a higher rate of serious mental illness.

2. Despite a higher proportion of clinical and social risk factors, MA beneficiaries have lower utilization of high-cost services such as hospitalizations and emergency room visits, and comparable average costs.

3. Dual-eligible beneficiaries in the MA plan (i.e., those who qualify for both Medicare and Medicaid) have lower expenditures per beneficiary.

4. Preventive services are generally comparable, except for breast cancer screening, which was somewhat higher among MA patients.

5. MA beneficiaries with diabetes have fewer serious lower extremity complications.

It should be reiterated that MA plans have been incentivized to enroll more dual-eligible patients, and more patients with disabilities and chronic illnesses through the Special Needs Plan supplemental payments. Thus, these differences in the composition of the patient population in MA and FFS are not surprising. That said, the results on reduced hospitalizations and expenditures are encouraging, although more data are needed on a broad spectrum of clinical outcomes.

As MA plans become more refined across time, their promise may indeed be realized. It is certainly logical to think that MA's capitation-based incentives foster an emphasis on preventive health interventions, better coordination of the care of patients with chronic medical conditions, and reduction in hospitalizations and other high-cost services. The achievement of such goals is always easier said than done, however (especially when providers are paid on a fee-for-service basis), and early supportive evidence has only begun to accumulate. More independent studies in the peer-reviewed literature will help answer the question of whether MA plans indeed provide a better quality of life for Medicare beneficiaries at lower cost. As we wait for this evidence, it is highly likely that MA as a share of the total Medicare program will continue to grow: the increase in MA enrollees by private health insurers and the recent infusion of private equity capital suggests that there is the potential for significant profitability in this program; moreover, CMS appears to be encouraging MA directly and indirectly,[23] and marketing for MA by its sponsors is becoming more extensive.

Accountable Care Organizations

Accountable care organizations (ACOs) have their roots in the health maintenance organizations of the 1980s and 1990s. HMOs were designed to bring together a broad range of medical services in coordinating the care of a defined population. Though the stated goals were lofty, there was a tendency to manage financial risk by using primary care gatekeepers and other measures that restricted access. This strategy failed to create lasting reform; only a few successful HMOs are still in operation. Ultimately, difficulties in obtaining access to specialist and other services created a patient backlash against HMOs that hastened their demise.

The immediate forerunner of the ACO model was CMS's Medicare Physician Group Practice Demonstration. This was a pilot program in which 10 large physician groups that were geographically dispersed throughout the country entered into contracts with CMS to create care processes that improved quality while reducing cost. If savings in Medicare expenditures exceeded a specified threshold, the physician group would share in the savings. Performance results after five years were reported in 2011.[24] The ten practice groups included 5,000 physicians and 220,000 Medicare beneficiaries in the fee-for-service program. Under the demonstration, physician groups continued to be paid under regular Medicare fee schedules and were eligible for performance payments based on savings in expenditures and improvements in a set of 32 quality measures. All of the physician groups improved quality scores in virtually all of the measures. Depending on the year of analysis, however, only four or five generated sufficient savings to qualify for a performance payment.

In the years leading up to the Affordable Care Act, the concept of an ACO gained traction.[25] The ACO model, consisting of providers across the care continuum who accept clinical and financial responsibility for the health care needs of a population, was scored favorably by the Congressional Budget Office and was included in the statutory language of the legislation (section 3022). ACOs have been supported by the CMS leadership in both Democrat and Republican administrations. The ACO model was supported by Don Berwick, the CMS administrator appointed by President Obama, as it captured the "Triple Aim" he articulated and popularized: "Improve the patient care experience, improve the health of populations, and reduce the per capita costs of health care."[26] ACOs continue under Seema

Verma, the CMS administrator appointed by President Trump, albeit with a redesign announced in the form of a final rule released on December 21, 2018.[27] This rule contains many changes intended to enhance competition, innovation, engagement, integrity, and quality. Most strongly, however, there is emphasis on moving toward "performance risk"—a two-sided contract in which ACOs would assume financial risk if expenditures were to rise as well as share in savings if they were to fall.

Up-to-date information on the full spectrum of ACOs are not readily available. The most comprehensive data are contained in a 2015 report by Leavitt Partners.[28] They identified 744 ACOs at that time, covering 23.5 million lives. ACOs were divided approximately equally between those led by physician groups, hospitals, and physicians plus hospitals. Most of the ACO contracts with government were with Medicare, although about 15 states had initiated (or were about to initiate) ACO-like programs for Medicaid. Commercial ACOs by that time were already equal to government ACOs in numbers of contracts, and they exceeded government ACOs in numbers of covered beneficiaries. Using data from national surveys of ACOs, Peiris et al. compared the performance of 228 commercial ACOs and 171 government ACOs.[29] They found that commercial ACOs were larger, showed more integration of physicians and hospitals, were more efficient with lower expenditures, and had higher quality scores.

The future sustainability of Medicare ACOs is uncertain. While most Medicare ACOs reduced costs in 2016, Medicare still lost $39 million on the program as a whole after accounting for administrative costs and performance payments.[30] Even the savings reported may be due more to a selection bias (i.e., the nonrandom pruning of high-cost patients and clinicians by ACOs).[31] Indeed, from the standpoint of health systems and their boards evaluating Medicare ACOs purely from the standpoint of fiduciary responsibility, the economic benefits are ambiguous due to a variety of factors: significant infrastructure start-up costs, lost revenue from reductions in utilization, patients attributed to their ACO but who obtain care in another system for which the expenditures are counted, and unknown levels of future benchmark resets by CMS. In May 2018, it was reported that 71 percent of existing Medicare ACOs are likely to leave the program rather than assuming downside financial risk.[32] For such systems, establishing a Medicare Advantage plan may be chosen as a better option.

Medicare Access and CHIP Reauthorization Act

Congress passed the Medicare Access and CHIP (Children's Health Insurance Program) Reauthorization Act (MACRA) in April 2015, establishing two new tracks for physician payment under fee-for-service Medicare: the Merit-based Incentive Payment System (MIPS) and advanced alternative payment models (Advanced APMs). It was projected that all but 4–5 percent of physicians would ultimately be paid under the MIPS track, as a substantial amount of revenue must be received through eligible alternative payment models to qualify for the APM track. Under MIPS, Medicare makes payment adjustments to physicians based on their composite score on four performance categories: a set of six quality metrics (mostly process oriented), cost (based on Medicare claims), a large number of clinical practice improvement activities (from which physicians can choose), and use of electronic health records for information exchange and interoperability. An equal number of providers receive upward adjustments and downward adjustments to maintain budget neutrality. Performance in one year determines payment adjustments two years later.

While some view MIPS as a positive step that aligns physician incentives with quality and efficiency, it has come under significant criticism. In October 2017, the Medicare Payment Advisory Commission voted to recommend repeal of MIPS because it weighs too heavily on process factors, such as whether they ordered appropriate tests or followed general clinical guidelines, rather than if patient care was ultimately improved by that provider's actions. In a March 2018 *Health Affairs* blog, the chair of MedPac and other colleagues summarized their concerns: "By trying to measure individual clinicians solely on their own activities and using this information to allocate payment for quality and efficiency at the national level, MIPS adopts a fragmented approach to quality measurement that is unfair and burdensome to providers, results in unreliable performance scores, and does not promote high-quality care in traditional fee-for-service Medicare."[33]

The Bipartisan Budget Act of 2018 delayed full implementation of MIPS until 2022, at which time the maximum payment adjustments are scheduled to be up to plus or minus 9 percent. At the present time, there is gradual implementation. Based on the most recent MIPS announcements, the maximum payment adjustment amount for performance in 2019 (i.e., the 2021 payment year) is plus or minus 7 percent.

Financial Status of Medicare Trust Funds

According to the 2018 annual report of the boards of trustees of the Medicare trust funds, in 2017 total Medicare expenditures were $710.2 billion and total income was $705.1 billion, producing a deficit for the year.[34] Based on an intermediate set of assumptions about projected costs and revenues, the trustees estimate that the Hospital Insurance Trust Fund, which had assets of $202 billion at the beginning of 2018, will be depleted by 2026. The Supplementary Medical Insurance Trust Fund is expected to be adequately financed over the next 10 years and beyond because premium income for Parts B and D, as well as general revenue income, are reset each year to cover costs. Looking further down the road, the trustees project that the number of workers per Medicare beneficiary will decline from its value of 3.1 at present to 2.4 in 2030. This inexorable demographic trend will pose a fundamental challenge for the future fiscal viability of the Hospital Insurance Trust Fund.

Summary

By 1965, a substantial share of the US population had employer-based health insurance but left out were the elderly and the poor. Medicaid and Medicare were enacted to provide access to health care for these two groups. From the beginning, private health insurers participated as fiscal intermediaries and across time began to participate actively through managed care products in both Medicare (Medicare Advantage) and Medicaid (Medicaid Managed Care).

The availability of medical services for Medicare and Medicaid beneficiaries at highly subsidized prices has contributed to the dramatic growth in expenditures that has occurred since 1965, paralleling the spending growth in the private health insurance sector. Because of the increased availability of health insurance with low co-pays, however, out-of-pocket spending by individuals as a fraction of their total health care costs has been reduced fivefold.

Although Medicare Advantage and Medicaid Managed Care are capitated at the plan level, providers are typically paid through private insurance according to a negotiated fee-for-service schedule rather than by subcapitation. This reinforces the fee-for-service payment methodology still used in most employer-based plans, thus presenting continued challenges to the prospect of constraining expenditure growth.

ACOs and MACRA are attempting to remodel the payment system for health care services by encouraging coordination/integration between hospitals and physicians and by modifying the fee-for-service system to include incentives and penalties around reporting, cost, and quality of care. Results to date have been mixed. Evidence regarding Medicare Advantage is early but encouraging of an enhancement in preventive services, reduction in hospital admissions, and improvement in some measures of health status.

Because of the aging baby-boom generation, in the coming decades there will be fewer workers per retiree contributing to the Medicare Hospital Insurance Trust Fund. Projected growth in Medicare expenditures will deplete the reserves in this fund in the coming decade unless some action is taken to increase contributions and/or reduce the draw from the fund.

11 MEDICAID

In contrast to Medicare, which was being developed essentially as a *de novo* program, Medicaid had strong roots in the New Deal and prior welfare legislation. Nonetheless, in the swirl of high-profile negotiations over Medicare, Medicaid—the third layer of Wilbur Ross's three-layer cake—initially took a back seat. As the legislative process unfolded, the concept of covering poor children, the disabled, and other needy individuals who could not afford private health insurance came to the front burner and garnered support. The Medicaid program now covers one in five Americans and is also the principal source of coverage for long-term care in the United States. In this chapter, we consider the historical context of Medicaid, rules for eligibility, characteristics of recipients, and financing. The impact of Medicaid on health status will be presented in chapter 20.

Historical Context

The 1950 amendments to the Social Security Act set the template for Medicaid.[1] These amendments authorized medical payments for individuals receiving public assistance through a program in which funds from federal general revenues matched state medical payments to providers. The Kerr-Mills Act in 1960 extended medical payments to a new population: individuals age 65 or over who were defined as "medically indigent" (i.e., persons who would not qualify for welfare, but whose incomes would be considered insufficient to pay for needed medical services).[2] The idea was that people would qualify not because they were eligible for public assistance if healthy, but because their payments for needed medical services would reduce their income below the poverty line. The Kerr-Mills legislation also included a straightforward and politically acceptable federal matching formula for state funds, which distributed payments based on each state's per capita income. States were given the responsibility for determining eligibility standards and benefit levels, as was the case with public assistance. Generally, the poorer the state, the less well funded was that state's welfare and medical assistance program.

Just as there was a groundswell of support for medical coverage of the elderly in establishing Medicare, there grew widespread support to provide medical care for children of poor families, who made up the single largest category of welfare beneficiaries. Mills was interested in expanding the thrust of the Kerr-Mills legislation to create state-based medical care programs for the poor as an extension of state-based public assistance programs. This interest was shared by federal officials in the Department of Health, Education, and Welfare, which created the Child Health and Medical Assistance Act as part of the administration's legislative proposal. Mills ultimately combined the administration's approach with requests from the American Medical Association and others to create the Title XIX (Medicaid) layer of the 1965 legislation.

Although they were part of the same bill and adopted at the same time, Medicare and Medicaid have been viewed differently by the population at large. Medicare has been broadly seen as an insurance program with nationally uniform standards: workers (and their employers) fund the Medicare trust fund through payroll taxes over a number of years and draw benefits from this fund after retirement. (This is true only for Part A, hospital services.) Medicaid, on the other hand, is viewed as an entitlement program and has the stigma of public assistance. (As noted in chapter 10, Medicare Parts B and D—physician and drug expenses—are partly financed by beneficiary premiums but largely by government general revenue. In this sense, Medicare is also an entitlement program like Medicaid and is often referred to as such.)

Medicaid varies widely in its standards for eligibility and benefits across states, as well as in its reimbursement rates to providers. Payments to physicians under Medicare Part B reflect their origins in "usual, customary, and reasonable" fees, while these fees are quite low under Medicaid. This discrepancy has translated into many more physicians accepting Medicare than Medicaid.

While much of the motivation for Medicaid was based on a desire to provide medical care for the poor, especially children and the disabled, Medicaid also offers benefits not normally covered by Medicare, like nursing home care and personal care services. As of September 2018, Medicaid (including the Children's Health Insurance Program, also known as CHIP) provided funding for the medical care of 72,966,000 low-income and disabled people.[3]

Eligibility

Medicaid recipients must be either US citizens or legal permanent residents and belong to one of several specific categories:

- Children in low-income households below a certain threshold
- Pregnant women
- Parents of Medicaid-eligible children who meet low-income requirements
- Low-income disabled people
- Low-income seniors 65 and older

Within these categories, states have the flexibility to define eligibility further; for example, in addition to income, eligibility is typically based on several other factors, including age, disability status, other government assistance, other health or medical conditions such as pregnancy, and in some cases financial resources (or assets). In addition to eligibility, each state has broad flexibility in determining provider reimbursement rates as well as the scope and types of services it will cover and the delivery mechanism by which health care services are provided. The federal Centers for Medicare and Medicaid Services (CMS) monitors the state-run programs.

Each year, modifications are made to the Medicaid program, whether by statute or by CMS policies. But there have been a number of select key milestones that have had noteworthy effects (see also table 11.1):

- Dental services in the Early and Periodic Screening, Diagnostic and Treatment (EPSDT) program for children under age 21 (an important early milestone) include pain relief, restoration of teeth, and maintenance for dental health.
- Disproportionate share payments to hospitals treating a high proportion of low-income patients have become important to safety-net hospitals as a means of partly offsetting the cost of treating such patients.

Table 11.1. Select Medicaid milestones

Year	Milestone
1967	Early and Periodic Screening, Diagnostic, and Treatment program for children under age 21. Includes dental, hearing. and vision.
1972	Federal Supplemental Security Income program gives states the ability to link to Medicaid for disabled residents.
1981	Disproportionate share payments by states to hospitals treating a high percentage of low-income patients. Payment limits revised in 1997.
1980s	Beginnings of Medicaid Managed Care.
1988	Qualified Medicare Beneficiary eligibility rule: coverage for payment to women and infants whose family income was less than or equal to 100% of federal poverty line (FPL). Threshold of FPL was raised to 133% in 1989.
1996	Welfare reform: link between Medicaid and welfare assistance was severed. Enrollment in Medicaid no longer automatic with receipt of welfare cash assistance.
1997	Children's Health Insurance Program (CHIP) established. Offers low-cost health coverage for children 18 years of age and younger; designed for families whose earnings exceed Medicaid thresholds but cannot afford to buy private insurance. CHIP reauthorized in 2009 with increased funding and a broader range of options and incentives.
2010	Patient Protection and Affordable Care Act (ACA) provided for expansion of Medicaid program by states, with optional participation based on 2012 Supreme Court ruling.

- Eligibility for pregnant women and infants with low family incomes and the Children's Health Insurance Program have been critical in assuring needed medical, obstetrical, and pediatric care for this population.

Since states have significant latitude in their administration of Medicaid and CHIP, eligibility rules vary widely. Thus, eligibility varies from state to state, and because someone qualifies for Medicaid in one state does not mean he or she will qualify in another. Thresholds for eligibility are expressed as a percent of the federal poverty line (FPL) (table 11.2). The FPL is higher in Alaska and Hawaii because of the higher cost of living in those two states.

Pregnant women are eligible for Medicaid if their household income is less than specified percentages of the FPL, ranging from 133 percent of the FPL in Louisiana and South Dakota to 375 percent in Iowa. Most states have eligibility thresholds for pregnant women in the range of 150 percent to 250 percent of the FPL. Similar ranges are seen for the eligibility of children, with somewhat higher thresholds for percentage of the FPL.

Table 11.2. Federal poverty levels for 48 states and District of Columbia, Alaska, and Hawaii ($), FY2018

Number of people in household	48 states and District of Columbia	Alaska	Hawaii
1	12,140	15,180	13,960
2	16,460	20,580	18,930
3	20,780	25,980	23,900
4	25,100	31,380	28,870
5	29,400	36,780	33,840
6	33,740	42,180	38,810
7	38,060	47,580	43,780
8	42,380	52,980	48,750
9 or more[a]	4,320	5,400	4,970

Source: "November 2018 Medicaid & CHIP Enrollment Data Highlights," Medicaid.gov, accessed December 14, 2018, https://www.medicaid.gov/medicaid/program-information/medicaid-and-chip-enrollment-data/report-highlights/total-enrollment/index.html

[a] Add this amount for each additional person.

Medicaid eligibility rules for parents (or other certified caretakers) of Medicaid-eligible children are more strict. Such parents are eligible for Medicaid only if they are in households that are below 20 percent of the FPL in seven states, between 20 and 29 percent of the FPL in five states, between 30 and 39 percent of the FPL in five states, and between 40 and 49 percent of the FPL in six states (table 11.3). Minimum-wage and other low-income workers—parents or not—would have income above these thresholds and therefore would not qualify for Medicaid. This group was a major contributor to the large number of uninsured Americans (about 48 million people) before enactment of the Affordable Care Act. As of December 2019, five states have CMS-approved work requirements for Medicaid recipients (usually 80 hours per month), although only one (Indiana) has been implemented. The approvals for three states were set aside by courts, and six more are pending.[4] A state-by-state review has indicated that implementation of Medicaid work requirements has been a challenging process.[5]

Characteristics of Medicaid and CHIP Recipients

Almost half of Medicaid/CHIP recipients are children, 13 percent are disabled (ages 19–64), and 11 percent are age 65 or older (table 11.4). Thus, children, older adults and the disabled account for 70 percent of all Medicaid/CHIP recipients. It is pertinent in understanding the dynamics of

Table 11.3. Income eligibility of adults, parents, or caregivers for Medicaid and CHIP, by state, 2018

Percentage of federal poverty level (%)[a]	State
10–19	Alabama, Arkansas, Indiana, Louisiana, Missouri, Texas, West Virginia
20–29	Florida, Idaho, Kentucky, Mississippi, Montana
30–39	Georgia, Kansas, Nevada, New Jersey, Pennsylvania
40–49	New Mexico, North Carolina, Oklahoma, Oregon, Virginia, Washington
50–59	Iowa, Michigan, Nebraska, North Dakota, South Dakota, Utah, Vermont, Wyoming
60–69	Colorado, New Hampshire, South Carolina
70–99	Delaware, Ohio, Wisconsin
100–133	Alaska, Arizona, California, Connecticut, District of Columbia, Hawaii, Illinois, Maine, Maryland, Massachusetts, Minnesota, Rhode Island, Tennessee

Source: "Medicaid, Children's Health Insurance Program, and Basic Health Program Eligibility Levels," Medicaid.gov, accessed October 18, 2018, www.medicaid.gov/medicaid/program-information/medicaid-and-chip-eligibility-levels/index.html.
[a] As defined by modified adjusted gross income.

Table 11.4. Characteristics of Medicaid and CHIP recipients, 2015

Category of participant[a]	Number in 2015	Percentage of total
Child/youth (under age 19)	30,419,902	45.8
Ages 65 and older	7,155,401	10.8
Disabled (ages 19–64)	8,781,327	13.2
Institutionalized (ages 19–64)	380,517	0.6
Recent mother (ages 19 and older)	1,040,193	1.6
Working full-time, year-round (ages 19–64)	4,678,142	7.0
Working part-time or part-year (ages 19–64)	3,319,811	5.0
Other	10,641,447	16.0
Total means-tested public health insurance	66,416,740	100.0

Source: Amanda Lee and Beth Jarosz, "Majority of People Covered by Medicaid, and Similar Programs, Are Children, Older Adults, or Disabled," Population Reference Bureau, June 29, 2017, https://www.prb.org/majority-of-people-covered-by-medicaid-and-similar-programs.
[a] Categories are mutually exclusive. Full time, year-round are those working 35 hours or more per week, 50 or more weeks per year. Part time includes those working at least 10 hours per week, at least 47 weeks per year, excluding full-time, year-round workers.

Medicaid that children comprise about 40 percent of enrollees but account for only 19 percent of expenditures, while the disabled comprise 15 percent of enrollees but account for 39 percent of expenditures (figure 11.1).

Because of the strict income criteria for eligibility of adults, only about 4.7 million adults ages 19–64 who were working full-time, year-round were

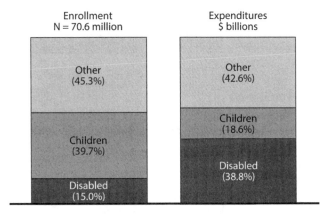

Enrollment
N = 70.6 million

Other
(45.3%)

Children
(39.7%)

Disabled
(15.0%)

Expenditures
$ billions

Other
(42.6%)

Children
(18.6%)

Disabled
(38.8%)

Figure 11.1. Distribution of Medicaid enrollees and expenditures, FY2016. Adapted from Christian J. Wolfe, Kathryn E. Rennie, and Christopher J. Truffer, *2017 Actuarial Report on the Financial Outlook for Medicaid* (Washington, DC: Centers for Medicare and Medicaid Services), figure 8, accessed December 12, 2018, https://www.cms.gov/Research-Statistics -Data-and-Systems/Research/ActuarialStudies/Downloads/MedicaidReport2017.pdf.

eligible for Medicaid in 2015, and only about 3.3 million in this age group who were working part-time or for part of the year were eligible (table 11.4). Most of these were parents of eligible children.

Another way of understanding the role that Medicaid plays among low-income individuals, families, and the elderly and disabled is to view the percentage of people in these categories who are enrolled in Medicaid.[6] About half of pregnant women are Medicaid beneficiaries, as well as 38 percent of all children and 83 percent of children in households below the federal poverty line (figure 11.2).

Additional insights into the characteristics of the Medicaid population ages 19–64 can be gleaned from comparisons of their demographic distributions in comparison with those who are beneficiaries of private health insurance. For example, there is a higher proportion of Medicaid/CHIP beneficiaries who are female and members of minority groups, and a lower proportion who completed college (table 11.5). These characteristics are those that would be expected based on the fact that private insurance is predominantly associated with employer-based, higher-wage positions.

Financing

Under Medicaid, states receive matching funds from the federal government to cover the costs of medical services provided to low-income residents

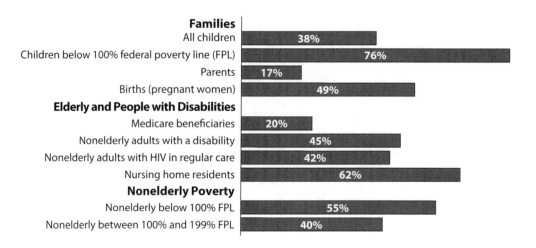

Families
All children — 38%
Children below 100% federal poverty line (FPL) — 76%
Parents — 17%
Births (pregnant women) — 49%
Elderly and People with Disabilities
Medicare beneficiaries — 20%
Nonelderly adults with a disability — 45%
Nonelderly adults with HIV in regular care — 42%
Nursing home residents — 62%
Nonelderly Poverty
Nonelderly below 100% FPL — 55%
Nonelderly between 100% and 199% FPL — 40%

Figure 11.2. Percentage of selected populations with Medicaid coverage. Adapted from Wolfe, Rennie, and Truffer, *2017 Actuarial Report on the Financial Outlook for Medicaid*, figure 4.

who meet the eligibility requirements defined by federal law and modified by the state. Under state-determined reimbursement rules, states pay providers according to negotiated fee scales or pay managed care plans according to negotiated capitation rates for the medical and administrative costs of providing care to Medicaid patients. States then report these payments to CMS, a percentage of which, called the Federal Medical Assistance Percentage (FMAP), is then reimbursed to states by CMS. FMAP is calculated annually for each state based on a formula that adjusts for state per capita income relative to the national average. By law, the FMAP cannot be less than 50 percent. The highest FMAP percentage in the nation for FY2020 is Mississippi at 76 percent.[7] The federal government also pays for a portion of each state's administration costs. Beneficiary premiums and cost sharing, such as deductibles or co-payments, are very limited in Medicaid.

Unlike some parts of Medicare, Medicaid's financial operations are not financed through a trust fund. With minor exceptions, revenue sources dedicated to Medicaid, like Medicare's payroll tax for the Hospital Insurance Trust Fund (i.e., Part A), do not exist. Federal and state general revenues are therefore used to paying for Medicaid on an as-needed basis. To pay for the state portion of the costs, states may also utilize local government revenues. Since federal and state funding to pay for Medicaid is authorized by annual legislative appropriations, overall Medicaid revenues and expenses are automatically in financial balance. Projections on future costs for Medicaid,[8]

Table 11.5. Selected demographic characteristics of Medicaid recipients, ages 19–64, in comparison with beneficiaries of private health insurance

	Selected coverage source at time of interview, age 19–64 (%)	
Characteristic	Medicaid or CHIP	Private
Gender		
Male	37.9	49.6
Female	62.1	50.4
Race		
Hispanic	25.2	13.2
White, non-Hispanic	46.3	68.5
Black, non-Hispanic	20.3	10.5
Other non-white, non-Hispanic	8.3	7.7
Education		
Less than high school	23.4	4.9
High school diploma/GED	34.5	19.7
Some college	33.6	33.0
College or graduate degree	8.5	42.4
Marital Status		
Married	30.0	60.7
Widowed	2.2	1.2
Divorced or separated	16.4	8.9
Living with partner	14.4	7.1
Never married	37.0	22.1

Source: Adapted from "Exhibit 2: Characteristics of Non-Institutionalized Individuals by Age and Source of Health Care Coverage, 2017," in *MACStats: Medicaid and CHIP Data Book*, 4–8 (Washington, DC: Medicaid and CHIP Payment and Access Commission (MACPAC), December 2018), https://www.macpac.gov/wp -content/uploads/2015/01/Exhibit-2.-Characteristics-of-Non-Institutionalized-Individuals-by-Age-and-Source-of -Health-Coverage-2017.pdf.

while not posing a formal actuarial challenge as with the Medicare trust funds, are nonetheless problematic for future federal and state budgets.

Payments by Medicaid to Hospitals and Physicians

Payments to Hospitals

In government fiscal year 2017, the latest data for which complete hospital data are available, Medicaid spent $177.5 billion on hospital care.[9] Payments to hospitals for Medicaid patients flow through the state, either directly on a fee-for-service (FFS) basis or indirectly through a Medicaid Managed Care (MMC) company. Although MMC companies receive a capitated payment from the state, they typically pay hospitals on a fee-for-service basis, usually related to diagnosis-related groups.

Under the general category of "FFS," Medicaid counts both the base payment to hospitals for a specific set of services as well as supplemental payments. CMS makes Medicaid Disproportionate Share Hospital (DSH) payments to hospitals that serve a high proportion of Medicaid or uninsured patients. In addition, there are several non-DSH supplemental payments made to states, mostly based on negotiated agreements that involve CMS waivers and the use of matching dollars from intergovernmental transfers within the state (e.g., a millage or sales tax within a municipality).

Half of the $177.5 billion paid to hospitals for Medicaid patients in FY2017 were made under FFS, and the other half through MMC (table 11.6). It can also be seen that a little more than half of the FFS payments were base payments for specific services while the remainder was for supplemental payments.

Medicaid DSH payments are statutorily required payments to hospitals that are designed to offset some or all of the financial shortfalls that result from caring for Medicaid or uninsured patients. State DSH spending is limited by federal allotments, which vary widely. In FY2017, the percent of Medicaid spending attributable to DSH ranged from less than 1 percent in ten states to 12 percent in New Hampshire.[10] The relative amounts of current DSH allotments to states can be largely traced back to each state's DSH spending in 1992, when DSH allotments were first established. With the advent of Medicaid expansion under the Patient Protections and Affordable

Table 11.6. Base and supplemental Medicaid payments to hospitals, FY2017

	Dollar amount in billions ($)	Percentage (%)
Total	177.5	100.0
Managed care	88.7	50.0
Fee-for-service:		
Base payments	46.2	26.0
Supplemental		
Disproportionate Share Hospital	12.4	7.0
Upper payment limit	12.4	7.0
Other[a]	17.8	10.0

Source: Adapted from MACPAC, Medicaid Base and Supplemental Payments to Hospitals, figure 1.[9]
  [a] Includes uncompensated care payments (5%), delivery system reform incentive payments (4%), and graduate medical education (1%).

Care Act (chapter 12), reductions in DSH payments are scheduled since they are less needed; however, implementation of the DSH reduction has been delayed thus far.

An upper payment limit (UPL) is designed specifically for Medicaid patients, not the uninsured. Under UPL rules, states can make up part or all of the difference between the FFS base payment "and the amount that Medicare would have paid for the same service."[11] Like DSH, the use of UPL varies widely across states. In FY2017, the percent of Medicaid spending attributable to UPL ranged from less than 1 percent in 28 states to 10 percent or more in four states (Alabama, Colorado, Illinois, Oklahoma).[12]

In a study of DSH hospitals nationally for the year 2011, Nelb et al. found that when supplemental payments were added to the base or standard Medicaid rate, and after accounting for the contribution that hospitals often make to the financing of Medicaid through state taxes or through local intergovernmental transfers, hospitals were reimbursed 85 percent of their costs of treating Medicaid and uninsured patients combined, including both FFS and Medicaid Managed Care payments.[13] Of this amount, 64 percent was from standard Medicaid payments, 11 percent from DSH supplemental payments, and 10 percent from UPL and other non-DSH payments. Within the 64 percent of Medicaid payments was 7 percent due to local governments through tax or millage revenues. In Appendix materials, Nelb et al. reported that children's hospitals had 6–7 percent higher reimbursement for Medicaid and uninsured patients than adult hospitals and overall hospital reimbursement varied widely by state; these are generally between 80 and 100 percent, but seven states are in the range of 65 to 79 percent.[14]

While these data may be applicable to hospitals on average across the nation, there is tremendous variation across states in Medicaid supplemental payments to hospitals. In FY2016, three states received 52.8 percent of the total supplemental hospital payments nationally: Texas (8.75 percent of US population) received 22.3 percent, California (12.1 percent of US population) received 19.6 percent, and New York (6.1 percent of US population) received 10.9 percent. By contrast, Florida (6.5 percent of US population) received 2.6 percent of total supplemental hospital payments, and Pennsylvania (3.9 percent of US population) received 2 percent of total supplemental payments.

Payments to Physicians and Other Medicaid-Approved Health Care Providers

States pay physicians and other Medicaid-approved health care providers directly in the FFS part of Medicaid according to a percentage of Medicare fees that varies by state or a fee schedule developed by the state based on local considerations. For patients who belong to a MMC plan, doctors typically receive a payment according to a negotiated fee-for-service schedule, although there is beginning to be a move toward subcapitation to physician groups who are willing to accept risk. (So far, this is a small minority.)

Nationally, in 2016 the ratio of Medicaid-to-Medicare physician payments for the same service was 0.72, with considerable variability across states.[15] In a few states, there is a physician supplemental payment that closes the gap between Medicaid and Medicare payments. However, physicians are reluctant to see Medicaid patients not only because of lower reimbursement rates but because it often takes considerable administrative time and effort to submit bills, a long time to receive payment, and a disproportionate share of physician time compared to other patients because of more complex medical, social, and behavioral problems.[16] In 2011, 33 percent of office-based physicians would not accept a new Medicaid patient, as opposed to 17 percent for Medicare patients and 18 percent for patients with private insurance.[17]

Payments to States

Wide variations across states in eligibility rules and in payments to hospitals and doctors are associated with equally wide variations in total Medicaid expenditures (table 11.7). When total Medicaid expenditures per recipient are categorized into increments between $4,000 and $11,000, there is approximately a twofold difference in per-recipient spending between states spending the lowest amount per Medicaid recipient ($4,000–$4,999) and the highest amount ($9,000–$10,999). Most states spent between $5,000 and $8,999 per Medicaid recipient. There are no high-quality analyses of whether there are different health outcomes for different spending amounts; such analyses would necessarily depend on observational data in which health status of a state's population would be highly cofounded by its social, demographic, economic, and cultural characteristics.

Table 11.7. Total Medicaid and CHIP expenditures per recipient, by state, FY2014

Range of expenditures per beneficiary ($)	States
4,000–4,999	Alabama, Colorado, Florida, New Jersey, South Carolina
5,000–5,999	Arizona, California, Idaho, Louisiana, North Carolina, Oklahoma, South Dakota, Utah, Washington, West Virginia, Wisconsin
6,000–6,999	Arkansas, Hawaii, Iowa, Kansas, Kentucky, Michigan, Mississippi, Montana, North Carolina, Oregon, Tennessee, Texas, Wyoming
7,000–7,999	Indiana, Maine, New Hampshire, Ohio, Virginia
8,000–8,999	Connecticut, Maryland, Minnesota, Missouri, New York
9,000–11,999	Alaska, Delaware, District of Columbia, North Dakota, Pennsylvania

Source: Kaiser Family Foundation, "Data Note: Variation in Per Enrollee Medicaid Spending," June 2017, http://files.kff.org/attachment/Data-Note-Variation-in-Per-Enrollee-Medicaid-Spending-Across-States.

Medicaid Managed Care

From the beginnings of the Medicaid program, there has always been a struggle at both the federal and state levels to provide adequate financing, assure sufficient provider participation, and promote quality in the care provided. Moreover, the FFS financing mechanism under which Medicaid commenced was open-ended and often led to total expenses exceeding projections, causing state budget shortfalls. This phenomenon was exacerbated because of federally mandated eligibility expansion in the late 1980s and increased service intensity due to evolving medical technology. Subjecting Medicaid to managed care seemed like a good way to promote high-quality care while putting a brake on spending. Patients would be assigned to a primary care provider who would guide them through an appropriate care plan more efficiently. A prepaid, capitated approach would also put a cap on a state's Medicaid budget.

Initially, it was thought that substantial savings would readily occur in Medicaid from conversion to managed care, generalizing from the experience in commercial insurance. But this generalization was not straightforward. Providers who accepted Medicaid were already receiving markedly reduced fees and were reluctant to reduce them further. As well, Medicaid was providing financial support to sustain the financial viability of safety-net hospitals; extracting price reductions from these institutions might jeopardize their ability to continue their operations.

Despite these barriers, some states (Oregon, Tennessee, Hawaii, and Rhode Island) were in the vanguard and obtained waivers from CMS to develop strategies to convert the acute care part of their Medicaid program to a prepaid approach.[18] As the structure of these Medicaid managed health care plans evolved and showed some evidence of success, more states obtained federal waivers to experiment with a variety of models and arrangements. Across time, commercial plans increasingly entered the market and accepted risk through capitation from the state. By 2002, 58 percent of Medicaid beneficiaries were enrolled in some type of managed care program;[19] by July 2016, this figure increased to 81 percent—65 million of the total 80.2 million Medicaid beneficiaries.[20]

Like Medicare Advantage, which is essentially Medicare Managed Care, private health insurers will enter the market if the capitated payments paid by states to Medicaid Managed Care companies are greater than the medical expenses of their members plus the costs of program administration. The opportunity for profitability varies by state, depending on eligibility rules, medical risk of the population covered, rules of engagement with the state, and of course the state's capitated rates. Currently, the overall environment appears to be more attractive than it has in the past. Goldsmith, Mosley, and Jacobs cite a 2012 CitiGroup study of earnings before interest, taxes, depreciation, and amortization (EBITDA), a measure of profitability, for different types of health care coverage.[21] Using an EBITDA of $28 per member per month (PMPM) for a commercial insurance policy as a reference point, CitiGroup estimated that certain subgroups of Medicaid have a high EBITDA ($20 PMPM for the aged, blind, and disabled; $90 PMPM for dual-eligibles). The EBITDA for straight Medicaid was estimated to be $7 per member—not very high, but still a positive number and one that can be averaged in with the higher-EBITDA groups. In California during 2014 and 2015, for example, the first two years of the Affordable Care Act, Medicaid Managed Care contractors generated profits of $5.4 billion. Based on statutory filings of the National Association of Insurance Commissioners, Goldsmith, Mosley, and Jacobs also report a wide variation in plan administrative overhead and financial reserves, which may reflect inefficiencies in the program.

Summary

Medicaid was passed in 1965 in conjunction with Medicare as amendments to the Social Security Act of 1935. It was modeled after 1950 amendments to the Social Security Act, and the 1960 Kerr-Mills Act, which created state-administered programs to provide medical payments to the poor using matching funds from the federal government. These matching payments, called the Federal Medical Assistance Percentage, is calculated annually for each state based on a formula that adjusts for state per capita income and other factors.

Eligibility and benefits vary greatly across states, but Medicaid beneficiaries are mainly children, low-income seniors, low-income disabled people, pregnant women, and the parents of children who are below low-income thresholds. One in five Americans are covered by Medicaid and it is the principal source of coverage for long-term care in the nation. Almost half of Medicaid recipients are children and an additional quarter are disabled or over age 65.

Disproportionate share payments to hospitals treating a high proportion of low-income patients (some with Medicaid and some uninsured) have become an important source of funding for safety-net hospitals as a means of partly offsetting the cost of treating such patients. The amount of federal DSH and other supplemental payments varies widely across states. In 2016, three states received over half of the total supplemental payments nationally.

Beneficiary premiums and cost sharing, such as deductibles or co-payments, are very limited in Medicaid. Moreover, there is no trust fund for Medicaid based on payroll taxes or other dedicated revenue sources; rather, payments are made on a pay-as-you-go basis from federal and state general revenues. In an attempt to constrain costs without impacting quality, Medicaid Managed Care plans have evolved. In MMC plans, insurers receive capitated payments (per recipient per month) from states, and then contract with providers and hospitals to provide medical services, usually on a fee-for-service basis. There are wide variations across states in their MMC plans' administrative overhead, medical payments, profits, and reserves.

Medicare and Medicaid are now mature programs that have filled important gaps in access to health care for older adults, children, and the disabled. In 2010, however, there remained 50 million people without health insurance. This gap in access was associated with a tremendous level of discussion and debate about providing some form of health care coverage for this population, culminating in passage of the Patient Protection and Affordable Care Act in 2010 (chapter 12).

12 THE AFFORDABLE CARE ACT

Prior to enactment of the Patient Protection and Affordable Care Act (ACA for short) in 2010, a collection of interwoven stakeholders evolved over the course of a century to create a US health care industry with a fee-for-service, private health insurance backbone. This structure was working for a large majority of Americans. In 2010, the US population was 306.1 million, of which 256.2 million had some form of health insurance. But that left 49.9 million, or 16.3 percent, uninsured. Medicaid and Medicare had filled important gaps in access for children and for those over 64 years of age, but of the 192 million Americans between the ages of 19 and 64 in 2010, there were 42 million people, or 22 percent, who were uninsured.[1]

Because of the wide latitude among states in eligibility rules for Medicaid (chapter 10), significant variations in the rates of uninsured individuals were present, especially among individuals with low incomes. In 2010–11 the uninsured rate among individuals with incomes less than 200 percent of the federal poverty line (FPL) varied among states from 20 percent to 50 percent (figure 12.1). (Outliers beyond this range were Massachusetts at the low end and Texas at the high end.) There was less variation in uninsured rates for higher-income individuals (i.e., those with *greater than or equal to* 400 percent of the FPL—from about 5 percent to 10 percent). The high rate of uninsurance among individuals with limited income was one of the two primary motivations for the ACA; but just as with enactment of Medicare and Medicaid, passage of the ACA was a contentious political process. Although starting with a modicum of bipartisan support, the bill ultimately received no votes from Republicans and required procedural maneuvering in Congress by Democrats through the budget reconciliation process to become law. Steven Brill provides an interesting account of the process by which ACA became enacted into law.[2]

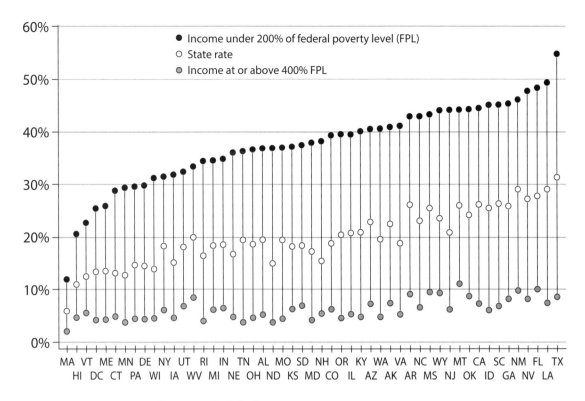

Figure 12.1. Percentage of uninsured adults by state, ages 19–64, 2010–2011. Cathy Schoen, David Radley, Pamela Riley, Jacob Lippa, Julia Berenson, Cara Dermody, and Anthony Shih, *Health Care in the Two Americas: Findings from the Scorecard on State Health System Performance for Low-Income Populations, 2013* (New York; Washington, DC: Commonwealth Fund, September 2013), Exhibit 7, https://www.commonwealthfund.org/publications/fund-reports/2013/sep/low-income-scorecard.

Basic Provisions of the Affordable Care Act

At the time of this writing in the winter of 2019, the constitutionality of the Affordable Care Act is under judicial review and may not survive the legal battles that are winding their way to the Supreme Court. Assuming that ACA survives more or less in its current form (which already incorporates a variety of restrictions to the original act), it will remain as far-reaching legislation that touches virtually all Americans through changes in the tax code, health insurance plan requirements, and other provisions.

Two key provisions of the ACA directed at reducing the number of Americans without health insurance are Medicaid expansion and the health care marketplace exchanges. Before addressing these two provisions, it should be noted that the ACA also affects existing insurance policies, whether obtained through an employer-sponsored group plan or purchased on the individual market. Specifically, the ACA calls for all insurance plans to cover adult children up to age 26; for insurers to spend at least 80 percent of premium dollars on medical expenses in individual and small-group plans, and 85 percent in large-group plans; for elimination of preexisting condition exclusions; and for elimination of annual and lifetime caps on coverage. In addition, a set of essential health benefits (EHB) are defined for new enrollees in all health insurance plans, as are maximum limits for out-of-pocket and deductible expenses.

Shown in table 12.1 are core provisions of the ACA pertaining to individual and employer mandates, health care marketplaces, Medicaid expansion, and dependent coverage. Table 12.2 lists core ACA provisions pertaining to insurers. A detailed but concisely stated summary of the entirety of the ACA's provisions has been published by the Kaiser Family Foundation.[3]

Table 12.1. Provisions of the Affordable Care Act: individual and employer mandates, health care marketplaces, and Medicaid expansion

Provision	Description
Individual mandate	Everyone not covered by an employer-sponsored health plan is required to buy insurance or pay a penalty (2.5% of taxable income in 2016).
Employer mandate	Employers with more than 50 full-time employees (>30 hours/week) must offer health insurance to more than 95% of employees.
Health care marketplaces	"Exchanges" established in all 50 states, administered by state or federal government.
Benefit tiers	Creates four benefit categories of plans (bronze, silver, gold, and platinum) with actuarial values of 50%, 70%, 80%, and 90% of the plan benefit costs. Out-of-pocket limits equal to health savings account limits, with reductions in limits according to income.
Subsidies	Households with incomes between 100% and 400% of the federal poverty line are eligible to receive federal subsidies (premium credits and cost-sharing subsidies) for policies purchased on an exchange.
Medicaid expansion	Expand Medicaid eligibility to children, pregnant women, parents, and adults without dependent children with incomes up to 133% of the federal poverty line.
Financing of Medicaid expansion	States receive federal funding to finance coverage of newly eligible Medicaid recipients: 100% in 2014, sliding to 90% in 2020 and subsequent years.

Source: "Summary of the Affordable Care Act," Kaiser Family Foundation.[3]

Table 12.2. Provisions of the Affordable Care Act: insurer responsibilities

Provision	Description
Guaranteed issue	Prohibits insurers from denying coverage because of preexisting conditions.
Community rating	Premiums must be the same for everyone of a given age.
Essential health benefits	A set of ten categories of health benefits must be provided consistent with that of a "typical employer plan." Also included are additional prevention services for women (existing policies can be exempted under grandfather rules).
Coverage caps	Bars annual and lifetime coverage caps on essential health benefits.
Fraction of premiums spent on medical care	Large group plans must spend at least 85% of premiums on medical expenses, and individual or small-group plans must spend at least 80%.
Medicaid expansion	Expand Medicaid eligibility to children, pregnant women, parents, and adults without dependent children with incomes up to 133% of the federal poverty line.

Source: "Summary of the Affordable Care Act," Kaiser Family Foundation.[3]

In terms of improving the balance of care, cost, and access, a key goal of the ACA was to increase access (i.e., reduce the uninsured rate) while ensuring high quality, comprehensive health benefits without adding to government budget deficits. It is pertinent to document at the outset the net effect of the ACA on the goal of reducing the number of Americans without health insurance. Historically, there was a significant decline in the uninsured rate in the United States that occurred after the implementation of Medicare and Medicaid, from almost 25 percent prior to 1965 to a low of about 12 percent in the 1970s. Between 1990 and implementation of the ACA, the uninsured rate was in the range of 14–16 percent. After implementation of the ACA, the uninsured rate declined to 8.6 percent in 2015,[4] reached a low of 7.9 percent in 2017, and increased to 8.5 percent in 2018.[5] It is likely that the uninsured rate will continue to inch up because of a variety of developments since the ACA was first implemented. These include the Supreme Court decision that made Medicaid expansion optional for states and various recent legislative actions and regulatory decisions that have undone many of the ACA's central provisions.

In addition to improving access, a second principal goal of the ACA was to constrain spiraling expenditures. The rate of growth in health care spending in the United States has indeed slowed since enactment of the ACA, but it is not clear that this "bending of the cost curve" can be attributed to the ACA. The effects of the 2008–2009 recession on the gross domestic product and prices no doubt played a significant role, as did the shifting of health care costs from employer to employee with the greater use of high deductible health plans and increased co-pays and coinsurance rates. Other provisions of the ACA intended to bend the cost curve are works in progress: Bundling of doctor-hospital payments by Medicare and other innovations are beginning to have some effect, but major ACA initiatives such as accountable care organizations, the Merit-based Incentive Payment System (MIPS) and advanced alternative payment models (APMs) (chapter 10) have yet to impact net expenditures favorably. Moreover, scheduled reductions in many of the payments to hospitals and physicians (e.g., the reduction in Disproportionate Share Hospital payments that were supposed to occur in conjunction with Medicaid expansion) have not yet been implemented.

Key Health Insurance Provisions under the Affordable Care Act

Coverage of adult children up to age 26, establishment of essential health benefits, and elimination of exclusions for preexisting conditions are key provisions of the ACA that affect existing health insurance policies, whether obtained through an employer-sponsored group plan or purchased on the individual market.

Coverage of Dependents below the Age of 26

Before the ACA, most health insurers could remove children over 18 from their parents' coverage because of their legal age as adults, regardless of whether they were a student or where they lived. Of the 49.9 million people without health insurance in 2010, 8.8 million were between the ages of 19 and 25.[6] Through the ACA, this demographic is now covered under parents' policies if parents have health insurance. Prior to the ACA, if these young adults were working at an entry-level job that didn't provide health insurance or had recently graduated from a college where they were covered by the student health service, the cost of an individual health care policy was typically unaffordable. Coverage under a parent's policy means that a young adult and the parent no longer have to worry about unanticipated medical expenses. In 2017, the number of 19-to-25-year-olds without health insurance dropped to 4.3 million, a reduction by about half.[7]

Essential Health Benefits

EHBs, which represent a floor on the benefit package for all ACA-compliant insurance policies, are becoming increasingly applicable to virtually all preexisting insurance policies as they evolve. To say that 16 percent of the population did not have health insurance coverage in 2010 is not to say that 84 percent had comprehensive or even adequate coverage. While Medicare and Medicaid have specific coverage provisions that are typically quite broad, many of the plans on the individual market, and some in the group market, had limited coverage. For example, only 12 percent of policies on the individual market covered maternity care.[8] Many plans did not cover preventive screenings, mental health and substance abuse services, or rehabilitative services and had limited formularies for prescription drugs.

In attempting to help with the "care" part of the care, cost, and access balance, health insurance plans under ACA must cover 10 categories of essential health benefits (box 12.1); however, the legislative language did not establish a single, nationally uniform package of health services. The Secretary of the Department of Health and Human Services (HHS) was given broad latitude in defining and implementing EHBs under the law. The Institute of Medicine

---

Box 12.1. Essential health benefits under the Affordable Care Act

---

- Ambulatory patient services, including hospital outpatient and physician services
- Emergency services
- Hospitalization (inpatient care)
- Maternity and newborn care
- Mental health and substance use disorder services, including behavioral health treatment
- Prescription drugs
- Rehabilitative and habilitative services and devices
- Laboratory tests
- Preventive and wellness services and chronic disease management
- Pediatric services, including oral and vision care

(now the National Academy of Medicine) was asked to assemble the Committee on Defining and Revising an Essential Health Benefits Package for Qualified Health Plans, which gathered extensive public input and analyzed data from a variety of sources. Its report provided guidance to the HHS Secretary on the critical issue of how to balance the comprehensiveness of benefits against cost. The committee's solution: "Build on what currently exists, learn over time, and make it better. That is, the initial EHB should be a modification of what small employers are currently offering. All stakeholders should then learn enough over time—during implementation and through experimentation and research—to improve the package."[9]

Most states have indeed used a small employer plan as the benchmark for EHB. In February 2013, HHS finalized its policies regarding EHB, in which the secretary gave broad discretion to the states in choosing an EHB benchmark from among 10 different types of state or federal health insurance plans. Nineteen of 24 states chose a small group plan that was already operating in their state, and the remaining 26 states were defaulted to a small group plan.[10] As would be expected, while this approach was well received by state officials and insurers, some consumer and provider groups were disappointed that the EHBs did not replicate the more comprehensive benefits of some large group plans.[11]

At the start of the ACA in 2010, many existing group and individual plans obtained "grandfather" status, which allowed them to be exempt from the provisions for preexisting conditions and essential health benefits, so long as individuals remained in the same plan. It is anticipated that fewer and fewer plans will retain grandfather status across time as they evolve. New federal rules under the present administration, however, allow association health plans and short-term limited duration plans to circumvent essential health benefits and guaranteed issue.

Guaranteed Issue

Of all the provisions of the ACA, guaranteed issue has had the most profound impact on the private health insurance industry, which, along with Medicaid expansion, comprise the backbone of the ACA coverage mechanisms. The details of how guaranteed issue impacts overall health insurance premiums and their affordability will be discussed later in the context of the individual mandate, but it is important to recognize that prior to the ACA, private insurers used underwriting to shape the health insurance risk pool to meet the competitive premium they were offering in the market. By not covering an array of preexisting conditions, premiums could be kept down and medical management by the insurer created a performance efficiency safety net. Underwriting was a key part of the actuarial process of insurers and profoundly impacted benefit design and coverage. After the ACA, underwriting limits for preexisting conditions were eliminated. This meant that insurers had to rethink and retool their approach to policy and benefit design as well as medical management.

Another impact of guaranteed issue was the rise in premiums for some individuals. Prior to the ACA, underwriting exclusions for people with preexisting conditions meant that the private insurance risk pool was artificially low when compared to the risk in the general population. That meant the healthy did not need to bear the burden of sharing risk with those who had significant illness. Once the risk pool was rebalanced to reflect the risk of the entire population and had the EHB requirements covered, premiums did go up for healthy people to reflect the actual risk in the population. The artificially low rates for healthy pools were gone and many were angry. This was a moral judgment and a key provision of the ACA.

Health Care Marketplace Exchanges

As noted, the combination of employer-based health insurance (including government and military employers), Medicare, and Medicaid provided health care coverage for 84 percent of the population in 2010. This left 16 percent, or 50 million people, uninsured. Under the ACA, about 5 million individuals younger than age 26 were covered as dependents, leaving about 45 million Americans uninsured. For those who were below 133 percent of the federal poverty line (about half), the ACA intended to provide health care coverage through Medicaid expansion. The other half had incomes above 133 percent of the FPL, but they were either self-employed and did not purchase health insurance, worked for employers that did not offer health insurance, or were offered employer-sponsored insurance but declined because of cost or other considerations.

The health care marketplace exchanges, which began in 2014, were designed to create a market environment in which private insurers offer insurance coverage with means-based subsidies funded by the federal government. These subsidies are provided according to a sliding scale. In Medicaid expansion states, the sliding scale begins with a generous subsidy at 138 percent of the FPL but is reduced to zero subsidy at 400 percent of the FPL. In nonexpansion states, the subsidy begins at 100 percent of the FPL. By way of example, in 2018, the FPL was $12,140 for an individual and $25,100 for a family of four (return to table 11.2 for reference). For a family of four with an income ranging from $30,000 to $90,000, the bronze plan has a lower monthly premium (for families with annual incomes of $30,000 or $60,000, the family cost is zero) (table 12.3), but the deductible is higher. In 2018, 11.8 million individuals purchased health insurance on the exchanges.[12]

To accomplish the goal of facilitating a private health insurance marketplace in which comprehensive yet affordable health insurance could be provided to uninsured individuals whose family incomes are between 100 percent and 400 percent of the FPL, designers of the ACA relied on four pillars:

1. Individual mandate: everyone not covered by an employer-sponsored plan must buy health insurance or pay a penalty.
2. Guaranteed issue: insurers are prohibited from denying coverage or raising premiums based on preexisting conditions.
3. Community rating: premiums must be the same for everyone of a given age (and tobacco use), regardless of health status.
4. Premium subsidies: makes health insurance affordable for those with limited incomes.

These four provisions are interrelated. In order for the health care marketplaces to function effectively, they must all be in force. ACA marketplaces function less effectively when these provisions are eliminated or diluted through legislation, court decisions, and regulatory pronouncements.

Table 12.3. Illustrative health care marketplace insurance policies for a family of four with two adults age 40 and two children, US average, 2018 plans

| | Silver Plan | | | | Bronze Plan | | |
| | Monthly premium cost ($) | | | Out-of-pocket annual limit | Monthly premium cost ($) | | |
Income ($)[a]	Total	Family	Subsidy		Total	Family	Subsidy
30,000	1,529	52	1,477	2.8% of income	1,088	0	1,088
60,000	1,529	398	1,131	7.96% of income	1,088	0	1,088
90,000	1,529	740	790	$7,900	1,088	298	790

Source: "Health Insurance Marketplace Calculator," Kaiser Family Foundation, accessed March 29, 2019, https://www.kff.org/interactive/subsidy-calculator.
[a] Modified adjusted gross income as reported on federal tax returns, which includes adjusted gross income, tax-exempt interest, untaxed foreign income, and nontaxable Social Security benefits.

Rationale for Individual Mandate, Guaranteed Issue, and Community Rating

To understand how the individual mandate works in lockstep with guaranteed issue and community rating, we will review the history of the mandate and explain why it was designed to work together with guaranteed issue and community rating to prevent adverse selection.

The idea of an individual mandate for the uninsured can be traced to 1989 when Stuart Butler, then director of domestic policy studies at the Heritage Foundation, proposed it as part of a proposal for national health care. In what Butler described as the Heritage Plan, all households would be mandated to obtain health insurance protection. Using a rationale that first draws analogies to mandating that passengers in automobiles wear seatbelts and the requirement that anybody driving an automobile must have liability insurance, Butler then states that, by contrast, "neither the federal government nor any state requires all households to protect themselves from the potentially catastrophic costs of a serious accident or illness. Under the Heritage Plan, there would be such a requirement."[13]

According to the Heritage Plan, based on a subsequent conference lecture given by Butler on the same topic, "We would include a mandate in our proposal—not a mandate on employers, but a mandate on heads of households—to obtain at least a basic package of health insurance for themselves and their families. That would have to include, by federal law, a catastrophic provision in the form of a stop loss for a family's total health outlays. It would have to include all members of the family, and it might also include certain very specific services, such as preventive care, well baby visits, and other items."[14] (In a very different political environment, Butler later asserted that his version of a health insurance mandate is different from that in the ACA, and he points to certain distinctions.[15] An opinion piece in the *Wall Street Journal* two days later refers to these distinctions as "hair-splitting" and expresses the view that the fundamental concept of the mandate under ACA is the same as the one advocated by Butler in 1989.[16] The reader can be the judge.)

Thus, the concept of a mandate for health insurance was, not long ago, endorsed as a critical building block across the political spectrum. And for good reason: the basis for a health insurance system that includes both an individual mandate and community rating is rooted in the fundamental concept of insurance as a means of spreading risk among a large number of individuals with varying risk profiles. An individual buys insurance to cover the risk that health care services will be needed, the probability of which is largely unknown. If a large number of such individuals each contribute a (relatively) small premium to a financial pool, then the cost of any one individual's emergency or unanticipated illness can be covered by drawing from the pooled premiums. The greater the number of individuals who contribute to the pool, and the more representative they are of a cross-section of the general population in terms of health risk, the more efficient the system becomes in creating an "average" premium that would be affordable by all members of the pool.

If the healthiest members of the pool are allowed to opt out, however, or are encouraged to purchase a carved-out policy with a low premium designed for healthy people, adverse selection occurs and the individuals remaining in the pool are then faced with higher premiums. To drive this point home, let's consider the actuarial arithmetic behind premium calculations. Across the entire insured population in a community, some individuals will have a higher baseline risk for needing medical services than others, based on medical history and other factors. The premium calculation under "community rating" is determined by taking into account the *total risk of an entire insured population*—including those who are unlikely to use health care services as well as those who are highly likely—and the total anticipated cost of such care. This premium will be higher if a broad array of health services are covered, and lower if the list of covered services is more restricted. The premium will also be higher if the deductible and co-pays are low (as this will increase utilization), and vice versa.

By contrast, under "experience rating," which has been a staple of commercial insurance plans but in which the Blue Cross Blue Shield plans have also participated for many years in the commercial market, premiums and other costs are not the same for individuals with different health risks. The cost of health insurance under experience rating will be based on the actuarially estimated cost of health care for people of different risk groups, based on their historical experience. It will be higher for older people, women of reproductive age, individuals with preexisting conditions or greater genetic risks, and so on. A young person with no significant medical history will be able to purchase insurance at low cost. An individual with chronic disease, or someone with a recent diagnosis of cancer who has a chance of recurrence, will be faced with a higher total cost of health insurance. Under experience rating, many plans in the past have denied coverage to those with preexisting medical conditions, or have set a premium for individuals with preexisting conditions that is so high as to be unaffordable.

With this as background, let's now do a thought experiment in which the premium that had been paid to an insurer by an employer for individual or family coverage under a community-rated group plan is instead paid to the employee. (This hypothetical example doesn't take into account that health insurance premiums paid by the employer aren't taxed, while such payments to employees as cash would be taxed. But let that nuance ride for the sake of the thought experiment.) Let's also assume that the plan is in actuarial equilibrium such that the premiums and other expenditures that employees and employers pay into the plan are exactly offset by the cost of care provided and the cost of administering the plan.

Now let's suppose that the employer has designed different plans for different kinds of employees and that employees could choose plans that seem "right for them" or not choose a plan at all. Thus, young, healthy employees might choose a plan with a restricted set of covered benefits, very low premiums, and a high deductible and pocket the difference if they use little or no medical care. Or they might pocket the entire amount provided by their employer and not purchase insurance at all. Older individuals with known chronic medical conditions requiring frequent physician visits and expensive medications would prefer a plan with a broad range of covered benefits and a low deductible.

What would happen under such a scenario? The employer would now be able to offer very low-cost plans to their young, healthy employees, but this would generate a very small amount of premium revenues. To remain in financial equilibrium, the same *total* premium revenues that were previously received under the group plan would still be needed to cover the health care costs of *all* employees, including those with significant illnesses. Such employees would therefore have to be charged a much higher premium to make up the difference. Depending on the extent and cost of the projected health care for these employees, the premium might be several multiples of the cash payment for health insurance received from their employer. To the extent that employees are divided into smaller and smaller subgroups according to health risk, the premiums for employees with the greatest health care costs would escalate significantly. In effect, the more refined this process becomes—in terms of subdividing employees into a large number of well-defined, health risk strata—the less this looks like insurance and the more it looks like paying directly for health care.

The above scenario describes what might happen at the extreme to illustrate the underlying forces at work. What *actually* happens depends upon behavioral factors having to do with the value people attach to having a comprehensive health insurance plan even if they do not have a significant medical history, the size of the penalty, and other considerations.[17] If there are few departures of individuals from the exchanges when given the opportunity, the exchanges should remain intact; if there are large numbers who leave the exchange plans, then premiums will rise dramatically and the viability of the exchanges will be tenuous.

Implications of Individual Mandate Penalty Repeal

The individual mandate provision of the ACA states that everyone not covered by an employer-sponsored health insurance plan is required to buy insurance or pay a penalty. In 2018, the penalty was $695 per adult (plus $347.50 per child under 18), up to a total of $2,085 or 2.5 percent of family income, whichever is greater. Hardship exclusions could be claimed based on low income or a high percent of family income that would be consumed by the lowest-priced insurance plan. In 2015, the last year for which IRS released data, 12 million tax filers claimed a hardship exemption and 6.7 million tax filers paid the penalty.[18] The average penalty was $462. Some health economists have expressed the view that these penalties were inadequate (i.e., much lower than other countries that have insurance-based national health insurance, such as Germany or Switzerland, and less strictly enforced).[19]

As of December 22, 2017, when the Tax Cut and Jobs Act of 2017 was signed into law, this issue became moot since the penalty associated with the insurance mandate was eliminated. As a consequence of the mandate penalty repeal, the discussion here so far suggests that the exchange premiums will increase and, potentially, cause a spiraling exodus from the plan. On the other hand, it may be that most of the people who would choose not to purchase insurance on the exchange have already made this decision and paid the penalty. A 2018 poll found that the mandate penalty ranks low as a reason for buying individual insurance: the major reasons for doing so were protection against high medical bills (75 percent), peace of mind (66 percent) or because a family member has an ongoing health condition (41 percent).[20] As well, among these individuals who buy individual insurance, the fact that government can provide financial help was endorsed as a major reason by 35 percent of those polled.

Some opponents of the ACA have argued that elimination of the penalty essentially "repeals" the individual mandate and thus disables the entire ACA, even though much of the ACA has little to do with the mandate and the exchanges can operate without it. On December 18, 2019, in a 2-to-1 majority opinion the Fifth Disrict Court of Appeals concluded that the mandate is unconstitutional if it doesn't raise money but did not rule on whether the mandate can be severed from the rest of the law.[21] Rather, the court just sent the severance issue back down to the lower court. This legal wrangling will likely take some time to wind through the courts and may ultimately be decided by the Supreme Court. One possibility is a final ruling that the mandate is unconsititutional but can be severed from the rest of the ACA. In that case, the other provisions of the ACA (such as Medicaid expansion, parental coverage from ages 19–26, essential health benefits, coverage despite preexisting conditions, the ban on lifetime caps, etc.) will remain. But there will clearly be a major upheaval if it is ruled that the mandate cannot be severed from the rest of the ACA, thus making the entire law unconstitutional.

Implications of New Regulatory Rules Regarding Association Health Plans and Short-Term Limited Duration Plans

In addition to the elimination of the individual mandate penalty, two 2018 federal regulations are presenting challenges to the ACA exchanges: the final rules for association health plans (AHP)[22] and for short-term limited duration (STLD) plans.[23] These rules authorize the sale of health insurance policies that are exempt from many of the consumer protections included in the ACA's guaranteed issue and community rating provisions. The final AHP rule states that it is expected that "a substantial number of uninsured people will enroll in AHPs because . . . the coverage will be more affordable than what would otherwise be available to them, and other people who currently have coverage will replace it with AHP coverage because the AHP coverage will be more affordable or better suit their needs."[24] AHP and STLD plans are now being offered by virtually all of the major health insurance companies.

It may very well better suit the needs of a young healthy male to purchase an AHP without maternity care coverage at a lower premium than would be available on the health care exchanges. But such decisions many times over will induce adverse selection for the exchanges. The AHP and

STLD plans provide lower monthly premiums for healthy individuals, but they do so by excluding the coverage of people with preexisting conditions; charging higher premiums based on age, gender, medical history, and other personal characteristics; covering a more restricted set of health benefits that can exclude maternity care, prescription drugs, and mental or behavioral health conditions, among others; require higher out-of-pocket cost sharing; and curtail coverage once claims reach an annual or lifetime cap set by the insurer. In general, the departures from ACA rules are greater under the STLD plans than the AHPs. The STLD plans can be renewed or extended for up to 36 months, but the insurer can simply not renew a member at the end of a short-term contract at the insurer's discretion based on medical utilization or other factors.

A recent study of existing STLDs nationally found that 0 percent of plans covered maternity care, 29 percent covered outpatient prescription drugs, and 38 percent covered treatment for opioid abuse or other substance abuse.[25] While monthly premiums are often considerably lower than the ACA exchange plans, especially for young, healthy people, the STLD plans have out-of-pocket maximums as high as $20,000–$30,000. According to data from the National Association of Insurance Commissioners, the three largest insurers offering STLD plans had "medical loss ratios" (i.e., the percent of total premium revenue spent on medical care) of 34 to 52 percent,[26] well below the 80 percent required for small group plans under ACA. Thus, such plans appear to be highly profitable.

Other recent federal actions also potentially undermine stability of the ACA exchanges. For example, the open enrollment period has been shortened and budgets for outreach and enrollment efforts have been reduced, including budget cuts to ACA Navigator organizations.

During 2018, cost-sharing subsidies to insurers by the federal government were terminated, so premiums were increased to offset this loss of revenue. This should be a one-time effect. Although the premium increase was passed on to enrollees, those receiving income-based subsidies saw their subsidy payments increase as well, restraining departures from the exchanges.

Despite these challenges, there is some evidence for improving stability in the individual market based on a study of the market environment in 10 states (seven with federal exchanges, two with state-run exchanges, and one hybrid).[27] Based upon detailed analyses of financial and enrollment data, as well as interviews with market participants and regulators, it was concluded that: (1) enrollment was strong in the ACA's subsidized exchanges, despite sharp cuts in the open enrollment period and in federal funds for marketing and enrollee navigation; and (2) state-operated exchanges had somewhat stronger enrollment and lower premiums; and (3) geographic gaps in coverage are being filled as insurers become more profitable.

The Congressional Budget Office (CBO) estimates that repeal of the mandate penalty will cause a decrease in enrollment in the nongroup health insurance market by 3 million in 2019.[28] However, Kaiser Family Foundation polling focused on behavioral factors suggests that the effect of the mandate penalty may be more muted,[29] as does another analysis that focuses on premium subsidies, state market reforms, mandate exemptions, and other factors.[30] A study from the Commonwealth Fund of the role of behavioral factors on the effect of eliminating the individual mandate projects a wide range of outcomes under different assumptions, with estimated declines in insured persons ranging from 2.8 to 13 million people when the mandate is eliminated, and a shift to the cheapest plan with the lowest actuarial value ranging from 3 to 13 percent.[31] In the 10-state study discussed earlier, the "dominant" view among market participants and regulators is that the adverse effect of the mandate penalty repeal will be less than originally thought due to two considerations: (1) in comparison to the cost of insurance, the mandate penalty was quite small to begin with; and (2) even without a mandate, demand for ACA exchange products is largely motivated by the fact that most of the exchange enrollees receive substantial subsidies.[32]

The CBO estimate and the studies cited do not take into account the effects of AHPs and STLD plans. On balance, the combined effects of repealing the individual mandate penalty, allowing AHPs and STLD plans to market and sell policies without ACA consumer safeguards, and continuing efforts to create obstacles to exchange enrollment, are likely to reduce enrollment and pose significant challenges to the stability of the ACA-compliant individual markets. While data from 2018 suggested some stability, with insurers having their most profitable year yet on ACA exchanges,[33] a gap is developing between those on the exchanges who are and are not subsidized; the former is growing and the latter is declining sharply. Between 2016 and 2018, the ACA marketplaces reported an enrollment drop of 2.5 million in unsubsidized individuals (who are not shielded from premium increases), an average drop of 24 percent.[34] Those receiving subsidies increased enrollment by 4 percent during this period. About 87 percent of those on the exhanges receive a subsidy.

Reduction in Number of Health Plans Participating in the ACA Health Care Marketplace

A number of the legal and policy decisions discussed above have fundamentally changed the structure and operation of the ACA exchanges. Repeal of the mandate, promotion of AHPs and STLD plans, cancellation of payments to insurers for cost-sharing subsidies, reduction in marketing budgets during open enrollment periods, and the temporary freezing of risk-adjustment payments have, collectively, led to many insurance companies exiting the ACA marketplace. The number of counties and percent of US population having a choice of at least three marketplace insurers was relatively stable in 2015 and 2016 (80 percent of counties and 93 percent of population), but in 2017 these figures fell precipitously (36 percent of counties and 60 percent of population).[35] By 2018, 30 percent of counties and almost 20 percent of the population had only one marketplace insurer. Counties with limited insurer competition tended to be those that were rural, had a high mortality rate, had greater retained insurer earnings (i.e., a low "medical loss ratio"), and were located in states that did not expand Medicaid.[36] The concentration of market power by a single insurer has the potential to adversely affect cost, the scope of medical coverage, and the quality of care.

Role of the ACA Exchanges in Solidifying the Basic Structure of the US Health Care Industry

While the various professional societies and other interest groups who lobbied on behalf of doctors, hospitals, insurance companies, and pharmaceutical companies were not happy with all of the provisions of the ACA, they and other stakeholder groups favored the ACA at the time of its passage. In ways that were even more fundamental than Medicaid and Medicare, ACA's exchanges solidified the essential elements of the US health care industry: a fee-for-service infrastructure with a transactional, claims-based, private health insurance backbone. All of the intrinsic forces putting upward pressure on both price and quantity that were described in chapters 2 through 6 are fortified under the ACA exchanges, as is the private health insurance infrastructure as described in chapters 8 and 9. These forces will be exacerbated in geographic areas where there is only a single insurer that can exert monopoly power. The ability to incentivize prevention, early diagnosis, and lower-cost ambulatory care is essentially absent under the exchanges.

And the increasing entry of AHPs and STLD plans into allowable nongroup health insurance allows further exploitation of the intrinsic imperfections in health care markets. Of course, if the ACA marketplaces are found to be unconstitutional in the absence of a penalty for ignoring the mandate to purchase insurance, these exchanges will disappear entirely.

Medicaid Expansion

In the original design of the ACA, it was anticipated that uninsured individuals above a specified family income threshold—about half of the total—would gain access to health insurance through the exchanges, while the remaining half with lower incomes would gain access by expanding the Medicaid program to include them. With regards to Medicaid expansion, it was anticipated that there would be a national standard in which anyone with income up to 138 percent of the federal poverty level could qualify.

The expectation of a national Medicaid expansion ended on June 28, 2012, when the Supreme Court ruled that states could opt out of the Medicaid expansion provision of the ACA. Initially, it was expected that only a few states would opt out, since the federal government would pay for 100 percent of the cost of newly eligible enrollees initially, with a glide path down to 90 percent by 2020 and thereafter. At the present time, Medicaid expansion has been adopted by 36 states and the District of Columbia (figure 12.2). This includes Idaho, Nebraska, and Utah, where voters approved ballot initiatives in November 2019 to expand Medicaid for adults with incomes up to 138 percent of the FPL. These voter-approved initiatives have not been implemented by the legislatures in these states.

The lack of nationwide Medicaid expansion led the CBO to reduce its projections regarding the impact of ACA on the percentage of uninsured adults 19–64 years of age. This rate was initially projected to decline from 18.2 percent prior to ACA to 7.6 percent in 2016, but was adjusted upward to 9.3 percent for 2016 to account for states not expanding Medicaid (figure 12.3). This adjusted projection turned out to be only about 1 percent shy of the actual 2016 figure.

Besides an overall dampening of the impact of ACA on uninsured rates nationally, the decision by some states not to expand Medicaid has led to marked differences in access between states. For the years 2013–2017, there was a 9.3 percent decline in rates of uninsured among individuals 19–64 years old living in expansion states, as compared to a 3.7 percent decline

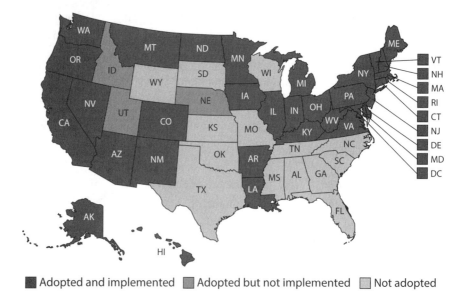

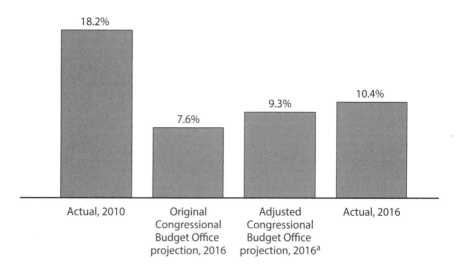

■ Adopted and implemented ■ Adopted but not implemented ☐ Not adopted

Figure 12.2. Status of state action on the Medicaid expansion decision, as of November 2019. "Status of State Medicaid Expansion Decisions: Interactive Map," Kaiser Family Foundation, last updated November 15, 2019, https://www.kff.org /medicaid/issue-brief/status-of-state-medicaid-expansion-decisions-interactive-map.

Figure 12.3. Uninsured rate for adults, 19–64 years of age. Aviva Aron-Dine, "CBO Correctly Predicted Historic Coverage Gains under ACA," *Off the Charts* (blog), Center on Budget and Policy Priorities, May 30, 2017, https://www.cbpp.org/blog/cbo-correctly -predicted-historic-coverage-gains-under-aca. [a] Congressional Budget Office projections adjusted for state decisions not to expand Medicaid.

in nonexpansion states.[37] Moreover, at any given starting rate of uninsured in 2013, states that expanded Medicaid had a greater rate of reduction in the statewide uninsured rate.[38]

Downward pressure on Medicaid enrollment—for both traditional and expansion programs—is emanating from the current HHS administration, which is encouraging states to apply for waivers that place new conditions on Medicaid eligibility as well as additional costs on beneficiaries in the form of premiums and co-payments at the point of service. With oversight from the Centers for Medicare and Medicaid Services (CMS), states are granted significant flexibility in how they run their Medicaid programs. Under a provision of the Social Security Act, Section 1115, the US Secretary of HHS can waive federal guidelines on Medicaid to allow states to pilot and evaluate innovative approaches to serving beneficiaries. Most waivers are granted by CMS for a limited period and can be withdrawn once they expire.

In November 2017, CMS posted revised criteria for Section 1115 waivers that, in contrast to previous administrations, did not include as a goal to "increase and strengthen overall coverage of low-income individuals in the state." In January 2018, additional guidance was posted that allowed waiver proposals to include a work requirement for Medicaid beneficiaries, which had never previously been approved.[39] According to the Medicaid Waiver Tracker of the Henry J. Kaiser Family Foundation, as of December 2019, five states have CMS-approved work requirements and the approvals for six more are pending.[40] The typical requirement is 80 hours per month. Thus far, available data contradict claims that people who lose Medicaid because of work requirements find jobs. Only a small fraction of these individuals find work—usually part-time without employee health insurance—and the vast majority become uninsured.[41] Other constraints on Medicaid enrollment include 15 states with approved and pending waivers for eligibility and enrollment restrictions, and 13 states with approved and pending waivers for benefit restrictions and imposition of co-pays and healthy behavior requirements.

States that have expanded Medicaid have incorporated newly enrolled patients into existing state Medicaid infrastructure, which has increasingly moved to Medicaid Managed Care (chapter 10). Since such managed care contracts for Medicaid patients are with private health insurers, Medicaid expansion has, like the exchanges, increased the prevalence of private health insurance in both employer-sponsored and government-sponsored health care programs.

Affordable Care Act Costs and Revenues

It is noteworthy that the Affordable Care Act includes the word "affordable" as the adjective modifying the word "care." One might guess there were two intended meanings: one related to the affordability of coverage to enrollees, whether through the exchanges or Medicaid expansion, and the other related to the overall affordability of the program to the nation. Regarding the latter meaning, the Congressional Budget Office made initial projections of the effects of the ACA on the federal budget deficit based on a series of assumptions regarding both revenues and costs.[42]

The cost of the ACA's expansion of coverage to the uninsured, standardization of essential health benefits, and other provisions were projected to be partly offset through reductions in existing payments: these included reductions in Medicare payments to physicians, hospitals, Medicare Advantage Plans, and drug companies as well as reductions in payments under the Disproportionate Share Hospital and upper payment limit programs as Medicaid expansion was implemented. In addition, there were projected increased revenues to pay for the ACA from higher payroll taxes paid by individuals with incomes exceeding $200,000 and married couples filing jointly with incomes exceeding $250,000 (an increase of 0.9 percent), as well as a 3.8 percent tax on net investment income for those exceeding these income thresholds. A variety of excise taxes on drug companies, medical devices, and "Cadillac" employer plans were also levied. Overall, projected revenues reported by the CBO in March 2010, and again in February 2011, exceeded projected expenses.

As explained in CBO materials, it is evidently not straightforward to determine the actual streams of revenues and costs that have actually occurred, because inflows and outflows related to many provisions of the ACA are embedded in overall categories of the federal budget, such as Medicare, and aren't carved out to be tracked separately.[43] In this respect, the CBO explains that the ACA is no different from any other legislation. As a measure of whether costs and/or revenues are in line with projections, the CBO *can* assess specific components of the ACA. For example, the projected federal subsidies for newly insured individuals through ACA (i.e., through Medicaid expansion or the exchanges) tracked the actual subsidies quite well for 2014 and 2015, and overestimated actual subsidies in 2016.[44] These projections would result in a greater reduction in the federal budget deficit for the years 2012–2019 than the amount forecasted (table 12.4). Most of

Table 12.4. Estimated budgetary effects of the enactment of the Afforable Care Act from the Congressional Budget Office, 2012–2019

	March 2010 estimate ($ billions)	February 2011 estimate ($ billions)
Insurance coverage provisions		
Gross cost	931	1,390
Net cost	778	1,042
Other provisions affecting direct spending	−498	−732
Other provisions affecting revenues	−412	−520
Net effect on federal budget deficit	−132	−210

Source: Adapted from Douglas W. Elmendorf, "CBO's Analysis of the Major Health Care Legislation Enacted in March 2010," testimony before the Subcommittee on Health, Committee on Energy and Commerce, US House of Representatives, March 30, 2011, https://www.cbo.gov/sites/default/files/03-30-healthcarelegislation.pdf.

this improvement was due to an overprojection in the cost of the ACA related to health care exchanges; Medicaid expansion projections were essentially on track.

Summary

Enactment of Medicare and Medicaid in 1965 led to a reduction in the percentage of uninsured Americans from 25 percent to 16 percent. Despite numerous challenges in the course of its implementation, enactment of the Affordable Care Act led to a further reduction in the rate of uninsured individuals to 9 percent in 2017. This was done by covering dependents up to the age of 26 on existing insurance policies, expanding Medicaid to cover adults with family incomes up to 138 percent of the federal poverty line, and establishing health care marketplaces, or "exchanges," in which private insurance companies offer coverage with subsidized premiums for families whose incomes are less than 400 percent of the FPL. The reduction in uninsured rates was constrained by the Supreme Court decision to allow states to opt out of Medicaid expansion; at present 14 states continue to opt out. Enrolling uninsured people who are currently eligible for coverage under Medicaid expansion, or for premium subsidies on the ACA exchanges, would further reduce the uninsured rate by one third.

The costs of ACA were designed to be offset by a group of spending reductions and revenue enhancements that were projected by the CBO to reduce the federal budget deficit. Streams of costs and revenues associated with ACA have not been carved out of the federal budget, so it is difficult to assess the net actual effect of ACA on the federal deficit, but available data track the projections reasonably well.

It is possible that the judicial branch of government will decide that the entire ACA is unconstitutional in the absence of a penalty for ignoring the health insurance mandate. It is also possible that the exchanges alone will be ruled unconstitutional, leaving the rest of the ACA in place. Even if the exchanges were ultimately found to be consititutional, several foundational provisions of the exchanges have already been eliminated or weakened. In addition to the destabilizing impact of eliminating the individual mandate penalty, the beneficial effects of the ACA's bans on excluding preexisting conditions and annual/lifetime caps, its requirement to charge uniform premiums for individuals of a given age, and its financial model have been diluted by new federal rules, relaxed medical loss ratios under certain types of high-deductible insurance products, and reductions in resources devoted to enrollment. Recent data indicate a reversal of the downward trend in uninsured rates.

PART III
CONTEMPORARY ENVIRONMENT

13 EVIDENCE-BASED PRACTICE

Ideally, people should receive health care that is known to work and not receive care that doesn't work. Physicians and other providers who help their patients follow this dictum are providing care according to evidence-based practice. In an ideal world, to the extent that there *is* benefit from the care provided, it should also be the case that the amount of benefit should justify its cost.

In a perfect market, the consumption of health care that is known to be effective at a price that justifies the benefit would occur automatically through the "invisible hand" of Adam Smith (chapter 2). Individuals with a particular illness would have perfect knowledge about the effectiveness of a recommended treatment. They would know if it is effective compared to doing nothing and if it is more effective than an existing treatment that might cost a lot less. If the recommended treatment is known to be effective, they would also know the *amount* of benefit that can be expected (e.g., reduction in pain, improvement in mobility, reduction in anxiety, extension of life) and the capabilities of the doctor and hospital in delivering that amount of benefit. And finally, they would know the exact price (total cost) of the entire episode of treatment, which had been determined in the market by a large number of people with the same illness interacting with a large number of doctors and hospitals.

On this basis, individuals could make judgments about whether the amount of benefit, if it exists, is worth it to them. These judgments would vary among individuals depending on their personal income and wealth. Even among individuals in the same financial strata, judgments about whether a particular treatment is worth the cost would vary depending on the value they personally attach to its benefit.

The nature of health care is such that the above scenario does not apply (as discussed in chapters 3–6). Patients do not have perfect information about the efficacy of a treatment or about the ability of their doctor to provide it. In addition, the perceived time sensitivity of a decision, the amount of social support available to help with the choice, and the fear of significant disability or mortality, all affect even the most knowledgeable patient's decision-making ability. Therefore, doctors ideally serve as the patient's agent in recommending a treatment, taking all circumstances and the patient's values into account. But physicians are also mindful that their own income may depend on the volume of care provided and/or a recommendation for a procedural treatment rather than a lower-cost option.

Information about the efficacy and risks of different treatments is also muddied by direct-to-consumer advertising of pharmaceutical companies and medical product manufacturers. And, instead of price being determined in the market by the interaction of a large number of buyers and sellers, predetermined prices are established by private health insurers and government, at levels that have been carried forward historically from a baseline of cost-plus reimbursement (hospitals) and usual, customary, and reasonable fees (physicians). Patients do not make decisions about whether a recommended treatment is "worth it" based on *these* prices, however; such decisions are made based on their out-of-pocket cost, which is typically a small fraction of the full price paid to providers.

When we move from a theoretical perfect market to the reality of our current health care industry, we lose much of the potential for automatic self-corrections. In a pure perfect competition environment, ineffective treatments would wane, treatments that are known to be effective but *not* being provided would be demanded by consumers, and prices that are too high to attract demand would decline. Rather, in our current health care industry, ineffective treatments continue to be chosen and provided; effective, low-cost treatments are often not provided; and the prices paid to hospitals and physicians, which are higher than would be the case if patients paid the full cost, are sustained.

In the absence of a perfect market, decisions about whether a health care service is covered by an employer- or government-sponsored health plan become a matter of interest to all who contribute financially to this coverage, whether as employees, employers, and/or taxpayers. In deciding whether a medical treatment should be covered, the obvious question is whether the benefit derived from the treatment is worth it, taking into account the types of benefits (survival, reduction in pain, etc.) and to whom the benefits accrue (self, family members, society). The answer to such a question, it turns out, is easier in theory than in practice.

Estimates of the effectiveness of medical and surgical treatments are based on clinical research findings, some of which are more definitive than others. Common sense dictates that only effective treatments that outweigh the risks should be provided and ineffective treatments withheld. But even if we knew which treatments are really effective, in a world of limited resources not *all* effective treatments should be provided. Employees paying into an employer's health plan, as well as taxpayers paying into government health programs, will have varying levels of enthusiasm about making such payments depending on a treatment's cost relative to its benefit. A $10,000 cancer treatment that extends life for an average of five years is one that virtually all would agree should be supported as a covered benefit. A treatment that is effective in extending life by an average of five days and costs $100,000, however, would probably not be supported by taxpayers, employers, or employees. There's a lot of room in between. Where do we draw the line? These questions can be addressed by cost-benefit and cost-effectiveness analysis.

To make a judgment about whether a treatment is worth it, there are three steps: First, we must know how effective it is in achieving a defined outcome. In the cancer example, this could be the number of life-years gained. Second, we must know the cost of the treatment. In the cancer example, we can calculate a cost per life-year gained. It's the third step that is the most difficult: at what cost per life-year gained does the treatment become "worth it."

Let's consider these three steps in turn. Here we delve into the first step—how to assess the effectiveness of a treatment. The latter two steps—related to cost—are considered in chapter 14. Even with 100 percent access to health care, if we don't provide effective treatments at costs that are justified by their benefit, care and cost will be out of balance.

Is a Treatment Effective?

How can we estimate clinical effectiveness? Again, in the cancer example, one measure is the number of life-years extended as a result of the treatment, often adjusted by the "quality" of those life-years. But each illness has its own outcome measure or measures. Treatment of hypertension can be measured objectively by the magnitude of reduction in blood pressure. Treatment of pain can be measured subjectively by patient self-report on a pain scale, and treatment of depression can be measured by improvement in mood on a depression inventory. Across the vast array of illnesses, the goal is to determine whether a treatment causes a beneficial clinical outcome. How well does a medication to treat migraine headaches cause them to go away or become less severe? Among people who have had a heart attack, how well can a medication prevent recurrence? To what extent does hip replacement in individuals with osteoarthritis improve their mobility and reduce pain? How well does a new variant of a surgical procedure improve its success rate? Does a weight-reduction program in diabetic patients lead to fewer complications from the disease? Does a behavioral treatment improve the anxiety of individuals with obsessive-compulsive disorder? The examples go on and on. In all of these cases, an additional important question is whether the new treatment not only does better than placebo in producing a desired result but also better than the current "gold standard" treatment. And finally, there may be different outcomes of interest depending on the age of the patient, the time frame (short term vs. long term), and other considerations.

Levels of Evidence

Patients generally expect that physicians can answer these questions about treatment effectiveness based on accurate information. They expect that only effective treatments will be provided and ineffective treatments withheld. This seems straightforward enough. But to fulfill this expectation requires that physicians are acting purely as the patient's agent without regard to the personal financial benefits of providing a treatment and that definitive information is available on the *causal* link between treatment and outcome. Both of these requirements are a challenge in our current health care environment. Some physicians may make recommendations based more on personal finance than as the patient's agent. Moreover, information on the causal link between treatment and outcome is not straightforward. An analysis of the the benefits and harms of 3,000 medical treatments summarized by Smith et al. concluded that 50 percent of medical treatments were found to be of unknown effectiveness.[1] Of the remaining 50 percent,

- 34 percent were found to be beneficial or likely to be beneficial,
- 7 percent showed trade-offs between benefits and harms,
- 6 percent were unlikely to be beneficial, and
- 3 percent were rated as likely to be ineffective or harmful.

In evaluating published research papers on treatment effectiveness, confidence in the results is influenced by the design of the study and the care with which it was conducted. A general categorization of "levels of evidence" has emerged. Let's consider these different evidence levels in terms of how informative they are for clinical practice.

Testimonials

Not included in the categorization of levels of evidence in clinical research is a category that is not based on evidence: that is, testimonials about the effectiveness of a product or service in marketing materials—whether TV, radio, print, or social media. Something like, "I used to suffer from tremendous muscle strains and pains. I couldn't do my job as a firefighter and couldn't even play with my children. But then I started using X cream, and it was a miracle. Now I'm back to work as good as ever, and my kids love to play football with me in the backyard every night before dinner. Take it from me—X really works!" Testimonials of a few people, whether actual consumers or paid actors, are clearly worthless in establishing efficacy but appear to be very effective in selling health-related goods and services that do not require approval by the Food and Drug Administration (FDA) or other regulatory agencies.

Expert Opinion

Expert opinion is considered to be the lowest level of evidence, and it is relatively uncommon to rely solely on such evidence in contemporary clinical practice. In the absence of data from clinical research, experts in a field sometimes provide an appraisal of a treatment (or potential treatment) as a theory based on knowledge of physiology, laboratory findings, or generalizations from "first principles" of comparable scientific and clinical research. While the opinions of experts may have preliminary value in addressing a clinical question about which there are limited research data, such opinion is subject to the biases of the expert and can lead to delays in incorporating new data into assessments of effectiveness.

Case Series

The next level of evidence, which is still published in the professional literature, is the uncontrolled "case series." A surgeon may report on a new variant of a common operation, or an endocrinologist may report on a new variant of a common protocol for treating people with diabetes. Detailed information is given about the patients receiving the treatment, and the results might *seem* quite good. But the data are difficult to evaluate because there may have been selection bias in choosing patients for the new procedure, and there are no control groups that would convey comparative information on what the outcomes would be if the standard treatment were used or if there were no (or placebo) treatment. In addition, the author is usually the physician reporting on his or her own cases, who also serves as the data collector and analyst. Biases, incomplete inclusion of cases, and conflicts in analyzing the data are concerns in case series reports. Nonetheless, case series sometimes provide the first hints that a particular intervention may have benefit and lead to studies using more informative methods.

Case-Control and Cross-Sectional Studies

The next level of evidence is more analytic, based on research designs that attempt to link an "exposure" with an outome. In case-control studies this is done by identifying cases (a group with the outcome) and controls (a group without the outcome) and then looking back retrospectively to compare the frequency of exposure in cases vs. controls. Cross-sectional studies more broadly attempt to link exposures and outcomes by statistical analysis of the variations in these variables across geographic areas or other units of observations. These types of studies cannot establish a causal link between exposure and outcome, but they can efficiently identify strong associations that could then be investigated using a causal design.

The exposure can be a risk factor (obesity, smoking, environmental exposure, etc.) or it could be a drug that was taken or a surgical procedure that had been performed. Outcomes could be a disease, but it could also be an adverse event associated with treatment or other outcome. For example, a case-control study may compare the prevalence of obesity among individuals who have diabetes (cases) and those who don't have diabetes (controls). If the prevalence of obesity were much higher among cases than controls, a link between diabetes and obesity can be inferred (but not proven). A cross-sectional study of the same question might correlate obesity rates in a cross-section of zip codes with the prevalence rates of diabetes in those zip codes.

In such studies, there are typically statistical adjustments to correct for differences between the groups in factors that might influence the outcomes (i.e., "confounding variables"). These are variables such as age, gender, race, severity or duration of disease, and family history. In a case-control design, a more rigorous strategy would be to match cases and controls according to one or more of the key confounding variables. While matching may strengthen confidence about an association between exposure and outcome, selection bias is still in play and statistical techniques are often inadequate to adjust for known and unknown confounding variables. Large case-control studies across multiple sites may have independent data collection and analysis, but frequently the authors of smaller case-control reports are also the health professionals directly involved in the care provided as well as the data collectors and analysts.

Longitudinal Cohort Studies

A level of evidence similar to that of case-control studies and cross-sectional analyses is the longitudinal cohort design. This type of design is used when a group of patients with a specific exposure (a "cohort") is followed across time to determine the incidence of a variety of outcomes. Longitudinal studies can be prospective or retrospective. In a prospective longitudinal study, the cohort is identified at a given point in time and then examined periodically to assess the outcome measures of interest. The retrospective longitudinal study takes advantage of a database that contains information on individuals going back many years who are evaluated periodically across time; data on exposures that were or were not present in the database at a baseline year is used to define a cohort of individuals, who are then "followed" in the database with respect to the occurance of outcomes across time.

Associations from longitudinal studies can be inferred when specified outcomes occur more commonly among those with certain exposures, but causality cannot be interpreted from this observational design. As in case-control studies, an attempt is usually made to control for differences between outcome groups with respect to various confounding variables using statistical methods. Whether prospective or retrospective, longitudinal cohort studies suffer from essentially the same types of selection biases affecting case-control studies. Like case-control studies, large-scale longitudinal cohort studies may or may not have independent data collection and analysis.

In recent years, there has been a growing literature that supports the use of "real world evidence," sometimes formalized as "pragmatic clinical trials," to address patient risk factors, treatment outcomes, or other clinical questions that have typically been addressed in longitudinal cohort studies. These observational studies take advantage of large longitudinal databases based on health insurance claims and/or electronic medical records. Cross-sectional observational studies that are "nested" within longitudinal databases are also possible using the real world evidence, or pragmatic clinical trials, approach. That said, such studies are subject to the biases of observational studies and are vulnerable to the limitations of how variables were collected and stored in the database, which may be different than how the information would be collected if the research question had driven the variable definition. It is rarely feasible to go back to patients in such databases to obtain additional information.

Randomized Controlled Trials

The highest level of evidence is the randomized controlled trial (RCT), an experimental design from which causal interpretations can be made. As applied to treatment efficacy studies, patients are assigned to either a new treatment or placebo randomly (and sometimes a treatment arm representing the current standard of care is also included). The randomization process equalizes variations between study groups in factors that may be known to affect outcome (like severity of disease, duration of disease, age, etc.) as well as unknown confounding variables. As a result of randomization, the distribution of these characteristics in the different study groups should essentially be the same, especially as the sample size increases. Major RCTs will have an independent committee to monitor safety as well as an independent statistical center to perform data analysis.

The experimental design of RCTs that leads to a causal interpretation of treatment outcome contrasts with observational studies in which the researcher observes what choices patients (and their doctors) make about their treatment and compares the outcomes of patients who have chosen one treatment rather than another (or sometimes no treatment). Thus, as already noted, the results of observational studies can only be interpreted in terms of an association, not causation.

Limitations of RCTs—including their complexity, cost, rigid inclusion and exclusion criteria, and the controlled research/clinical settings of these studies that might limit generalizabililty—are discussed in chapter 21.

Pictorial Display of Levels of Evidence

Levels of evidence in clinical research are typically illustrated as a pyramid, suggesting that as the quality of evidence increases as one moves up the pyramid, the amount of evidence (e.g., numbers of published papers) declines. Expert opinion is shown at the base of the pyramid, case studies on the next rung up, and so on. A pyramid is misleading, however, in illustrating the relative frequency of studies. At the base of the pyramid, expert opinion without supportive clinical research is *not* the most common type of report; it is now quite infrequent. Similarly, case studies are not the second most common type of research report, since published studies usually contain some type of control group. Instead, the categorization of evidence is more of a "normal curve," with the most common types of studies having some sort of control group (albeit nonrandomized), such as case-control or longitudinal cohort studies (figure 13.1).

Dashed lines between case-control and longitudinal cohort studies, and between RCTs and meta-analysis of RCTs, indicate that even though one is shown "above" the other, the validity of evidence is often about the same, depending on the specific studies involved. In some categorizations of levels of evidence, a meta-analysis of RCTs (i.e., estimating the effect of a treatment using aggregate information from several RCTs) is placed at a higher level than that of the single RCT. If individual RCTs have limited sample size but use the same methodology (i.e., type of random assignment, use or not of placebo, lack of knowledge of group assignment by treating providers, list of inclusion and exclusion criteria, etc.), then combining several randomized clinical trials will yield a more accurate estimate of the effect of the treatment being studied, with a smaller error distribution around the estimate. The methodologies employed by different RCTs of a particular treatment may differ, however, and often the treatment itself is not the same

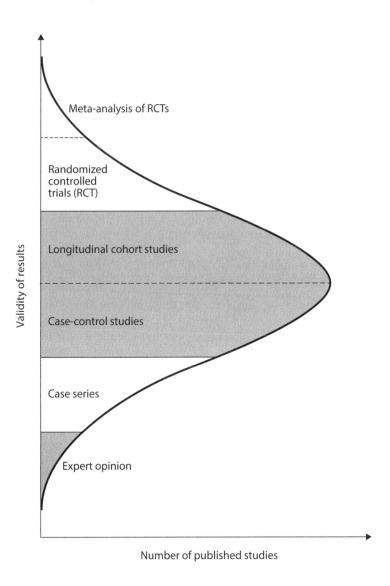

Figure 13.1. Levels of evidence from clinical research

Meta-analysis of RCTs

Randomized controlled trials (RCT)

Longitudinal cohort studies

Case-control studies

Case series

Expert opinion

Validity of results

Number of published studies

in all respects. In such cases, combining studies in a meta-analysis may lead to misleading results, and a single, methodologically sound RCT with a large sample size is more valid.

Large-scale randomized controlled trials that enroll a sufficiently large number of participants to make statistically meaningful conclusions require enormous resources and time. Therefore, while they provide the most definitive causal information about the efficacy of a treatment, many clinical questions involving alternative treatment options do not have the benefit of such research and must be addressed using the best information available, usually from case-control and/or longitudinal cohort studies. The *Cochrane Database of Systematic Reviews* is an excellent warehouse of information about the effectiveness of a wide variety of medical treatments; it can be found online at www.cochranelibrary.com.

Use of Evidence in Clinical Practice

An estimate of how well a new treatment works in producing a desired outcome is sometimes referred to as a measure of *treatment efficacy,* as distinguished from the *clinical effectiveness* of the treatment in real-world practice. This is because participants in published studies belong to specific patient groups with particular inclusion and exclusion criteria, are treated in a highly standardized manner, and conform to other restrictive requirements of the study that may not be present in the real-world environment of clinical practice. For these reasons, the clinical effectiveness of a treatment may differ from the pure measure of its efficacy obtained from RCTs.

Thus, use of the best available evidence in clinical practice does not imply a rote approach to patient care based solely on efficacy from research studies. The particular clinical characteristics and social/cultural/economic circumstances of a patient may differ to some degree from the research participants, and the values and desires of the patient and his or her family must be taken into account.

From this vantage point, what is often referred to as "evidence-based practice" means that the clinician ideally serves as the patient's agent, basing recommendations mainly on the best evidence from rigorous clinical research but also taking into account his or her own clinical experience and the patient's expressed values, desires, and circumstances. Physicians sometimes give more weight to their clinical experience based on a desire to tailor or "personalize" treatment. In comparison with best evidence, decisions based on clinical experience tend to underestimate harms and overestimate benefits.[2] When anecdotal personal experience replaces the best evidence in the literature, the health care provided, on balance, is of lower quality.

Given the competing influences that govern health care decision-making and utilization, it is not surprising that (1) some procedures and medical treatments have been overused and/or misused, and (2) major health care industry stakeholders and politicians have opposed the creation of national, evidence-based recommendations regarding coverage.[3] There is tremendous potential to improve the quality of health care by substantially reducing the amount of unnecessary or ineffective treatments currently being provided while increasing the utilization of health care that is effective in preventing or treating illness. That said, the reality of medical decision-making is nuanced and complex. From this perspective, research evidence and clinical practice can be categorized according to three scenarios:

1. Clinical practice evolves appropriately in accordance with the evolution of credible evidence: effective treatments are adopted and ineffective treatments are discontinued.
2. Clinical practice ignores credible evidence: a treatment continues when it is shown to be ineffective or is not implemented despite evidence of efficacy.
3. For a wide variety of clinical situations, there is limited evidence upon which the physician can base a strong recommendation one way or the other; in these cases, a joint patient-physician decision is made, taking into account an assessment of the diverse and imperfect information available.

Let's consider each of these scenarios in turn.

Evidence That Changes Clinical Practice: The Adoption of Effective Treatments

The most common example of this scenario is when RCTs demonstrate efficacy and usher in broad acceptance of a new treatment paradigm. Among a very long list of RCTs that have established efficacy for a variety of treatments are the following examples of transformative medical innovations (many of which were described in chapter 1):

- Antenatal and newborn strategies involving surfactant, steroid, and antibiotic treatments that improve survival of premature babies
- Evolution of chemotherapy strategies for childhood acute lymphoblastic leukemia and many other cancers, as well as the more recent successes with targeted therapy and immunotherapy
- Medical treatment of AIDS
- Oral direct-acting antiviral medications for the treatment of hepatitis C as well as numerous medical and surgical interventions in hypertension, heart disease, and stroke
- Vaccines

Evidence That Changes Clinical Practice: Discontinuation of Ineffective Treatments

There are also examples in which common treatments were provided for many years based on the best evidence available but were discontinued after RCTs showed a lack of efficacy and evidence of harm. Two prominent examples are hormone replacement therapy for menopausal women and bone marrow transplant therapy for women with metastatic breast cancer.

Hormone Replacement Therapy in Menopausal Women

Menopause represents a cessation of menstrual cycles due to the depletion of oocytes (eggs) in ovarian follicles. In a normal menstrual cycle, the growing follicle that is destined to ovulate its egg produces estrogen. But in menopause, since there is no longer growth of estrogen-producing ovarian follicles each month, circulating estrogen levels fall, producing a variety of physiologic changes, including symptoms such as hot flashes and night sweats. Based on the low rate of cardiovascular disease in premenopausal women and the favorable effect of estrogen on lipids, the potential benefit of preventing heart disease by taking estrogen after menopause took hold. Although initially approved by the FDA for menopausal vasomotor symptoms, estrogen began to be prescribed as protection against heart disease, as well as for other potential benefits such as prevention of osteoporosis and treatment of depression, dementia, genital atrophy, and other conditions.

Comparing women who took estrogen after menopause with those who did not, a large number of observational studies concluded that estrogen replacement therapy provided protection against heart disease, the leading cause of death in women. A 1998 meta-analysis of studies on the risk of coronary heart disease in estrogen users vs. nonusers yielded a relative risk of 0.70 (i.e., estrogen users were estimated to have 30 percent less risk for heart disease than nonusers).[4]

On the basis of the underlying scientific logic, the weight of observational studies concluding that estrogen protected against heart disease, and other observational studies showing beneficial effects in the prevention of osteoporosis and other conditions (and, some would add, because of aggressive marketing to physicians and menopausal women by pharmaceutical companies), physicians became confident about the overall net beneficial effects of estrogen replacement therapy. For women who did not have a hysterectomy, some form of progesterone was added to estrogen to protect against uterine endometrial cancer. This is hormone replacement therapy.

Between 1995 and 2001, menopausal hormone therapy prescriptions increased from 58 million to 91 million. In 2001, 42 percent of women between the ages of 50 and 74 in the United States were taking hormone therapy.[5] In 2000, Premarin, the leading estrogen tablet, was second only to Lipitor in the number of dispensed prescriptions.[6]

All of this growth in menopausal hormone therapy occurred despite the absence of a large-scale, placebo-controlled randomized trial demonstrating benefit with respect to cardiovascular protection. There were other concerns, especially the finding in case-control studies that hormone therapy was associated with an increased risk of breast cancer. In 1997, the Collaborative Group on Hormonal Factors in Breast Cancer published an analysis of data from 51 epidemiological studies of 52,705 women with breast cancer and 108,411 women without breast cancer. They found, in aggregate, an association between hormone therapy and breast cancer, the strength of which increased with increasing duration of use. The estimated risk of breast cancer was about 35 percent higher for women who used hormone therapy for at least five years vs. women who never used hormone therapy. It was also found that the association between hormone use and breast cancer was reduced after cessation of hormone use.[7]

In order to obtain more definitive evidence about the benefits and risks of menopausal hormone replacement, in 1991 the National Institues of Health (NIH) initiated the Women's Health Initiative (WHI) under the leadership of cardiologist Bernadine Healy, MD, who served as director of the NIH at that time. While there were other components, with respect to heart disease the WHI consisted of two randomized, placebo-controlled, double-blind trials: in one trial, women who had undergone hysterectomy were randomized to estrogen alone vs. placebo, and in the other trial, women who had not undergone hysterectomy were randomized to estrogen plus an analogue of progesterone (a "progestin") vs. placebo. The medications used were products of Wyeth-Ayerst, now a part of Pfizer, and were donated to the WHI.

Over the course of the WHI, more than 160,000 postmenopausal women aged 50–79 years (at time of study enrollment) were enrolled over 15 years. The WHI was one of the largest publicly funded clinical trials in US history; its $625 million budget was allocated as a line item by Congress separate from the base NIH budget.

While the WHI was in progress, there were some early signals that the protection against heart disease suggested by the observational studies was not correct. In 1998 the Heart and Estrogen/progestin Replacement Study (HERS), a randomized, blinded, placebo-controlled trial of hormone replacement therapy in women with established coronary disease found no difference between the treatment and placebo groups in the occurrence of subsequent myocardial infarction.[8]

On May 31, 2002, when the WHI had been enrolling patients into the trials for five to six years, the trial of estrogen plus progestin (E + P) vs. placebo was stopped because the relative incidence of breast cancer in the treatment vs. placebo arms exceeded the "stop" threshold and the overall index of net benefit indicated that risks exceeded benefits.[9] The risk ratio for breast cancer for women in the treatment arm of the E + P trial was 1.24, which was statistically significant. (The corresponding estimate for estrogen alone was 0.80, which was not significantly different from 1.00.) Hip fracture and total fracture rates were significantly lower for women in the treatment arms of both the E + P and only estrogen (E-alone) trials. Stroke, pulmonary embolism, and deep vein thrombosis all occurred more frequently among women in the treatment arms of both the E + P and E-alone trials compared to placebo (table 13.1). The risk of coronary heart disease was significantly elevated in women taking E + P but not in women taking estrogen alone.

In retrospect, it may not seem logical that so many physicians would have counseled their patients to take estrogen and that so many patients would have agreed. But many thoughtful and distinguished epidemiologists,

Table 13.1. Cardiovascular outcomes in the estrogen plus progestin and estrogen-alone randomized controlled trials of the Women's Health Initiative

Endpoint	Estrogen + progestin Hazard ratio (95% CI)[a]	Estrogen alone Hazard ratio (95% CI)
Coronary heart disease[b]	1.18 (0.95–1.45)	0.97 (0.78–1.14)
Stroke	1.37 (1.07–1.76)	1.35 (1.07–1.70)
Pulmonary embolism	1.98 (1.36–2.87)	1.35 (0.89–2.05)
Deep vein thrombosis	1.87 (1.37–2.54)	1.48 (1.06–2.07)

Source: Adapted from Barbara V. Howard and Jacques E. Rossouw, "Estrogens and Cardiovascular Disease Risk Revisited," Current Opinion in Lipidology 24, no. 6 (2013): 493–99, doi:10.1097/mol.0000000000000022.

[a] Hazard ratio refers to a type of risk ratio that adjusts for time of exposure. Hazard ratios are calculated in studies where patients are followed across time to event endpoints. Each trial also reported a 95 percent confidence interval (CI) for the estimated hazard ratios, shown in parentheses.

[b] Coronary heart disease includes silent myocardial infarction and coronary heart disease death.

cardiologists, reproductive endocrinologists, and gynecologists believed in the weight of the observational studies supporting cardiovascular protections. The WHI taught an important lesson: statistical adjustment in observational studies may not adequately "control" for differences between individuals who decide to take a medication and those who don't. Adjusting statistically for the greater exercise, more careful diet and lower smoking rates of the women who chose to take estrogen did not evidently capture the fact that they were, overall, more health-minded in their day-to-day life. Ultimately, the women who chose to take estrogen in the observational studies probably may have had less heart disease than those who didn't make this choice because of their *other* cumulative behaviors that were "heart-healthy." Randomization eliminated this bias.

Two years after release of the WHI results, annual prescriptions for oral estrogens in the United States declined from about 50 million to 30 million, and for oral estrogen plus progestin from about 20 million to 10 million.[10] Following the announcement of the WHI results regarding the effect of E + P on breast cancer, one report indicated a significant decrease in breast cancer incidence among WHI E + P participants after discontinuing hormone therapy,[11] and another reported an overall decrease in breast cancer incidence nationally.[12] A 2015 report with additional follow-up of E + P participants confirmed a steady increase in breast cancer over the time period they were taking hormonal therapy and a sharp decline after E + P was discontinued.[13] The same report documented a lower risk of invasive breast cancer in the estrogen-alone arm of the WHI (i.e., for women without a uterus). On the positive side, medical events don't necessarily translate into mortality if effective treatment is provided; after cumulative follow-up of 18 years, all-cause mortality was no different in the intervention groups than placebo, and there was also no difference in mortality from cardiovascular disease or cancer.[14]

The WHI is an example where medical practice fundamentally changed in response to the results of a randomized clinical trial. Nuances in the results with longer follow-up, especially related to age when starting hormone therapy, and whether the patient is a candidate for estrogen-alone treatment, has led to informed recommnedations and practice. Ten years after the WHI results, three prominent medical organizations (North American Menopause Society, American Society for Reproductive Medicine, and the Endocrine Society) issued a joint statement, based on evidence from the WHI and subsequent studies, delineating specific patient categories, modes of administration, and time periods for when hormone therapy might be considered and recommended.[15]

Bone Marrow Transplant Therapy in Women with Metastatic Breast Cancer

In 1998, the wife of a colleague (we'll call her Joan), a vibrant woman in her 40s, was diagnosed with metastatic breast cancer. Oncologists from several major US cancer centers were consulted. Joan made her decision about what type of treatment to undergo based on a discussion of alternatives with these oncologists and taking into account her own values and desires. She knew she would die without treatment and wanted to do whatever she could to live, even if it meant undergoing a form of treatment with severe effects and the possibility of death from the treatment itself. Joan chose to proceed with the most aggressive treatment: high-dose chemotherapy plus autologous bone marrow transplant (HDC-ABMT).

HDC-ABMT is a treatment that allows the patient to withstand very high doses of chemotherapy that would otherwise be lethal. It does this by first extracting blood-cell-making stem cells from the patient's bone marrow or blood and then reinfusing (transplanting) them back into the patient after chemotherapy to regenerate mature blood cells. In this way, chemotherapy drugs at doses that destroy the patient's immune system can be administered, since the regenerated white blood cells from the ABMT restores the patient's ability to fight infection.

In the 1960s and 1970s, a lifetime of study of stem cells and their therapeutic potential led Dr. E. Donnall Thomas and his team to cure patients with leukemia by using ABMT in conjunction with levels of radiation and high-dose chemotherapy that would otherwise be lethal.[16] This pioneering work would be recognized in 1990 by the Nobel Prize in Physiology or Medicine. Subsequently, some oncologists thought that a similar approach might work for patients with solid tumors; uncontrolled early-phase studies suggested that it might be of potential value in patients with breast cancer.

The enthusiasm for HDC-ABMT for patients with breast cancer was reflected in acronyms such as STAMP (Solid Tumor Autologous Marrow Program) at the Dana-Farber Cancer Institute. As a medical procedure, and not a new drug, HDC-ABMT did not need to go through the FDA regulatory approval process. Patient advocacy groups convinced some legislatures (e.g., Massachusetts) to mandate insurance coverage for HDC-ABMT for breast cancer. Patients were successful in winning big verdicts against health maintenance organizations that did not cover HDC-ABMT when the HMO withheld coverage on the grounds that it was experimental (i.e., without evidence from randomized, controlled clinical trials). By the 1990s, despite the absence of RCT evidence, most major medical centers were offering HDC-ABMT to patients with metastatic breast cancer and more than 41,000 women in the United States received this treatment.[17]

Joan was one of those 41,000 women. She survived the treatment, but barely. Experiencing this treatment was a full-time job in terms of medical appointments, but the major challenge was combating its extremely severe side effects on a daily—really, hourly—basis. She succumbed to her cancer in 1999. In April 2000, Edward Stadtmauer and his colleagues reported the results of a large, randomized trial of HDC-ABMT in the treatment of patients with breast cancer and found no survival advantage in comparison with standard-dose chemotherapy.[18] The three-year survival was 32 percent in the transplant group and 38 percent in the conventional treatment group. These results corroborated the finding of no benefit in four other randomized trials published in 1999 and 2000,[19] three of which were presented at the 1999 annual meeting of the American Society of Clinical Oncology.

Initially, as reported by Howard et al., many professional groups reacted cautiously to the finding of no benefit from HDC-ABMT.[20] In 1999, the American Cancer Society continued to "strongly support" insurance coverage for such treatment, arguing that there is insufficient evidence to determine its efficacy and a need for additional clinical trials. But the cumulative evidence from the five carefully done randomized trials took hold. An editorial accompanying the report by Stadtmauer et al. concluded that "this form of treatment for women with metastatic breast cancer has been proved to be ineffective and should be abandoned."[21] By May 2000, the number of HDC-ABMT procedures for women with metastatic breast cancer was 20 percent of its March 1998 peak; by May 2001, only a few hospitals were still performing this procedure.[22]

It is understandable that a woman with metastatic breast cancer, who is sure to die of her disease, might grasp for any treatment that can provide her with hope of a cure, no matter how small the chance and how severe the side effects. It is also understandable that physicians who devote their professional careers to care for such patients will want to believe in the value of a new treatment, especially one that was awarded a Nobel Prize for its proven benefit in other areas of oncology and has promising data from early uncontrolled patient series. The story of the rise and fall of HDC-ABMT for metastatic breast cancer has been reported as a cautionary tale in the medical literature[23] and in a book entitled *False Hope: Bone Marrow Transplantation for Breast Cancer*.[24]

There are at three clear lessons to be learned from the saga of HDC-ABMT: First, a lesson of caution about observational studies, especially when the treatment involved has significant morbidity, mortality, and cost. Second, a lesson of caution regarding the inevitable combination of patient advocacy groups, doctors, lawyers, insurance companies, and politicians who can create an environment in which emotions overwhelm science and data. And third, a lesson in the importance of high-level evidence from carefully done RCTs and the need to invest in such research.

Ignoring the Evidence: Continuing Ineffective Treatments

Among the many reasons for choosing to enter a health profession, "wanting to help people" is high on the list of most students. So why would physicians continue to perform procedures that have been shown to be ineffective or even harmful?

As discussed in the context of induced demand in chapter 5, information asymmetry between patient and doctor means that the physician should act as the patient's agent in making treatment recommendations. But in a fee-for-service environment, economic models of physician behavior logically theorize that while they derive professional satisfaction from serving as the patient's agent in recommending the best treatments relative to their cost, physicians also take into account their own income. Moreover, in the mental calculation of the cost-benefit ratio to the patient, the physician generally considers the out-of-pocket cost to the patient, not the overall cost to society. Thus, during the decade or so when there was no clear evidence about the efficacy of HDC-ABMT for metastatic breast cancer, physicians would recommend this treatment when there was insurance coverage and low out-of-pocket cost to the patient, not considering the huge cost to society (through insurance premiums and Medicare trust expenses) for treatments that cost $100,000 or more.

Although oncologists ultimately abandoned HDC-ABMT for metastatic breast cancer in response to the negative results of several RCTs, it is sometimes the case that treatments continue despite evidence from RCTs that they are ineffective. Two examples are arthroscopy for knee osteoarthritis and stents for coronary artery disease.

Arthroscopy for Knee Osteoarthritis

Arthroscopy for knee osteoarthritis is similar to menopausal hormone therapy and HDC-ABMT in one respect: it did not require FDA or other regulatory approval to take hold as a common treatment. Arthroscopy for knee osteoarthritis, like other modifications of surgical procedures, requires no evidence of efficacy. From a practical standpoint, it just requires insurance coverage. Both HDC-ABMT and knee arthroscopy were being used by physicians and hospitals and covered by insurance plans for other indications besides metastatic breast cancer and osteoarthritis.

The rationale for arthroscopic treatment of osteoarthritis was based on logic that would be categorized as the lowest level of evidence (expert opinion) in figure 13.1. It would make sense—anatomically and physiologically—that the debris released by osteoarthritic cartilage, the degeneration of meniscal cartilage, and the proliferation of the soft synovial tissue that lines the joint space lead to inflammatory changes that produce pain and impaired mobility. Thus, it would also make sense that "cleaning up" the inflammatory debris and crystals in the knee produced by osteoarthritis, and surgically repairing or resecting torn menisci, would reduce its associated pain and improve mobility. On this basis, and with supportive results from uncontrolled case series (the second lowest level of evidence), knee arthroscopy for osteoarthritis grew to become a common orthopedic operation.

Knee arthroscopies represented about half of the total 985,000 orthopedic procedures performed in freestanding ambulatory surgery centers in 2006; moreover, the rate of knee arthroscopy per capita in the United States was more than twofold higher than in England or Ontario, Canada.[25] Based on data from nine states, 29.2 percent of these arthroscopies were for osteoarthritis;[26] extrapolating from these two studies, there were about 288,000 knee arthroscopies for osteoarthritis in 2006. This does not count arthroscopies performed in hospital-based outpatient surgical facilities, for which there are no national data but which are substantial in number. At a cost of $10,000–$20,000 per arthroscopy, knee arthroscopy for osteoarthritis costs the nation many billions of dollars, not counting the discomfort and absence from work due to several weeks of postoperative recovery.

Of note, the 288,000 cases in 2006 were performed after a well-publicized RCT in 2002 that showed no benefit of knee arthroscopy for osteoarthritis in comparison with sham surgery.[27] Led by J. Bruce Moseley, this truly remarkable RCT randomized Veterans Benefits Administration patients into three groups after stratifying by severity of osteoarthritis: (1) arthroscopy with rinsing by at least 10 liters of fluid; (2) arthroscopy with rinsing by at least 10 liters of fluid *plus* surgical debridement of rough articular cartilage, removal of loose debris, and trimming of torn or degenerated meniscal fragments; and (3) sham surgery in which a standard arthroscopic debridement procedure was simulated. Of 324 consecutive patient who met study criteria, 44 percent declined to participate; the remaining 180 patients were randomized to the three groups. All three groups showed a slight reduction in pain after two weeks (with the greatest in the placebo group), which was approximately sustained. There were no statistical differences between the three groups in pain scores at any point of evaluation after surgery. Measures of mobility were also not different between the three study groups, with little improvement from baseline in any of the three groups.

As was the case with the menopausal hormone therapy and breast cancer bone marrow transplant trials, the initial reaction in the orthopedic community to the Moseley RCT was guarded. Concerns were expressed about several methodologic issues (e.g., pain measurement instrument, sample restricted to veterans who were mainly male, eligibility criteria). In reading the commentaries, there was the usual reaction of clinicians who "believed" that knee arthroscopy helped *their* patients based on *their* personal clinical experience: opinions were expressed that flaws in the study meant that the results weren't definitive and shouldn't preclude individual physicians performing this operation based on an assessment of a particular patient's medical history and clinical presentation.

Based on the survey of nine states for which data on knee arthroscopy for osteoarthritis were available, the rate of these procedures declined slightly in the United States after the negative 2002 RCT reported by Moseley et al., but the rate of arthroscopy for osteoarthritis plus meniscal tear increased.[28] (Note: the category "osteoarthritis plus meniscal tear" was not broken down to indicate how many of these were acute, traumatic meniscal tears.) Internationally, a similar picture emerged. In both Finland and Sweden, where knee arthroscopy for osteoarthritis was separated from arthroscopy for traumatic meniscal tears, the rates of osteoarthritis arthroscopies remained roughly constant between 1997 and 2007.[29] A similar finding occurred in New South Wales, Australia.[30] In other words, practice did not change in the United States or internationally for several years after the compelling 2002 RCT using sham-surgery controls.

To address the methodologic concerns of the 2002 RCT, a group at the University of Western Ontario led by Alexandra Kirkley conducted an RCT of arthroscopy for knee osteoarthritis in which 188 patients were randomized to either surgical lavage and arthroscopic debridement together with optimized physical and medical therapy or physical and medical therapy alone. A well-validated measure of pain, stiffness, and physical function related to osteoarthritis was used as the outcome measure and patients were followed for two years after surgery. In their 2008 publication, Kirkley and her colleagues reported that both groups showed a decline in the osteoporosis symptom measure after treatment; this was slightly greater in the arthroscopy group at three months, but the two study groups experienced the same amount of improvement at all measurement intervals from six months through two years of follow-up.[31]

The data from Finland and Sweden showed a reduction in the rates of arthroscopy for knee osteoarthritis procedures beginning in 2007.[32] It is not known whether these procedures have declined in the United States as a whole, since the last National Survey of Ambulatory Surgery, which had been conducted by the Centers for Disease Control and Prevention at regular intervals, was in 2006. One encouraging sign is that knee arthroscopy in the state of Florida, while still high, has declined from a peak of about 460 per 100,000 population in 2007 to 350 per 100,000 in 2015.[33] An additional sign for the future can be found in the practice of young orthopedists. Based on an examination of the American Board of Orthopaedic Surgery database, which includes six-month case logs for each examinee sitting for Part 2 of a two-part board certification examination for 1999 to 2009, showed that the number of knee arthroscopies for osteoarthritis declined by 40 percent.[34] National data, however, still show an upward trend among practicing orthopedists; based on data from the Dartmouth Atlas Custom Rate Generator of "total/unicompartment knee arthroscopy per 1,000 Medicare beneficiaries with osteoarthritis/joint pain in the lower leg," in 2005 this national rate was 246 of 1,000 symptomatic beneficiaries, and in 2014 it was 520 of 1,000.[35]

In 2010, a review of the evidence published in *Best Practice & Research: Clinical Rheumatology* concluded that "arthroscopy, while shown to be promising in uncontrolled studies, has now been convincingly demonstrated to not be efficacious for the treatment of osteoarthritis. It should not be carried out to help patients with osteoarthritis except perhaps if there is evidence of recent trauma and a symptomatic meniscal tear."[36] By 2016, a guest editorial in *Acta Orthopaedica* was more definitive: it concluded that "available evidence supports the reversal of a common medical practice. It is time to abandon ship."[37]

In 2016, another randomized trial of arthroscopy, this one comparing exercise therapy vs. arthroscopic surgery for degenerative (i.e., not traumatic) meniscal tears, concluded that there was no difference in clinical outcome between exercise therapy and arthroscopy.[38] Later in 2017, an expert panel published a "Rapid Recommendation" paper in the *British Medical Journal*. Based on a systematic review of 13 randomized trials for benefit outcomes and 12 observational studies for complications, the expert panel made a "strong recommendation against the use of arthroscopy in nearly all patients with degenerative knee disease."[39] This recommendation applied to knee osteoarthritis with or without associated meniscal tears.

The long-term effect that these recommendations will have on the rate of knee arthroscopies for osteoarthritis will become apparent over time; thus far, large numbers of these operations are still being performed.

Coronary Stents for Patients with Stable Coronary Artery Disease

One of the marvels of modern medicine was the development of technology that allowed a damaged blood vessel to be visualized and a catheter to be placed in a peripheral vessel and advanced to the point of the damage. A major application of this technology was coronary angiography, which involved snaking the catheter into the coronary arteries that supply the heart muscle to see if there is any obstruction of blood flow (usually from atherosclerosis, or hardening of the arteries due to deposition of fatty plaques). Subsequently, stents of various types were developed that could be threaded through these catheters to try to recreate and maintain patency of the coronary arteries. Called "percutaneous coronary intervention," or PCI, a major medical achievement was the RCT demonstration that this procedure reduced the probability of mortality and morbidity in patients having an acute myocardial infarction (MI).[40]

Like arthroscopy for the knee, however, interventional cardiologists generalized this finding to other applications before solid evidence was available.

PCIs evolved from use in patients having an acute MI to common use in patients who had "stable angina" (i.e., they had chest pain that would come and go when the heart muscle was getting less oxygen from the coronary arteries than it needed, but medical evaluation would reveal no acute MI).

The beneficial effects of lifestyle modification became a cornerstone of counseling and management of patients with stable angina, and medical therapies—statins, antihypertensive drugs, and daily aspirin—became increasingly effective. Nonetheless, by 2012, Rita Redberg, editor of *Archives of Internal Medicine* wrote, "More than 1 million stents are implanted annually in the United States to treat coronary disease, in the continuing hope that they are more effective than medical therapy in preventing heart attacks and prolonging life, despite abundant evidence to the contrary."[41]

What happened? Cardiologists and their patients believed that PCI would help prevent heart attacks, stroke, and premature death, and it seemed logical that if you could visualize a blockage of the coronary artery, physically opening up the blockage would help. This is similar to an orthopedist visualizing inflammatory debris and crystals in the knee joint and presuming that removing the offending substances would help the inflammatory pain. On the other hand, coronary artery physiology being likened to household plumbing is not consistent with the current consensus that coronary artery disease is a systemic inflammatory disorder of the arteries that cannot be successfully treated by surgical intervention at a particular site on one artery. In 1995, Topol and Nissen anticipated these issues by arguing "that we may benefit from shifting the current focus and preoccupation with coronary luminology to achieving the desired clinical end point: promoting survival and long-term freedom from myocardial infarction and the disabling symptoms of coronary heart disease."[42]

In 2007, a large RCT was published that found no benefit from PCI in patients with stable coronary disease.[43] Whether patients were treated with medication and lifestyle interventions ("optimal medical therapy") or optimal medical therapy plus PCI made no difference in their clinical outcome. This RCT, called the COURAGE (Clinical Outcomes Utilizing Revascularization and Aggressive Drug Evaluation) trial, involved randomization of 2,287 patients with significant coronary disease at 50 US and Canadian centers. During a follow-up period of 2.5 to 7.0 years, adding PCI to optimal medical therapy did not reduce the rates of death or nonfatal MI in patients with stable coronary disease.

In 2012, a meta-analysis of RCTs conducted by Kathleen Stergiopoulos and David Brown concluded that "initial stent implantation for stable coronary artery disease shows no evidence of benefit compared with initial medical therapy."[44] In an interview with the *New York Times*, Dr. Brown stated, "More than half of patients with stable coronary artery disease are now implanted with stents without even trying drug treatment." The reason, he continued, was financial: "When you put in a stent, everyone is happy—the hospital is making more money, the doctor is making more money—everybody is happier except the health care system as a whole, which is paying more money for no better results."[45] Also interviewed in the *Times* article was Dr. Harlan Krumholz, a cardiologist and professor of medicine at Yale who was not involved in the study. His take: "When people are making decisions, it's important to disclose to them that this procedure—outside of an emergency—is not known to be lifesaving or to prevent heart attacks. The vast majority of people who have this procedure have the expectation that it will help them live longer. That belief is out of alignment with the evidence."

The COURAGE trial appeared to have some impact on PCI rates after it was published. A study comparing the rate of PCI in the United States for patients with stable angina before and after the COURAGE trial found that there was a 17 percent reduction after the trial.[46] In 2014, however (the latest data available), based on data from national cardiovascular disease registries of the American College of Cardiology, only about half of the PCI procedures performed on patients without acute coronary syndrome were considered appropriate.[47]

Newer technologies have emerged. Stents have been developed with a polymer coat containing drugs that are slowly released to block cell proliferation. The hope is that these "drug-eluting" stents will reduce the rate of restenosis in comparison with the standard stents. On the other hand, the drug-eluting stents are associated with increased thrombosis and require longer periods of time in which patients need to take blood thinners. To date, there is no randomized trial comparing drug-eluting stents with standard stents for patients with stable angina. If physicians "believe" that the drug-eluting stents will be effective, they might play down the evidence from RCTs of standard stents in counseling patients with stable angina. Instead, they can convey that although there is no evidence from RCTs, the logic of the drug-eluting stents suggests that it *may* reduce their likelihood of a future MI and/or death. Technology marches on, physicians and patients want to "believe," and private insurance plans and Medicare cover the procedure.

Ignoring the Best Evidence: Not Performing Recommended Tests or Treatments

Each medical specialty and subspecialty has an associated professional society that develops guidelines for practice based on the best evidence available. Physicians who work in these fields have spent many years obtaining specialized training after medical school, and they continue to maintain their knowledge through regular grand rounds, formal experiences in continuing medical education, attending regional and national meetings of their specialty and subspecialty, and reading professional journals and other pertinent materials. While they cannot possibly keep up with the medical literature in general, or even come close to reading all the published papers in their field, they *know* the basic guidelines for practice in their specialty.

And yet, when the essential recommendations of these guidelines, based on best evidence, are compared with the actual provision of medical care, only about half of patients receive recommended care. The most comprehensive analysis of this phenomenon was conducted by Elizabeth McGlynn and her colleagues in a study funded by the Robert Wood Johnson Foundation and reported in 2003.[48] In this remarkable study, 13,275 adults from 12 metropolitan areas in the United States participated in a telephone interview regarding their health history pertaining to 25 acute and chronic conditions. Of these, 12,412 had visited a health care provider in the previous two years, 7,528 of whom provided written consent to provide access to their medical records. The mean age of participants was 45.5 years, 60 percent of whom were female and 19 percent nonwhite. The mean years of education was 14. At least one chronic condition was present in 45 percent of participants and 36 percent experienced at least one acute condition for which they sought medical attention.

The basis for "recommended care" was derived from the RAND Corporation's Quality of Care Assessment Tools system, from which were selected acute and chronic conditions that represented the leading causes of illness, death, and health care use in each age group, as well as preventive care related to these causes. These items were modified by four nine-member multispecialty panels of physicians nominated by their specialty societies according to standardized methods of consensus building. Data from the telephone interviews and medical records were compared to recommended standards of care. Overall, participants received 54.9 percent of recommended care. This percentage held across the board, with 54.9 percent of recommended preventive care, 53.5 percent of recommended acute care, and 56.1 percent of recommended chronic care. The range was from 10 percent recommended care for alcohol dependence to 79 percent for senile cataract, with a broad group of eight conditions between 50 and 60 percent, such as asthma, osteoarthritis, and depression. Funding for an update of this study has not been forthcoming, and there are no other reports that are as comprehensive.

Clinical Decisions with Imperfect Information

Many clinical decisions are straightforward. A patient's signs and symptoms can be diagnosed accurately and treated effectively. For example, pain from symptomatic gallstones can be treated by removing the gallbladder. An infection due to a specific organism can be treated with an antibiotic to which the organism is sensitive. A symptomatic inguinal hernia can be surgically repaired. Blood pressure and circulating cholesterol above certain levels can be reduced with medications that are effective in accomplishing those objectives. A broken bone can be reset and casted. And so on.

Even these straightforward clinical decisions, however, have some nuances. How will the surgery be performed (laparotomy, laparoscopy, or robotic)? Which antibiotic among several effective ones will be given? Which medication for hypertension or high cholesterol will be prescribed? What type of cast will be used? Such nuances will be resolved by a discussion between doctor and patient that takes into account the medical history and physical examination of the patient, the experience of the doctor, cost, and other considerations.

Other clinical situations are less straightforward. The patient's symptoms may raise the possibility of a variety of causes, for which a diagnostic evaluation is conducted. Some of the results of this evaluation—whether an imaging study or laboratory test—may be interpreted differently by different clinicians, leading to disparate treatment recommendations. Even when a diagnosis and its cause are clear, there may be incomplete information about which treatment would be best, since there are many clinical situations for which there is no large-scale, randomized controlled clinical trial to provide guidance. In these situations, the patient has a specific problem for which he or she has decided to see a doctor to find out what's wrong and get the problem solved. The patient wants and expects something to be done. The doctor, having entered a healing profession because he or she wants to help people, and having been trained for many years in medicine in general and then further in a particular medical or surgical specialty, also wants to fix the patient's problem. The tendency in these situations, especially when the patient will bear only a small fraction of the cost, is to do *something* (i.e., to order tests, make diagnoses, and perform treatments—sometimes to a fault).

Thus, the forces at work in the presence of uncertainty are toward overuse—overtesting, overdiagnosis, and overtreatment. Much has been written about this phenomenon in recent years. The prominent journal *JAMA Internal Medicine* contains a regular series called "Less Is More" where they ask the reader to explore a series of reports "documenting the ways that overuse of medical care fails to improve outcomes, harms patients, and wastes resources."[49] Several books on the subject have been written.[50] And chapter 5 herein explained that although much of the reason that per capita utilization is higher in one geographic area than another is due to variation in patient health status, a major factor responsible for higher utilization is a medical practice style that entails more tests and treatments.

The problem of overtesting, overdiagnosis, and overtreatment is eloquently described by Atul Gawande in a *New Yorker* article titled "Overkill."[51] Dr. Gawande draws on national data, but mainly focuses on stories from friends and family. He also relates examples from patients seen in his own practice, who present to him having had unnecessary tests, resulting in overdiagnosis of a condition that would not be a true health problem, and then to an unnecessary treatment. In a self-revelatory passage at the end of his article, Dr. Gawande describes a patient with a tiny microcarcinoma in her thyroid gland. As a general surgeon specializing in thyroid tumors, he knew that this small tumor would not have been recognized were it not for an imaging study performed elsewhere and that it would almost certainly not have caused her problems in the future. And yet, because of his patient's anxiety about doing "too little," he obliged her request and knowingly did "too much" from a medical perspective by proceeding to remove her thyroid gland. Despite a surgical complication, the patient recovered well and was pleased with the outcome. Dr. Gawande relates this story in a way that conveys the complexity of clinical practice and doctor-patient decision-making, which takes into account the objective medical facts, but also the patient's desires, her psychological state, and her financial picture (the procedure was covered by her insurance plan).

A frequently cited example of how uncertainty about diagnosis and treatment translates into overuse is the evaluation and management of low back pain. Almost all of us will suffer from an episode of low back pain at some point in our lives. It is among the most frequent reasons that people see a primary care provider.

Magnetic resonance imaging (MRI) of the spine allows high-resolution, three-dimensional imaging of neuronal structures and the surrounding vertebral bones and intervertebral discs. MRI offered the promise of a better understanding of the etiology of low back pain, with an eye toward hopefully defining optimal treatments, but studies of the relationship between MRI findings and low back pain have been inconsistent and often irreproducible. The use of MRI for low back pain without associated neurologic symptoms or signs of infection or malignancy increases the use of invasive procedures but does not result in improvement of clinical outcomes, either short-term or long-term.[52] Perhaps most unsettling, studies in asymptomatic volunteers reveal an age-dependent pattern of what were once thought to be pathophysiologic MRI findings.[53]

While MRI advanced the diagnosis and treatment of many spinal conditions (e.g. tumor, infection, spinal injury), its use in the evaluation of low back pain created uncertainty, leading to overdiagnosis and overtreatment. Visualization of MRIs of the spine that would not be normal in a young adult, but which are common in asymptomatic older adults, leads naturally to older patients with low back pain—and their physicians—believing that surgery will help. In a fee-for-service environment, even when the physician serves (partly) as the patient's agent, more surgeries will occur to correct diagnostic findings that may not be responsible for the patient's low back pain.

As early as the 1990s, in an international comparison of 11 countries, the rate of back surgery in the United States was found to be at least 40 percent higher than in any other country, and it was more than five times those in England and Scotland.[54] In addition, it was found that rates of back surgery across countries increased almost linearly with the per capita supply of orthopedic surgeons and neurosurgeons.

Over the past few decades, coinciding with the emergence and refinement of MRI, surgery for back pain increased severalfold. The rate of lumbar fusion surgery, for example, increased from 0.3 per 1,000 Medicare enrollees in 1992 to 1.1 per 1,000 enrollees in 2003.[55] Moreover, there was a twentyfold range in the rate of lumbar fusion surgery per enrollee across different hospital referral regions, far in excess of what one would expect to be the variation in the underlying prevalence of spinal conditions for which surgery was medically indicated.

Summary

When specific symptoms prompt a visit to a physician or other health professional, it is reasonable to expect that the health care provider will perform appropriate tests if needed, make a diagnosis, and only recommend treatments that are known to be effective. This is easier said than done. The different types of research methods that lead to a graduated assessment of the efficacy of a test or treatment fall along a continuum. When placed on this continuum, the gold standard of strength of evidence regarding the efficacy of a test in making a diagnosis, or a medication or procedure in treating a disease, is the randomized clinical trial. Regardless, the use of evidence in clinical practice plays out in three scenarios: (1) when clinical practice changes in accordance with credible new information regarding efficacy, (2) when clinical practice ignores new credible evidence, and (3) when there is uncertainty regarding a test, diagnosis, and/or treatment.

While a large fraction of medical care is straightforward, with readily recognized and accurate diagnoses managed with effective treatment, and while there are many examples of new, useful treatments being rapidly adopted after RCTs have established efficacy, there are other examples of medical and surgical practices that continue despite evidence demonstrating a lack of efficacy as well as recommendations based on high-level evidence not being followed. There are also a wide variety of medical conditions about which there is significant uncertainty regarding the utility of diagnostic testing and treatment, which tends to result in overtesting, overdiagnosis, and overtreatment.

Physicians and others who care for those afflicted with a wide variety of illnesses are producing a large number of studies that seek to clarify clinical decisions in the face of uncertainty. More of this work is needed, as is the funding of large-scale RCTs for the most important clinical questions. Once efficacy is established and quantified for a particular treatment, the next step is to make a judgment about whether it is worth the cost. The methods for making this assessment will be considered in the next chapter.

14 COST-BENEFIT, COST-EFFECTIVENESS, AND COST-UTILITY ANALYSIS

Is a new treatment worth it? In an idealized competitive market, each person with a particular illness would answer that question on an individual basis. With perfect knowledge of the treatment's efficacy, side effects, and price, individuals with that illness would decide whether to pay for the treatment given their personal budget constraint and the value that they would derive from the treatment's benefit relative to other uses of their income.

For treatments provided under employer-based health insurance or government programs, however, individuals do not make personal decisions based on the efficacy and price of these treatments. Rather, a set of benefits are defined as "covered" by employer and employee premiums and government programs. Under these conditions, health insurance benefits become more like public goods: that is, once a treatment becomes a covered benefit for everyone in the plan (e.g., the essential health benefits of Affordable Care Act–compliant plans, or the defined benefits of Medicare and Medicaid plans), individuals cannot effectively be excluded from use of the health benefit, and one individual's use of the benefit does not reduce its availability to others. Like other public goods, society's collective resources should, ideally, only be allocated for tests or treatments if their benefits outweigh their costs.

The gold standard for determining whether a public program is "worth it" is to perform a cost-benefit analysis. This involves placing a dollar value on both the benefits and costs of the program or treatment (both tangible and intangible). The benefit-to-cost ratio can then be calculated: a ratio greater than one would imply that the treatment is "worth doing."

Measuring the benefits of health care outcomes is not straightforward, however. For health care outcomes that extend lives, this requires putting a dollar value on a life (or a life-year), which many are reluctant to do. For outcomes that reduce morbidity from an illness, this requires putting a value on an outcome such as pain reduction or mobility improvement, which is difficult to accomplish.

When the goal is not to determine the absolute ratio of costs and benefits for a particular program or treatment but instead to compare it to another program or treatment, a *cost-effectiveness analysis* can be performed. In a cost-effectiveness analysis of a medical therapy, the cost of two treatments that achieve the same level of benefit (e.g., the same number of life-years gained, the same amount of pain reduction) can be calculated without having to place a dollar value on the benefit.

Often alternative treatments of a disease (e.g., drug A vs. drug B or medical vs. surgical treatment) may have varying effects on more than one type of health outcome. For example, both medical and surgical treatments of heart disease may extend lives but differentially impact the quality of those extra life-years in terms of pain, activity level, the complexity of maintenance treatments, and other considerations. Analysis of their comparative effectiveness requires a blended measure of averted mortality and quality of life. *Cost-utility analysis* accomplishes this by using an outcome measure such as "quality adjusted life-years" (QALYs) gained. Between two alternative drugs, treatment with the one that has a lower cost per QALY gained would be preferred. Whether *either* drug treatment would be considered "worth it" it from a societal/taxpayer standpoint depends on whether the cost per QALY gained is below the dollar value that society attaches to a QALY. A cost per QALY of $10,000 may seem like excellent value, while a cost of $1 million per QALY may be considered too much. Once the cost-utility analysis of cost per QALY is compared to a threshold of acceptable societal dollar value, the cost-utility analysis begins to blend with cost-benefit analysis.

Cost-Benefit Analysis

Water projects in the United States during the 1930s were the first initiatives subjected to formal cost-benefit analysis, and the UK began to use this method in the evaluation of road and rail transportation alternatives around 1960.[1] In the case of health care, cost-benefit analysis has been used for programs of public benefit, such as immunization against a communicable disease and air pollution standards, and it can theoretically be justified in evaluating treatments covered by public programs such as Medicare, Medicaid, and other areas of safety-net funding as well as in evaluating biomedical and population health research.

The rationale for communicable disease immunization and environmental safeguards is that they entail externalities. In the case of immunization, there are positive externalities in the sense that benefits accrue to persons other than those who are vaccinated (i.e., a "herd effect"). Escaping the disease by one person confers an indirect benefit on some other individual, when the latter does not catch it from the former. In the case of pollution control, the benefit is the reduction in negative externalities that accrue to an entire local population when a private manufacturing plant reduces its emissions. The cost-benefit rationale for research is that individuals as consumers, rather than as citizens, will often have a short-term perspective and not value potential benefits for future generations as much as short-term consumption. Scientific discovery entails the externality that the production of knowledge by a scientist benefits many others, and it also represents a non-zero-sum enterprise in that more knowledge for individual A does not mean less for individual B.

The question for such programs, and by extension for the public funding of the medical diagnosis and treatment of specific diseases, is whether the benefits to society (including indirect benefits and externalities) outweigh the costs.

Estimating Costs and Benefits: General Approach

The purpose of cost-benefit analysis is to quantify the dollar value of the costs and benefits of programs that are candidates for public funds so as to provide a basis for decision-making about whether they should be supported.

Estimating the cost component of a medical treatment is straightforward in principle, if not always in practice, because of the level of detail involved. It involves identifying the many elements of the treatment, along with its dollar cost. Estimating the benefit component is more challenging. The benefits of a medical intervention are the costs of the disease now being borne that would be averted if the intervention were successful. Since the success rate of the intervention is virtually always less than 100 percent, potential benefits are smaller than the total costs of the disease now being borne.

Once the concept of benefits as averted costs is appreciated, two important steps remain in valuing the benefits:

1. *Measurement of efficacy:* A link must be established between the intervention and health outcomes. Is the prevention or treatment intervention efficacious? If so, which health outcomes are improved and by how much?
2. *Valuation:* How much value can be attached to the various health outcomes that have been quantitatively estimated?

Both of these steps entail significant challenges. Data on efficacy and their quantification for a wide variety of interventions and treatments are rarely crystal clear and often quite murky (chapter 12). Moreover, in order for the benefit/cost ratio to be expressed in an apples-to-apples manner, benefits must be measured in the same numeraire as costs (i.e., in dollars). But how does one attach a dollar value to the benefits of a medical treatment when it includes such intangibles as averted pain and suffering, reduced disability, or averted death?

Early in the development of this field, a threefold classification of benefits was delineated:[2]

1. *Direct, tangible benefits (DTB):* Medical resources, such as health personnel and medication, currently being devoted to the diagnosis and treatment of a disease that would be saved if the disease were wholly or partly averted. Averted direct nonmedical costs to patients and their families associated with treatment (e.g., travel, child care, etc.) can also be included. DTB can be measured in dollars.
2. *Indirect, tangible benefits (ITB):* Earnings, lost as a result of morbidity and premature mortality, that would continue if the disease were wholly or partly averted. ITB can be measured in dollars.
3. *Intangible benefits (IB):* Grief associated with mortality and pain and discomfort associated with morbidity that would be avoided if the disease were wholly or partly averted. It is difficult to attach a dollar value to intangible benefits.

Both benefits and costs accrue over time, but for each category of benefits and costs, the dollar stream has a different time course. Recognizing this, the time value of money needs to be accounted for, since a dollar is not worth as much in the future as it is today. Therefore, a "present value" calculation is needed. For each benefit and cost, this gives the current dollar value of a future stream of dollars that are discounted at a specified rate.

Reviewing the literature on the appropriate discount rate for the analysis of benefits and costs in the health field, Cutler and Meara use 3 percent in their study of neonatal care.[3] If desired, a sensitivity analysis can be performed using different discount rates. The higher the discount rate, the lower the present value of the future dollars.

Understanding that all benefits and costs are expressed in present values, the benefit/cost ratio can therefore be written as follows:

$$\frac{\text{Benefits}}{\text{Costs}} = \frac{\$DTB + \$ITB + \$IB}{\$Costs}$$

If the dollar value of tangible benefits ($DTB + $ITB) exceeds the dollar cost of a program, then without even considering the value of intangible benefits ($IB) it makes sense to proceed with the program on purely economic terms. In that case, the benefit/cost ratio would appear to constitute a lower bound that exceeds 1.0. (It has been argued that the dollar value of indirect, tangible benefits, when added to direct benefits, does not constitute a lower bound, since a case can be made that consumption should be deducted from earnings in such a calculation.)

If the dollar value of tangible benefits is about equal to the cost in dollars, then any modest value attached to intangible benefits would make the benefit/cost ratio greater than 1.0, also favoring project funding. But if costs exceed tangible benefits, then the value attached to intangible benefits becomes critical in deciding whether to proceed with the project. The question becomes: "Is the value of the intangible benefits of avoiding pain, suffering, and grief greater than the amount by which costs exceed the tangible benefits?" In this regard, the key question is, in fact, "What is the value of a life?"

One answer to this question might be "priceless." But if cost-benefit analysis is used as a way of determining whether a health-related project is worthy of funding, or in creating a list of projects rank-ordered by the benefit/cost ratio, the issue of "pricing the priceless"[4] must be addressed.

Valuing a Life: Ethical Considerations

Is it ethical to put a value on life in order to determine whether a medical treatment should be covered by insurance plans or government programs?

If medical treatment of an extremely preterm baby results in survival, or if a cancer treatment can be shown to cure a patient long-term, we can measure the number of lives "saved" as a result of treatment. While not straightforward in practice, such estimates can be made without concern about the ethics of doing so. But attaching a dollar value to such lives raises fundamental ethical considerations. Is the value of a life-year for one person equal to that of all others, or does its value change from one person to another based on age, sex, economic productivity (as measured by indirect, tangible benefits), or contribution to society in other ways?

Most commentators would agree that the very notion of attaching a higher intangible value for some lives than for others is ethically jarring, regardless of people's differential contribution to the social, cultural, or economic fabric of society.[5] But even if it were agreed that the intangible value of life is not different from one person to another, it is difficult to skirt the issue of valuing a life *per se* in decisions about the expenditure of society's resources on new medical treatments. As Richard Hirth and his coauthors have pointed out, "Only finite resources are available with which to both save lives and pursue myriad other goals. Thus, resource allocation decisions with respect to life are unavoidable."[6]

Indeed, it remains the case that the valuation of life is often explicitly included in resource allocation decisions in the United States, especially for public projects in the transportation and environmental sectors. Under Executive Order 12866, cost-benefit analysis is required by the Office of Management and Budget (OMB) for any "significant" proposed regulation.[7] And under OMB Circular No. A-94, cost-benefit analysis "is recommended as the technique to use in a formal economic analysis of government programs or projects."[8] The benefits of most major government program, such as a transportation or environmental project, takes into account the saving of lives and includes a dollar value placed on each life saved. The exception is health care: for a variety of historical and political reasons, the economic costs and benefits of medical interventions are not included in reports of federally funded research or in policy decisions.

Valuing a Life: Methodologic Considerations

The headline of a 2017 *Bloomberg* article by Dave Merrill states: "No One Values Your Life More than the Federal Government." For example, the Environmental Protection Agency (EPA) values a life at about $10 million. This value is significantly higher than other measures that have intuitive appeal (figure 14.1).

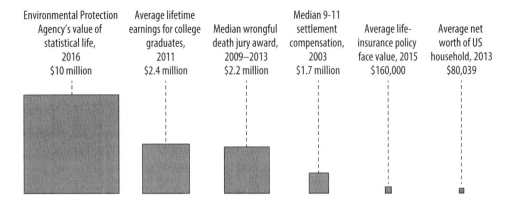

| Environmental Protection Agency's value of statistical life, 2016 $10 million | Average lifetime earnings for college graduates, 2011 $2.4 million | Median wrongful death jury award, 2009–2013 $2.2 million | Median 9-11 settlement compensation, 2003 $1.7 million | Average life-insurance policy face value, 2015 $160,000 | Average net worth of US household, 2013 $80,039 |

Figure 14.1. Measures of the value of life. Adapted from Dave Merrill, "No One Values Your Life More than the Federal Government," *Bloomberg*, October 19, 2017, https://www.bloomberg.com/graphics/2017-value-of-life.

As another example, a 2016 memo from the acting general counsel in the Office of the Secretary of Transportation provided an estimate of $9.6 million for the value of life to be used when "valuing the reduction of fatalities and injuries by regulations or investments."[9] The reason that the EPA and Department of Transportation figures are so high is that they calculate a value of a statistical life (VSL) by extrapolating the value that individuals place on a hypothetical, very small change in the likelihood of their death. This statistical extrapolation is quite different from the value of an actual life or the price that someone would pay to avoid certain death. VSL estimates fall into the general category of what is called a "willingness to pay" or "contingent valuation" approach to valuing a life. An example of the EPA's methodology is provided on their website. In these calculations, the estimated value of a life does not change depending on sex, economic productivity, or other factors:

> Suppose each person in a sample of 100,000 people were asked how much he or she would be willing to pay for a reduction in their individual risk of dying of 1 in 100,000, or 0.001%, over the next year. Since this reduction in risk would mean that we would expect one fewer death among the sample of 100,000 people over the next year on average, this is sometimes described as "one statistical life saved." Now suppose that the average response to this hypothetical question was $100. Then the total dollar amount that the group would be willing to pay to save one statistical life in a year would be $100 per person × 100,000 people, or $10 million. This is what is meant by the "value of a statistical life." Importantly, this is not an estimate of how much

money any single individual or group would be willing to pay to prevent the certain death of any particular person.[10]

An earlier take on the valuation of a life, which employed a willingness-to-pay approach but used observed data rather than a hypothetical abstraction, was contributed by Richard Thaler, who received the 2017 Nobel Memorial Prize in Economic Sciences for his contribution to behavioral economics. Thaler developed a model for the valuation of a life as his doctoral thesis and published a distilled version with his thesis mentor, Sherwin Rosen, in a volume published by the National Bureau of Economic Research in 1976.[11]

Thaler begins with the statement, "The value of a life is the amount members of society are willing to pay for it." His model estimates one "important component" of the value of a life, the value people attach to their own safety, but doesn't address "the amount that others (family and friends) are willing to pay to insure the safety of particular individuals." Thaler uses a strategy in demand theory called "revealed preference," and in his application of this strategy, the value that people attach to safety is "revealed" by wage differences in risky jobs. Different jobs have different work-related probabilities of death. The extra wage associated with a riskier job is viewed as the amount that compensates for the value that workers associate with the increased risks of working in that job.

In developing his revealed preference approach, Thaler creates a mathematical model in which "marriages between jobs and applicants at each level of risk are represented by common tangents of acceptance wage [by workers] and offer wage [by employers] functions" (bracketed phrases added). He estimates this model statistically using 1967 actuarial data on the extra risk of death associated with 36 hazardous occupations that have average death rates five times the baseline risk. For example, the number of extra deaths above baseline per 100,000 policy years of truck drivers was 98 in 1976 and 114, 203, and 204 for teamsters, railroad conductors, and ironworkers, respectively. Using this approach, Thaler's overall estimate for the value of life was approximately $200,000 in 1967 dollars, or about $1.5 million in today's dollars, based on the US Bureau of Labor Statistics inflation calculator.[12] This was a conservative estimate since it doesn't account for the value of a person's life to family and friends, and since people who don't work at risky jobs (i.e., most people) might attach a greater value to risk avoidance than those that do.

Cost-Effectiveness and Cost-Utility Analysis

Evaluation of new projects in water supply, transportation, energy, and other large public programs routinely incorporate cost-benefit analysis into planning. By contrast, few if any decisions about coverage for a medical treatment are made using a full cost-benefit analysis in which the value of a life is explicitly taken into account. This is where cost effectiveness and cost utility come in.

Cost-effectiveness analysis estimates the efficacy of two treatments in achieving a common outcome and their related costs. The calculation of the costs of each treatment is often technically tedious and laborious. Extensive manuals and guidelines have been written with commentary on a variety of methodologic considerations.[13] While tedious, however, this step is relatively straightforward. The more difficult step is estimating a common measure of efficacy for each of the competing treatments of the same illness. We learned in the last chapter how difficult it is to obtain unambiguous data on treatment efficacy, and while cost-effectiveness analysis can provide data on the comparative economics of two treatments in achieving a specified common outcome, it is silent on the question of whether either treatment is worth the cost on an absolute basis.

Furthermore, with many diseases, the measurement of a single outcome such as pain, mobility, or depression may be inadequate. A comprehensive measure of efficacy that reflects a variety of outcome dimensions is often needed. A patient with end-stage renal disease, for example, who takes a variety of medications for medical problems and undergoes hemodialysis several times per week, may experience extra years of life but not "healthy life-years." In view of these considerations, methods have been developed to "standardize" a healthy life-year by adjustments based on the perceived quality of life. Specifically, cost-utility analysis is an extension of cost-effectiveness analysis in that it can account for several outcomes, including both mortality and morbidity, by incorporating quality adjusted life-years.

QALY measurements take into account the effect of a treatment on both length of life and quality of life. The quality of life is assigned a "utility value" between 0 (dead) and 1 (perfect health). A year of life lived in perfect health is worth 1 QALY (one year of life × one utility value). A year of life lived requiring hemodialysis several times per week is worth less than 1 QALY; if the utility value for this situation were assessed as 0.5, for example, one year of life lived with renal disease and dialysis would be worth 0.5 QALYs

(1 year × 0.5 utility value). Half a year lived in perfect health would also be worth 0.5 QALYs using this approach. The first written reference to the notion of incorporating quality of life into the economic analysis of health programs was by Klarman, Francis, and Rosenthal in 1968, who when comparing patients with end-stage renal disease to those undergoing chronic hemodialysis commented that the transplant patients "enjoy a differential in the quality of life, which may be quantified as a fraction of each life-year gained."[14]

The use of QALYs and cost-utility analysis has increasingly become an accepted approach in the evaluation of new treatments, particularly in the United Kingdom and many other nations where technology appraisals using QALY measurements have become a routine part of the evaluation of treatments to be covered under a national health system.

Once data on the cost and efficacy of each treatment is known using a common metric (e.g., a QALY), cost-utility analysis can estimate the cost per QALY for each treatment and/or the *incremental* cost-effectiveness ratio (ICER), which is defined as the ratio of the difference between treatments in costs (incremental cost) divided by the difference in QALYs (incremental effect). On this basis, the utility-adjusted outcomes of the two treatments can be compared in relation to their costs. In recent years, estimation of ICER has become, internationally, a standard approach for reporting the results of cost-effectiveness (or more specifically cost-utility) analyses, whether in the medical literature or by government agencies.

A number of limitations of QALYs (and therefore cost-utility analysis) have been identified. These include ethical concerns (e.g., is the life of someone who is wheelchair-bound less valuable than someone who isn't?) and a variety of methodologic limitations (e.g., measurement from survey instruments, difficulty of generalizing utility values from disabilities associated with one disease to another, and differences between populations in assigning utility values to the same disability).[15] In addition, data from one study suggest that the preferences of individuals regarding the probabilities of four health states (no physical disability, limps, walks with crutches, and needs a wheelchair) and three life-year spans (5, 10, and 15 years) are not consistent with the assumptions underlying the validity of the QALY model using utility values.[16] All that said, the QALY has become an accepted standard for cost-utility analysis.

Cost-Utility Analysis and the Threshold Value of a Life-Year

Under cost-utility analysis, calculation of the cost per QALY of two treatments and the incremental cost-effectiveness ratio between them provides complementary information. Suppose that a standard treatment for a form of cancer (drug A) is being compared with a new treatment (drug B) (table 14.1). Randomized trials for each treatment against placebo yield estimates of quality adjusted life-years gained for each treatment, which is 2.5 QALYs for drug A and 3.0 QALYs for drug B. After determining the cost of an average treatment course for each drug, the cost per QALY for each drug can be calculated, which is $10,000 for standard treatment with drug A and $20,000 for the new treatment with drug B. Although a head-to-head randomized trial of A vs. B was not done (as is the current reality in most cases), estimation of the incremental cost-effectiveness ratio associated with the new treatment can be calculated from the two separate randomized trials, assuming that the demographics and clinical staging of patients in the two studies were similar. The estimated ratio associated with the new treatment is ($60,000 for drug B – $25,000 for drug A) ÷ (3.0 QALYs for drug B – 2.5 QALYs for drug A), or $70,000 per QALY.

In this hypothetical example, drug A is the standard treatment: it has already been approved for use by the Food and Drug Administration (FDA) as safe and effective, and the Centers for Medicare and Medicaid Services (CMS) has included drug A it in its national coverage determination as "reasonable and necessary." Assuming that the new treatment with drug B has met the FDA threshold for safety, its randomized trial vs. placebo that yields 3.0 QALYs gained would also warrant approval. Accordingly, CMS would likely deem it as "reasonable and necessary." Drug A would be available through Medicare and employer-sponsored insurance plans for $25,000 and result in an average extension of life by 2.5 QALYs. Drug B would be available for $60,000 and result in an average extension of life by 3.0 QALYs. The out-of-pocket cost to patients would be a small fraction of the

Table 14.1. Hypothetical comparison of standard treatment for cancer (drug A) vs. new treatment (drug B)

Treatment	Cost	Quality adjusted life-year (QALY)	Cost ÷ QALY	Incremental cost-effectiveness ratio
Drug A	$25,000	2.5 years	$10,000	($60,000 – $25,000) ÷ (3.0 – 2.5) = $70,000
Drug B	$60,000	3.0 years	$20,000	

price paid by Medicare or the employer health plan. The deductible would be exhausted under both treatments, so the difference in out-of-pocket costs between the two drugs is likely to be small. Under these circumstances, drug B would almost certainly take over the market because it adds six months of quality adjusted life-years. From a societal perspective, however, how much redistribution of resources through tax dollars is acceptable to achieve the extension of life associated with the new treatment over the standard treatment. Is it "worth" $70,000 per QALY? Suppose the incremental cost-effectiveness ratio per QALY was $500,000?

Once cost-utility analysis moves from calculation of a cost per QALY or an ICER to a comparison of those results against a societal threshold for "willingness to pay" for a QALY, cost-utility analysis begins to merge with cost-benefit analysis. In cost-benefit analysis, the estimated value of life is entered directly into the denominator, while in cost-utility analysis it is being compared as a threshold value to an estimate of the incremental cost-effectiveness ratio. In both cost-benefit analysis and cost-utility analysis, attaching a dollar value to a standardized healthy life-year is imprecise at best, and opinions about whether six months of extra life is worth some threshold value of ICER will vary greatly.

An early approach to gauging the threshold value of extra life was based on an analysis of individuals with end-stage renal disease who received chronic renal dialysis. This rationale was based in part on the 1972 decision of the US government to include coverage under Medicare for the costs of dialysis in patients with end-stage renal disease. The results of the cost-effectiveness study by Klarman, Francis, and Rosenthal was available to policy makers at that time. It might be inferred that the perceived societal benefits of dialysis for patients at the time of this decision, which included the value of longer lives, was at least equal to the calculated cost of treatment and thus met the societal threshold for the benefit/cost ratio under the budget constraints at the time.

Taking this inference as a reasonable approach, there have been several studies over the years on the value of the life-years added by dialysis in patients with end-stage renal disease. In a systematic review of 13 such studies between 1968 and 1998, Wolfgang Winkelmayer and his collaborators found that the estimated cost of treatment in hemodialysis centers was within a narrow range of $55,000 to $80,000 per life-year in virtually all pertinent studies, with a mean of $65,300, despite considerable variation in methodology and imputed costs.[17] Applying to this mean cost a utility value of 0.8, which was cited in this study as the highest (and therefore the most conservative) among published assessments, yields a QALY value of $81,600 in 2002 dollars. This would be equivalent to $116,700 in 2019 dollars.

In a 2009 update to the study by Winkelmayer et al., researchers used large data sets from several sources: the US Renal Data System on outcomes for more than 500,000 dialysis patients between 1996 and 2003, Kaiser Permanente on disease progression in more than 1.1 million patients during the same period, and direct inquiries of patients with different severities of the disease regarding their assessment of utility values.[18] Using computer simulation models and sensitivity analyses of different model assumptions in an attempt to converge on best estimates, Lee, Chertow, and Zenios concluded that the incremental cost of dialysis per quality adjusted life-year gained was $129,000 in 2009 dollars (or $154,700 in 2019 dollars). This estimate provides a de facto shadow value for a QALY, recognizing that dialysis for end-stage renal disease is, to this day, the only medical treatment specifically covered by Medicare and that other treatments with lower costs per life-year gained might not currently obtain approval were they brought forward for coverage.

In his 2004 book entitled *Your Money or Your Life*, economist David Cutler uses $100,000 as his value for a QALY as a conservative analysis of the data available at that time, which is equivalent to $136,200 in 2019 dollars. The World Health Organization (WHO) has a rule of thumb that was adopted by the WHO-CHOICE (Choosing Interventions that are Cost Effective) project: interventions that cost up to three times average per capita income per QALY are considered cost-effective.[19] Since current per capita income in the United States is about $60,000, this would imply a threshold of $180,000 per QALY for cost effectiveness of health care interventions. Taking into account all of these approaches, in the United States the value of a QALY in 2019 would appear to be in the range of $136,000 to $180,000. Conceptually, taking the midpoint of this range, if analysis shows that a new treatment costs less than $155,000 to $160,000 per life-year gained, it would meet this benchmark for funding. In practice, however, if CMS ever gets to the point of taking cost-utility analysis into account in approving new treatments, it is possible that they may take into consideration the QALY thresholds in other countries, which are much lower.

Table 14.2. Estimated cost per quality adjusted life-year (QALY) for selected medical interventions (in 2019 dollars)

Intervention	Cost ($) per healthy year (QALY)
Tetanus booster	
Booster at age 65	17,748
Boosters every 10 years	1,104,558
Aspirin to prevent heart disease	
Men 45, 10-year risk = 2.5%	15,330
Mammography for breast cancer	
Women, 50–79, screened every two years	40,715
Screening for diabetes	
Age 55: high blood pressure vs. no screening	68,096
All adults aged 55 vs. adults with high blood pressure	715,059
Screening once for HIV	
HIV prevalence = 1.0%	46,159
HIV prevalence = 0.1%	90,969
Diet and exercise to prevent diabetes	
Adults at high risk	254,819
Adults with diabetes	63,081
Smoking cessation	
15 programs weighted by percent enrolled	6,943
Neonatal care for premature infants (< 1500g birth weight)	5,758
Treatment of end-stage renal disease	
Transplant, living donor, human leukocyte antigen compatible	40,909
Dialysis	74,237

Sources: Adapted from Louise B. Russell, "The Science of Making Better Decisions about Health: Cost-Effectiveness and Cost-Benefit Analysis," Agency for Healthcare Research and Quality Archive, last updated September 2015, https://www.ahrq.gov/professionals/education/curriculum-tools/population-health/russell.html; David A. Axelrod, Mark A. Schnitzler, Huiling Xiao, William Irish, Elizabeth Tuttle-Newhall, Su-Hsin Chang, Bertram L. Kasiske, Tarek Alhamad, and Krista L. Lentine, "An Economic Assessment of Contemporary Kidney Transplant Practice," *American Journal of Transplantation* 18, no. 5 (2018): 1168–76, doi:10.1111/ajt.14702.

A number of studies have provided estimates for the cost per healthy year (i.e., cost per QALY) of a variety of interventions (table 14.2). Of course, cost per QALY is but one input into the policy decision-making process. From a societal standpoint, the impact of different mixes of interventions on other social goals, as well as the total budget for public funding of health care innovations, will likely reduce the threshold level in practice. In the UK, for example, the threshold for recommending health care technologies as cost-effective is £30,000 per QALY, or about $38,000 per QALY under current exchange rates.

Constraints on the Use of Cost-Benefit and Cost-Effectiveness Analysis

The rationale for cost-benefit and cost-effectiveness analyses would appear to be straightforward and noncontroversial: in a world of finite resources, if public funds are to be used for health care tests or treatments, the benefits should outweigh the costs. And when two or more treatments are effective in improving health outcomes, the one that costs the least for a given outcome should be chosen.

In the United Kingdom, where most health care is provided under the auspices of the National Health Service (NHS), a National Institute for Health and Care Excellence (NICE) advises NHS leadership on the use of health technologies. Since 2013, NICE has used "£ per QALY" in their appraisals.[20]

Between March 1, 2000, and December 12, 2019, NICE made 925 recommendations on a wide cross section of drugs and technologies. Of these, 475 were recommended, 208 were refined or "optimized" for specific subgroups and for very detailed clinical characteristics, and 129 were not recommended.[21] In 2018, for example, a medication for neurotrophic keratitis was not recommended: "At the time of appraisal, the technology was not considered to be an appropriate use of NHS resources for routine commissioning based on the data available."[22] And, as another example, a medication for treatment of atopic dermatitis was given an "optimized" recommendation "as an option for treatment of moderate to severe atopic dermatitis in adults, only if: the disease has not responded to at least one other systemic therapy . . . or these are contraindicated or not tolerated."[23] Perusal of the NICE website reveals an extensive investment in assessing a broad range of drugs, technologies, and other innovations.

NICE recommendations are explicitly influenced by its findings regarding cost per QALY. A cost of £20,000 per QALY or less usually warrants that an intervention is adopted. At costs between £20,000 and £30,000 per QALY, further considerations must support the intervention (e.g., whether it adds additional benefits not captured by the improvement in QALYs). An intervention with a cost above £30,000 per QALY requires an increasingly stronger case with regard to additional factors supporting the intervention. In special cases, such as rare diseases, the cost per

QALY threshold can be higher.[24] These thresholds for cost per QALY are clearly much lower than the implied value of a QALY as determined by an assessment of dialysis funding or willingness-to-pay calculations in the United States. If a policy of including cost considerations in recommendations regarding coverage for new health care treatments in the United States were implemented, perhaps the threshold would be higher. But having *no* threshold, based on fears of rationing and "death panels," leads inexorably to greater utilization of ineffective treatments and higher prices.

The British rationale for implementing such a system of health care recommendations based on cost per QALY is indicative of the fundamentally different mindset that it represents than that in the United States. In response to a suggestion that the threshold for recommending new health care treatments be moved even lower—to £13,000—based on empirical research that estimated a QALY is forgone by other NHS patients for approximately every £13,000 spent on new technologies,[25] NICE's chief executive Sir Andrew Dillon said,

> Over the last 16 years, we think we've found a balance that reflects what the public expect the NHS to do. Our independent committees use a threshold for recommending treatments of between £20,000 and £30,000 per quality adjusted life year. We think it represents a reasonable compromise between ensuring everyone has fair and equitable access to the NHS and enabling access to new and innovative treatments.
>
> At this threshold, NICE currently recommends 8 out of 10 drugs or other technologies that it appraises, including 6 out of 10 cancer drugs. So we are careful about protecting, as much as we can, the interests of those who don't benefit from the newest treatments.
>
> Unless you believe that drug companies would be prepared to lower their prices in an unprecedented way, reducing the threshold to £13,000 per QALY would mean the NHS closing the door on most new treatments.
>
> At the other end of the spectrum, we obviously can't just say yes to anything and everything. . . . And we need to think carefully about what's being valued. Concentrating only on QALYs means we are in danger of losing sight of other things that people, health systems and the government value very highly. This includes encouraging an innovative UK research base, or perhaps valuing more highly specific treatments that may be the only option for people with certain conditions. These aspects are not captured by the QALY which is why our committees have never used QALY as the sole determinant in their decisions.[26]

Like the UK, but perhaps not with the same level of depth and breadth, most other countries have created agencies or other entities that make assessments of health care medications, technologies, or other treatments from the standpoint of whether the balance between efficacy and cost warrant recommendation. For example, the Canadian Coordinating Office for Health Technology Assessment was created in 1989. The Swedish Agency for Health Technology Assessment has been in operation as a governmental agency since 1992. In Switzerland, new health care drugs or technologies are added to the approved list only after evaluation and approval by the Federal Coverage Committee. Australia has several different advisory committees on drugs, devices, medical practices, and prostheses in which assessments are made utilizing efficacy and cost information. In 2004, Germany created the Institute for Quality and Efficiency in Health Care, and France created the National Health Authority. And in 2016, Japan started a pilot phase for economic evaluation of new health care technologies.

In the United States, a counterpart to NICE and similar agencies of other governments is the Institute for Clinical and Economic Review, a nonprofit organization funded by nonprofit foundations, grants, contracts, and other sources, including some pharmaceutical companies. The institute assesses the value of drugs and other technologies using cost-effectiveness analysis and other considerations that contribute to long-term value.[27] However, unlike NICE in the UK and similar agencies in other countries, which were created by legislation and are accountable to their respective governments, the Institute for Clinical and Economic Review has no authority and can only provide guidance. Indeed, while the pharmacy benefit manager CVS-Caremark has been attempting to use institute analyses and a cost-per-QALY threshold as a framework for allowing clients to exclude drugs from their formularies, this initiative has been slow to gain traction with customers and has been fiercely opposed by patient advocacy groups.[28]

Historically, the political process in the United States, entwined with the various entrenched stakeholders and their lobbyists, has prevented meaningful implementation of cost-benefit and cost-effectiveness analysis in making coverage decisions. Not long ago, there was reason to be optimistic that this would occur. In 2007, the nonpartisan Congressional Budget Office released a report entitled *Research on the Comparative Effectiveness of Medical Treatments: Issues and Options for an Expanded Federal Role*. In this report, a definition of comparative-effectiveness research included the notion of including both costs and benefits: "As applied in the health care sector, an analysis of comparative effectiveness is simply a rigorous evaluation of the impact of different options that are available for treating a given medical condition for a particular set of patients. Such a study may compare similar treatments, such as competing drugs, or it may analyze very different approaches, such as surgery and drug therapy. The analysis may focus only on the relative medical benefits and risks of each option, or it may also weigh both the costs and the benefits of those options."[29]

After defining comparative effectiveness, the report includes cost-benefit analysis as a "related term." In the preface to this report, then CBO director Peter Orszag framed the issue this way: "Only a limited amount of evidence is available about which treatments work best for which patients and whether the added benefits of more-effective but more-expensive services are sufficient to warrant their added costs . . . generating better information about the costs and benefits of different treatment options—through research on the comparative effectiveness of those options—could help reduce health care spending without adversely affecting health overall."[30]

To this day, however, cost considerations are not taken into account in official US government processes and procedures. The FDA certifies that a drug is "safe and effective" without taking cost into account. This has led to high-priced "me-too" drugs with little if any incremental efficacy. And once a drug is approved, it can be used for off-label indications without appraisal of cost and efficacy in comparison with existing treatments for those indications. Standards of evidence are even lower for medical devices. They do not require demonstration of efficacy from randomized, controlled trials; showing that a device is "substantially equivalent" to an existing device on the market is sufficient. And physicians who develop new medical procedures or protocols with existing drugs and devices have no regulatory oversight.

In contrast to the national coverage decisions in other countries based on detailed technology assessments, Medicare covers any treatment that it believes is "reasonable and necessary." In 2000, Medicare issued a "notice of intent" that it was planning to propose a definition of "reasonable and necessary" in which new treatments would have to provide "added value" defined in cost-effectiveness terms.[31] Due to political opposition, however, Medicare never issued the proposed rule. As a practical matter, therefore, under current policy and law, Medicare generally covers any treatment in which it is thought that the medical benefits outweigh the harms, independent of its effectiveness or cost in comparison with alternative therapies.

A recent example of the US mindset with regards to the use of cost in comparative-effectiveness analysis was in the creation of the Patient-Centered Outcomes Research Institute (PCORI) as part of the Affordable Care Act (ACA). The legislative architects of ACA were aware of the gaps in information about efficacy in health care and created PCORI as a private, nonprofit 501(c)(1) organization with a clear mandate to carry out the funding of comparative clinical effectiveness research. The statutory language is clear that such comparative-effectiveness research should not place a lower value on outcomes in individuals who are older, near end of life, or disabled. Although the CBO defined comparative effectiveness as including analyses that take costs and benefits into consideration and viewed cost-benefit analysis as a term related to comparative-effectiveness research, the ACA statutory language specifically prohibits PCORI from developing or employing "a dollars-per-quality adjusted life year . . . as a threshold to establish what type of health care is cost effective or recommended." In addition, it immediately continues, "the Secretary [of the Department of Health and Human Services] shall not utilize such an adjusted life year (or such a similar measure) as a threshold to determine coverage, reimbursement, or incentive programs under title XVIII."[32]

PCORI has an extremely valuable mission: it "helps people make informed health care decisions, and improves health care delivery and outcomes, by producing and promoting high integrity, evidence-based information that comes from research guided by patients, caregivers and the broader health care community."[33] Moreover, it attempts to achieve this mission in part by funding "pragmatic" clinical trials using large data sets obtained in real-world clinical circumstances, which is a strategy that can complement data from classic randomized controlled trials. The prohibition against using cost in the comparative assessment, however, runs counter to the policies in other countries and to the straightforward rationale stated in the first paragraph of this section. The United States may indeed be unique in this prohibition.

How did the United States get to these seemingly counterproductive circumstances regarding comparative-effectiveness research and cost-effectiveness analysis? Tom Allen, who represented Maine in the US House of Representatives from 1997 to 2009, provides perspective:

> The cost and quality of health care will continue to be a critical public issue, and good information is still the foundation for sound public policy. Obstacles

exist. Some are specific to CER/EBM [comparative-effectiveness research and evidence-based medicine] and some are a general product of our current political dysfunction. . . .

CER and EBM are still unlikely to move voters because they are complicated to explain and debate productively with the public at large. Second, organized providers of health care services or products will still watch out for their private interests, sometimes in ways that make productive change more difficult. Third, organized proponents will have diverging reasons for supporting a renewed effort to promote the use of medical evidence, depending, among other things, on whether their primary interest is drugs, devices, or medical procedures. . . .

The congressional dysfunction obstacles are serious. . . . I [have] argued that two competing world views, one grounded in individualism and the other in community, are the principal factors driving America's political polarization. The hardening of these incompatible world views makes compromise on most significant proposed legislation almost impossible. Individualism and community are core American values; our national tragedy is that they have been set against each other in a political struggle that masks the importance of each to our national identity.

Our intense polarization creates serious impediments to collaborative policy-making.[34]

In their book *Unhealthy Politics: The Battle over Evidence-Based Medicine*, Eric Patashnik, Alan Gerber, and Conor Dowling argue that programs like PCORI are no different than a large number of previous attempted initiatives: "Past federal efforts to promote evidence-based practices through medical research and clinical guideline development have crumbled under pressure from doctors, drug companies and the medical device industry."[35] They focus on three "sets of actors: physicians, politicians and the public" and use a blend of policy analysis and political science to understand what they describe as the "deep-seated economic and cultural forces sustaining the status quo" in opposing both limits on the supply or consumption of medical technologies and attempts to use objective analyses that weigh both treatment efficacy and cost in making or implementing policy.[36]

Patashnik and his coauthors make the case that our current reality with regards to evidence-based practice and cost-benefit/cost-effectiveness analysis is a combination of

1. delegation of authority to doctors in their role as the patient's agent, given asymmetric information between doctors and patients;

2. the public's misperception of doctors as trustworthy agents of their health and medical care, which extends to the public's trust of medical societies; and

3. the weak incentives for politicians to address the status quo when it threatens "not just the incomes of business groups (such as the medical products industry) but also the autonomy and authority of trusted professionals, such as doctors."[37]

Although approached from a different angle, analysis of the economic and historical underpinnings of the US health care industry in parts 1 and 2 of this book leads to very similar conclusions. The United States has developed an industry deeply rooted in concepts of physician autonomy, the sanctity of the physician-patient relationship, and the physician acting as the patient's agent in a setting of asymmetric information. Layered onto these fundamental concepts is the desire among providers and politicians for a "free market" environment unfettered by regulation. This has been implemented through a private health insurance backbone in which patients pay only a fraction of the full price that is received by providers of health care goods and services.

Industry stakeholders are not consistently incentivized to support evidence-based practice and cost-benefit/cost-effectiveness analysis. While there is potential benefit for patients and the national cost of health care to assess the entry of potential new treatments in terms of how effective they are in comparison with gold-standard treatments, or how expensive they are in comparison with treatments of comparable efficacy, the impact on the individual stakeholder tends to be in the opposite direction. Thus, the instinct on the part of any stakeholder who might be adversely affected by such a broad assessment of a new treatment is to cry foul, and the path of least resistance on the part of government is to stand on the sidelines, or even formally restrict analyses that might raise questions about the cost effectiveness of a particular treatment. The net result is reduced quality of care and reduced efficiency. Some treatments are provided that are not effective or are more expensive than treatments of comparable efficacy, while effective treatments are often not provided.

Summary

In a health care world of perfect competition, each individual would decide whether a proposed medical treatment for a particular illness is worth the cost. This decision would be made based on the full market price of the treatment, knowledge of treatment efficacy, and a personal income constraint. In our current reality, individuals do not make such decisions because employers, insurers, and government fundamentally influence them. Given this reality and finite resources, it makes sense to assess, as broadly and accurately as possible, the costs and benefits of a proposed treatment in comparison with other treatments or no treatment. In traditional cost-benefit analysis, both the costs and benefits are measured in dollar terms. The benefits are averted costs (i.e., the averted direct medical costs of treating the illness, averted lost earnings, and averted intangible costs of morbidity and mortality).

If, for ethical or political reasons, there is caution about valuing averted mortality (i.e., valuing life), cost-effectiveness analysis can be performed. In that case, two or more treatments with a specified, objective outcome can be compared in terms of the cost of achieving that outcome. When it is decided that there is a need for health care technology assessment in the allocation of public funds, however, it is hard to avoid attaching some value to the benefit of averted mortality. This has been done in the United Kingdom and many other countries using cost-utility analysis, in which the cost per quality adjusted life-year gained is compared to a threshold of societal willingness to pay, but political barriers have prevented implementation of such a process in the United States.

15 HEALTH CARE LAW

James M. Roberts and David S. Guzick

Like all areas of commerce in the United States, the health care industry is governed by a general set of federal, state, and local laws and also by specific statutes that pertain to its particular domain. Many of the specific statutes related to health care services and products are discussed throughout this book. Examples include the statutory language in the Affordable Care Act that prohibits the Patient-Centered Outcomes Research Institute from conducting cost-effectiveness analyses (chapter 14) and the statute in the Medicare Modernization Act that prohibits Medicare from negotiating price with drug manufacturers (chapter 19). Indeed, Medicare, Medicaid, and the Affordable Care Act, while presented in chapters 10–12 from the standpoint of how they affect health care and health, are essentially discussions of specific health care laws.

A granular review of other health-related laws would include a myriad of topics such as state and federal licensing requirements of health professionals, medical malpractice, and the laws governing various categories of health delivery sites, such as laboratories, ambulatory surgery centers, and hospitals. For our purposes, however, we will focus on far-reaching laws that profoundly influence health care on a day-to-day basis. These laws arose from critical features of the health care industry. Specifically,

- the US system of fee-for-service claims with third-party payments has given rise to laws that are focused on fraud and conflict of interest;
- the lack of access to needed health care by uninsured individuals has led to laws requiring hospitals to evaluate and stabilize any individuals when they present to the emergency room for care, regardless of their insurance status; and

- the importance of the integrity, portability, and privacy of personal health information, along with the many untoward implications when privacy is breached, have led to laws that govern and protect these data.

Fraud: The False Claims Act and "Qui Tam" Relators

The claims-based, fee-for-service health insurance backbone of the US health care industry has led to enormous administrative complexity. Providers must ensure that the code for each billing claim (among the tens of thousands of possible health care codes) is appropriately documented in the medical record and meets the requirements for medical necessity and all the other criteria for payment. Adding to the complexity is that these criteria often vary from payer to payer. As we will see in chapter 18, billing and insurance-related administrative costs, which are absorbed by both providers and payers, consume about 25 cents of every insurance premium dollar. Even with elaborate systems and large numbers of dedicated personnel who want to do the right thing, audits may uncover a small percentage of claims in which the clinical documentation and billing codes don't match, or in which other aspects of the process are out of compliance. These mismatches are often recognized as inadvertent and resolved, albeit with yet more administrative expense.

The complexity and automated nature of the claims-based billing process, however, invites the potential for fraud and abuse. For those who intend to profit from cracks in the system that can be creatively exploited, there are many opportunities to engage in health care fraud. Some of the more common examples are

- performing medically unnecessary or unindicated diagnostic studies or procedures strictly to generate insurance payments,
- misrepresenting noncovered treatments as medically necessary to generate insurance payments,
- "upcoding" (i.e., billing for more expensive procedures than were actually provided), and
- fabrication of entire claims for services that were never rendered, sometimes using stolen identities, or padding a claim for a provided service with charges for procedures that did not take place.

Fraud under the last bullet is typically clear on its face. For the first three bullets, some examples of fraud are also clearly evident, but in other cases billing inconsistencies are more ambiguous; in such cases, "fraud" is often in the eyes of the beholder. Clearly, the opportunity for true fraud is inherent in the complexity of the system, and the scope of fraud is significant. In *License to Steal*, Malcolm K. Sparrow shows how well-orchestrated attacks on a system that was designed simply to find and correct billing errors can overcome the industry's meager electronic defenses. Following the simple dictum, "bill your lies correctly,"[1] Sparrow shows how fraud perpetrators can steal millions of dollars with impunity.

The National Health Care Anti-Fraud Association estimates conservatively that fraud costs the United States about 3 percent of health care expenditures annually, while others put the figure at three times that amount.[2] At the current level of national health care expenditures, these estimates imply that about $100 billion to $300 billion annually is lost to health care fraud.

Internationally, the European Healthcare Fraud and Corruption Network (EHFCN) has been formed to confront fraud in the various European Union country-specific health systems. The EHFCN estimates the annual loss from fraud and corruption in the European Union at about €56 billion,[3] or approximately $64 billion dollars at current exchange rates. Thus, the level of health care fraud among European countries—with varying provider reimbursement models—would suggest that the predominant US fee-for-service payment mechanism is not the *only* cause for the health care fraud perpetrated in the United States.

Government authorities identify only a small fraction of health care fraud. The Office of the Inspector General (OIG) and Department of Justice (DOJ) typically pursue potential fraud for US federal health care programs, seeking penalties specified under the False Claims Act (FCA). The original FCA (often referred to as the "Lincoln Act") stemmed from Civil War times as a law to deter individuals from defrauding the Union government by presenting bills for nonexistent or deficient supplies for the war effort. Later amendments enacted in 1986 provided that whistleblowers ("qui tam relators") were entitled to 15–30 percent of any financial recovery by the government.[4] Furthermore, companies and other entities that defraud the government were made liable for treble damages and a fine for each false claim.

As of 2017, per-claim fines were set from $10,957 to $21,916.[5] Court opinions have reduced thresholds for establishing liable conduct simply to showing gross negligence on the part of defendants—there is no need to show actual knowledge or specific intent—and these opinions have substantially increased recoveries by the government and relators. Of the $3.7 billion in judgments and settlements recovered by the DOJ in 2017, $2.5 billion came from the health care industry.[6] Of this amount, 85 percent was attributable to qui tam cases initiated by whistleblowers. Whistleblowers have standing to proceed even if they were participants in the alleged fraud in an organization's revenue cycle or compliance departments, so long as they possess information not available to the general public. Only where they are criminally convicted in the underlying fraud are they precluded from any recovery.

Provisions under the False Claims Act are typically part of the penalty calculations for a variety of health care law infractions. For the first half of 2018, there were 49 settlements with providers under the act (figure 15.1). Following the aims of the FCA that strictly apply to federal government programs, commercial insurers embed in their provider agreements contractual provisions that aid in their recovery for claims that were either techni-

Figure 15.1. Number of settlements under the False Claims Act, January–June 2018, by allegation type. Gibson Dunn, "2018 Mid-Year FDA and Health Care Compliance and Enforcement Update—Providers" (client letter), July 26, 2018, https://www.gibsondunn.com/wp-content/uploads/2018/07/2018-mid-year-fda-health-care-compliance-and-enforcement-update-providers.pdf.

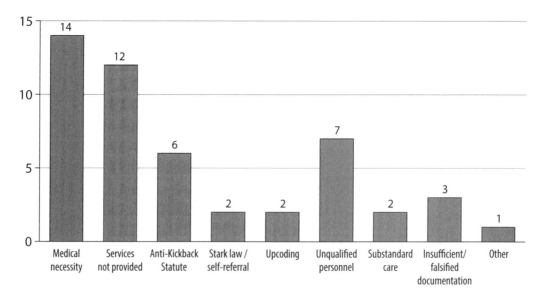

cally deficient or misrepresented. In comparing awardable penalties and fines—whether contractual, brought in an independent fraud case, or pursued by the OIG and the DOJ under the False Claims Act—those of the FCA are typically the most potent.

In summary, the complexity of the billing claims process invites the potential for fraud, which may amount to as much as 3–9 percent of all health care expenditures. Our current system of whistleblowers and post-hoc, retrospective audits, however, identifies only a small fraction of the large amount of fraudulent activity that exploits the "bill your lies correctly" rule. Moreover, this system financially incentivizes whistleblower insiders (vendors or employees), who sometimes bring forward billing infractions that are technical and ambiguous in nature for personal financial gain. What is needed, conceptually (although some rudimentary forms are in practice today), is substantially enhanced artificial intelligence and information technology that could enable real-time audits and much earlier identification of outliers, whether by claim or ordering provider. This technology, when and if it becomes available, could identify the bulk of billing fraud and thereby significantly reduce the scale of its impact. An effective system of this type would also proactively inhibit those who commit fraud by "billing their lies correctly." It also goes without saying that pursuing other types of reimbursement/payment systems that are not as dependent on a per-claim-submission basis would have a positive impact as well.

Conflicts of Interest: The Anti-Kickback Statute and Stark Laws

Because physicians are the principal decision-makers about medical treatments, due to their role as the patient's agent in the context of asymmetric information (chapter 5), their ability to refer patients to other physicians, hospitals, and other health care facilities invites the potential for "kickback" payments from these receiving parties. Moreover, the nonindependence of supply and demand in health care, combined with imperfect and asymmetric information, can lead to induced demand (chapters 3, 5, 13, and 17), which invites the potential for self-referrals to facilities in which physicians have an ownership stake and from which they derive passive income. From one perspective, these behaviors represent nonbilling examples of fraud and abuse, largely addressed by two laws—the Anti-Kickback Statute and the Stark law. From another perspective, aggressive pursuit of recovery under these laws, while reflecting the complexity and limitations of claims reimbursement, is sometimes done without assessing how these laws undermine clinical collaboration and coordination that can reduce cost and enhance quality.

Anti-Kickback Statute

The origins of the anti-kickback law can be found in the Copeland Act of 1931, which was enacted in response to attempts by Depression-era employers to circumvent mandatory wage provisions in federal contracts by requiring employees to make kickbacks.

After the enactment of Medicare and Medicaid in 1965, which granted health care access and financial support for millions of Americans, many examples of referral kickbacks involving patients enrolled in these programs were observed. To curtail this behavior, in 1972 Congress passed the Anti-Kickback Statute (AKS) as an amendment to the Social Security Act. The main provisions of the AKS made it a misdemeanor to "furnish items or services to an individual for which payment is or may be made [through Medicare or Medicaid]," where the provider "solicits, offers, or receives any (1) kickback or bribe in connection with furnishing of such items or services or making receipt of such payment, or (2) rebate of any fee or charge for referring any such individual to another person for furnishing of such items or services."[7]

The penalties under the AKS were further strengthened in 1977 when Congress amended the statute to make violations of it felonies punishable by up to five years of imprisonment. Current penalties under AKS violations include imprisonment of up to five years, fines of up to $25,000 per violation or twice the alleged gain or loss, exclusion from participation in federal health care programs, and civil penalties of up to $50,000 per kickback plus treble damages (three times the amount of remuneration).[8] In addition, the Affordable Care Act established that a violation of the AKS could render all claims submitted in conjunction therewith as false or fraudulent claims under subchapter III of chapter 37 of Title 31 (the False Claims Act).

The AKS is an intent-based statute; in prosecutions, proving intent is a key component of exacting settlements or judgments. Most federal circuit courts have adopted the "one purpose" test first expressed in *United States vs. Greber.*[9] Regardless of other motivations for any payment made, if one purpose of the payment is to incentivize the physician to refer patients, then the AKS would be deemed violated. The Affordable Care Act additionally amended the intent portion of the AKS to state that a person "need not have actual knowledge of this section or specific intent to commit a violation of this section."[10] As a result, the government can now meet the intent requirement by simply demonstrating that, under the facts, the "reasonable man" should have known.

Original AKS statutory provisions, subsequent judicial pronouncements, and OIG clarifications of various fact scenarios have led to a host of published exclusions from the application of this statute. These exclusions are collectively referred to as "safe harbors" (box 15.1). Many of these provisions reflect the influence of various interest-group lobbying efforts. Some of the safe harbors that are most often used by health care providers as exemptions from prosecution under the Anti-Kickback Statute include

- referrals made as part of an employment or professional services arrangement (where as a condition of employment, for example, referrals for physician specialty services are required to be within the employer physician group);
- payments made for the lease of equipment or of office space (where undercharging for these items could be an indirect way of paying kickbacks to referring physicians); and
- certain payments made for the purposes of health practitioner recruitment (again, where substantial above-market payments made to recruit practitioners in high demand would appear to influence the physician's future referral patterns).

In each of these safe harbor exemptions, there are stipulated, but sometimes vague, requirements that must be met to satisfy the safe harbor and be immune from prosecution.

Even with all these seemingly explicit safe harbors, frontline hospital and physician practice administrators grapple with every provider-to-provider transaction, never being sure whether the facts of particular physician-to-physician or physician-hospital relationships, or other collaborations among other health care providers, would fall under these safe harbors or pass muster under desired business or compensation arrangements. As a consequence, the AKS has had the effect of requiring transactional parties to undertake intense administrative and legal scrutiny of

Box 15.1. List of safe harbors under the Anti-Kickback Statute

- Investment interests in publicly traded companies
- Space rentals
- Equipment rentals
- Personal services and management contracts
- Sale of a practice
- Referral services
- Warranties
- Discounts
- Employees
- Group purchasing organizations
- Certain Medicare Part A waivers of coinsurance and deductibles
- Investment interests in group practices composed exclusively of active investors who are licensed health professionals
- Increased coverage, reduced cost-sharing amounts, or reduced premium amounts offered by certain health plans (managed care)
- Price reductions offered to certain health plans
- Investment interests in underserved areas
- Rural practitioner recruitment incentives
- Investment interests in ambulatory surgery centers
- Obstetrical malpractice insurance subsidies
- Referral agreements for specialty services
- Cooperative hospital service organizations
- Ambulance replenishment arrangements
- Electronic prescribing and electronic medical records
- Federally qualified health centers

Source: "Anti-Kickback Statute Safe Harbors," Anti-Kickback Statute: Information on Penalties and Legal News, accessed January 29, 2019, http://www.antikickbackstatute.com.

prospective business arrangements where professional services are to be rendered and various forms of compensation are to be paid.

This scrutiny does not come cheap. An American Hospital Association report published in 2017 estimated that providers spend nearly $39 billion a year solely on the administrative activities related to regulatory compliance in the regulated areas of the Centers for Medicare and Medicaid Services, the Office of Inspector General, the Office for Civil Rights, and the Office of the National Coordinator for Health Information Technology.[11]

Increasingly, fair market valuation determinations in compensation arrangements have become focal points in many AKS government investigations and litigation, with disagreements about the basis and appropriateness of fair market valuation comparisons. If a provider organization fails to undertake a credible (and professional) fair-market-value assessment, the government can more readily argue that amounts paid were not market value and were intended as kickbacks for referrals.

Given the severity of AKS penalties, including a 2015 DOJ memo from its deputy general counsel expressing an intention to prosecute participating corporate administrators (referred to as the "Yates memo"),[12] there exists a healthy respect for complying with the AKS. Sometimes the desire for compliance (i.e., the desire to avoid risk) rises to the point where it inhibits physician-hospital collaborations in pursuing "value" arrangements that improve health care while reducing cost. This is true despite the ability of the would-be collaborators to solicit an advance "advisory opinion" from the OIG on the legality of an intended arrangement. Many organizations are concerned that despite a promise of anonymity from the OIG, these types of opinion requests could trigger further inquiries by the DOJ and the OIG into the general business dealings of the organization, with often limited confidence that the specifics of every AKS (or any other federal health care regulatory) requirement would be met. As a consequence, many well-intentioned arrangements to improve the delivery of health care, which likely would have passed muster under an advisory opinion, go unsubmitted and unimplemented.

The desire for risk avoidance under the AKS is particularly acute because of the severity of the penalties. As noted, the recent change under the Affordable Care Act that permits the additional assessment of "per claim" FCA financial penalties has enlarged AKS penalty recoveries. For example, in 2016, the Tenet Healthcare Corporation paid $513 million to resolve criminal and civil kickback claims.[13] And on March 1, 2016, the DOJ announced that Olympus Corporation of the Americas, the nation's largest manufacturer of endoscopes and related equipment, had agreed to a $623.2 million settlement to resolve criminal charges and civil claims relating to a scheme to pay kickbacks to doctors and hospitals. This settlement, which has been characterized as the largest total amount paid in US history for violations involving the AKS by a medical device company, included many of these enhanced penalty components.[14]

In comparison to the False Claims Act, where qui tam relators are independently incented to bring actions, the inherent policy and regulatory needs to prevent kickback schemes that result in the delivery of unjustified health care services appears on its face unassailable. As with the FCA, however, there are similar problems with vague standards and the need for continuing amendments and judicial clarifications. In addition, despite some enhanced safe harbors for collaborative arrangements, the chilling effect of the severe penalties under the AKS naturally can inhibit collaborations between providers that can enhance care and reduce cost. The Centers for Medicare and Medicaid Services has acknowledged this dilemma, as evidenced in its 2018 rule-making request for information submission, stating,

> The Office of Inspector General (OIG) seeks to identify ways in which it might modify or add new safe harbors to the anti-kickback statute and exceptions to the beneficiary inducements civil monetary penalty (CMP) definition of "remuneration" in order to foster arrangements that would promote care coordination and advance the delivery of value-based care, while also protecting against harms caused by fraud and abuse. *Through internal discussion and with the benefit of facts and information received from external stakeholders, OIG has identified the broad reach of the anti-kickback statute and beneficiary inducements CMP as a potential impediment to beneficial arrangements that would advance coordinated care.*[15] (emphasis added)

On balance, the AKS has been effective in deterrence and in recovery of monies paid for tainted services. Part of the dilemma of the AKS lies with some of its seemingly inexplicable safe harbors, which have long been critiqued for actually sanctioning known kickback arrangements. One prominent example is the safe harbor for group purchasing organizations (GPOs). By some estimates, GPOs control purchasing of over $300 billion annually in drugs, devices, and supplies for the nation's health care system. Congress sanctioned these organizations' "kickback" business practices in the 1980s in reaction to intense lobbying by GPOs. The rationale for creating the safe harbor was simply to sanction that which was already known to occur, namely that device and drug manufacturers had been paying kickbacks to GPOs (to preserve their sole-source or volume-guaranteed positions). Thus, what otherwise could have been criminal behavior for overt kickbacks received a pass under this AKS safe harbor. A viewpoint in *JAMA* reviewing the safe harbor permitting kickbacks to GPOs concluded that "to protect consumers from bearing the cost of vendor fees and kickbacks, policy makers should reevaluate the safe harbor laws exempting GPOs from anti-kickback statutes. More choices with honest prices and fair market practices promoting competition could result in lower prices, help reduce critical drug and supply shortages, and bring more innovative products to the bedside."[16]

One approach to deciding whether further reformations of the AKS are needed would be to undertake empirical analyses of the expected cost and quality goals of a specific desired collaboration in comparison with the value of the statute's financial recoveries and deterrent impact of avoiding referral/kickback schemes. If it were found that the clinical and financial benefits of such a proposed collaboration outweighed the potential for overutilization and increased cost, then consideration should be given to establishing an additional safe harbor. Also, to be consistent, the same logic should apply to existing safe harbors. That is, if overutilization and cost under an existing safe harbor were shown to exceed the benefits of the arrangement for which a safe harbor was granted, then consideration should be given to removing that safe harbor.

Stark Law

The origin of Stark law was the bill for the Ethics in Patient Referrals Act, sponsored by Fortney "Pete" Stark, a longstanding California congressman. Enacted in 1989, the original bill was straightforward. Congressman Stark (retrospectively) put it this way: "Basically it says anyone who takes a bribe or a split or a commission or a kickback in exchange for referring services gets five years or a $50,000 fine."[17] Since its initial enactment, however, the original Stark law has evolved into a complex set of federal laws that prohibit self-referral by physicians (unless an exception applies). Specifically, it prohibits a referral by a physician of a Medicare or Medicaid patient to an entity providing designated health services (DHS) if the physician (or an immediate family member) has a financial relationship with that entity.

Across time, provisions under Stark have been incorporated into the Omnibus Budget Reconciliation Acts of 1989 ("Stark I"), 1993 ("Stark II"), and final implementation (sometimes referred to as "Stark III") under amendments in 2001, 2004, and 2007. The Stark laws have gone well beyond Congressman Stark's original language and intent, such that he now advocates repeal.[18] Under the various amendments, 35 exceptions have been crafted, each with their own specific requirements, along with other additional provisions. An "overview" of Stark law, published by the American Medical Association, itself amounts to 79 pages.[19]

Initially, designated health services focused on laboratory services. The scope of what currently constitutes DHS, however, now includes

- clinical laboratory services;
- physical therapy services;
- occupational therapy services;
- radiology services, including magnetic resonance imaging, computerized axial tomography scans, and ultrasound services;
- radiation therapy services and supplies;
- durable medical equipment and supplies;
- parenteral and enteral nutrients, equipment, and supplies;
- prosthetics, orthotics, and prosthetic devices and supplies;
- home health services;
- outpatient prescription drugs;
- inpatient and outpatient hospital services; and
- outpatient speech-language pathology services.

Penalties for violations of Stark law include

- denial of payment for the DHS provided;
- refund of monies received by physicians and facilities for amounts collected;
- payment of civil penalties of up to $15,000 for each service that a person "knows or should know" was provided in violation of the law, and three times the amount of improper payment the entity received from the Medicare program;
- exclusion from the Medicare program and/or state health care programs, including Medicaid; and
- payment of civil penalties for attempting to circumvent the law of up to $100,000 for each circumvention scheme.

Additionally, Stark law currently contain a number of exceptions to what otherwise would be disallowed DHS transactions. Among these are

- physician services,
- in-office ancillary services,

- rental of office space and equipment,
- a bona fide employment relationship, and
- services provided by an academic medical center as a result of a physician's referral, as long as certain conditions are met.

Unlike the Anti-Kickback Statute, no showing of intent is required. Stark is tantamount to a strict liability statute, meaning that it doesn't consider motive or knowledge of the law. Engaging in a financial transaction for a DHS and failing to meet the requirements of an exception exposes one to its penalties. As with the AKS, however, certain enacted exceptions to Stark have been noted to have a basic policy inconsistency. Why would there be an in-office ancillary services exception when the most predictable behavior of physicians pursuing their financial interests would be to order those services provided through either their own individual or group practices? In recent published comments by the American Physical Therapy Association (APTA) before the Health Subcommittee of the House Committee on Ways and Means, they noted, "One of the biggest loopholes that result in abusive financing arrangements that are created solely for profit without regard to the best interest of the Medicare beneficiary is the in-office ancillary services (IOAS) exception of the Stark Law. . . . As Congress moves to increase flexibility and explore additional exceptions under the Stark Law, APTA recommends the establishment of meaningful protections to ensure that the original intent of the law remains intact."[20]

The fact that Stark law expressly permits such IOAS financial transactions undermines the integrity assumptions regarding Congress' intent. As is true with the limitations of most laws, however, the content of Stark exceptions reflects the realities of effective lobbying and the general political compromises that occur with the enactment of any legislation.

Similar to the problems that have developed under the AKS, prohibitions of the Stark law have become increasingly inapposite for, and a significant impediment to, newer "value-based" payment models in which physicians and hospitals are paid not entirely by the volume of services they provide, but also by their efficiency and the quality of their processes and outcomes. Reducing the risk of overutilization of health care services, which was a central motivation in the passage of the Stark law, can potentially be addressed in many value-based payment models that are problematic under Stark.

The impact of Stark was considered in two "Convener on Stark Law" gatherings in 2009. Health care industry members across all branches of government, academia, health care lawyers, patients, and consumers issued a report in which the executive summary reported pros as the law having "encouraged compliance programs, restricted investment, and aided enforcement" and cons as "increased complexity and unintended consequences, impediment to changes in health care delivery and payment, inevitable noncompliance, and disproportional consequences."[21]

Stark law has come a long way since the simple framing intended by Congressman Stark in his initial legislation, which was focused on bribes and kickbacks for referrals. Stark now represents a complex set of laws intended to prevent self-referrals and the associated induced demand and incremental costs, but which also imposes restrictions on a variety of clinical and business relationships that, if they were allowed, could improve quality and reduce costs. Under the report's heading of "Impediment to Changes in Healthcare Delivery and Payment," the consensus conclusion of the convener group was "the Stark Law's requirement that any financial relationship between an entity and a physician fit within an exception can serve as an impediment to the development of new delivery and payment systems. Arrangements such as pay-for-performance, shared savings and bundled payments are frequently problematic under the Stark Law because they may not fit squarely within any existing exception."[22]

Congress has recognized some of the law's limitations, including the point that alternative payment models would be difficult or impossible to establish in a regulatory scheme that was crafted in response to a fee-for-service payment environment. As a result, section 3022(f) of the Affordable Care Act granted the Health and Human Services (HHS) Secretary the authority to waive those requirements of sections 1128A and 1128B and Title XVIII of the Social Security Act. These waivers can include certain requirements of the AKS and a few pertaining to Stark law. Under that authority, among others, the HHS Secretary has issued waivers from fraud and abuse laws for participants in the Medicare Shared Savings Program, the Bundled Payments for Care Improvement Initiative, the Comprehensive Care for Joint Replacement, and other accountable care organization programs.

One notable example of employing HHS Secretary waivers to enhance collaborative care was under the provisions of the 2015 Medicare Access and CHIP Reauthorization Act (MACRA) (chapter 10). MACRA reformed two important provisions related to "gainsharing," an arrangement in which a hospital agrees to share with a physician or group of physicians the value

of any decreases in the hospital's costs or increases in revenues that are attributable to their efforts. Specifically, MACRA included a directive requiring the HHS Secretary to develop options for amending existing fraud and
abuse laws and regulations to permit certain gainsharing arrangements,
and made modifications of the circumstances under which a gainsharing
arrangement would trigger a civil money penalty.[23]

Access and Medical Record Portability: Emergency Medical Treatment and Active Labor Act

In 1987, David Ansell and Robert Schiff reported a marked increase in "patient dumping" in many US cities. Defining "dumping" as "the denial of or
limitation in the provision of medical services to a patient for economic reasons and the referral of that patient elsewhere,"[24] the authors reported that
such patient transfers increased in Dallas from 70 per month in 1982 to more
than 200 per month in 1983; from 169 to 930 in Washington, DC, between
1981 and 1985; and from 1,295 to 5,652 in Chicago between 1980 and 1984.

This analysis followed a 1986 report in which the circumstances of 467
patients transferred to Cook County Hospital in Chicago were summarized.
The conclusion was that "patients are transferred to public hospitals predominantly for economic reasons, in spite of the fact that many of them are
in an unstable condition at the time of transfer."[25] Indeed, 87 percent were
transferred because they lacked adequate medical insurance, 24 percent
were clinically unstable at the time of transfer, and the proportion of transferred patients who died was 9.4 percent, two and a half times higher than
the mortality rate of those who were not transferred.

These two articles reflected ongoing concerns about patient dumping in
the larger health care community. Congress undertook debates and public
hearings to confront the problem, resulting in legislation to prohibit financial discrimination and the transfer of uninsured and Medicaid patients
from private to public hospitals. This was accomplished by the 1986 Emergency Medical Treatment and Active Labor Act (EMTALA),[26] which was
enacted as part of the Consolidated Omnibus Reconciliation Act. While
only facilities that participated in Medicare and Medicaid were subject to
EMTALA's requirements, almost all US hospitals participate.

EMTALA describes hospital and physician obligations as they relate to
an emergency medical condition, defined as:

(A) a medical condition manifesting itself by acute symptoms of sufficient severity (including severe pain) such that the absence of immediate medical attention could reasonably be expected to result in—

 (i) placing the individual's health (or, with respect to a pregnant woman, the health of the woman or her unborn child) in serious jeopardy,

 (ii) serious impairment to bodily functions, or

 (iii) serious dysfunction of any bodily organ or part, or

(B) with respect to a pregnant woman who is having contractions—

 (i) that there is inadequate time to effect a safe transfer to another hospital before delivery, or

 (ii) that the transfer may pose a threat to the health or safety of the woman or the unborn child."[27]

Under EMTALA, hospitals are required to

- provide appropriate medical screening examinations that are sufficient to either identify or exclude the existence of an emergency medical condition;
- stabilize patients with emergency medical conditions to a level commensurate with the hospital's capabilities;
- provide timely consultation, treatment, and hospitalization for the emergency medical condition within the "capacity" of the treating hospital and medical staff;
- transfer unstable patients to a higher level of care if benefits outweigh the risks of transfer; and
- report known violations by hospitals and physicians receiving such transfers.[28]

Adding to the prospects of new civil suits, severe monetary penalties were also built into the EMTALA law. If hospitals and physicians negligently violated EMTALA, they would be subject to a civil monetary penalty of up to $50,000 (or not more than $25,000 in the case of a hospital with less than 100 beds) for each such violation. The enforcement language included the prospect of additional fines related to the presentation of reimbursement claims when the above screening, stabilization, or transfer requirements were violated.[29] In addition to fines, patients who were injured are permitted to bring civil actions against the hospital, allowing them to pursue damages available for personal injury under the law of the state in which the hospital is located.[30]

In general, hospitals have been in good compliance with EMTALA. Over the 13-year time period of 2002–2015, the Centers for Medicare and Medicaid Services conducted about 6,000 investigations, of which about 2,500 were found to have merit as EMTALA violations.[31] This may sound like a large number, but 2,500 cases represent a tiny fraction of the hundreds of millions of emergency room visits that occurred throughout the nation over this time period. Of the 2,500 cases with merit, there were 192 settlements, with fines totaling $6.4 million.

When viewed from an enforcement perspective, EMTALA seems like a relatively minor law compared with the large recoveries obtained by the government under the AKS and Stark laws. But viewed from the perspective of promoting access and equity, EMTALA has been extraordinarily important as a comprehensive law guaranteeing nondiscriminatory access to emergency medical care and hospital services.

At the same time, since it was and is an unfunded mandate, US hospitals—primarily safety-net hospitals, but almost all hospitals to some extent—have provided uncompensated care to large numbers of patients. Indeed, those who are opposed to Medicaid expansion, and to federal subsidies for people who seek individual health insurance policies in the exchange marketplace, argue that uninsured patients already have access to health care through emergency rooms and that hospitals are substantially compensated for their care from a variety of federal, state, and local sources. While this statement is largely correct, the question remains as to whether this overall scenario is the best way to provide medical services for the uninsured. When a patient presents to an emergency room for a problem that could be easily addressed in a primary care clinic, there is inefficiency, high cost, and a mismatch of resources; and when care is delayed until the underlying medical condition becomes acute or advanced, there is unnecessary morbidity and mortality. Moreover, public funding only partly reimburses the costs of such uncompensated care, and the availability of funding from local municipalities, state subsidies, and federal programs, such as Disproportionate Share Hospital payments and upper payment limits, are extremely variable across hospitals depending on the state and local environment in which they are located.

Health Insurance Portability and Accountability Act

In the early 1990s, an increasing number of physician practices and hospitals began to utilize an array of computerized methods for electronically storing medical records. Because of concerns about the safety and privacy of these records, and also the difficulty that employees faced in keeping their health care insurance coverage intact when moving from one employer to the next, the benefits of creating a uniform computerized medical record system became apparent. Thus, a framework developed for creating a law that required uniform standards for the capture, storage, and sharing of medical record data in conjunction with new privacy protections. Moreover, this capture and storage framework was envisioned in the context of the content moving through a more robust and portable record-sharing environment via electronic data interchanges, which were initially formed in large health care systems and appeared under state government creation, facilitating state-funded Medicaid and other health programs.

As the deliberations about these issues unfolded, two distinct sections emerged. The first was the portability portion, which addressed standards that would ensure that employees would be able to maintain their health insurance when changing employers. The second part of the legislation dealt with aspects of accountability that mandated the creation and adoption of standards regarding the electronic exchange, privacy, and security of administrative and financial data relating to protected health information (PHI). Ultimately, the Health Insurance Portability and Accountability Act (HIPAA) was passed on August 21, 1996, with Ted Kennedy and Nancy Kassebaum as the act's two lead sponsors.

In 1999, the initial Privacy Rule was proposed, with multiple intakes and modifications thereafter. In August 2000, the Transaction and Code Sets Final Rule was published, creating industry-wide standards that the same codes and identifiers would be used across the board. The Privacy Final Rule was published in December 2000, protecting individual patient data, relating not only to name and medical information but also such data as home and email addresses, social security numbers, photographs, and other personal data. Enforcement Rule specifications were finalized in 2006.[32]

Subsequent amendments and modifications to HIPAA have continued on roughly an annual basis. An important provision was added to the 2009 American Recovery and Reinvestment Act, which created the Health Information Technology for Economic and Clinical Health Act. This provision required hospitals, physicians, and other entities covered under HIPAA to disclose to those whom the breach affected. In January 2013, HIPAA was updated via the Final Omnibus Rule. The most significant changes related to the expansion of HIPAA requirements to cover "business associates." This addition represented a large and significant group well beyond the prior covered entities of mostly physicians and hospitals. A business associate became defined as "a person or entity, other than a member of the workforce of a covered entity, who performs functions or activities on behalf of, or provides certain services to, a covered entity that involve access by the business associate to protected health information." Furthermore, "business associate includes a subcontractor that creates, receives, maintains, or transmits protected health information on behalf of the business associate."[33]

In addition, the 2013 Final Omnibus Rule updated the definition of "significant harm" to an individual in the analysis of a breach. This update provided more scrutiny with the intent of requiring disclosure of breaches that previously were unreported. Before this update and prior to needing to disclose, an organization needed proof that harm had occurred, whereas organizations today must prove that harm has not occurred.

The need for defining comprehensive terms was also an important part of fulfilling the intent of the law. "Health information" was statutorily defined as "any individually identified health information including demographic information that relates to the individual's past, present, or future physical or mental health condition or any other identifying information that can be used to identify the individual."[34] Without listing them here, a large number of specific identifiers are considered PHI and must be protected by from unauthorized disclosure.

HIPAA law applies to those defined as "covered entities" (table 15.1), as created by the Office of Civil Rights. By way of exclusion, a religious organization not involved in health care delivery, reporters and editors, police and fire departments (except emergency medical technicians), patients and their relatives, and clubs and associations (which are not health care providers) are among those not considered covered entities.

The legislative intent for HIPAA reflected progressive goals pertaining to the standardization of medical record data capture and their movement through electronic records, as well as assuring the protection of employee and patient privacy rights. The sheer complexity of the law's provisions, however, and the nature of the data that would be construed as potentially identifying

Table 15.1. Covered entities under the Health Insurance Portability and Accountability Act

Health care providers	Health plans	Health care clearinghouses
• Doctors • Clinics • Psychologists • Dentists • Chiropractors • Nursing Homes • Pharmacies	• Health insurance companies • Health maintanence organizations • Company health plans • Government programs that pay for health care, such as Medicare, Medicaid, and the military and veterans health care programs	This includes entities that process nonstandard health information they receive from another entity into a standard format (i.e., standard electronic format or data content) or vice versa.

Source: Office for Civil Rights, "Covered Entities and Business Associates," Health Information Privacy, US Department of Health and Human Services, accessed March 1, 2019, https://www.hhs.gov/hipaa/for -professionals/covered-entities/index.html.

affected individuals, have required precise definitions and protocols. While the language that has been crafted attempts to balance deeply held privacy concerns with the need for portability of information and the potential benefits of addressing clinical research questions with deidentified electronic records, there have emerged many difficulties and controversies. Some current examples include the inability of parents to access needed medical records of their adult children, the difficulty that medical researchers often encounter in obtaining data to answer important clinical questions, and difficulties police often have in obtaining needed distinguishing information for "people of interest," including data on those who they may plan to arrest.[35]

The law's impact on health research has been a distinctive problem. The Institute of Medicine's Committee on Health Research and the Privacy of Health Information assessed the impact of HIPAA on research. The committee concluded that "the HIPAA Privacy Rule does not protect privacy as well as it should, and that, as currently implemented, the HIPAA Privacy Rule impedes important health research. The committee found that the Privacy Rule (1) is not uniformly applicable to all health research, (2) overstates the ability of informed consent to protect privacy rather than incorporating comprehensive privacy protections, (3) conflicts with other federal regulations governing health research, (4) is interpreted differently across institutions, and (5) creates barriers to research and leads to biased research samples, which generate invalid conclusions."[36]

A survey conducted by the Association of American Medical Colleges confirmed a number of these negative effects of HIPAA on research, including

- reduced patient recruitment,
- increased likelihood of selection bias,
- increased costs of conducting research by requiring more paperwork and complicating the IRB approval process,
- increased errors in research due to the complexities of accurately accounting for deidentified information,
- increased difficulty in conducting multisite trials because IRB interpretations of HIPAA rules vary, and
- abandonment of research projects because compliance with HIPAA rules required too many resources.[37]

Legitimate concerns about the fine and penalty aspects of HIPAA have also been raised. The Office of Civil Rights is charged with enforcement of HIPAA regulations and available civil and criminal fines and penalties for privacy breaches have made noncompliance a significant consideration. In 2018, total fines paid for HIPAA violations amounted to $28,683,400, with a mean of $2,607,582 per violation. The methods for privacy breach fines include an assessment on a per-medical-record basis. The underlying causes for imposition of the range of such fines and settlements include consideration of such matters as

- risk analysis failures,
- impermissible disclosure of electronic personal health information,
- lack of policies covering electronic devices,
- lack of encryption,
- insufficient security policies,
- insufficient physical safeguards,
- filming patients without consent,
- insufficient reviews of system activity,
- failure related to response to a detected breach, and
- insufficient technical controls to prevent unauthorized ePHI access.[38]

The incidence and magnitude of HIPAA fines has been rising steadily over the past decade (figure 15.2). Initially, costs for HIPAA implementation

Figure 15.2. Trends in Health Insurance Portability and Accountability Act (HIPAA) penalties. "Summary of 2018 HIPAA Fines and Settlements," *HIPAA Journal.*[38]

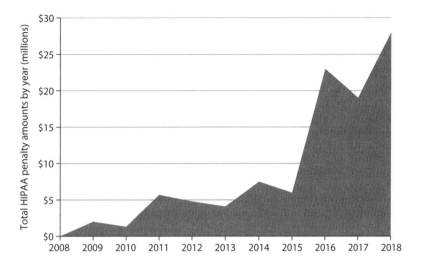

were projected to be quite high. For the period 2003–2012, the Department of the Health and Human Services estimated that the net costs of implementation would be roughly $17.5 billion.[39] Savings were expected to come from efficiency gains and improved clinical guidelines, allowing treatments to be standardized for various medical conditions. Few if any studies have been able to validate these earlier cost and savings estimates.[40] Most hospital and physician practice administrators would argue, to the contrary, that HIPAA has been a drain on efficiency.

The Health Insurance Portability and Accountability Act has been transformational in ensuring the privacy of personal health information and the portability of medical records when individuals change their insurance plans. On the other hand, the rapid evolution of electronic medical records spawned in part by HIPAA has not resulted in the level of uniformity that would be ideal from the standpoint of data exchange across health systems, and it has created significant financial and operational burdens on health care providers. Although meeting the various HIPAA privacy requirements may be viewed as onerous and unnecessary by US health care providers and their business associates, one only has to look to the Europeans to see how important privacy rights are perceived. In May 2018, a European Union law titled the General Data Protection Regulation came into effect and covers any company that has EU residents' personal data. HIPAA penalties pale by comparison.[41]

Summary

All health care services are governed by a set of federal, state, and local laws. Several specific laws arose in response to distinctive characteristics of health care services in the United States, and they each have their own rationale, success in achieving regulatory goals, and untoward effects.

The False Claims Act was designed to combat billing fraud perpetrated by those who choose to exploit the complex and highly automated nature of the claims-based billing process in the United States. By "billing their lies correctly," providers engaging in this activity can receive large amounts of fraudulent payments for a variety of diagnostic studies, visits, and procedures. It is estimated that $100 billion to $300 billion is lost to billing fraud annually, of which only a small fraction is recovered. At the same time, the complexity and nonuniformity of the claims-based billing process create enormous administrative costs, estimated at 25 percent of health insurance premiums, while also generating considerable provider frustration and discontent. Ideally, a streamlined and uniform system of claims and billing, with enhanced information technology, could result in real-time audits that would sharply curtail billing fraud while at the same time significantly reduce administrative billing and insurance-rated costs. Current trends toward more capitated and value-based reimbursement models also should lessen dependency on employing the False Claims Act.

The US system of fee-for-service claims with third-party payments has also given rise to the Anti-Kickback Statute and Stark laws designed to prevent physician self-referrals and kickback payments for referrals to and from other entities. Across time, in part as a result of significant lobbying by interest groups, a large number of exemptions have been granted in the form of safe harbors. Some of these seem appropriate (e.g., employed medical school faculty who practice and refer patients to hospital facilities that are integrated with the medical school as part of an academic health center), while others would appear to be clearly counter to the intent of these laws (e.g., specialty physicians referring to specialty lab, imaging, or surgical centers in which they have an ownership stake, or drug and device manufacturers paying kickbacks to group purchasing organizations for including their products).

The lack of access to needed health care by uninsured individuals led to the Emergency Medical Treatment and Active Labor Act, requiring hospitals to evaluate and stabilize any individual when they present to the emergency room for care, regardless of their insurance status. Enactment of EMTALA and the broad-based legal interpretation in subsequent court opinions have created an enduring and powerful statement about the evolving societal commitment to health care as "sort of a right" in the United States. As an unfunded mandate, however, hospitals carry the burden of a large amount of uncompensated care, largely borne by safety-net hospitals for which they are only partly reimbursed by public funding sources. Regardless, there are better ways to deliver nonemergent health care to the uninsured, from both a cost and quality standpoint, than through the emergency rooms of hospitals.

The importance of the integrity, portability, and privacy of personal health information, and the many untoward implications when privacy is breached, led to enactment of the Health Insurance Portability and Accountability Act. One part of HIPAA ensured that employees would be able to maintain their health insurance when changing employers. The second part related to privacy, specifically mandating the creation and adoption of standards regarding the electronic exchange, privacy, and security of administrative and financial data relating to protected health information. Like EMTALA, the evolution of HIPAA after its enactment has created an impact on health care services far more profound than initially envisioned. HIPAA has been transformational in ensuring the privacy of personal health information and the portability of medical records, but it has also created significant financial and operational burdens on health care providers. Like the False Claims Act, the benefit/cost ratio of this legislation would be weighted much more toward "benefit" if the technology of electronic medical records can achieve their promise from the standpoint of database uniformity and the ease and security of data exchange across health systems.

16 THE SAFETY AND QUALITY OF PATIENT CARE

At its best, health care in the United States is the finest in the world. For a large percentage of the population, patients obtain medical care from experienced and evidence-based physicians who serve as their true agent in making clinical recommendations. Such practitioners treat their patients based on state-of-the-art knowledge with well-honed technical skill. Patients and their doctors access what they need for such treatments in health systems dedicated to safety, quality, hospitality, and service. They take full advantage of the extraordinary advances that have occurred in pharmaceuticals, laboratory tests, imaging diagnostics, medical devices and products, electronic transfer of information, and other technological innovations. This is not a uniform experience across the population, however:

- Ten percent of Americans still have no access to health care through insurance coverage and have as their main resort an emergency room, where they will be seen in accordance with EMTALA (chapter 15).
- An increasing number of Americans have a limited scope of coverage due to their purchase of a low-premium, high-deductible health plan.
- Some nonefficacious treatments are being provided, as are high-cost treatments that are no more effective than lower-cost treatments.
- Many best-practice treatments are often not provided.
- Patients in hospitals and nursing homes experience system-related medical errors that accompany high variability in clinical practice.
- Individuals and corporations who pay taxes and health insurance premiums are adversely impacted by high national spending on health care.

Many forces have been at work in producing this state of affairs in which care, cost, and access are out of balance—a state of affairs in which the quality of care can be superb for some but not for others due to inequities in access, and in which the cost of care is uniformly high. This is the conundrum of US health care: high cost without commensurate levels of quality and access. In his monograph *The Quality Cure*, economist David Cutler refers to cost, access, and quality of care as the "three horsemen of the apocalypse"[1] In his textbook on health policy, Donald Barr refers to these three core issues as the points of an equilateral triangle.[2] He explains that as soon an attempt is made to address one of these issues, the others are affected, usually adversely.[3]

When assessing the current status of care, cost, and access in terms of specific areas that are most out of balance, and which therefore would have the most favorable impact if they were successfully addressed, we should always remain mindful of their interrelationships. The focus on imbalance is not intended to detract from the excellent work and impressive outcomes that are being accomplished by hard-working, well-meaning people throughout the industry. Those responsible for various components of health care all try to help their nonprofit institution or corporate firm be successful in achieving various missions—financial and otherwise—with the added benefit of working in a field where the noble goal of improved health is the *raison d'être*.

But in doing these jobs, myself included, we contribute to the hardwiring of the industry's underlying structure and therefore to the imbalance of care, cost, and access. Wittingly or unwittingly, in satisfying our fiduciary responsibilities and pursuing the goals of our own piece of the health care industry, we exploit the market imperfections that historically became protected by statute and cultural norms and further solidify the structure of an industry in which all the key stakeholders—doctors, hospitals, insurers, pharmaceutical companies, employers, employees—are doing sufficiently well to be (understandably) resistant to change.

Each stakeholder, of course, sees itself as being in a state of constant change. The rising cost of health insurance premiums, for example, has caused employers to shift more of the financial burden to employees. Hospitals and doctors are striving to improve quality while reducing cost. Insurers and pharmaceutical companies also see themselves as always working to add value. These stakeholders, while doing all of the above each day and also believing that they are being "mistreated" in some respects, are doing so within an industry that, overall, is treating them well. While they *are* in a constant state of change, the overall structure of the industry is not something they would like to change in a fundamental way.

The Tension between Professional Autonomy and High Reliability

"The patient comes first." This is a core value in the mission statements of physician practices, hospitals, and other health care providers. Implicit in this statement is what does not come first: not the doctor, nurse, or other health professional; not the computer screen, documentation, or coding; and not the financial implications of providing care one way rather than another.

"Because I want to help people." This is the answer given by most applicants to medical school in answer to the question: "Why do you want to become a doctor?" Similar sentiments motivate people to enter other health professions. Thus, virtually everyone who becomes a physician does so with a strongly held view—in fact, the very reason for choosing the profession—that the patient comes first.

Just as it is a short distance from "because I want to help people" to "the patient comes first," most health professionals readily translate "the patient comes first" to a desire to provide the highest-quality health care possible. This translation is not simple, however. After long periods of training, and years of clinical experience, physicians naturally develop beliefs about how best to approach the clinical circumstances of their patients. However, their approach may or may not be consistent with the best evidence available and with their specialty's recommendations and guidelines (chapter 13). The professional autonomy of the physician, which in the advocacy language of the profession is often described as the "sanctity of the physician-patient relationship," is important, but as a society we have to ask ourselves about the limits of autonomy when the variability in clinical decision-making impairs quality. As the years pass from completion of training, intuitive decisions made by physicians based on their "clinical experience" may or may not be informed by current medical literature. In hospital practice, clinical outcomes are not optimized when the varied intuitions and clinical experiences of a dozen specialists in a particular field lead to a dozen different ways to approach the care of a given patient. Thus, there is an ongoing tension between professional autonomy and high reliability.

During my childhood and adolescence, the physician who treated all members of my family, Dr. Berman, was a general practitioner (family medicine was not yet a specialty). Dr. Berman had a small office with no receptionist. A nurse assisted him on some visits, but he took our temperature and blood pressure and drew our blood himself. He saw to the routine health care needs of our family, but he also set my arm in a cast when it was fractured during a high school basketball game and diagnosed early breast cancer in my grandmother. (I vividly recall that he admitted her to the hospital, chose the surgeon, and made post-op rounds in the hospital and subsequent visits to our home.) Dr. Berman, to me, exemplified the "patient comes first" view of high-quality health care and profoundly influenced my choice of medicine as a career.

Half a century later, the health professions are not the same. Explosions in scientific knowledge and medical technology have occurred. People are living longer and often develop more complex conditions affecting many organ systems at once. And health care teams are required to provide care that can best take advantage of new and constantly evolving knowledge and technology. Patients appropriately expect evidence-based decision-making, with documentation of what was done and why. The few scratches that Dr. Berman made in his chart would not now pass muster, and in retrospect our family had no way of knowing whether his decisions about treating (or not treating) a condition, and how to do so, were correct based on the best scientific evidence. We trusted him, and I like to think that we did so with good reason.

In a 2009 article by David Leonhardt in the *New York Times Magazine*, the appeal of physician autonomy is nicely put: "Doctors have a degree of professional autonomy that is probably unmatched outside academia. And that is how we like it. We think of our doctors as wise men and women who can combine knowledge and instinct to land on just the right treatment. Our fictional doctor heroes, from Marcus Welby to House, are iconoclasts who don't go by the book. They rely on intuition, and intuition is indeed a powerful thing, be it in medicine or other parts of life."[4]

Indeed, across generations of medical students and house officers, continuing to the present, variations among attending physicians in practice "styles" have been accepted and even celebrated. While there are many ways of performing a certain surgical procedure or providing care to a particular type of medical patient, there always seems to be an "institutional way." Moreover, within each institution there is variation between attending physicians. Being trained in a surgical field, I learned that each of my teachers had their preferred draping method, their favorite instruments, their personalized set of steps in a surgical sequence, their individual variants in performing each step, their own variation on pre-op and post-op orders, and so on. As a resident, you learned the institutional way and then the modifications of the various faculty surgeons.

All of these variations appeared to work reasonably well, although experientially some *seemed* to work better than others. Thus, each surgeon-in-training builds on the basic way of doing different operations at his or her institution of training and then chooses what he or she perceives as the very best combination of surgical techniques from a myriad of experiences under different attending surgeons, making that unique combination his or her own. Similarly, each pulmonary care specialist develops his or her own style of adjusting the settings of a ventilator for patients in an intensive care unit, each endocrinologist develops his or her own style of adjusting insulin for their diabetic patients, and so on.

Alongside the science of medical and surgical practice, this reflects the "art" of medicine. In many respects, it will remain alive and well, as it should. In certain areas, however, we must ask ourselves whether the desire for professional autonomy must be balanced against the need for high reliability to achieve optimal patient outcomes.

Lack of High Reliability Leads to System Errors

As an example, here is a story about the management of sepsis at the University of Florida Health, the academic health center where I had responsibility as its president.

Sepsis is a potentially life-threatening condition caused by the body's extreme response to an infection. Sepsis occurs when an infection that is already present—in the lungs, urinary tract, skin, or elsewhere—triggers a chain reaction affecting all organ systems. The depletion of intravascular volume caused by sepsis, along with depression of the heart's function and increased metabolism, leads to an imbalance between the need for oxygen by tissues throughout the body and its ability to deliver that oxygen through the bloodstream. Untreated, this process can lead to global tissue hypoxia, multiorgan failure, shock, and death.

Individuals with infection who are at greatest risk for transition to sepsis are those who are over 65 years old or less than 1 year old, are immunocompromised, and/or have chronic diseases. The transition from infection to sepsis to septic shock occurs during the critical "golden hours" when the earlier the recognition and treatment, the better will be the outcome. These golden hours may elapse in the emergency room, hospital ward, or intensive care unit. In 2001, a randomized clinical trial demonstrated markedly improved outcomes with the early recognition and treatment of sepsis before the patient lands in the intensive care unit.[5] Since then, dozens of randomized clinical trials and other studies have reaffirmed this central conclusion and clarified the best approach to early recognition and treatment. Health care personnel working in hospitals and other facilities where sepsis might occur learned that they needed to "think sepsis" (know signs and symptoms to identify and treat patients as early as possible), "act fast" (once identified, treat early with recommended interventions), and "reassess" (check patient progress frequently to change therapy as needed). In 2008, international guidelines appeared as part of the Surviving Sepsis Campaign, which specified the protocols for early diagnosis, treatment, and reassessment. These guidelines, updated in 2012, have become widely known and adopted.[6]

In the fall of every year, a national consortium of hospitals receives information on their performance with respect to a wide variety of quality measures. These data are expressed as hospital performance metrics; they are shown as trend lines across time within hospitals and also relative to other hospitals. In October 2016, although our hospital received good news on our performance in many areas, the data on sepsis told us that we were going in the wrong direction. In our sepsis quality-of-care metrics, we were not performing at the highest percentile in comparison with other hospitals, which is where we wanted to be for all quality measures.

When we looked into the matter, it turned out that when it came to the evaluation and treatment of sepsis, our system was set up to respect professional autonomy more than high reliability. Each nurse and each doctor was making decisions consistent with their professional role in the hospital and doing what they thought was best for every patient, but this resulted in a large variation in clinical practice that was not always consistent. Nurses were familiar with the signs and symptoms of sepsis but not fully empowered to call a "sepsis alert" themselves, which would immediately bring together a team to evaluate the patient; instead, they contacted the physician on call, who may have been busy with other patients. Early identification was often difficult. Depending on which physician was called, there was variability in diagnosis since some physicians chose not to follow the increasingly recommended diagnostic criteria but instead made a diagnosis based on their overall clinical impression. They took the international criteria into account, codified by our institutional processes, but gave more weight to their clinical experience. Thus, diagnosis was often delayed until the patient was further along on the sepsis continuum and therefore more difficult to treat successfully. Once the diagnosis was made, there was, again, professional variation by physicians in treatment with varying degrees of divergence from the international guidelines and our institutional guidelines. These variations were based on the individual physician's view of the clinical situation at hand. Sometimes physicians were reluctant to follow certain aspects of the guidelines without consultation with a subspecialist, further delaying treatment. For example, a general internist might be reluctant to give a large fluid bolus—part of the guidelines—to a patient with heart disease for fear of other complications, and would want to consult with a cardiologist.

Improving this type of longstanding embedded culture is never easy. It takes much more than bringing together the people in leadership roles for the various clinical services, who would then hopefully follow the same guidelines and ensure that others on their service would do the same. Nursing and physician behavior are the products of years of training and cultural assimilation. And there are many hundreds of nurses and physicians that would individually have to buy in to the idea of following a more refined standard process even if, deep down, they disagreed with certain elements. We instituted structured process improvement rules: nurses had the clear authority and, indeed, an overt expectation to call a sepsis alert at the earliest time that the patient's signs and symptoms warranted it. Once the diagnosis was made, the standard treatment process should be rapidly implemented; timely reevaluation should then occur, with adjustment of treatment as needed, per consistent guidelines. It took six months of "two steps forward and one step back" to reach a point where the sepsis recommendations and new processes were followed in a reasonably uniform fashion. All of our quality metrics related to sepsis improved—time to diagnosis, need for intensive care admission, time in hospital, need for readmission, mortality rates, and others.

To Err Is Human

Our experience with sepsis is but one example of a system challenge. These experiences across all medical centers do not reflect a lack individual expertise, good intentions, or hard work among health care professionals. Rather, challenges in patient safety and overall quality of care typically result from some level of dysfunction in a system of care, partly from the tension between professional autonomy and high reliability, and partly from the sheer complexity of delivering care through patient care teams to large numbers of patients who present with a wide range of clinical urgency. Such dysfunction can occur in a complex system such as a hospital, a less complex but still multilayered system such as a physician's office, or something in between, such as a nursing home or outpatient surgicenter.

In 1998, the National Academy of Medicine (then called the Institute of Medicine) established the Committee on Quality of Health Care in America, which was charged with developing "a strategy that [would] result in a *threshold improvement* in quality over the next ten years."[7] Their first report, *To Err Is Human: Building a Safer Health System*, focused on patient safety, the first domain of quality. Funded largely by endowments from the Howard Hughes Medical Institute and an endowment established for the National Research Council by the Kellogg Foundation, the committee identified a high prevalence of adverse events due to medical errors and published this report as a call to action: "It is simply not acceptable for patients to be harmed by the same health care system that is supposed to offer healing and comfort. . . . A comprehensive approach to improving patient safety is needed. . . . To err is human, but errors can be corrected. Safety is a critical first step."[8]

The broad goal of *To Err Is Human*, including its eight detailed recommendations, was to create an environment in which hospitals and other health care entities would be incentivized to build a culture of safety that would substantially reduce medical errors. Upon its release, however, attention was riveted not to this broad objective but to a sentence on the very first page of the report: it was stated that between 44,000 and 98,000 deaths due to medical errors in hospitals occurred in 1997.[9] There is reason to believe that this estimate was a significant overstatement, but the report proved to be an important turning point; in particular, it was a wake-up call for hospitals, which have truly changed their care processes in fundamental ways since then.

Medical errors are sometimes broadly defined as acts of omission or commission that may or may not lead to patient harm. Linking deaths to medical errors, however, implies that the deaths would not have occurred in the absence of the error, or somewhat more strongly, the deaths would not have occurred if optimal care had been provided. Some hospitalized patients who are otherwise healthy die in hospitals because of a serious medication error (i.e., wrong drug or wrong dose) or due to a major medical or surgical error. These tragic cases should occur extremely rarely if at all, like airplane accidents. Most patient deaths in hospitals, however, occur in patients who are already quite sick and not from any event within the control of a health care professional. Any medical action in a sick patient is associated with some risk. In the best of hands, every surgical procedure is associated with a measurable, nonzero risk of injury. In the best of hands—with full knowledge of the patient's history, physical exam, and lab findings—every medication also has a known frequency of side effects and adverse outcomes.

When an unanticipated death occurs in a hospital, a "root cause analysis" is typically performed in which a senior medical officer convenes the personnel who were involved in the patient's care, as well as local experts in the type of illness involved, to go through the chronology of events in detail so as to understand what had occurred and to learn whether care processes can be improved. While such reviews might yield a clear and unmistakable link to a specific medical learning moment, the situation is usually more complex with many factors involved, especially in sick patients who have a number of concurrent medical problems.

To Err Is Human based its estimates of the number of deaths due to medical errors by extrapolating data from two studies, one from Colorado and Utah and the other from New York. These studies yielded estimates of the proportion of hospitalizations that result in adverse events as well as the proportion of adverse events that were associated with death. Reporting that "over half of these adverse events resulted from medical errors and could have been prevented,"[10] the committee estimated the proportion of deaths per hospitalization due to medical errors in these two studies and then extrapolated to the number of hospitalizations nationally. The linkages of a medical error with an adverse event and death in the studies cited were made on the basis of peer review using structured review instruments.

In 2001, Hayward and Hofer report on a study that illustrates the limitations of interpreting medical error statistics and extrapolating their implications for patient outcomes such as death.[11] Specifically quoting the Institute of Medicine committee's statements about deaths due to medical errors as a motivation for their study, Howard and Hofer investigated the reliability of such adverse-event reviews and the reproducibility of the committee's extrapolations by engaging 14 board-certified internists trained in the use of structured review instruments to review 111 hospital deaths at seven Department of Veterans Affairs medical centers. The inter-rater reliability of these reviews was low: if one reviewer rated a death as "definitely or probably preventable," the likelihood that the next reviewer examining the same case would agree (16 percent) was about the same as the likelihood that he or she would rate the case as "definitely not preventable" (18 percent). Moreover, the mean of reviewer ratings about whether a death could have been prevented was skewed upward due to outliers. While the estimate of preventability was 6 percent if a mean was used, it was only 1.3 percent if the median reviewer estimate was used. Furthermore, if the question was not whether optimal care could have prevented a death, but rather whether optimal care would have been expected to extend that patient's life by three months or longer with good cognitive health, the estimate declined to 0.5 percent of all deaths. Howard and Hofer conclude that, based on the review of deaths by the 14 board-certified internists and adjusting for skewness, optimal care in all cases would have resulted in about one additional patient out of every 10,000 admissions living at least three months longer in good cognitive health.

The Hayward and Hofer study points out that the care of patients with advanced complex illness often leads to outcomes that are difficult to tie back to a specific event with consensus. It also supports the argument made by McDonald, Weiner, and Hui that quantification of the link between an error and a death should take into account the expected risk of death in the absence of medical error.[12] Thus, the methodology used by the Committee on Quality of Health Care in America in generating their extrapolations most likely led to an exaggeration of the number of deaths caused by medical errors. All that said, the committee's report was indeed a wake-up call for hospitals to promote a culture of safety and to examine their care systems more carefully to ensure the highest safety of their patients. After all, even if the number of deaths caused by medical errors was much less than 48,000 to 98,000, there is plenty of room for improvement. As illustrated by the sepsis example, there are opportunities to create care systems that improve patient outcomes, including reduced mortality, in the absence of a

specific a priori "error" of a nurse or doctor. The goal for every hospital—
and by extension, every health care facility and practice—is to create systems of care that, at a minimum, do no harm, and ideally provide efficient
diagnosis and effective treatment in a healing environment that respects
patients' preferences, needs, and values.

Following the publication of *To Err Is Human*, organizations such as the
Institute for Healthcare Improvement became more prominent and actively
collaborated with hospitals and other health care facilities to accelerate the
progress of their patient safety and quality programs. Increasingly, hospital and medical center leaders and their boards took ownership of safety
and quality outcomes as well as invested resources in personnel and various digital and other tools to help monitor and improve their processes.

To Err Is Human made a substantial impact on subsequent nationwide
efforts to improve patient safety. As stated by Donald Berwick in 2004, then
president of the Institute for Healthcare Improvement, "The names of the
patients whose lives we save can never be known. Our contribution will be
what did *not* happen to them" (emphasis added).[13] Data on improved mortality rates come from the Healthcare Cost and Utilization Project of the
Agency for Healthcare Research and Quality (figure 16.1). Significant declines in mortality can be seen in each of the highly prevalent conditions of
stroke, acute myocardial infarction, pneumonia, and congestive heart failure between 2002 and 2012, and overall national hospital mortality has
mirrored these trends. Between 2000 and 2015, hospital admissions were
about the same (35.3 million in 2000 vs. 35.8 million in 2015), but the number of deaths declined from 834,802 in 2000 to 681,740 in 2015.[14] That's a
decline of over 150,000 hospital deaths per year. Put differently, between
2000 and 2015 the estimated mortality rate in hospitals (deaths per 100
admissions) declined almost 20 percent, from 2.36 in 2000 to 1.90 in 2015.

Ensuring Safety
Accreditation, Licensing, Certification, and Credentialing

Beginning with the report on medical education by Abraham Flexner in
1910 (chapter 8), an emphasis on education and training that blends scientific education with clinical training steadily evolved in all the health professions. Exacting standards of accreditation, licensing, board certification,
and hospital privileging were established. While such a rigorous regulatory
process is inconsistent with the perfect market assumption of free entry, it

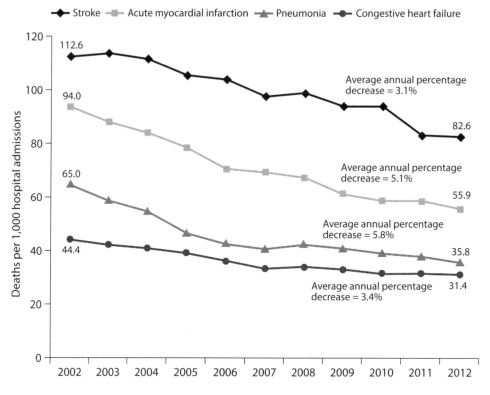

Figure 16.1. Trends in observed inpatient mortality rate per 1,000 hospital admissions for four high-volume conditions, 2002–2012. Anika L. Hines, Kevin C. Heslin, Joanna Jiang, and Rosanna Coffey, "Trends in Observed Adult Inpatient Mortality for High-Volume Conditions, 2002–2012," Statistical Brief #194 Healthcare Cost and Utilization Project, Agency for Healthcare Research and Quality, July 2015, https://www.hcup-us.ahrq .gov/reports/statbriefs/sb194-Inpatient-Mortality-High-Volume-Conditions.jsp.

provides an important safeguard for patients. US colleges of medicine, dentistry, pharmacy, nursing, and other health professions must pass a rigorous process of accreditation and periodic reaccreditation.

In medicine, dentistry, and pharmacy, professional education of four years occurs after four years of undergraduate preparation, followed by several to many years of additional training for those interested in practicing a specialty/subspecialty. Individuals in the fields of clinical psychology, physical therapy, and others take four-plus years to obtain a PhD, also typically followed by internships, fellowships, and/or postdoctoral positions before they practice independently. Each specialty and subspecialty has their own board certification (or equivalent) process, and additional safeguards occur at the level of state licensing and hospital privileging. In cases where regulatory oversight is lax, as in recent reports of rogue midwifery practices, significant patient harm can result.[15]

Assessment of Drug Safety

The Food and Drug Administration (FDA) has its roots in drug safety. At the turn of the twentieth century there were few effective drug treatments (chapter 8), and the first legislation that addressed drug safety was the Pure Food and Drug Act of 1906. This act was patterned after consumer product laws, focusing on provisions such as halting the sales of a drug if it were found to be hazardous to patients once on the market.

The requirement that manufacturers of a drug needed to show that it was safe *before* it could be sold did not occur until the Food, Drug, and Cosmetic (FD&C) Act of 1938. The FD&C Act was enacted in response to the deaths of more than 100 people in 15 states who took the antibiotic sulfanilamide, which had been used for many years in pill form to treat sore throat, in a new raspberry-flavored elixir; it turned out that the elixir was an analogue of what today would be called antifreeze.[16] The new law required drug companies to show evidence of a drug's safety (although under less rigorous standards than today). Although better than no requirement for the demonstration of safety, this law was still weak because the burden of proof was on the FDA. Unless the FDA found the drug to be unsafe on the basis of its own testing, marketing could begin as soon as 60 days after submission.[17]

In the early 1960s, thousands of European children were born with limb defects to mothers who had taken thalidomide, prompting a 1962 amendment to the FD&C Act, shifting the burden of proof of safety from the FDA to the drug company.[18] In addition, for the first time, applications from drug companies to the FDA needed to demonstrate "effectiveness" in addition to safety. Effectiveness was measured against no treatment or placebo, however, and not an existing treatment. Cost was not a consideration.

Since the FDA no longer did its own testing and relied on drug companies to demonstrate safety, it developed statutory guidelines that provided incentives for these firms to provide the needed data. As pointed out in a National Academy of Medicine report, these incentives are in the form of patents, patent extensions, or periods of market exclusivity "in exchange for data on new drugs, new indications for old drugs, and new information about the action of old drugs in special populations such as children."[19] If the safety of a drug is assured, the granting of patent extensions or market exclusivity for new indications or special populations on the basis of efficacy (typically vs. placebo) has led to market distortions related to pharmaceutical pricing (chapter 19).

Drug development occurs after researchers at "sponsors"—usually universities, research institutes, or pharmaceutical companies—identify potential compounds that may be helpful in treating a disease. The first step is to conduct preclinical research, in which data on the potential for harm (toxicity) are obtained from laboratory animals. These studies must follow highly regulated methods and processes known as "good laboratory practices," which delineate standards and requirements for researchers, facilities, equipment, and so on. An Investigational New Drug Application is then submitted to the FDA showing the results of preclinical testing in laboratory animals and what the sponsor proposes to do for human testing. At this stage, the FDA's Center for Drug Evaluation and Research (CDER), which provides oversight on the entire process for drug approval, decides whether it is safe for the company to move forward with testing in humans.

If it is concluded from the evaluation of such experiments that the new drug is safe to test in humans, and if a proposed clinical study is approved by a local Institutional Review Board (IRB), the first phase of clinical trials can begin. Healthy volunteers are usually the participants in a Phase 1 trial, the main goal of which is to determine the frequency and severity of the drug's side effects. The IRB, a panel of scientists and nonscientists, oversees the clinical research. This panel reviews and approves its study protocols (informed consent, schedule of tests and procedures, medications and dosages, study length, etc.) to ensure that the researchers have taken appropriate steps to protect study participants from harm.

Phase 1 studies are designed to confirm the safety of the drug at specified dosages; if safety is confirmed, the next phases of clinical trials can occur. These are directed at the drug's efficacy as well as the continuing assessment of its safety through collection of data on adverse effects. While the use of any drug is associated with some measure of risk, at the end of this assessment process, CDER will call a drug "safe" if its overall health benefits are judged to exceed its risks. This process has stood the test of time in producing an excellent safety record for FDA-approved drugs. The limitations of this approval process relate to the FDA's reliance on clinical trials that often compare a new drug with placebo rather than with existing effective medications as well as the absence of cost considerations (chapter 17).

Assessment of Medical Device Safety

While modifications to the approval process for medical devices are now underway,[20] the current assessment of the safety of medical devices is much less rigorous than that of drugs. In *An American Sickness*, physician-journalist Elisabeth Rosenthal points out a troublesome irony: new devices are scrutinized by the FDA far less carefully than new drugs, despite the fact that many devices become permanently implanted in the body while most drugs can be discontinued quickly if necessary.

Three different classes of medical devices were defined in a 1976 amendment to the 1938 FD&C Act. Rosenthal describes the three classes this way:

> Class 1 included equipment like tongue depressors that required little if any scrutiny. Devices whose impact as "life threatening or life sustaining," such as pacemakers, were included in Class 3. Class 2 devices were those in between, which were governed by a new program called 510(k). To gain access to the market via the 510(k) route, companies had only to claim that their new device was "substantially equivalent" to a product already sold in the United States and used for the same purpose. The program defined "substantially equivalent" in vague terms . . . : "Not intended to be so narrow as to refer only to devices that are identical to marketed devices, nor so broad as to refer to devices which are intended to be used for the same purposes as marketed devices."[21]

It is apparent from these standards that approval of safety and efficacy by the FDA is potentially much easier for devices than for drugs. Drug approval requires a multiphase process of steps, progressing from discovery to animal studies of toxicity, to human studies of safety, to randomized clinical trials (usually two) demonstrating efficacy, and to a summary judgment of net benefit over harm. This process takes several to many years. Device approval requires only documentation of "substantial equivalence" to an existing product (a "predicate device"). Moreover, the level of data documenting substantial equivalence is far stringent less for approvals through the Class 2 510(k) route than Class 3, and a fast track was created for Class 2 approvals within 90 days.

It has been reported that in contrast to the 1,200 hours spent on Class 3 requests, the FDA spent about 20 hours on 510(k) requests, only 10 percent of 510(k) applications included clinical data, and only 8 percent were submitted for outside review.[22] It is not surprising, therefore, that the vast majority of applications are now Class 2. By 2011, there were only 30–50 Class

3 approvals.[23] By contrast, in 2017 month-by-month listings of 510(k) approvals were in the range of 250–300.[24] This compares with a total of 46 novel drug approvals for all of 2017.[25]

Not only is the number of approvals of medical devices quite large, but the FDA's ability to obtain data on device-related complications is not centralized and compulsory but dependent on a wide assortment of registries to which patients, doctors, and manufacturers can report problems voluntarily. Device manufacturers could continue to sell Class 2 products even when the predicate device had been recalled because of patient harm.[26]

In 2017, there were 49 FDA recalls of medical devices.[27] At the time of this writing, there are at least 12 open class-action lawsuits involving medical devices over a wide range of applications: hernia and transvaginal mesh; bone cement; hip, elbow, and knee implants; inferior vena cava filters; intraoperative warmers; breast implants; and others.[28] While it is not known whether there would be any fewer recalls or lawsuits if more scrutiny were given to a subset of 510(k) applications at high risk for harm, concerns regarding the process of approval for such a wide range of medical devices under this program has captured the attention of the FDA leadership. A modernization plan has recently been announced by the FDA.[29]

Crossing the Quality Chasm

In 2001, the Committee on Quality of Health Care in America released its second and final report, *Crossing the Quality Chasm: A New Health System for the 21st Century*.[30] This report expanded on the first quality domain—safety—to encompass quality of care across all domains. The committee concluded that a "higher level of quality cannot be achieved by further stressing current systems of care. The current care systems cannot do the job. Trying harder will not work. Changing systems of care will."[31]

The committee proposed six aims for quality to address what it concluded were the key dimensions in which care systems were functioning at "far lower levels than it can and should be."[32] Specifically, they proposed that health care should be:

- *Safe*: avoiding injuries to patients from the care that is intended to help them.

- *Effective*: providing services based on scientific knowledge to all who could benefit, and refraining from providing services to those not likely to benefit [avoiding underuse and overuse, respectively].
- *Patient-centered*: providing care that is respectful of and responsive to individual patient preferences, need, and values, and ensuring that patient values guide all clinical decisions.
- *Timely*: reducing waits and sometimes harmful delays for both those who receive and those who give care.
- *Efficient*: avoiding waste, including waste of equipment, supplies, ideas, and energy.
- *Equitable*: providing care that does not vary in quality because of personal characteristics such as gender, ethnicity, geographic location, and socioeconomic status.[33]

For our local health system and many others across the nation, these six overarching aims have stood the test of time in guiding efforts to improve our quality of care. In providing an organizing framework for the activities and goals in hospitals and other health care facilities, it defines true north. As applied to a specific example such as sepsis, shortcomings in performance against these aims can be identified by leadership in a given hospital, remedies in the care system can be designed and implemented, and improvements measured. As applied to the US health care industry as a whole, the same process can occur and is occurring.

Following on the heels of *To Err Is Human*, *Crossing the Quality Chasm* caused a serious inwardly directed review of care systems by the leadership of the various entities that make up the health care industry—not only hospitals but all the other health care constituencies as well. This quality journey is ongoing nationally. As already discussed, progress is being made by health care institutions to upgrade care processes in a manner that improve the safety of care (i.e., avoiding injuries or harm). This applies not only to mortality (figure 16.1) but also to other areas of patient care safety to avoid harm. The effectiveness of such efforts has been demonstrated by the Partnership for Patients (PfP) campaign of the Center for Medicare and Medicaid Innovation, which was created by the 2010 Patient Protection and Affordable Care Act (ACA). The PfP campaign created 16 Hospital Improvement Innovation Networks and funded 17 state, regional, national, and hospital system organizations as Hospital Engagement Networks, which were integrated with the 18 sites of the ACA's Community Care Transitions Program and the goals of decreasing both preventable hospital-acquired conditions and preventable complications during a transition from one care setting to another. One of the measures for the latter goal was reduction in hospital readmissions. Data from 2010 were used as a baseline, and an interim report on the PfP campaign showed impressive national results.[34] Overall, it was estimated that there were over 1.6 million fewer adverse events during 2011–2013, as compared with the 2010 baseline. Expressed as a percentage reduction in rates per 1,000 hospital discharges, improvements ranged from 3.6 percent for ventilator-associated pneumonia to 49.2 percent for central line–associated blood stream infection. Overall, there was an average 16.8 percent reduction in adverse events nationally. Importantly, these reductions were observed to be of approximately the same magnitude in hospitals that did not participate in the Hospital Engagement Networks and those that were part of the network. Thus, the broad impact of the national quality movement brought about by *To Err Is Human* and *Crossing the Quality Chasm*, and championed by the Institute for Healthcare Improvement and other organizations, has been demonstrably effective.

Along similar lines, in January 2019, the Agency for Healthcare Research and Quality (AHRQ) released data on trends in 28 measures of hospital-acquired conditions (HACs) for the years 2014 to 2017 (table 16.1). Updating its methods and including a larger fraction of hospital inpatients

Table 16.1. National estimates of hospital-acquired conditions per 1,000 hospital admissions, 2014 and 2017

Hospital-acquired condition (HAC)	2014	2017	Percentage change, 2014 to 2017 (%)
Adverse drug events	33.7	24.2	−28
Catheter-associated urinary tract infections	5.7	5.4	−5
Central line-associated bloodstream infections	0.29	0.27	−6
Clostridioides difficile infections	2.9	1.8	−37
Falls	8.0	7.6	−5
Obstetric adverse events	2.3	2.2	−5
Pressure ulcers/pressure injuries	21.7	23.0	6
Surgical site infections	2.5	2.5	0
Ventilator-associated pneumonias	1.2	1.0	−13
(Post-op) venous thromboembolisms	0.9	0.7	−17
All other HACs	19.6	17.2	−12
Totals (rounded)	99.0	86.0	−13

Source: Adapted from Agency for Healthcare Research and Quality (AHRQ), *AHRQ National Scorecard on Hospital-Acquired Conditions: Updated Baseline Rates and Preliminary Results 2014–2017*, (Rockville, MD: AHRQ, January 2019), https://www.ahrq.gov/sites/default/files/wysiwyg/professionals/quality-patient-safety/pfp/hacreport-2019.pdf.

nationally, the baseline 2014 rate of HACs was 99 per 1,000 hospital admissions. This fell to 86 HACs per 1,000 admissions in 2017, a decline of 13 percent. Based on the HAC reductions that the AHRQ tracked for 2015, 2016, and 2017, it was estimated that 910,000 fewer HACs occurred nationally than if the 2014 rates had persisted, leading to approximately 20,500 HAC-related inpatient deaths averted during this time period.

Formal quality programs in health care facilities and practices are now routinely taking steps to improve the overarching aims identified in *Crossing the Quality Chasm*. In addition to mortality and other safety issues, timeliness and patient-centeredness have become core goals in most health care facilities and are often integrated into branding and business plans. With regards to the three other quality goals—effectiveness, efficiency, and equity—progress is also being made, but there are structural impediments in some areas due to an inherent lack of alignment in the industry. Along these lines, we will consider "effectiveness" and "efficiency" under the general heading of "cost" in chapters 17–19 and "equity" under the general heading of "access" in chapter 20.

Summary

The US health care industry has arrived at a point in which care, cost, and access are out of balance. Regarding patient care (i.e., the safety and quality of care), important regulatory safeguards are provided by the accreditation, training, licensing, and credentialing requirements of health professionals and the institutions that train and/or employ and host them. The Food and Drug Administration administers a rigorous approval process pertaining to drug safety. The safety oversight of medical devices has been less rigorous, but an upgrade to this process is underway.

Physicians and other health care professionals are key drivers of safety and quality through the care decisions they make with their patients, but they operate in complex systems that also contribute to patient care outcomes. Professional autonomy that is deeply rooted in training and experience can sometimes interfere with highly reliable, favorable outcomes in such systems. System dysfunction also attributes to undesired outcomes.

Two publications from a committee appointed by the National Academy of Medicine, *To Err Is Human* and *Crossing the Quality Chasm*, prompted a serious inwardly directed assessment of care processes and quality outcome metrics in hospitals and other health care entities throughout the nation. Spurred by these reports, and with formal institutional quality programs being championed by national organizations such as the Institute for Healthcare Improvement and by the Partnership for Patients campaign of the Center for Medicare and Medicaid Innovation, there has been a marked reduction in rates of hospital mortality and other measures of patient harm. Structural barriers remain, however, in quality metrics related to effectiveness, efficiency, and equity.

17 THE COST CONUNDRUM I
UTILIZATION

In assessing the current balance of care, cost, and access in the United States, cost weighs down the scale disproportionately, without commensurate outcomes in quality of care and access. Oft-cited international comparisons, showing poorer access and health outcomes in the United States despite much higher expenditures, reflect America's fundamental conundrum in health care. Let's draw on some of the concepts and findings of previous chapters while taking a deeper dive into the reasons for the high cost of US health care, beginning with a framework for deconstructing the growth in health care spending into its components of utilization and price, and then considering each of these two components in turn.

Starting with the fundamental economic identity,

$$\text{Expenditures} = \text{Price} \times \text{Quantity}$$

we remember that price and quantity of health care in the United States have been impacted by subsidized prices and induced demand (chapters 2 and 3). Subsidized prices increase the quantity of health care utilized by movement along the demand curve of consumers, while induced demand shifts the demand curve outward, increasing both price and quantity (figure 17.1). Since expenditures equal price (P) times quantity (Q), spending associated with the baseline case (i.e., no price subsidy and no induced demand) is shown by the light gray rectangle associated with baseline P_C and Q_C. The increase in expenditures associated with a producer price subsidy of $P_I - P_S$ is shown in dark gray, and the additional increment in expenditures due to induced demand is shown by the hatched rectangle.

Thus, greater expenditures due to price subsidies and induced demand are the result of higher utilization (this chapter) *and* higher prices (chapters

Figure 17.1. The effect of price subsidies and induced demand on expenditures

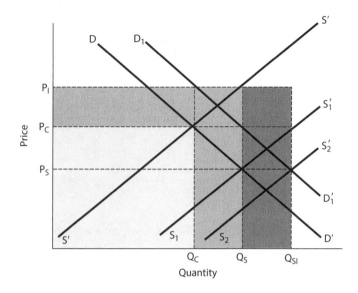

18 and 19). The relative contribution of utilization and price to expenditure growth was about the same in the 1960s, was weighted more toward price beginning in the 1970s, and has been almost entirely weighted toward price since the 1980s. While utilization per capita has been relatively constant in recent decades, service mix can be much improved. However, the mix of services used can be much improved. Low-value services should be reduced and high-value services should be increased.

Organizing Framework

For a better understanding of these components, we can create a framework that parses the relative contribution of utilization and price in accounting for expenditure growth. For the nation as a whole, total personal health care expenditures (E) is identically equal to population size (POP) times expenditures per capita (EPC). In turn, EPC equals average medical care price (P) times health care utilization per capita (UPC):

(1) $E = POP \times EPC = POP \times P \times UPC$

Using data from 1960–2017 (table 17.1), the growth in total personal health care expenditures in the United States can be been accounted for by its component parts: population, price, and utilization per capita. Two databases are particularly important in the parsing of expenditures:

Table 17.1. Decomposition of the growth in the US healthcare expenditures, 1960–2016

	1960	1970	1980	1990	2000	2010	2017
Amounts or indices							
1. Population size (in millions)	178.9	203.9	226.6	248.7	281.1	308.7	324.5
2. Per capita personal health care expenditures ($)	125.0	300.0	942.0	2,425.0	4,119.0	7,108.0	9,106.0
3. Total personal health care expenditures (E), in $billions	23.3	63.1	217.0	615.3	1,161.5	2,196.0	2,961.0
4. Medical care price index (P)	21.9	32.7	71.5	155.9	255.5	382.7	471.9
5. Consumer price index (CPI)	29.3	37.8	77.8	127.4	168.8	216.7	242.8
6. Gross domestic product (GDP), in $trillions	0.5	1.1	2.9	6.0	10.3	15.0	19.5
Compounded annual growth rates (%)[a]							
7. Per capita personal health care expenditures (EPC)		9.15	12.12	9.92	5.44	5.61	3.60
8. Medical care price index (P)		4.09	8.14	8.11	5.06	4.12	3.04
9. Utilization per capita (UPC)		5.06	3.98	1.81	0.38	1.49	0.56
10. Population		1.32	1.06	0.93	1.23	0.94	0.72
11. Calculated personal health care expenditures		10.41	13.18	10.85	6.67	6.55	4.32
12. Actual personal health care expenditures		10.47	13.15	10.98	6.56	6.58	4.36
13. CPI		2.58	7.49	5.06	2.85	2.53	1.64
14. GDP		7.08	10.33	7.62	5.57	3.87	3.82

Sources: Lines 1, 4, 5, 6: Federal Reserve Bank of St. Louis (FRED) Economic Research tables "Population," "Consumer Price Index for All Urban Consumers, Medical Care in US City Average," "Consumer Price Index for All Urban Consumers, All Items," and "Gross Domestic Product," accessed December 19, 2018, https://fred.stlouisfed.org. Lines 2 and 3: "National Health Care Expenditures Data," Historical, NHE Tables (zip file), Table02 (Excel data sheet), Centers for Medicare and Medicaid Services, accessed December 19, 2018, https://www.cms.gov /Research-Statistics-Data-and-Systems/Statistics-Trends-and-Reports/NationalHealthExpendData/NationalHealthAccountsHistorical.

[a] Calculated over the years in the previous interval. Rates for line 11 equal line 7 plus line 10. Rates for line 12 are based on data in line 3.

- The "medical care" component of the Bureau of Labor Statistics consumer price index (CPI), which is one of eight major categories of the CPI. It comprises both medical services (e.g., professional, hospital, and health insurance) and medical commodities (e.g., drugs, devices, and supplies) and reflects changes in total payments for each made by private insurers and Medicare as well as by patients (i.e., their co-pays and deductibles).[1]
- Personal health consumption expenditures, both national and per capita, which come from the National Health Expenditure Data tables reported by the Centers for Medicare and Medicaid Services (CMS).[2] These figures differ slightly from those shown in tables 10.1 and 10.2,

in that the *personal* expenditures in table 17.1 do not include spending on government administration, insurers' profits and administrative costs, and government public health activities, which are thought to represent costs that for the most part are not reflected in the medical care price index.

The growth rate of a product of two or more variables is the sum of the growth rates of each variable. As applied to equation (1), this result yields

(2)   Growth rate of E = Growth rate of POP + Growth rate of EPC

and

(3)   Growth rate of EPC = Growth rate of P + Growth rate of UPC

Overall, we have

(4)   Growth rate of E = Growth rate of POP + Growth rate of P + Growth rate of UPC

The compounded annual growth rate (CAGR) of utilization per capita is not observed but can be calculated as a residual amount from the observed CAGRs of expenditures per capita and price. Using the CAGR for the decade 1960 to 1970 as an example, the growth rate of expenditures per capita (line 7) was 9.15 percent, while the growth rate for price (line 8) was 4.09 percent. Therefore, from equation (3) the imputed growth rate for utilization per capita (line 9) was 9.15 − 4.09, or 5.06 percent. Thus, in that decade the growth in price and utilization contributed almost equally to the overall growth in expenditures, with price contributing about 45 percent. It should be noted that the residual term UPC is not a pure measure of utilization, as it represents not only changes in service volume over time but also changes in the intensitiy of service (e.g., when major surgicy that required an inpatient admission can now be done as an outpatient using minimally invasive methods).

How can the validity of this model be assessed? If equation (4) were valid, the sum of variables on the right side of the equation would yield a *computed* value for the growth rate of national personal health care expenditures that would agree with the growth rate of *actual* expenditures. Indeed, a comparison of lines 11 and 12 show that the computed and actual values for each decade are very close.

Here are some takeaways from the CAGR data:

- *National personal health care expenditures*: In the decades of the 1960s, '70s, and '80s, these expenditures (line 3) grew at a very high rate, with growth rates (line 12) in the 10 to 13 percent range. In the 1990s and 2000s, the growth rate declined to about 6.5 percent. In the 2010s, the growth rate of expenditures declined further, to an average of 4.4 percent, largely due to the aftermath of recession.
- *Population growth*: In all decades since 1960, population growth contributed about 1 percent to the compounded annual growth rate of national personal health care expenditures. There is a recent trend downward.
- *Relative contribution of price and utilization to per capita expenditure growth*: In the 1960s, the growth rate of per capita personal health care expenditures reflected almost equal contributions of price and utilization growth. In the 1970s, the growth of prices became more important, contributing about two-thirds of the growth rate in per capita expenditures. Since the 1980s, per capita expenditure growth has become even more linked to price and less to utilization, with medical care price inflation contributing 73 to 93 percent of the growth in personal health care expenditures.
- *Comparison with gross domestic product (GDP)*: For each decade from the 1960s onward, the growth rate for personal health care expenditures (line 11) exceeded the growth rate for the gross domestic product (line 14), which explains why health care spending is consuming an increasing fraction of national income. This difference appears to have been reduced since 2010, but a projected uptick in medical prices (chapter 18) is likely to push the growth in health care spending further ahead of GDP growth. It is also noteworthy that the growth rate of the medical care price index (line 8) has been consistently above the growth rate of the overall consumer price index (line 13) since 1960.

Results in Context of Previous Findings

As a way of framing the discussion of the cost conundrum for health care, it is instructive to consider the CAGR results in the context of findings in previous chapters:

- Using an econometric model estimated with a variety of robust datasets for the years 1996 to 2013, Dieleman et al. concluded that all of the growth in health care expenditures during this period was due to price rather than utilization.[3] It is remarkable that a similar conclusion is reached from the analysis of Bureau of Labor Statistics and CMS databases using very different methods: that is, price has been much more important than utilization in explaining the growth in medical expenditures in recent decades.

Regarding price, in previous chapters we reviewed the high and rising pharmaceutical prices in comparison with peer nations. This also holds for medical device prices. Administrative overhead was also found to be severalfold higher than in peer nations. Regarding utilization, specific diagnostic imaging studies and procedures were highlighted in several studies as having particular potential for provider-induced demand.

- A significant share of geographic variation in health care utilization and expenditure is unexplained by health status and supply-side factors such as practice styles (chapter 5). Residual, unexplained variation in spending might be due to unmeasured variables associated with health status, patient preferences, practice styles, or other pertinent factors. Residual unexplained variation also implies that some of the high costs of medical care may be due to inefficiencies, including inadequate use of evidence-based practice and inadequate care systems in hospitals and other health care service sites.

Ezekiel Emanuel has calculated health care costs for the United States, Germany, the Netherlands, and Sweden on a per capita basis,[4] using data from the 2018 Papanicolas, Woskie, and Jha paper.[5] Consistent with the thrust of the other findings, he concluded that two drivers of utilization (imaging studies and high volumes of selected procedures) and two drivers of price (drug prices and administrative overhead) account for almost two-thirds of the higher health care costs in the United States.

With this framework as background, we will now consider the utilization component of medical spending.

Utilization

Health care utilization increased throughout most of the twentieth century. Few now die at a young age from the infectious diseases that took the lives of so many during the first half of the twentieth century, but living longer

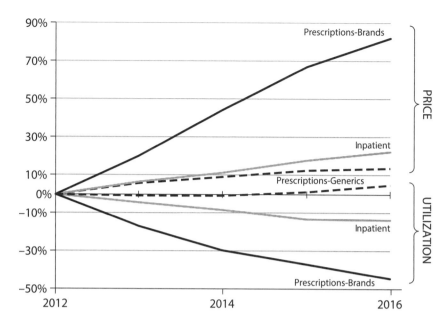

Figure 17.2. Percentage change in the US health care price and utilization, 2012–2016. Adapted from Health Care Cost Institute, *2016 Health Care Cost and Utilization Report* (Washington, DC: Health Care Cost Institute, January 2018), table A3, https://drive.google.com/file/d/1vi3S2pjThLFVwB7OtYwFmOiLVPTFl_wk/view.

means a greater prevalence of lifestyle-related diseases such as type 2 diabetes, heart disease, and stroke and of age-associated afflictions such as cancer and neurodegenerative diseases. The increased prevalence of these diseases, coupled with the emergence of effective treatments that could be purchased at highly subsidized prices, drove the increase in health care utilization during most of the second half of the twentieth century.

From the standpoint of overall health care utilization, this process appears to have played itself out by the 1980s, as noted earlier. Recent data on price and utilization in the employer-sponsored, insured sector of the health care industry bear out these trends. Data compiled by the Health Care Cost Institute for the years 2012 to 2016 show flat or declining utilization for all components but generic prescription drugs, and increasing prices in all components, especially branded prescription drugs (figure 17.2).

In addition, harkening back to chapter 6, our almost twofold-higher health care expenditures per capita in comparison with other high-income nations can also be attributed to price, since overall utilization is comparable. Since the comparator countries have universal coverage with low or no co-pays, it may seem counterintuitive that utilization is not lower in the United States, where there are significant deductibles, co-pays, and coinsurance. As noted in chapter 4, out-of-pocket expenditures per capita in the United States is twice as high (or almost twice as high) as they are in Canada, Denmark, France, Germany, Italy, Japan, the Netherlands, Spain, and the United Kingdom.[6] Other things being equal, higher out-of-pocket expenditures would predict lower utilization in the United States. The observed similar levels of actual utilization are likely due to offsetting forces:

- *Lower* utilization in the United States of medical services that are reduced by co-pays or deductibles—for example, a per capita mean of 4 physician visits per year in the United States vs. about 6.5 for other high-income countries, and 125 hospital discharges per 1,000 population in the United States vs. 150 per 1,000 population for the other countries;[7] versus
- *Higher* utilization in the United States of medical services that are potentially subject to provider-induced demand—for example, the highest or second-highest rates of coronary angioplasty, coronary artery bypass surgery, cataract surgery, total knee replacements, CT scans, and MRIs.[8]

The ideal objective in a health care industry based on health insurance with co-pays and deductibles is to create benefit designs that strike the right balance regarding out-of-pocket costs: they should be low enough to ensure that people in need of highly effective medical care do not forego treatment because of cost while not so low as to encourage discretionary or ineffective treatments that become overused. It benefits the individual and the society for patients in need of effective health care to obtain it at an affordable price (e.g., the diabetic in need of insulin, the stroke victim in need of emergency endovascular treatment, and the sexually active teenager in need of contraception). It does not benefit the individual and society, however, to subsidize the cost of treatments that, depending on the clinical circumstances, would not hold up to peer-review scrutiny regarding effectiveness.

"Value-based insurance products" for patients, in parallel with "value-based reimbursement" for providers, attempt to achieve this finely-tuned balance through benefit design. Value in health care is in the eye of the beholder, but for our purposes we will follow a standard definition in the literature, which defines value as the health outcomes achieved per dollar spent.[9] For patients, the idea is to incorporate a low (or no) co-pay for effective tests or treatments and high co-pays for treatments with little demonstrated efficacy. For physicians and other providers, the idea is that compensation should be enhanced for high-value services and reduced for low-value services.

Value-based insurance products are in an early stage of development. Most current plans do not distinguish between low- and high-value services and drugs with respect to patient co-pays or provider reimbursement. Thus, prevailing insurance practice poses two key challenges vis-à-vis the ideal of encouraging the use of needed health care while discouraging unneeded use:

1. With respect to the use of needed medical care at affordable prices, financial barriers are posed by increasing out-of-pocket costs. Currently, patients are facing increasing prices for many drugs and other services, for which there is often a fixed percentage rate of coinsurance above the deductible. Out-of-pocket costs are also on the rise due to the increasing use of high-deductible health plans.
2. Overuse can occur when, in a setting of highly subsidized prices, demand can be induced. Partly related to the practice styles and beliefs of physicians and other health care professionals, and partly by financial gain, medical overuse continues to result in health care utilization that is not supported by the best evidence. The recent growth of direct-to-consumer advertising has also contributed to overuse.

These two challenges adversely affecting value-based utilization will now be considered in turn.

Effect of Increasing Out-of-Pocket Costs on Utilization

In recent years, out-of-pocket costs have been increasing due to higher drug costs and changes in health plan benefit design, including higher co-payments, coinsurance rates, and/or deductibles. The use of insulin by patients with diabetes is a good example of the adverse impact of increasing drug prices on the utilization of needed medications. Acccording to the American Diabetes Association, the cost of insulin rose almost 600 percent between 2001 and 2015.[10] The average annual spending for insulin among

Type 1 diabetics increased from $2,864 to $5,705 between 2012 and 2016.[11] The cost of insulin has continued its rapid rise since 2016, which particularly affects those with above-aveage insulin needs. (The reasons for the price increase are reviewed in chapter 18.) For the individual with diabetes whose health plan has a coinsurance rate for drugs that is a fixed percentage of the list price, higher insulin prices translate into higher out-of-pocket costs. Patients with limited incomes may cut back on their insulin dosages until they have acute symptoms like dizziness. Such a scenario may lead to episodic emergency room visits, poorer glycemic control across longer periods of time, and therefore more severe long-term sequelae involving the blood vessels, heart, eyes, nerves, and kidneys. There are many examples of this phenomenon for medications used in neurology, cardiology, pulmonology, hepatology, and other areas of medical care.

High-Deductible Health Plans

High-deductible health plans (HDHPs) have increasingly become a reason for greater out-of-pocket costs. Whether through employers or individual policies purchased from association health plans or short-term limited duration plans, individuals purchasing these plans tend to be younger, healthier, and/or have lower incomes. But if there is an accident or serious illness, a large set of medical bills subject to the high deductible will appear all at once. These bills represent a significant challenge for a large fraction of the population since, according to the Federal Reserve, 40 percent of adults cannot cover an unexpected expense of $400 without selling something or borrowing money.[12]

Although a serious accident or unexpected illness is an unusual event, an HDHP may also impact more "routine" medical problems. For example, someone who has symptoms of what is perceived as a minor illness (e.g., a cold or flu) may delay care under a high-deductible plan until the underlying condition evolves into something that is more serious and difficult to treat (e.g., pneumonia). Indeed, delay in care has been documented in a natural experiment of patients with diabetes whose employer changed their health insurance from a low-deductible to high-deductible plan. J. Frank Wharam and his collaborators used a commercial claims database to create a cohort of private firms that made such a switch; comparable firms that continued with a low-deductible plan were used as controls.[13] They were able to identify 33,957 patients with diabetes who were employed by firms that switched from low-deductible to high-deductible plans and 242,942 diabetic patients who were matched on a variety demographic characteristics and employed by firms that maintained a low-deductible plan. Patients were followed up to four years. In the high-deductible group, there was a mean delay of 1.5 months in seeking care for the first major symptom, 1.9 months for the first diagnostic test, and 3.1 months for the first procedure-based treatment, most commonly associated with coronary artery disease.[14]

Notwithstanding these findings, the direction for health insurance in the United States is clearly toward HDHPs. In 2018, 29 percent of employees in a nationwide sample of private firms were enrolled in HDHPs, as compared to 9 percent a decade earlier.[15] Using dollars saved by reduced premiums, some employers deposit part of these savings in health savings accounts (HSAs) for employees, which can be used to defray incurred medical expenses. HDHPs could be a good thing if ineffective health care services were discontinued because of the high deductibles and effective services were retained. Based on the best evidence available, however, this has not occurred. Zarek Brot-Goldberg and his colleagues leveraged six years of detailed patient-provider data in another natural experiment: a large self-insured firm transitioned from "free" (zero premium and zero deductible) health care to an HDHP for its employees and their families, numbering more than 100,000 people.[16] They found a reduction in utilization across the full spectrum of health care services—a decline in both potentially effective care, including preventive services, and in potentially wasteful care. There was no evidence of price shopping after two years in the high-deductible plan.[17]

A systematic review of 28 methodologically rigorous studies that compared HDHPs and traditional health plans also showed an across-the-board impact of the HDHP in most studies; that is, there was a reduction in *both* inappropriate and appropriate care, including preventive services.[18] Using claims from a large commercial insurer, Reid, Rabideau, and Good compared the change in spending on 26 "low-value" services for patients switching from a traditional health plan to a HDHP plan. Specific low-value services were chosen based on extensive previous research and included procedures such as screening for carotid artery disease in an asymptomatic adult, a brain wave measure or head imaging for uncomplicated headache, and stress testing for stable coronary artery disease. Although there was an average $232 reduction in annual outpatient spending overall, no significant reductions were observed for the low-value services. The authors concluded that HDHPs may be "too blunt an instrument to specifically curtail low-value health care spending."[19]

Major employers that have implemented high-deductible plans have taken note that their employees reduce both needed and unneeded care under HDHPs. For example, as reported by *Bloomberg*, Jamie Dimon, CEO of JPMorgan, stated, "We all thought high deductibles are going to drive people to get involved—'skin in the game.' [Instead] they didn't get the surgery they needed, when they needed it, because they can't afford the high deductible in one shot."[20] Also according to *Bloomberg*, JPMorgan effectively eliminated the deductible for employees earning less than $60,000 per year.[21] And when CVS Pharmacy switched its 200,000 employees and their families to a high-deductible plan, some employees stopped taking their prescribed medications; therefore, CVS now offers their employees a group of generic drugs for free, including insulin.[22] This approach has been formalized into a framework called a "high-value health plan," which is an HSA-HDHP coupled plan combined with exemptions for services that have proven benefit.[23] Recognizing that HDHPs (whether coupled or not with HSAs) will play an increasingly important role in US health insurance plans, it will be instructive to learn from actions like those taken by JPMorgan and CVS in their efforts to find a "sweet spot" of coverage options for their employees.

The high-deductible health plan, especially when combined with a health savings account, is potentially a powerful idea if employees are provided with safeguards for needed medications and services, and if they have ready access to high-quality information (and potentially other tools) to avoid low-value services. We must be careful, however, for situations in which the language often associated with HDHPs, like "consumer directed health care," is not a euphemism for shifting the cost of health care from employers to employees. This topic will be discussed further in chapter 20.

Value-Based Insurance Design: Out-of-Pocket Costs

Value-based insurance design (VBID) derives from the principle of encouraging the use of high-value clinical services by reducing or removing out-of-pocket costs for these services, and reducing the use of low-value services by raising their out-of-pocket costs. Based on a consumer's age and risk factors, VBID in principle aligns his or her out-of-pocket costs with clinical services, based on the relative value of these services given his or her demographic and clinical characteristics.

Most of the implementation of VBID has thus far focused on the reduction or elimination of cost sharing for high-value services, such as primary and preventive care; generic drugs; and medications that target control of asthma, high blood pressure, high cholesterol, and diabetes, among others. Fewer programs have increased cost-sharing for low-value services, including specified subspecialty diagnostic studies and interventional treatments. A number of states are experimenting with pilot VBID programs, as are Blue Cross Blue Shield and commercial plans.[24] While modest benefits have been reported in the component of VBID focused on reducing cost-sharing for high-value services,[25] most employers have been reluctant to increase cost-sharing for low-value services. Results from the experience of the few employers who have done so are accumulating.

Effect of Induced Demand on Utilization

Utilization is influenced not only by subsidized prices, but by induced demand. Demand can be induced directly by providers, but also by pharmaceutical companies, medical device manufacturers, and hospitals through marketing or other means (chapter 5).

Although the concept of "induced demand" sounds pejorative, some types of induced demand are appropriate and warranted. Patients may be recommended a new treatment by their physician, for example, that has good evidence of better outcomes and fewer side effects, but about which they would otherwise not be aware. In this regard, the physician is acting as the patient's agent, doing good and avoiding harm. In some cases, however, physicians and other providers may recommend treatments that are inconsistent with best evidence but follow a set of practice styles and beliefs that are deeply rooted in their training, clinical experience, and standards of local practice. This phenomenon, which has come to be known as "medical overuse," leads to increased health care expenditures due to the provision of too much low-value care. Additional induced demand for services that are ineffective but costly, or minimally more effective than standard treatments but much costlier, may be motivated by conscious or unconscious conflicts of interest and personal financial gain. This behavior represents unwarranted physician-induced demand. Finally, demand may be influenced by drug company marketing, whether to patients, physicians, or both. Marketing to physicians by medical device manufacturers can also create utilization of a new technology before definitive outcome data are available.

In chapter 10 we discussed some specific examples of unwarranted induced demand in terms of specific medical services that continue to be provided despite randomized clinical trials failing to demonstrate effectiveness. Here we provide a broader overview of medical overuse and the impact on utilization of direct-to-consumer advertising.

Medical Overuse

The "Less Is More" series in *JAMA Internal Medicine* publishes articles that document "the ways that overuse of medical care fails to improve outcomes, harms patients, and wastes resources."[26] In announcing the launch of this series in 2010, Deborah Grady and Rita Redberg stated cogently the many reasons why more medical care may be provided than is needed: "These include payment systems that reward procedures disproportionately compared with talking to patients, expectations of patients who equate testing and interventions with better care, the glamour of technology, the fact that it may be quicker to order a test or write a prescription than explain to a patient why they are not being treated, and of course, defensive medicine. Another reason is 'technology creep.' After a device is approved for use with a high-risk population in which there is a proven benefit, its use often expands to lower-risk groups in which the benefit does not outweigh the risk."[27]

In 2013, a paper published by Lipitz-Snyderman and Bach in the "Less Is More" series created a helpful conceptualization.[28] These writers identified three different dimensions of overuse:

- *Benefit-harm*: Overuse occurs when the potential harms exceed the potential benefits. Examples given were unnecessary colorectal cancer screening for average-risk individuals and futile therapy in terminally ill patients.
- *Benefit-cost*: Overuse occurs when the magnitude of potential benefits is small relative to the costs. Examples given were bone scans for groups at low risk of osteoporosis and high-cost chemotherapy when the expected increased survival is minimal.

- *Consideration of patient preference*: Overuse occurs when patients' values and preferences are not taken into account in a shared decision-making manner. An example given was initiation of dialysis in a situation involving survival and quality-of-life tradeoffs.

Many other examples can be given in each category. Under benefit-harm, for example, antibiotic overuse in inpatient settings has been found to lead to antibiotic resistance and *Clostridium difficile* infection,[29] and 45 of 274 patients seen in consultation by a senior neurosurgeon had been told they needed spine surgery despite the lack of abnormal neurological and radiographic findings.[30] Under benefit-cost, it has been estimated that 26 percent of advanced imaging[31] and 12 percent of cardiac catheterizations for nonacute indicataions[32] are unnecessary or inappropriate. And under patient preference, aggressive treatment is sometimes used near the end of life for patients with cancer and other chronic illnesses, even when the intensity level does not match patients' preferences.[33]

In January 2018 and February 2019, *JAMA Internal Medicine* published its fourth[34] and fifth[35] annual updates on medical overuse. From a structured review of the literature, it is a telling commentary on the maturation of the field that they were able to identify 777 articles published in 2016 and 910 in 2017 that addressed the issue of medical overuse in the care of adults, even after discarding editorials, letters, case reports, and review papers. From these articles, the updates consisted of describing the 10 most important studies each year, as judged by consensus according to quality of methods, magnitude of clinical impact, and number of patients potentially affected. A somewhat different organizational scheme was used than the one proposed by Lipitz-Snyderman and Bach: papers were categorized by overtesting, overdiagnosis, overtreatment, and methods to reduce overuse.

- *Overtesting* was documented in the evaluation of stroke, pulmonary embolism, upper respiratory symptoms, the detection of asymptomatic carotid stenosis, and unnecessary electrocardiograms in low-risk asymptomatic adults that may lead to a cascade of downstream services. For example, a study of patients with respiratory symptoms showed that use of the CT scan in emergency rooms increased dramatically between 2001 and 2010 without improving patient management or outcome.[36]

- *Overdiagnosis* was documented in a study of physician-recommended interventions for an asymptomatic thyroid finding that was suspicious for cancer of a type that would not be harmful.[37]
- *Overtreatment* was documented in patients with localized prostate cancer and chronic obstructive pulmonary disease, and in the overuse of nutritional support in medical inpatients, calcium and vitamin D supplementation, medications for sciatica, and robotic-assisted surgery for radical nephrectomy. For example, a meta-analysis of 33 randomized trials involving 51,145 adults over the age of 50 showed that calcium and vitamin D supplementation did not reduce bone fracture risk compared to placebo or no treatment.[38]
- *Methods to reduce overtreatment* included the use of antibiotics for upper respiratory tract infections (URI), cardiac imaging for patients with chest pain, and guidelines to use spirometry for stepping down asthma treatment when patients achieve good control of their disease. For example, in a study of antibiotic use for URI, an intervention involving peer comparison led to a reduction in inappropriate antibiotic prescribing from 19.9 percent to 3.7 percent.[39]

The problem of overuse is not only being studied more extensively in the medical literature, but it is now being disseminated to a broader audience. H. Gilbert Welch, a primary care physician and epidemiologist at Dartmouth Medical School, has written three books on the subject.[40] As Jane Brody wrote in her *New York Times* review of Welch's last book, *Less Medicine, More Health*, "Dr. Welch submits that too many people are being tested for too many things, being subjected to treatments they do not need and, in the process, being exposed to procedures that may do more harm than good."[41] In a highly accessible fashion, Welch uses epidemiologic concepts to make the point that lowering the threshold of "positivity" for tests that screen for disease, especially those with a low underlying prevalence, will yield a large number of false positive tests. Given multiple tests with low positive thresholds, most people will be positive for *something*. Asymptomatic people then become "patients" and are given diagnostic labels, medications, and potentially invasive procedures. Welch applies this paradigm with great insight to a wide variety of conditions, ranging from hypertension to diabetes, osteoporosis, gallstones, bulging discs, damaged knee cartilage, cancer, and others.

It is encouraging that many physicians now acknowledge that overuse indeed occurs in medical practice. Lyu et al. surveyed 2,106 physicians from a random sample of 3,318 members of an American Medical Association online educational community.[42] The surveyed physicians reported that, in their judgment, a median of 21 percent of overall medical care was unnecessary, including 22 percent of prescription drugs, 25 percent of diagnostic tests, and 11 percent of procedures.

Recognizing that an emphasis on overuse challenges the status quo in medical practice, it is not surprising that there has been published criticism of the "overuse" literature. Lisa Rosenbaum, cardiologist and national correspondent for the *New England Journal of Medicine*, characterizes it as a "crusade" and an "oversimplification."[43] She concludes by stating that "until we learn how to better manage the uncomfortable uncertainties inherent in clinical care, 'less is more' may be an aphorism better suited to telling coherent stories than to the complex decisions faced by doctors and patients."[44] Responses to this criticism have emphasized the implications of *not* reducing unnecessary care from the perspective of both patient care and societal cost. John Mandrola, who states that he "lives and breathes less-is-more thinking" in his practice, expresses the view that "to simplify care . . . to heal and comfort with fewer drugs and procedures . . . defines elegance in medicine," and argues against Rosenbaum's view that a desire for information may be misperceived as greed. Rather, he opines that "medical waste is easily defined, due mostly to greed, and fixable with few tradeoffs."[45] Woloshin and Schwartz address each of Rosenbaum's arguments one by one, concluding that "we will not get to better health care by standing still."[46]

Readers can evaluate these three well-written papers and decide for themselves who makes the best case. I agree with Rosenbaum's statement that "perhaps the most accurate conclusion is that sometimes less is more, sometimes more is more, and often we just don't know."[47] Taking all of the evidence into account, however, a strong case can be made that reduction in the overuse of low-value health care services (as well as an increase in the underuse of high-value services) is not only possible but represents an essential step in improving US health care—by creating better matches between medical needs and medical care, and between clinical research and clinical practice.

Value-Based Insurance Design: Provider Reimbursement

Just as insurers are attempting to reduce utilization of low-value services by increasing consumer co-pays in value-based insurance design, they are also attempting to reduce such utilization by a variety of methods directed at providers. Some of these, such as the creation of accountable care organizations, payment bundling, the Merit-based Incentive Payment System and advanced alternative payment models, were created by CMS (chapter 10). Other value-based CMS programs that attempt to constrain expenditures through reduction in utilization (while also fostering high-quality care) include its Hospital Readmission Reduction, Hospital-Acquired Conditions Reduction, and Hospital Value-Based Purchasing programs.

Similarly, an increasingly common approach by which commercial payers are attempting to reduce utilization and in other ways increase the overall value of care is to shape the practice styles of providers in their plans through narrow and tiered networks. In narrow networks, physicians who deliver high quality care and outcomes are included in a restricted network for which consumers pay a lower premium and/or lower deductibles in comparison with the traditional broad network of physicians. In tiered networks, a large open traditional network of providers is offered but the deductibles are different between tiers of physicians, hospitals, and other providers. Those delivering higher value care (greater quality, outcome, and patient experience per dollar spent) may have lower or no deductible costs for the patient, whereas those in the lower tiers may have higher deductibles. A major component of providing higher-value care is the avoidance of low-value services. Payers can also incentivize providers to provide high-value care by giving them "green lights" through most of the pre-approval process, while requiring those providing a large amount of low-value care to stop and fully document the rationale for treatment at each stage of the pre-approval process.

This approach to controlling costs and improving the value of care has been facilitated by the emergence of resources that provide information to payers about the practice style of providers as defined by their mix of high-value and low-value services. For example, RowdMap (acquired by Cotiviti) uses the CMS database on physician claims to dive deeply into the practice decisions of individual physicians to categorize them according to their use of tests and procedures relative to value-based benchmarks. Insurers can then build their physician networks based on these data. When compared with procedure-specific benefit designs, these physician-assessment resources have made value-based reimbursement a more practical way to control health care costs by reducing the utilization of low-value services (i.e., reducing induced demand), reducing administrative costs, and encouraging the use of high-value services that enhance quality.

Direct-to-Consumer Advertising

Direct-to-consumer advertising (DTCA) by the pharmaceutical industry has increased dramatically in the United States over the past several decades. According to data from Competitive Media Reporting, DTCA increased from $55 million in 1991 to $2.5 billion in 2000, at which point some drugs had advertising budgets that eclipsed familiar brands like Pepsi, Budweiser, Dell, and Nike.[48] Since then, DTCA spending has continued to climb, reaching $5 billion in 2016, primarily driven by television spending.[49] The only other country in the world that allows DTCA of prescription drugs is New Zealand.

Most commentators date the initiation of growth in DTCA in the United States to an August 1997 clarification of broadcast regulations by the FDA. Until then, FDA regulations for pharmaceutical advertising required a "summary" of contraindications, side effects, effectiveness, and a "fair balance" of risks and benefits. In print ads, this required summary often meant the inclusion of a large amount of additional language in the advertising space, which would be unrealistic for broadcast media. That changed in August 1997 when the FDA allowed broadcast ads without the full summary. The brand name and treated conditions could be specifically stated so long as the ad includes in-broadcast disclosure of major side effects and a few other details, referred to as the "adequate provision requirement."[50]

A decade ago, most of the DTCA was for medications that treat conditions affecting large numbers of people, such as allergies, gastric ulcers, high cholesterol, hypertension, diabetes, and depression. More recently, however, there has been a shift to DTCA for drugs that treat conditions affecting a relatively smaller number of people, but with expensive prices.

The data on the five drugs with the highest DTCA expeditures in 2016 (table 17.2) reflect the net results of the positive and negative features of the US health care industry as applied to drug development and commercialization. On one hand, there is innovation and medical progress; on the other, there is high cost due to monopoly pricing and overutilization from DTCA-induced demand. We will consider innovation and cost in turn.

Table 17.2. Direct-to-consumer advertising (DTCA) expenditures: top five brands, 2016

Brand	Indication	2016 DTCA expenditures ($ millions)	Change from 2015 (%)	2016 drug sales ($ billion)	Change from 2015 (%)
Humira	Rheumatoid arthritis, psoriasis, ulcerative colitis, other	439	20.0	16.1	14.7
Lyrica	Neuropathic pain	392	19.0	5.0	2.7
Eliquis	Prevention of vascular complications in atrial fibrillation and post surgery	296	17.0	3.3	79.7
Xeljanz	Rheumatoid arthritis (RA), psoriatic RA	258	37.0	0.9	77.0
Opdivo	Advanced cancer unresponsive to conventional chemotherapy	168	32.0	3.8	301.0

Sources: Jon Swallen, "The Complex and Evolving DTC Advertising Landscape," *Kantar Media*, May 3, 2017, https://www.kantarmedia.com/us /thinking-and-resources/blog/the-complex-and-evolving-dtc-advertising-landscape; "Product Sales Data from Annual Reports of Major Pharaceutical Companies, 2016," Pharmacompass, accessed December 20, 2018, https://www.pharmacompass.com/data-compilation/product -sales-data-from-annual-reports-of-major-pharmaceutical-companies-2016.

Innovation

A market economy entails the earnings of short-term profits by producers who enter the market with a novel product (chapter 2). With free entry, however, these profits are eroded as more producers enter the market. When the assumption of free entry does not hold, supernormal profits can be sustained. This occurs when a patent is granted to a pharmaceutical company or device manufacturer: that is, producers are essentially granted monopolies for the duration of the patent. When FDA delegated to manufacturers its responsibility for conducting studies that assess the safety and efficacy of drugs and devices, the patent was the quid pro quo.

The perfect market is efficient but static. However, there may be "dynamic efficiencies" in a market economy that can justify sustained supernormal profits when there are innovations in technology, including drug development, that produce better health outcomes for people with serious illness. Firms that support the costs of a pharmaceutical innovation that improves health, and of obtaining a patent and bringing it to market through the FDA process, are rewarded with sustained profits. This incentive assures progress in biomedical science and clinical treatments, since drug development is a risky undertaking for the pharmaceutical industry.

The cost of bringing a drug to market from discovery to pharmacy is lengthy and expensive (chapter 14). The preclinical testing process, in which the manufacturer completes synthesis and purification of the drug and conducts limited animal testing, can take from two to six years; of the thousands of compounds tested each year, only a small fraction make it through this process and are selected for clinical testing; and as clinical testing unfolds in Phase 1 through Phase 3 trials, typically another six to nine years, the number of drugs that make it through each step is reduced further. Ultimately, relatively few new drugs are submitted for FDA approval.

Estimates of the cost of this process have varied widely. In a study from the Tufts Center for the Study of Drug Development, an industry-supported center, the average out-of-pocket cost per approved new compound was estimated to be $1.40 billion (in 2013 dollars).[51] This estimate was based on a survey of 106 randomly selected but unspecified drugs produced by 10 "multinational pharmaceutical companies," the details of which were governed by confidentiality agreements. The estimated out-of-pocket cost is converted to a capitalized cost of $2.6 billion, but this is at a real discount rate of 10.5 percent, which seems quite high as an estimated cost of capital.

The Tufts group's cost estimate of drug development for large pharmaceutical companies stands in contrast to a median figure of $648 million obtained in a study of smaller firms. This lower estimate was obtained by Prasad and Mailankody, who focused on biotech start-ups with no drugs on the US market prior to receiving FDA approval for a cancer drug from 2006 through 2015.[52] Ten such companies were identified and data on cumulative research and development spending were obtained from publicly available Securities and Exchange Commission 10-K filings. The $648 million median figure (mean = $720 million) was calculated from a range of expenditures that varied from $157 million to $1.9 billion. While there have been critical analyses of the methodologies used by both research groups,[53] it is possible that a significant part of the large difference in their average estimates is due to the types of drug companies and drugs being studied in the two investigations.

For our purposes in understanding the forces that drive health care utilization, the exact cost of drug development and commercialization is less the issue than the fact that the process *is* lengthy and expensive, and it has an uncertain outcome. Moreover, based on the Tufts data, which have been analyzed using a consistent methodology across time, the process of drug development is becoming more expensive—almost double what it was 10 to

15 years ago.[54] Given these substantial costs, and the reality that pharmaceutical executives have a fiduciary responsibility to their shareholders, their responsibility is to create a business model that overcomes these costs. In the aggregate, taking the cost of drug development into account, their business model needs to produce a rate of return on their capital that will be sufficient to satisfy their investors. This may mean, for example, attempting to reduce the cost of drug development by buying companies with promising early stage products rather than doing this work in-house or forging partnerships during the development process; approximately 70 percent of new sales by major pharmaceutical houses now accrue via this route.[55] But it also means choosing drugs for investment based on their potential price and market size.

The translation of innovation to a patent with monopoly pricing results in substantial health care costs that are largely paid not by individual patients but collectively by taxpayers, employers, and employees. There is consequently an appropriate public interest in ensuring that the level of supernormal profits are not exaggerated or unduly persistent. Of note in this regard is the finding that relative to its GDP, the fraction of globally produced new molecular entities (NMEs) is *not* disproportionately higher in the United States as compared with the number of NMEs produced by 18 other countries that are innovators in drug development but have regulated drug pricing.[56] The United Kingdom is responsible for the development of 12.5 percent of the NMEs but accounted for 4.7 percent of the GDP among innovator countries. Similarly, Switzerland, Belgium, Sweden, Denmark, Israel, and Finland innovated proportionately more than their GDP would predict. In these countries, regulated drug pricing was evidently not a deterrent to innovation. The US contribution to global discovery of NMEs was roughly proportional to its GDP, although the size of the US economy means that on an absolute basis both GDP and NMEs are the largest in the United States.

Cost and DTCA-Induced Utilization

Given the 1997 change in broadcast regulations that allows pharmaceutical companies to expand their market through television advertising, their boards and executives will have a fiduciary responsibility to exploit this method of generating utilization. In this regard, drug companies are behaving in accordance with their objectives in a market-based economy. It's just that they are doing so in a system (some of which was handed to them and some of which they had a hand in creating) that has led inexorably to the current US pharmaceutical environment of high list prices and DTCA-induced demand. In order for DTCA to induce demand,

1. it must result in a consumer being motivated to request the drug from a physician,
2. the physician must respond by prescribing the drug, and
3. the drug must be affordable to the patient.

Let's consider each of these steps in turn.

Consumer Response to DTCA

It will not be surprising that consumers respond to DTCA. As early as 2003, primary care patients in Sacramento who were exposed to DTCA made drug requests in 7.2 percent of visits.[57] More recently, it has been reported that granular information on the demographics of the audience watching particular television shows are being used to target the ad buys. For example, viewers of the television show *The Big Bang Theory* are 44 percent more likely to suffer from arthritis than the general public; consequently, arthritis medications account for a large share of the $22.5 million in total pharmaceutical ad spending allocated to *Big Bang Theory* air time.[58]

Physician Response to Patient DTCA Requests

Are physicians influenced by patients who request a medication by brand name? In surveys, most doctors think not. But in practice, there is evidence that they are indeed influenced. In a 2005 study, Kravitz et al.[59] addressed this question using a research design that took advantage of the "standardized patient" (SP) technique that is now an integral part of the curricula for medical students and other health profession students. In this educational method, "actors" are given "scripts" of different medical histories, symptoms, and signs, and students are expected to figure out the diagnosis, order appropriate tests, and so on. Kravitz and his colleagues designed the study using a variant of this model by introducing the SPs covertly into actual primary care practices. Specifically, SP roles were created for two conditions: half of the SPs simulated patients suffering from depression, describing lengthy periods of sadness, low energy, poor appetite and sleep, and early-morning awakening. An antidepressant or referral for behavioral treatment is indicated for these patients. The other half of the SPs described having suffered a career upheaval and having fatigue and stress—an "adjustment disorder" scenario that did not warrant treatment.

Each of these two conditions were played out in three scenarios: one involved the SP telling the doctor that she had seen a TV ad for Paxil and asking for that specific medication, another involved asking about medications in general, and the last involving no request for medication. Primary care physicians in three cities who agreed to participate in the trial knew they would receive unannounced visits from SPs. The process was randomized in such a way that each of the 152 physicians who participated saw one SP with depression and one with adjustment disorder. The results showed that patients' requests were very influential in physician prescribing. Whether or not the SP had symptoms of depression, if she requested Paxil she got an antidepressant about half the time, and over half of those prescriptions were for Paxil. The rate of prescribing in the "adjustment disorder" condition went from 10 percent when there was no request to 55 percent when the SP made a request for Paxil.

Using a similar research design, McKinley et al.[60] conducted a study with 192 primary care physicians in six states who were exposed to two video scenarios: one was an undiagnosed "patient" with symptoms strongly suggestive of sciatica pain, and the other was a "patient" with already diagnosed chronic knee arthritis. In half of the sciatica videos, the patient specifically requested oxycodone (an opioid narcotic) and in half of the knee arthritis videos, the patient asked for Celebrex (a nonsteroidal anti-inflammatory drug). In the remaining videos, the patients simply asked for "something to help with pain." Among the sciatica patients requesting oxycodone, almost 20 percent received the prescription compared to 1 percent making no specific request. Among the knee arthritis patients requesting Celebrex, about half received the prescription compared to about a quarter making no specific request.

Based on a survey of 2,938 randomly selected physicians in seven specialties across the nation, of whom 1,891 participated, it was found that 37 percent "sometimes or often" prescribed a brand-name drug when the patient asked for it, despite the availability of an equivalent generic.[61]

While patients requesting a brand-name pharmaceutical as a result of DTCA seems to be a major factor in physician behavior, the fact that the income of physicians usually depends on service volume (whether in private practice or through a salary plus bonus compensation plan) adds complexity. Since physicians are incentivized to move patients through the office for revenue and to stay on time, a lengthy discussion of why the branded drug being requested is not better and may have a higher out-of-pocket cost for the patient does not fit the business model. Many physicians find it easier to say yes and move on to the next patient.

In general, television ad spending—even when a specific brand name is used—tends to increase the overall size of the market for that *category* of drug; the expanding size of the market boosts sales of the branded product and also the sales of other drugs in that category.[62] For any given drug in which a drug company invests in DTCA, there are presumably internal analyses that project greater net revenues from DTCA than the cost of ad production and media buys. With data from one year's DTCA results, the appropriate level of investment for the following year can be refined. The DTCA expenditures and sales data in table 17.2 suggest the success of this process, although of course there are a variety of factors that influence sales besides marketing. The effectiveness of DTCA in driving sales is supported by research data: for example, in a study of DTCA for two statin drugs in which ad exposure varied widely across 75 designated market areas between 2005 and 2009, each 100-unit increase in ad viewership was associated with a 2.22 percent increase in statin sales.[63]

Affordability

For the DTCA business model to work for pharmaceutical companies, the prescription triggered by the ad needs to be filled. For this to happen, it must be affordable to the patient. The question of affordability of specialty drugs like those shown in table 17.2 brings us back to the effect of out-of-pocket costs on utilization. Affordability for patients is based not on the full price but on out-of-pocket cost. For Medicaid patients, although benefits vary by state, most of the FDA-approved high-priced drugs are covered in full, subject to meeting clinical criteria. For commercial-pay patients, coinsurance payments for high-priced drugs can be substantial ($20,000 or more per year) but are often paid in large part through patient co-pay coupons or by rebate cards provided by foundations that are typically funded by the pharmaceutical companies (and for which they can take a charitable tax deduction). In the absence of a rebate, the cost of these drugs is covered once the patient's out-of-pocket maximum is reached, which is variably affordable depending on patient income and type of plan (i.e., traditional vs. HDHP).

To offset out-of-pocket costs for Medicare patients, those with incomes up to 400 percent of the federal poverty line can often participate in a "pharmaceutical assistance program" through foundations funded by pharmaceutical companies. These programs are illegal, however, for Medicare beneficiaries whose incomes exceed four times the federal poverty line. Such beneficiaries are therefore often subject to the largest out-of-pocket payments for specialty drugs. The Medicare Part D prescription drug plan (which is also provided by most Medicare Advantage Plans) has variable cost-sharing requirements across the coverage year. Patients pay a deductible (up to $405 in 2018), followed by an initial coverage phase in which most high-priced drugs ($670 or more per month) are placed in a "specialty tier" that is subject to coinsurance of up to 33 percent. (Beneficiaries whose incomes are below 135 percent of the federal poverty line may be eligible for a low-income subsidy, called "Extra Help").

Once total (patient plus plan) prescription spending hits an initial coverage limit ($3,750 in 2018), beneficiaries enter a coverage gap (a.k.a. a "donut hole"). Originally, beneficiaries were responsible for 100 percent of their drug costs during the coverage gap, but the Affordable Care Act reduced this obligation across time to the current rate of 25 percent. Above a "catastrophic coverage limit" of $5,000 in out-of-pocket expense, beneficiaries pay a 5 percent coinsurance rate for the remainder of the year without limit.

Under this system, annual out-of-pocket costs to Medicare beneficiaries can be substantial for specialty drugs. For the most frequently used specialty drugs to treat rheumatoid arthritis (RA), multiple sclerosis (MS), and chronic myeloid leukemia (CML), for example, total out-of-pocket costs are about $5,300, $6,700, and $9,000, respectively.[64] While expensive, this compares to the annual cost for these drugs paid by Medicare: $58,000 (RA), $86,400 (MS) and $138,000 (CML).[65]

Thus, the prospect of a breakthrough drug has created incentives for innovation in drug development, but at a cost: monopoly pricing through the granting of patents and high (and potentially cost-ineffective) utilization because of price subsidies and direct-to-consumer advertising. Drug approvals by the FDA, while extremely expensive, are based on safety and efficacy without considering cost effectiveness. In other countries, taking cost and comparative efficacy into account has led to a mix of approvals and denials. Picking two drugs from table 17.2 as examples, based on public hearings and detailed analysis of available data on efficacy and cost effectiveness, the National Institute for Health and Care Excellence of Great Britain approved Humira for psoriatic rheumatoid arthritis of a particular severity level, but not rheumatoid arthritis *per se*, and Opdivo for metastatic melanoma but not for metastatic lung cancer.[66]

Summary

The total expenditure on health care equals the quantity of services utilized times the price of those services. From a model of expenditures that allows decomposition into its price and utilization components, and from the econometric literature, it was concluded that utilization and price both played important roles in the dramatic spending growth during much of the 1960s and 1970s. Beginning in the 1980s, however, most of the spending growth has been due to price rather than utilization.

The fact that utilization has been relatively flat in recent years does not mean that utilization is unimportant in its impact on care, cost, and access. To the extent that effective health care services are *not* being used, there would be benefit from increased utilization, and to the extent that ineffective services *are* being used, they should be reduced or curtailed. Further, the suppressive effects of increased out-of-pocket costs on the utilization of effective care, and the stimulatory effects of induced demand on the utilization of services that have limited or no efficacy, are perversely offsetting. Examples of both phenomena are provided. To improve the balance of care, cost, and access, we must address the factors constraining effective care and those that foster the continuation of cost-ineffective care. Ideas for how this might be accomplished are provided in chapter 22.

18 THE COST CONUNDRUM II
PRICE: ADMINISTRATION, INSURERS, PHYSICIANS, AND HOSPITALS

Utilization is one part of the cost conundrum. Price is the other. The cumulative effect of general inflation has been a 1,600 percent increase in the consumer price index (CPI) between 1936 and 2016 (figure 18.1). While overall that is quite substantial, growth in the medical care component of the CPI has been far greater (figure 18.2).

The medical care index is one of eight major groups that make up the CPI. Table 18.1 lists the subcategories of the medical care price index and their relative weights. Decade-by-decade growth rates in the subcategories of the medical care price index are shown in figure 18.3. Some subcategories of the medical care CPI have been broken out since 1956; others, like hospital services, had been incorporated into the overall index across time and were more recently broken down into inpatient and outpatient services (and made distinct from nursing home services).[1] Of note, health insurance

Figure 18.1. US consumer price index and medical care price index, 1935–2018. "Databases, Tables & Calculators by Subject," US Bureau of Labor Statistics, accessed January 3, 2019, https://www.bls.gov /data.

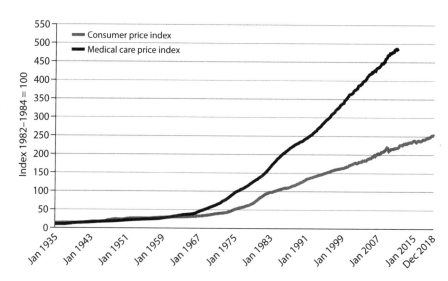

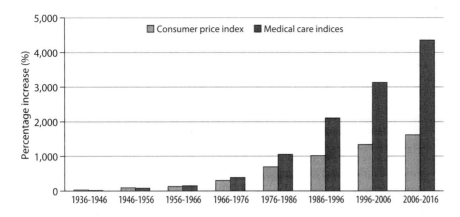

Figure 18.2. Cumulative growth in consumer price index and medical care indices, by decade, 1936–2016. "Databases, Tables & Calculators by Subject," US Bureau of Labor Statistics, accessed January 3, 2019, https://www.bls.gov/data.

Table 18.1. Bureau of Labor Statistics medical care indices and relative importance, as of December 2017

Item	Percentage of the medical care index (%)
Medical care commodities	20
Medicinal drugs	19
Prescription drugs	15
Nonprescription drugs	4
Medical equipment and supplies	1
Medical care services	80
Professional services	38
Physicians' services	20
Dental services	9
Eyeglasses and eye care	4
Services by other medical professionals	5
Hospital and related services	30
Hospital services	27
Nursing home and adult day care services	2
Care of invalids, elderly, and convalescents in the home	1
Health insurance[a]	12

Source: Adapted from "Measuring Price Change in the CPI: Medical Care," US Bureau of Labor Statistics.[2]

[a] Measures "retained earnings," which includes administrative costs and profits.

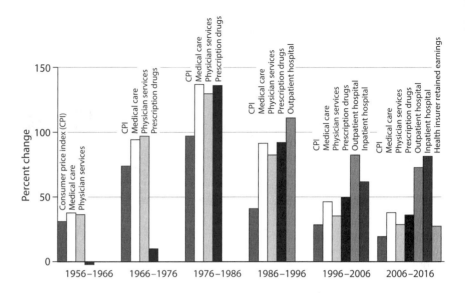

Figure 18.3. Percentage change in categories of medical care price index, by decade, 1956–2016. "Databases, Tables & Calculators by Subject," US Bureau of Labor Statistics, accessed January 3, 2019, https://www.bls.gov/data.

pricing (which reflects retained earnings, not premiums)[2] was broken out only since 2005.

Here and in the next chapter, we examine the primary role of price in health care expenditure growth. In this chapter, we begin with a consideration of billing and insurance-related administrative costs and then discuss monopolistic pricing as it applies to hospital and physician services. The pricing of pharmaceuticals and medical devices, which also reflects monopolistic elements, will be considered in chapter 19.

Billing and Insurance-Related Administrative Costs

When hospitals, physicians' offices, and insurance companies price their products, administrative costs are included. The Bureau of Labor Statistics (BLS) defines the price of health insurance as administrative costs, including profits, which they call "retained earnings." This is the difference between what insurers receive in premiums and pay out for medical care. Such an approach makes sense, since the economic activity provided by insurance companies pertains to the transaction costs of processing claims. The remaining share of the insurance premium is a pass-through payment for the costs of actual medical care.

For hospitals and physicians, almost two-thirds of administrative costs are due to billing and insurance-related (BIR) activities. For pharmaceutical costs, there has been a constellation of discounts and rebates administered through middlemen or intermediaries that have incentivized higher drug prices. These extra costs might also be viewed as administrative, but they will be considered separately in the next chapter since they are unrelated to billing and insurance-related administrative costs.

Overall Magnitude of Billing and Insurance-Related Administrative Costs

Medicare and Medicaid incur administrative costs directly but also indirectly through their fiscal intermediaries (private insurance companies). Insurers that operate commercial health insurance plans incur administrative costs as part of retained earnings, as noted earlier. Insurers also serve as third-party administrators to employers with self-insured health plans, who pay the insurer for their administrative transactional costs of processing claims plus a profit margin. Total administrative costs for government programs tend to be one third to one half the costs of private insurers. All told, the blended administrative costs of government and insurers in health care have been estimated to absorb about 8 percent of health care expenditures in the United States.[3]

Significant administrative costs are also incurred by providers, including hospitals, other health care facilities, physicians, and other health care professionals. These costs are incurred in the process of generating bills to patients and claims to payers (i.e., private insurers, Medicare and Medicaid). Ensuring compliance in the clinical documentation needed to support those claims necessitates additional administrative cost. The entire process is extremely nonstandardized and is different for each insurer and clinical service.

At a congressional hearing in 2014, the insurance industry provided estimates of retained earnings for traditional commercial health plans. For each dollar of insurance premium, they estimated retained earnings of about 13 cents: 10 cents for "claims processing, consumer services, provider support, compliance," and related activities, and 3 cents for profit.[4] This would imply a medical loss ratio (i.e., the fraction of premiums that the insurer pays for medical care) of 87 percent. It was noted in the testimony, however, that the Securities and Exchange Commission (SEC) filings by the six largest publicly traded health insurers reported lower medical loss ratios, ranging from 81.5 percent to 84.8 percent.[5] As we shall see, when provider billing and insurance-related costs are added to the retained earnings of insurers, total administrative costs for private health insurance absorb 20 to 25 cents of each premium dollar.

Complexity of Billing and Insurance-Related Activities and Their Origin

What started more than a century ago as a simple transaction between physician and patient—a fee for a medical service—has evolved into an extraordinary complex system of billing and insurance-related activities. The diagnostic coding system currently in use (*International Classification of Diseases*, Version 10, or ICD-10) has 68,000 codes, which in the United States is mapped to 10,000 distinct clinical services using the American Medical Association's Current Procedural Terminology (CPT) codes. Hospital and physician billing systems must accurately translate the information in the medical record to one or more of the diagnostic codes that defines the patient's medical problem and one or more of the services that describes what was done to address the problem. These services generate a set of charges. (In Medicare and some commercial plans, codes are often bundled into a "diagnostic-related group," or DRG, which forms the basis for the charge. The basic structure of the system is still the same.)

Importantly, each of the services charged must be justified by the diagnostic code, which in turn must be justified by the patient's underlying medical condition as documented in the electronic chart. The term "compliance" is given to the integrity of the chain that runs from medical evaluation and treatment as described in the chart, to determination of medical necessity and diagnostic code, to procedure code, to charge.

The ICD system is an international effort that was originally developed to collect mortality data for nations. It has since evolved to include data on disease morbidity, epidemiologic surveillance, and other matters pertaining to the general health of a nation's population. In some countries, it is also used for insurance and medical service reimbursement. It is safe to say, however, that the United States is the only country in the world that uses a system of detailed ICD-10 and CPT coding so extensively as the fundamental basis for financial transactions in health care. This reflects the fact that

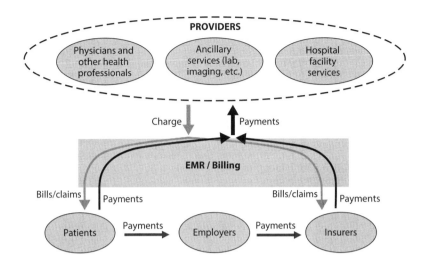

Figure 18.4. Billing and insurance-related activities under employer-based health insurance and an integrated health system with single electronic medical record (EMR)

the United States is the only country that relies so heavily on a claims-based fee-for-service health insurance model, whether through private or government sponsors.

Conceptually, the coding and billing system is straightforward (figure 18.4). In practice, however, it can be extraordinarily complex and frustrating for all concerned. The flow of claims and payments for an employer-based health plan and a participating health care system in which physicians, hospitals, and ancillary services all use the same electronic medical record proceeds along the following lines: The employer makes premium payments to an insurer, part of which it receives from their employees in the form of pre-tax contributions from earnings. Then every time a service is performed by a provider, it is coded correctly and billed accordingly. The charge follows a path through the electronic medical record (EMR), generating a payment "claim" to the insurer and a bill to the patient. (The bill to the patient depends on whether the deductible has been reached and takes into account co-pay and coinsurance amounts.) If there are no questions about these claims or bills and the system is running smoothly, payments are made by patients and insurers back to the providers, as shown by the black line.

There are many opportunities for the system not to work smoothly, however. A detailed, step-by-step description of the BIR process at a major academic medical center (Duke Health) with an integrated EMR across physicians, hospitals, and ancillary services was described by Tseng et al.[6] The process begins with registration, a clinical encounter, and the creation of a charge based on the nature of the clinical service provided. Although the system uses an electronic hub, the first step after the clinical encounter is performed by a team of trained coders who confirm the clinical information in the EMR and translate it into a billing code that will be the basis for the claim to the insurer. (The exception to manual confirmation is that "simple" clinic visits go through a first-pass automated coding system, but even these are rerouted for manual coding when the automated system fails.) This is a key step because the provider's goal is to make sure that the code captures the maximum level of complexity reflected in the patient's medical condition and services provided (i.e., maximize the amount to be billed) while the insurer's goal is to make sure that this level of complexity was not overstated (i.e., minimize the payment to be paid).

An entire industry of consultants has emerged to help providers with EMR clinical documentation and coding practices to maximize payments in a compliant fashion. Consultants are also extensively used by employers to assist them in choosing an insurer or to help them with actuarial and other data needed to create a self-insured plan and choose a third-party administrator. These represent additional administrative BIR cost not included in the computations above.

In the BIR system reported by Tseng et al., these initial codes are then run through an algorithm within the EMR that compares them with the electronically captured clinical information; in 17–20 percent of claims, this process triggers error warnings about inconsistencies that require manual intervention (i.e., "claims editing").[7] The next stage of processing is a review of the edited claims by third-party software ("claims scrubbing"). Third-party products are generally used because the EMR vendors have not yet developed accounting systems that reliably keep up with frequently changing insurer rules; in contrast, claims scrubbing software is updated several times per week. When the scrubbing process reveals potential errors (12 percent of claims for hospitals and 3 percent for physicians), more manual intervention is needed. Finally, the claim is submitted to the insurer. Despite all of the above efforts, in the Tseng et al. study, 8 percent of physician claims and 7 percent of hospital claims were initially denied by the insurer. This requires additional effort, which is quite time consuming for both provider and insurer (and frustrating for the patient), to straighten out the claim.

The BIR system described by Tseng et al. is as good as it gets. In many systems, patients receive separate bills from physicians, hospitals, imaging centers, labs, and others, each of which may use different EMR and billing systems. Such systems are inherently less efficient than a large integrated system that can take advantage of economies of scale and reduce redundancies. Moreover, the process illustrated in figure 18.4 is for a private health insurer. If Medicare or Medicaid is substituted for "insurer," the claims review and denial process can take on a different tone, since clinical documentation that is inadequate to justify a billing code (i.e., noncompliant) can be viewed by Medicare or Medicaid as fraudulent and be subject to legal proceedings and penalties (chapter 15). To protect against such proceedings and penalties, specialized compliance officers and lawyers who focus on billing compliance for government programs are hired by providers and contribute to additional administrative cost.

Most of these BIR administrative costs in the United States are due to the claims-based health insurance transactions that have become the backbone of our health care industry. Whether the insurer of figure 18.4 is a private health insurance company or a government program, detailed information is needed to satisfy their interest in making sure that the service for which a payment is requested is medically necessary and that the codes used for billing purposes are justified by clinical documentation. Medicare and Medicaid are increasingly being served by Medicare Advantage and Medicaid Managed Care (i.e., by private insurers), and while these insurers receive capitated payments from the government, they generally contract for medical services (physician and hospital) on a fee-for-service basis. Thus, the insurance-based, fee-for-service payment structure is becoming even more entrenched, as are the associated BIR administrative costs.

Estimates of Insurer and Provider Administrative Costs

An early study of administrative costs by Woolhandler, Campbell, and Himmelstein provided estimates for insurers and a variety of providers, including hospital, physicians, nursing homes, and home care.[8] The results for the year 1999 (table 18.2), along with comparable estimates for Canada (in which each province runs what is essentially a single-payer system; a small amount of health care is provided privately) estimated that administrative costs for health care in the United States were $294.3 billion, or $1,059 per capita. This was 3.4 times higher than the per capita administrative cost in Canada. Using the BLS medical care price index, the per capita cost of $1,059 in January 1999 would be equivalent to $2,090 in November 2018. After excluding from both the numerator and denominator those health care expenditure

Table 18.2. Costs of health care administration in the United States and Canada, 1999

Cost category	Spending per capita (US $)	
	United States	Canada
Insurance overhead	259	47
Employers' costs to manage health benefits	57	8
Hospital administration	315	103
Nursing home administration	62	29
Administrative costs of practitioners	324	107
Home care administration	42	13
Total	1,059	307

Source: Woolhandler, Campbell, and Himmelstein, "Costs of Health Care Administration in the United States and Canada."[8]

categories for which data on administrative costs were unavailable (e.g., retail pharmacy sales, medical equipment and supplies, and others), Woolhandler, Campbell, and Himmelstein calculated that administrative costs accounted for 31 percent of health care expenditures in the United States in 1999. These estimates include both administrative costs related to BIR and also to general administration. Thus these estimates of overall administrative costs are higher than if just BIR costs were considered.

Subsequent studies have focused on the BIR component of administrative costs. Khan et al. estimated that BIR costs in 2001 were 14 percent of physician revenue and 6.6 to 10.8 percent of hospital revenue.[9] Sakowski et al. and Casalino et al. both estimated that BIR costs in 2009 were between 10 and 13 percent of revenue.[10] Using BIR as a percent of revenue for providers and insurers from published studies, James Kahn, in a report for the National Academy of Medicine, multiplied these estimates by CMS health expenditure data to estimate annual BIR costs nationally for 2009 (table 18.3). The percent of revenues allocated to BIR for physicians, hospitals, and insurers are similar to the three studies cited in this paragraph.

Using a similar methodology, but updating the estimates of percent revenues spent on BIR with additional published studies, Jiwani et al. estimated "added" BIR costs in the United States, defined as "the cost of BIR activities that exceed those in systems with simplified BIR requirements,"[11] to be $471 billion in 2012. Of note in Jiwani's study is the use of SEC reports to obtain data on retained earnings by private insurers, similar to the methodology used in the congressional hearings on medical loss ratios noted

Table 18.3. Estimate of billing and insurance-related (BIR) costs in the US health care system, 2009

	Annual national health expenditures ($ billions)	Percentage for BIR costs (%)	Annual BIR costs ($ billions)
Physician care	539	13.0	70
Hospital	789	8.5	67
Subtotal			137
Other providers	771	10.0	77
Cumulative subtotal			214
Private insurers	854	12.3	105
Public programs	1,191	3.5	42
Cumulative total			361

Source: James G. Kahn, "Excess Billing and Insurance-Related Administrative Costs," in *The Healthcare Imperative: Lowering Costs and Improving Outcomes,* ed. Pierre L. Young, Robert S. Saunders, and LeighAnne Olsen, 142–51 (Washington, DC: National Academies Press, 2010).

above. Using this approach, it was estimated that insurers' administrative costs as defined by retained earnings were 18 percent.

The most detailed analysis of administrative costs associated with physician billing and insurance-related activities was reported by Tseng et al.[12] Introduced earlier in the discussion of claim processing, this study employed a time-driven, activity-based costing methodology. This approach combines process mapping from industrial engineering with activity-based cost estimation from accounting. A time-driven cost was estimated for each of the steps in the path of a medical bill through the revenue cycle. For each step, this required an estimate of the time required to complete the activity and the cost of the personnel doing the work. In addition, overhead was applied for functions such as human resources, utility bills, and information technology (including the EMR) on the basis of minutes-of-labor used for each activity. Using this methodology, the estimated BIR costs for the types of services studied (and the percent of professional revenue collected for that service) is as follows:

Primary care visit: $20.49 (14.5 percent)
Emergency department visit: $38.88 (25.2 percent)
General inpatient stay: $50.70 (8.0 percent)
Ambulatory surgery: $141.54 (13.4 percent)
Inpatient surgery: $141.54 (3.1 percent)

Given the average number of primary care visits per physician, it was estimated that BIR costs amounted to almost $100,000 per physician. The percent of revenue accounted for by BIR was much less for an inpatient surgery than for a primary care visit, but there are far fewer of such procedures than primary care visits.

It is likely that the BIR costs reported by Tseng et al. are underestimates. As the authors point out, and as further highlighted in an editorial by Lee and Blanchfield,[13] the BIR estimates included only the *operating* costs of the EMR, but not the allocated amortization of its *capital* costs, which are in the hundreds of millions for a large medical center. Various other overhead costs were also not included. Moreover, the detailed accounting of provider BIR costs by Tseng et al. doesn't take into consideration a large group of other expenses that support BIR activities—the parallel industry of educational institutions that have emerged to train highly specialized coders; consultants who advise providers, insurers, and employers on a wide variety of operational strategies and algorithms to enhance their efficiency and revenue production; and outside legal counsel retained by each provider, insurer, and employer to prevent or respond to government compliance concerns or to sue one another about a variety of complaints pertaining to charges and payments.

Not counting these additional costs, but taking into consideration the results of the studies discussed so far as a whole, we can construct a rough estimate of the fraction of health insurance premiums that are accounted for by billing and insurance-related costs. Insurer-related administrative costs account for about 13 percent (industry estimates) to 18 percent (SEC filings) of premium dollars counting insurer profits. According to insurance industry estimates,[14] about 20 percent of the remaining premium dollar is spent on inpatient hospital care and about 42 percent is spent on physician services and outpatient care. Based on Kahn's estimates that BIR accounts for (a midpoint of) 8.5 percent of inpatient costs and 14 percent of physician and outpatient costs, we can calculate additional BIR costs of 7.6 percent for providers:

Inpatient providers: 8.5% BIR cost of 20% of premium = 1.7% of premium dollars, plus

Outpatient providers: 14% BIR cost of 42% of premium = 5.9% of premium dollars.

Thus, we estimate that the sum of insurer and provider BIR expenses account for 13 + 7.6 = 20.6 percent (industry estimates) to 18 + 7.6 = 25.6 percent (SEC filings) of health insurance premiums. This 20 to 25 percent of premiums represents a floor on BIR expenses, with amortized capital expenses, the overhead of the EMR, consultants, and attorneys adding to BIR costs.

In addition to BIR administrative expenses, the major drivers of price in recent years have been insurers, physicians, hospitals, prescription drugs, and medical devices. The pricing of drugs and medical devices is presented in chapter 19. Considered here are insurers, physicians, and hospitals. Although we focus on "physicians" and "hospitals," the same concepts apply to other health care providers and other types of health care facilities.

Insurers

The contribution of insurers to the price of medical care is, in the language of the Bureau of Labor Statistics again, their "retained earnings" (i.e., both administrative costs and profit).

As noted earlier, if the medical loss ratio is 85 percent, this means that 85 percent of premiums are paid to providers for medical care as a pass-through, and 15 percent are retained for administrative expenses and profit. Also as noted, estimates of such costs are in the range of 13 percent (based on insurance industry estimates) to 18 percent (based on SEC filings). For plans compliant with the Affordable Care Act (ACA), retained earnings can be no more than 15 percent for large group plans and 20 percent for small group plans. For high-deductible, association health plans or short-term, limited duration plans, retained earnings are not capped and can be much higher. According to data from the National Association of Insurance Commissioners, the three largest insurers offering short-term, limited duration plans spent only 34 to 52 percent of premiums on medical care,[15] well below the 80 percent required for small group plans under the ACA. Thus, such plans appear to be highly profitable.

There are a number of ways in which insurers can contribute to price increases for health care:

1. Large insurers can exert market leverage and raise health care prices by entering into other aspects of the industry. This can include providing medical services directly or owning (or partnering with)

intermediaries in the pharmaceutical supply chain, such as pharmacy benefit managers and pharmacies.

2. As prices for drugs, physicians, and hospitals increase, even if utilization (number of claims) is the same, premiums increase. A constant *percentage* of premium going to retained earnings will increase retained earnings by an amount proportional to the increase in drug, doctor, and hospital prices. An increase in retained earnings is an increase in the price of health care.

3. Shifting more medical costs to patients can be done using a high-deductible benefit design, increasing co-pay amounts and coinsurance rates, changing the rules by which drug rebate coupons (chapter 19) apply to deductibles, or other means. Insurers can accomplish this directly in their individual plans or indirectly through employer-sponsored plans.

4. The part of retained earnings that represents insurer profit contributes to the price of medical care. For example, if medical claims are reported as 85 percent of total premium collections, leaving 15 percent as retained earnings, and if 3 percent of premiums are reported as profit, profitability of the insurance plan on an operating basis (i.e., the percent of all costs incurred in delivering the insurance-related functions, not counting the pass-through costs of medical care) is 3 divided by 15, or 20 percent. But if only 80 percent of premiums are paid for medical care (as is the case under ACA-compliant small group plans), or if only 50, 60, or 70 percent of premiums are paid for medical care (as is the case in many individual high-deductible plans), profit margins on the operating budget become much higher. This is because there is proportionately little additional administrative expense in the small-group and individual plans. Under these scenarios, the premium remains the same but less of it is used to pay for medical care and more is retained by the insurer as profit. The greater the profit, the greater the retained earnings and therefore the greater the price of medical care.

Insurers can enhance retained earnings by assigning certain profit centers that may be considered both administrative and medical service (e.g., disease management programs, case management and other "quality improvement" activities) to the "medical care claims" numerator under their allowable medical loss ratio. This shifting of cost from administrative to medical increases the share of allowable retained earnings that go to profit. Insurers can also enchance retained earnings by outsourcing administrative services to wholly owned subsidiaries that build a profit margin into the invoice they bill back to the insurance company for "claims processing."

The most efficient system of claims processing would theoretically be one in which the insurance company doesn't exist and patients paid the hospital or doctor directly. In this sense, any amount of health plan premiums not spent on medical care but retained by the insurer for administrative costs and profits increases the price of medical care generally. The more efficient the system (i.e., the lower the retained earnings), the less that insurers contribute to the overall price of health care. The reality is that reliance on private insurance in the United States is increasing, especially with Medicaid Managed Care (including Medicaid expansion patients), Medicare Advantage, and the marketplace health care exchanges. (Chapter 22 describes strategies for reducing billing and insurance-related administrative costs.)

Physicians and Hospitals

In chapter 3, we explained that imperfections in the market for physician and hospital services lead both to greater utilization *and* higher prices than would occur in a competitive market. Increased utilization is due to the fact that consumers make purchase decisions based on their low out-of-pocket costs, which are subsidized by health insurance plans or government programs like Medicare and Medicaid. Further increases in utilization can result from induced demand, especially in selected procedures and diagnostic studies. Physician and hospital prices are higher because they are not determined by the intersection of supply and demand in a market with many well-informed buyers and sellers but rather by negotiations between a much smaller number of insurers and health systems.

Monopoly Pricing

Physician and hospital prices that result from these negotiations reflect monopolistic characteristics of physicians and hospitals that have been longstanding. Let's take a step back to review the characteristics of a monopoly and then return to physician and hospital pricing.

The producer in a competitive market with many buyers and sellers is a "price taker;" that is, the producer sells its product at the price set by the intersection of market supply and demand. By contrast, monopolists are in a position to be "price searchers," setting the highest price that each buyer (segment of the market) will bear. In the case of a pure monopoly, the single firm is the industry and the industry is the firm—they are the same.

Pure monopolies emerge under circumstances that match the following characteristics:

1. There is one seller.
2. There are no close substitutes for the seller's product.
3. There are significant barriers to entry.

One circumstance often associated with these characteristics is economies of scale: in some industries, low average costs are only obtained through very large-scale production, restricting entry of new entrants. A "natural monopoly" like a public utility that supplies a community with electricity, gas, or water is an example. Another reason is that legal barriers may be put in place, such as the granting of a patent, a license, or a Certificate of Need.

Unlike a competitive market in which profitability draws more firms into the market, thereby shifting the supply curve outward and reducing price closer and closer to average cost and zero profit in the long term, pure monopolists can charge prices that persistently exceed their costs. An important characteristic of monopolistic pricing that relates to hospitals and physicians is the ability to price discriminate (i.e., charge different prices to different sets of consumers for the same service). At the extreme, perfect price discrimination would be when the monopolist charges the absolute highest price that each and every customer would individually be willing to pay. More pertinent for hospitals and physicians is price discrimination among buyers (i.e., when the monopolist charges a different price to different buyer segments, such as different health plans). As a consequence of monopoly pricing, in contrast to the allocative efficiency between consumer and producer surplus (chapter 2), monopoly produces allocative inefficiencies in that producer surplus becomes persistently greater than consumer surplus.

Historically important monopolies that ultimately produced antitrust legislation included the Carnegie Steel Company (which became US Steel),

Standard Oil Company, the American Tobacco Company, and AT&T. In the economy today, there are companies that have important monopoly characteristics but which are not pure monopolies. Examples are Apple, Facebook, Google, and Amazon. Periodically there are calls for antitrust action to split up these firms, but nothing has gained traction yet. In local communities, some firms, such as cable television operators and airlines, can express monopolistic characteristics in terms of pricing.

In the context of hospitals and physicians, price discrimination among buyers (mainly insurers, but also individual patients) reflects distinctive monopolistic characteristics. Prior to widespread health insurance, when physicians discounted their "usual, customary, and reasonable" fees to lower-income patients, one view of this behavior is that it was altruistic. Another view, however, is that it reflected almost perfect price discrimination—the physician was exerting monopoly power in charging what each patient could afford (i.e., what the market would bear). In current practice, the market leverage of large health systems that negotiate on behalf of hospitals and/or physicians results in different negotiated fee schedules for different insurers. This is typically expressed as a schedule of list prices that is set at several multiples of the Medicare fee schedule, from which contractual discounts are given to various payers based on historical precedent and the payer's weight and leverage in the market. Large insurers that will deliver more patients will get better prices.

Hospital Pricing

A hospital's schedule of list prices is referred to in the industry as a "charge-master." Historically, the Medicare fee schedule for hospitals was developed as a percent of charges, or a "cost-to-charge ratio." Contracted fee schedules negotiated between hospitals and commercial payers, however, are often substantially higher than the Medicare schedule. Maeda and Nelson used a 2013 commercial database from three large private health insurers to compare the prices paid to hospitals by commercial plans and Medicare Advantage (MA) plans.[16] The authors restricted their sample to acute care hospitals in metropolitan statistical areas that used Medicare's Inpatient Prospective Payment System (IPPS). With a few other minor restrictions, they were able to obtain a sample of about 593,000 MA hospital stays and 621,000 commercial stays. In addition to the prices for each MA and commercial stay, the amount that the Medicare fee-for-service program would have paid for each stay in the sample (including the beneficiary cost sharing amount) was computed by applying the IPPS payment rules to the services making up the diagnosis on the claim. Defining price as the total amount allowed paid on the claim (i.e., the amount paid to the hospital by both the insurer and patient), they found that payments on commercial claims averaged 189 percent of Medicare claims. A 2019 RAND study found even higher payments: on average across 25 states from 2015 throught 2017, case-mix-adjusted hospital prices as negotiated by commercial insurers were 241 percent of Medicare.[17]

Medicare Advantage showed better alignment: the average MA price per discharge across all hospital stays was $10,667, which was nearly identical to the average (computed) Medicare fee-for-service price for those stays of $10,716. When hospital stays were broken down according to medical or surgical stays, the MA and fee-for-service prices per discharge remained similar.

The use of cost-to-charge ratios has incentivized hospitals to increase their charges across time. This is because some types of commercial insurers (e.g., automobile insurers) will pay the full chargemaster price, which has grown over the years to be in the range of three to five times actual Medicare payments for nonprofit hospitals, and often much higher multiples for investor-owned hospitals. (In addition, at some brand-name institutions, a few international "self-pay" patients without insurance will pay the list price.)

To investigate this issue, Bai and Anderson subdivided the commercial market into health maintenance organizations (HMOs), preferred provider organizations (PPOs), and "other insurers," such as casualty (automobile) insurers, workman's compensation, and travel insurers.[18] Using data from Florida, they found that the median price paid by HMO and PPO insurers for hospital services was 2.5 times the Medicare price in 2016, while the median price paid by other insurers was 3.8 times the Medicare price. Within the other insurer segment, there was wide variability across hospitals. The median price paid by other insurers to nonprofit hospitals was about three times Medicare, but payments to the 20 highest priced hospitals were 7.8 to 14.1 times the Medicare rate. These 20 hospitals were all owned by a single for-profit hospital corporation. Despite treating a relatively small fraction of patients covered by "other insurers," these 20 hospitals generated about a quarter of their commercial net revenue from this category of payers.[19]

This degree of price augmentation is derived from market power, which increases when hospitals merge and expand their influence over a market. Mergers and acquisitions among hospitals are on the rise, resulting in higher prices: it has been estimated in several studies that hospital mergers can result in increased prices by 11 to 54 percent.[20]

The operating margins for most hospitals depend on profits generated from commercial payers. Even with safety-net funding (chapter 10), hospitals incur financial losses in the care of uninsured and Medicaid patients. Medicare patients are break-even at best, given the current cost structure of most hospitals. Thus, the operating margins for US hospitals is generally driven by the percentage of their patients who are commercially insured, their chargemaster (i.e., "list" prices), and the level of list-price discounting given to commercial payers.

Because they generally draw a high percentage of commercial patients, for-profit hospitals and community hospitals that are geographically situated in well-insured areas will have high operating profits. Academic (university-based) hospitals, which typically care for a mix of commercial and uninsured/Medicaid patients can also generate a healthy operating margin depending on their share of commercial-pay patients. Public hospitals that see predominantly uninsured and Medicaid patients must largely depend on community support (if any) from sales taxes and property taxes and on safety-net funding from federal and state sources. Their financial status will depend on the aggregate level of public support that they obtain, which varies widely across the municipalities and states in which these hospitals are located.

Based on data from BLS consumer price indices (figure 18.3), the growth rate of hospital prices since 1996 has been two- to threefold higher than the growth of physician prices. This conclusion is supported by the results of a study by Cooper et al., which used a claims database from private health insurance firms capturing 28 percent of Americans with employer-sponsored health insurance for the years 2007–2014.[21] During that period, the prices paid for inpatient care grew 42 percent for hospitals and 18 percent for physicians, while prices for outpatient care grew 25 percent for hospitals and 6 percent for physicians.

Physician Pricing

Physician prices since 1996 have grown 50 percent faster than the overall consumer price index (figure 18.3). Breaking down physician prices into commercial and government payers, the same phenomenon is found as with hospital services: prices paid to physicians by commercial payers are substantially higher than those paid by Medicare. A report from the Congressional Budget Office used the same claims database used in the study by Cooper et al. for the year 2014.[22] In this claims database, price is defined as the amount paid to the physician by the insurer plus the cost-sharing and deductibles amounts paid by the patient. Commercial prices paid to physicians, expressed as a multiple of the Medicare price, varied widely depending on the type of service. On average, commercial prices for office visits were about 120 percent of Medicare, surgical and other procedures were 150 to 200 percent of Medicare, and various imaging studies and radiation therapy was 200 to 250 percent of Medicare. Importantly, there was tremendous variation in commercial prices across metropolitan statistical areas (MSAs): commercial prices were 1.7 to 2.6 times higher in the 90th percentile MSA than in the 10th percentile. Even within MSAs there was significant variation among providers: commercial prices paid to the 90th percentile provider were 1.6 to 2.7 times higher than payments to the 10th percentile provider.

Two interrelated phenomena have influenced the growth of physician prices in recent years: one is a persistent shortage of physicians relative to expanding aggregate demand, and the other is a trend is toward physician employment, usually by a hospital/health system or a venture capital/private equity firm rather than private practice. In addition, the actions of State Medical Boards support monopolist policies on behalf of physicians,[23] reflecting similar behaviors on the part of state and national medical societies.

Hospital acquisition of physician practices is the other side of the consolidation coin noted above in relation to hospital mergers. Thus, the physician shortage has created a strong market price for physicians that is expressed in salary offers by hospitals and health systems and/or by practice monetization offers from venture capital and private equity firms, which often exceed the amount of professional collections that can realistically be generated in private practice. While procedural physicians can still earn substantial incomes in traditional, physician-owned private practice, especially those that have an ownership stake in imaging or surgical facilities that generate passive income, many other physicians have found that their value in the marketplace exceeds the amount they can collect on a fee-for-service basis in private practice.

As modeled by IHS Markit Ltd for 2017–2032 in a report prepared for the Association of American Medical Colleges, there is ambiguity and uncertainty about both current and future supply and demand.[24] That said, most of the forces at work constrain supply and augment demand. Constraining supply, IHS Markit reports the factors at work include:

- The increasing average age of the physician workforce and their projected retirement rates. More than one-third of all currently active physicians will be 65 or older within the next decade. (In the "2016 Survey of America's Physicians: Practice Patterns and Perspectives," 47 percent of respondents plan to accelerate retirement plans.)[25]
- Reduction in the number of hours worked per week. If the pattern of hours that younger physicians worked in 2016 is extrapolated to the age-adjusted workforce in 2030, there will be 32,500 fewer full-time equivalent physicians in the national supply from this factor alone.
- Constraints on the number of residency positions. Particularly in surgical fields, this limits the growth in physician supply that can offset retirements.

Augmenting demand, the factors at work include:

- Growth and aging of the US population. Between 2016 and 2030, the US population is projected to grow by close to 11 percent, from about 324 million to 359 million. The population under age 18 is projected to grow by only 3 percent, while those aged 65 and over, who are the greatest users of health care, are projected to grow by 50 percent.
- As has occurred over the past century, continued scientific discoveries—and their translation into new drugs, devices, and other technologies. These advances will continue to create novel treatments that are not currently available and extend lives into ages brackets that will require greater care by physicians.
- The trend toward employment of physicians by hospitals, and especially practice purchases by private equity or venture capital firms.

Potentially mitigating an increase in demand would be greater use of true capitation payments to physician groups to manage care and increasing the statutory scope of practice of nurse practitioners and physician's assistants.

Under a wide variety of scenarios that incorporated these and other factors, IHS Markit modeled future supply-demand gaps. They concluded that there was a physician shortage of 20,400 in 2017 and projected that physician demand will grow faster than supply, leading to a projected total shortfall between 29,000 and 42,900 physicians in 2020 and between 46,900 and 121,900 physicians by 2032 (the ranges come from the 25th and 75th percentile of projections, respectively).

While there have been contrary ideas about whether a shortage truly exists, the contrarian view is based on a series of assumptions regarding visits per year by the "average patient," the number of patient visits per hour, clinical hours per day, and days worked per year for each full-time equivalent physician.[26] While such calculations suggest a surplus of physicians if these assumptions were taken on face value, in our current real-world environment, the market has spoken. According to the 2018 Medscape Physician Compensation Report, which is based on responses from a sample of over 20,000 physicians, mean physician income across 29 specialties increased from $205,000 to $299,000 between 2011 and 2018, a compounded annual growth rate of 5.6 percent.[27] This compares to an average annual income growth rate of 2.1 percent for all workers nationally during this time period.[28] The growth in physician income (already high in 2011) at twice the rate of the rest of the US workforce would not have occurred if there were a surplus of physicians. Rather, physician salaries have been bid up by their shortage relative to demand as reflected by the following factors:

- *Price increases exceeding that of the CPI* (figure 18.2). Physician groups could not readily negotiate such price increases with insurers if there were a surplus.
- *Downstream value to hospitals in the form of surgical, imaging, and other ancillary hospital fees*, which results in salary offers that often exceed professional collections by a wide margin. This is especially true in many of the pediatric procedural subspecialties and several adult surgical specialties. The subsidies embedded in the physician salaries become part of the hospital's cost report, which is translated into higher hospital pricing. Hospitals can also obtain higher prices based on facility fees and other activities if the physician practices in a

"hospital clinic" rather than a private physician office. Thus, it is not surprising that increased spending on hospital outpatient services after physician practices acquisition is almost entirely due to price increases, since utilization changes are minimal.[29] The phenomenon of physician employment by hospitals is increasingly taking hold in recent years: in July 2012, 25 percent of physicians were employed by hospitals, but this figure increased to 42 percent of physicians by July 2016.[30]

- *Monetization of practices by venture capital and private equity firms.* This has especially occurred in specialties such as dermatology,[31] ophthalmology,[32] orthopedics,[33] and others that have the opportunity for induced demand and for ancillary income from laboratories, imaging centers, surgicenters, or other revenue sources that can be owned by the firm.

Summary

In recent decades, the growth in health care spending in the United States has been due primarily to price increases. The administrative cost of billing and insurance-related matters make up a large part of the price of health care services. This is due to the fact that the entire industry, both public and private, is driven by claims-based transactions. When such administrative costs incurred by insurers and providers are added together, they account for 20 to 25 percent of health insurance premiums. Taking into account the lower administrative costs of Medicare and Medicaid, for the US population as a whole, billing and insurance-related costs are in the range of $2,000 per person. When hospitals, physicians' offices, and insurance companies price their products, these administrative costs are embedded.

In addition to the role of administrative costs, the price of health care is influenced by insurers, physicians, and hospitals. Insurers can contribute to price increases by shifting more medical costs to patients, by assigning profit centers that can be considered both administrative and medical service to "medical care costs," by outsourcing administrative services to wholly owned subsidiaries that build in a second profit margin, and by entering into other aspects of the industry such as direct provision of medical services or acquisition of pharmacies and/or pharmacy benefit managers. Physicians and hospitals can influence price by exercising monopoly power and engaging in price discrimination. Commercial plans pay hospitals and physicians substantially more than Medicare for a given medical service. Physician pricing had its roots in the "usual, customary, and reasonable" fees that were a legacy of commercial plans and initially baked into Medicare fees. In recent years, the value of physician services to hospitals and private equity/venture capital firms, especially in certain specialties that can generate ancillary passive revenue, has exceeded the collections that physicians can obtain from traditional professional billing in private practice. The acquisition of physician practices by such entities is yet another factor putting upward pressure on prices for health care.

THE COST CONUNDRUM III
PRICE: PHARMACEUTICALS AND MEDICAL DEVICES

Pharmaceuticals and medical devices have played a major role in the extraordinary advances that have occurred in biomedical science and technology, but they have also contributed significantly to rising health care spending in the United States. As we shall see, there are a number of parallels between pharmaceuticals and medical devices with respect to oversight by the Food and Drug Administration (FDA), pricing opacity, numbers of intermediaries, and the potential for monopoly and oligopoly pricing.

Growth in Pharmaceutical Pricing

The growth in pharmaceutical pricing was about double that of the consumer price index (CPI) for each of the three decades between 1986 and 2016 (chapter 18). These differences compounded over time; for this 30-year period as a whole, the CPI increased by 116 percent while pharmaceutical prices increased by 290 percent.

Moreover, while the overall rate of increase in pharmaceutical prices was double that of the CPI, price increases have been much greater for patients with private health insurance than for Medicare patients. According to Magellan Rx Management's *Medical Pharmacy Trend Report*, the per-member-per-month (PMPM) pharmacy cost under commercial health plans increased by 21.2 percent from 2015 to 2016, which was significantly greater than the average 13 percent annual increase during the interval of 2012–2016.[1] Since there was a 5.4 percent *decline* in the utilization of prescription drugs during 2016 by members of commercial health plans, the 21.2 percent increase in PMPM pharmacy cost was due to an even greater increase in price.[2] This dramatic increase in PMPM pharmacy cost for

Table 19.1. Increases in selected drug prices, 2014–2017

Drug	Indication	Price ($) 2014	Price ($) 2017	% increase
Rebif	Relapsing multiple sclerosis	40,183	86,179	215
Byetta	Type 2 diabetes	3,503	8,019	229
Enbrel	Rheumatoid arthritis	23,527	57,746	245
Humira	Rheumatoid arthritis	23,305	57,736	248
Percocet	Pain management	66	197	296
Wellbutrin XL	Antidepressant	1,187	7,074	595
Evzio	Opiod overdose	575	3,750	652

Source: "Out-of-Control Prices: The Side Effect Big Pharma Never Mentioned," AHIP, July 7, 2018, https://www.ahip.org/then-vs-now.

commercial plans is quite remarkable when compared with the 2 percent increase in the CPI during 2016. By contrast, among Medicare patients there was only a 3 percent increase in PMPM pharmacy costs during 2016. This reflected a significant increase in price (7.9 percent), which offset a 5.1 percent reduction in utilization.[3]

Against this backdrop of substantial price increases in overall pharmaceutical pricing, especially for those with commercial health insurance, there has been a trend toward even higher pricing in a number of drug categories. In particular, there has been rapid growth in the price of some medically critical drugs in widespread use, such as the tripling of insulin prices during the decade from 2003 to 2012,[4] and even greater price increases in many specialty drugs (table 19.1).

The rate of prescription drug use per capita is about the same in the United States as in other high-income nations, but per capita expenditures is much greater in the United States. Like medical care in general, this implies that differences between the United States and other countries in prescription drug expenditures is mainly due to differences in price, not utilization. Through the mid-1990s, per capita pharmaceutical spending was no different in the United States than other countries (figure 19.1). During the 1990s, however, drug spending (mainly prices) began to rise at a faster rate in the United States than in other countries, a trend that has continued. International differences in drug pricing are present across the board—both for specialty drugs as well as more common drugs that are used in primary care. In a study of primary care prescription drugs in the United States compared with 10 peer nations, the US spent 203 percent more per

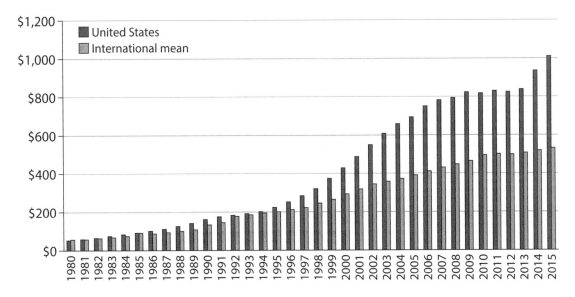

Figure 19.1. National trends in per capita pharmaceutical spending, 1980–2015, compared to international means (data from Australia, Canada, France, Germany, the Netherlands, Norway, Switzerland, and the United Kingdom). Dana O. Sarnak, David Squires, Greg Kuzmak, and Shawn Bishop, "Paying for Prescription Drugs Around the World: Why Is the US an Outlier?" (issue brief), Commonwealth Fund, October 2017, https://www.commonwealthfund.org/sites/default/files/documents/___media_files_publica tions_issue_brief_2017_oct_sarnak_paying_for_rx_ib_v2.pdf.

capita on primary care drugs (e.g., for hypertension, lipid lowering, ulcer/ heartburn treatment, noninsulin diabetes treatments, and others), despite purchasing 12 percent fewer days of therapy. The difference, again, was due to price.

In parallel with the underlying forces at work in the US health care industry generally, pharmaceutical pricing has evolved in a way that benefits the major stakeholders—in this case, drug companies, wholesale distributors, pharmacies, pharmacy benefit managers (PBMs), providers, and (increasingly) insurers—but with an adverse impact on overall patient care, cost, and access because of the tremendous variability in a drug's affordability to individual patients. As is understandable, each of the key stakeholders has tried to exploit market imperfections to enhance profitability. Sometimes, the actions of one stakeholder prompt retaliatory actions by another. More recently, consolidation among stakeholders has created perverse alignments such that PBMs, pharmacies, insurers, and providers all benefit from higher prices. Employers and patients are caught in the middle, facing higher costs that impact access and care.

Several factors have contributed to the growth in pharmaceutical pricing and expenditures in the United States: supply-chain intermediaries (wholesalers and PBMs), rebate coupons and charitable foundations for co-insurance, Medicare Part D, consolidation of supply-chain stakeholders, and the exploitation of patents. These each will be considered in turn.

Supply-Chain Intermediaries: Wholesalers and Pharmacy Benefit Managers

A simple, make-believe world of financial transactions for a prescription drug would involve a drug company, a pharmacy, a health plan, and a patient. The pharmacy would fill a patient's prescription by purchasing the drug directly from the drug company. It would price the drug at its cost plus a reasonable markup and be paid this price by the health plan and/or patient.

But the world is not that simple. There are other players in the flow of prescription drugs and dollars—for example, wholesalers and pharmacy benefit managers (figure 19.2). For the purposes of the discussion here, the pharmaceutical supply chain reflects the outpatient pharmacy system. The costs of inpatient pharmaceuticals are reflected in hospital inpatient pricing, which is discussed in chapter 18.

Wholesale distributors receive medications from the drug company at the wholesale acquisition cost, which becomes the list price. The wholesalers

Figure 19.2.
Pharmaceutical supply chain: flow of prescription drugs and dollars from drug company to patient

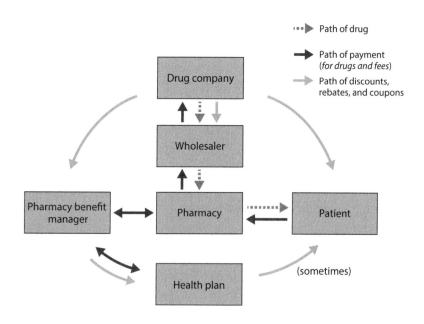

then distribute the drugs to retail pharmacies or specialty pharmacy providers as needed. The PBMs are middlemen who process prescription drug claims for insurance companies and health plan sponsors. Initially, the major rationale for PBMs was that their large market power could be used to negotiate prices with pharmaceutical manufacturers. As drug coverage expanded, however, with the inception of the Medicare Part D program in 2006 and the Affordable Care Act in 2010, so did the scope of PBMs. In addition to drug claims processing, they now conduct drug utilization reviews, decide which drugs should be in their formulary and which pharmacies should be in their network, and (opaquely) define the "spread" between the amount they reimburse pharmacies for a drug and the amount they charge their clients such as health plans. Large PBMs also operate mail order and specialty pharmacies.

Both wholesalers and PBMs evolved in response to the needs of a system characterized by a large number of health insurance plans, each one different, but each providing prescription drugs on a fee-for-service (in this case, "payment-for-drug") basis. The idea that PBMs could use their sizable aggregated demand as leverage to reduce drug prices and pass the savings to consumers is sound in principle. The problem is that the wholesalers and PBMs are incentivized toward higher list prices for brand-name drugs, just like drug companies and pharmacies, and are engaged in a system of discounts and rebates that partly reach health plans and patients but also increase PBM profits. Prices are inflated as a result of this process, and unequal access is fostered. Consolidation of insurers, PBMs, and pharmacies, a process that is currently reaching maturity, has created more concentrated market power that has solidified this price-inflating system.

The one straightforward path in the flow of the physical drugs, payments, and discounts/rebates (figure 19.2) is that of the physical drugs: it goes from manufacturer to wholesaler to pharmacy to patient. The complexity in the pharmaceutical supply chain—which has led to opacity, inefficiency, and high prices—resides in the system of payments, discounts, rebates, and co-pay coupons. Manufacturer discounts (price reductions that go to PBMs and pharmacies) and rebates (payments to PBMs that can be thought of like an after-purchase refund on a box top) vary for each drug of each pharmaceutical company, as does the percolation of these discounts and rebates to pharmacies, health plans, and patients. Manufacturer co-pay coupons go directly to patients. This practice lowers the price to the patient (sometimes to zero or close to zero), but it also distorts the relative price of low-cost alternatives. A generic, for example, may have a much lower list price, but the out-of-pocket cost to the patient is lower for the branded drug with the coupon, so the branded drug is chosen.

The byzantine and opaque nature of this pharmaceutical supply chain is itself a signal that the individual links in the chain can be exploited for enhanced profits and thus added health care costs. The arrows in figure 19.2 showing the flow of prescription drug payments, discounts, and rebates provide a general idea of how dollars flow, but there are many variations. (For example, in some cases like mail order pharmacies, manufacturers may work directly with pharmacies, bypassing the wholesalers.) For our purposes, the major takeaway is that the current system of discounts and rebates incentivizes all of the major players—drug companies, wholesalers, PBMs, providers, pharmacies, and insurers—toward higher list prices. Here's why:

- *Wholesalers*: Three companies account for 92 percent of all revenues from drug distribution in the United States (about $425 billion in 2017): AmerisourceBergen, Cardinal Health, and McKesson Corporation.[5] In return for their drug warehousing and distribution services, the wholesalers receive fees from the drug manufacturer, as well as bulk purchasing discounts; these revenues are a percentage of the brand-name drug's list price (usually about 2 to 5 percent). As the list price of a drug goes up, the wholesaler's revenues therefore also go up. For specialty drugs, especially oral medications requiring no special handling, the discrepancy between the cost of distribution and payment for a percentage of list price becomes apparent. For example, an oral specialty drug may have a list price of $400 per tablet and is packaged in 30-count bottles. If the wholesaler is paid 3 percent as a distribution fee, revenues for "distributing" (i.e., receiving and mailing) the bottle of pills would be $360, or $12 per pill.
- *Pharmacy benefit managers*: Through their formulary power and size, PBMs would ideally choose the lowest-cost drugs for their formularies, obtain price concessions from drug companies through rebates, and pass on the bulk of these savings to health plans. The health plans would then pass on the savings to their members (employers or individuals) through lower premiums and/or more generous benefits. In reality, this happens only to a limited extent. Since the PBMs will try to hold onto as much of its revenue as they can, it is expected that

although some of the price rebates is passed on to health plans, much of it is retained as income. The pricing spread between what a PBM will charge clients (everything from an insurer to a county jail) and what it pays pharmacies can be manyfold.[6] Even in Medicare and Medicaid, concerns have been expressed that PBMs are not choosing the lowest cost drugs for their formularies[7] and are charging much more for generic drugs from health plans or government programs than they are paying pharmacies.[8] For example, PBMs pay pharmacies about $85 for a tablet of a generic cancer drug (Gleevac) but often receive $200–$300 per tablet from Medicaid Managed Care plans, depending on the state.[9] In general, the higher the starting list price, the greater the opportunity for the PBM to retain a greater share of the difference between what it receives for a drug and what it pays.

- *Providers:* Hospitals and physicians who administer drugs earn profits not only from facility and professional fees but also from the difference in price between what they pay for the drugs and what they bill. This is referred to as "buy and bill" profit. As list prices increase, even if the *percentage* difference between buy and bill is the same, the higher the list price of a drug, the higher the profit.

- *Pharmacies and insurers:* In recent years, the major pharmacy chains have each consolidated with PBMs and insurers. CVS Pharmacy, which owned the PBM Caremark, purchased the insurer Aetna. Walgreens has partnered with the PBM Prime Therapeutics, which in turn is owned by 18 Blue Cross Blue Shield plans with over 20 million members nationwide. Cigna has purchased Express Scripts. Thus, the pharmacy, PBM, and insurer are becoming one and the same, with the integrated corporate entities benefiting from higher prices. The process of consolidation squeezes smaller independent pharmacies with respect to their inclusion in PBM networks and the amount of reimbursement they receive for drugs that they purchase.

- *Drug companies:* Although the PBMs exact concessions when drug manufacturers raise their list prices in terms of increased rebates, and although wholesalers also benefit from rising list prices as noted earlier, higher list prices also enhance drug company revenues. This has been reflected in the growth of prescription drug expenditures (figure 19.1) and strong drug company profitability. Between 2006 and 2015, the annual average profit margin of the 25 largest drug companies fluctuated between 15 and 20 percent, which compares favorably with the annual average profit margin for the 500 largest nondrug companies globally, which fluctuated between 4 and 9 percent.[10]

Drug Company Co-payment Coupons and Charitable Foundations for Coinsurance

Co-payment Coupons

Patients with commercial health insurance often receive coupons from drug companies for the full or partial cost of their co-pays on prescription drugs, especially high-priced specialty medications. This began as a retaliatory action by drug companies to undermine insurers' ability to increase the utilization of generics or other lower-price drugs through formulary tiers. For example, Dafny, Ody, and Schmitt found that coupons increased the sales of branded drugs by over 60 percent through reducing sales of bioequivalent generics, which became more expensive than the branded drugs after coupon discounts.[11] Currently, however, coupons are mainly used for high-priced specialty drugs or branded drugs for which there is no generic alternative. If patients were fully responsible for the co-pay, many would use lower-cost alternatives. But by eliminating or reducing co-pays so that out-of-pocket patient costs become lower than generic alternatives, these coupons allow drug companies to maintain a strategy of increasing the list prices of already costly drugs.

The use of co-pay coupons would generally be against the interest of insurers, who have an intrinsic interest in constraining premium increases. However, with the consolidation of insurers, PBMs, and pharmacies, the consolidated corporate entity may now benefit as a whole from the increasing list prices of specialty and branded drugs. The losers in this evolving coupon system are patients who don't have access to co-pay coupons, self-insured employers who have little leverage with the combined PBM/pharmacy entities, and all employers, employees, and individual purchasers of individual health plans who pay higher premiums due to rising pharmaceutical costs.

Ordinarily, it would be illegal to write off the co-pay or coinsurance of a patient who has private health insurance. If a physician were to write off coinsurance payments, it would be in violation of most contracts between physicians and health plans. Similarly, when drug companies write off co-pays with coupons, this could be viewed legally as "tortuous interference" designed to "disable" the cost-sharing provisions of health plan formularies that would foster lower-cost alternatives.[12] In effect, the drug company may be functioning as an unauthorized secondary insurer[13] that is enticing patients away from lower-cost drugs on the formulary (as required under the health plan contract) to that company's higher cost drug, without the patient having to meet the health plan contract's higher cost "sharing obligation" (i.e., the coinsurance payment).

Drug company co-pay coupons currently sit in a legal safe harbor, and as consolidation proceeds between insurers and PBMs there is less reason for insurers to bring legal action. Even though the coupons increase premiums, the consolidated corporate entity (which now includes the pharmacy and PBM as well as the insurer) can benefit from the higher list prices for specialty and branded drugs. As of this writing, there is some momentum to change federal rules around the safe-harbor provisions of the Anti-Kickback Statute that currently permit the use of coupons, rebates, and other discounting mechanisms. This is an evolving area.

Charitable Foundations

With respect to co-pays, Medicare functions differently from commercial insurance. If the co-pay of a physician's fee for a Medicare patient were written off, this would be a violation of the Anti-Kickback Statute, and would be subject to criminal penalties and civil fines. As a work-around, the pharmaceutical industry contributes to charitable foundations that make grants to individuals for the cost of co-pays that give patients access to high-priced drugs that they could not otherwise afford. These "patient assistance programs" are typically incorporated as nonprofit charitable foundations and therefore must certify that it has means-tested the patients it serves. The threshold for the means testing is commonly four times the federal poverty line, but it can vary. Most of the individuals receiving assistance are Medicare patients. The patient assistance program picks up the co-pay, but Medicare pays the remainder of the price to the drug company.

According to 2017 analyses by investment banking firm Bernstein, patient assistance foundations accounted for 10 of the largest 20 charities in the United States.[14] Recently, there has been increased scrutiny of these programs by the Office of the Inspector General, which has argued that donations to such foundations by pharmaceutical companies for the purpose of covering coinsurance payments for high-priced specialty and brand drugs violate the Anti-Kickback Statute by "inducing patients to purchase certain products and forcing federal health care programs to subsidize the costs of such products."[15] This surge in government enforcement has led to a number of high-profile settlements and the implementation of meaningful compliance controls and safeguards by drug companies. It remains to be seen how much this enforcement activity and increased compliance complexity will impact the amount of donations made by drug companies to these foundations.

Medicare Outpatient Drug Pricing

The Medicare program enacted in 1965 covered hospital (Part A) and physician (Part B) services. In most cases, prescription drugs were not covered, except when administered as part of an inpatient admission or to pay for drugs that were dispensed and administered in a physician's office and not self-administered at home. The Medicare Modernization Act of 2003 created Part D, the outpatient drug benefit.

Medicare Part B

Part B drug coverage pertains mostly to drugs that are administered in a physician's office by intramuscular injection or intravenous infusion, mostly cancer chemotherapy, but also including some drugs administered for ophthalmologic, rheumatologic, and other conditions. For many years, oncologists derived a substantial share of their income from the difference between their "buy and bill" drug prices. This created an incentive to use more expensive cancer drugs because of the greater profit margin between buy and bill. Part B physician-administered drug coverage was created largely to prevent the hospitalization of patients just so they would be eligible for drug coverage; it was never envisioned that Part B payments for physician-administered drugs would be transformed into profits from the sale of high-priced drugs used for chemotherapy. This arrangement carries with it some degree of professional conflict and the potential for physician-induced demand. The Medicare Modernization Act, however, lowered the margin between buy and bill to 6 percent, which was further reduced to 4.3 percent by the 2013 federal budget sequestration. Other factors related to drug prices have now effectively reduced the average oncologist's Part B drug margin to about 2.3 percent.[16] While some commercial payers have followed Medicare's lead, most still pay a significantly higher price to oncologists than does Medicare. United Healthcare, for example, makes payments to private practices for cancer drugs that are about 22 percent higher than Medicare.[17]

The reduction in Part B Medicare payments to physicians has led to a shift in chemotherapy toward hospital outpatient clinics in recent years. Data from the Medicare Payment Advisory Commission (MedPAC), the independent agency that advises Congress on matters related to Medicare, show that between 2005 and 2008, Medicare Part B spending increased only modestly in physicians' offices (from $9.1 billion to $9.8 billion) and hospital outpatient departments (from $2.8 billion to $3.1 billion). After 2008, however, Part B spending increased substantially due to the growth in chemotherapy prices, especially in hospital outpatient departments. Between 2008 and 2015, Part B spending increased at a 3.4-fold greater rate in hospitals outpatient departments (from $3.1 billion to $10.4 billion, a 236 percent increase) than in physicians' offices (from $9.8 billion to $16.6 billion, a 69 percent increase).[18]

While physician profits have been squeezed because of the reduction in Part B buy-and-bill drug margins, hospitals can charge facility fees and have access to lower prices for drugs through the "340b" program, which was enacted in 1992 with bipartisan support. This program was designed for hospitals and clinics that serve large numbers of high-risk, high-need individuals, mainly Medicaid patients. Approximately 40 percent of hospitals now participate. In the field of oncology, the market value of physicians is now often greater as hospital employees than as private practitioners. At United Healthcare, for example, while payments to private practices are 24 percent higher than Medicare, payments to hospitals for the same treatment average 146 percent higher.[19] Thus, oncologists are increasingly being employed by hospitals, which can afford to pay them higher incomes because of facility fees and 340b pricing.

In January 2018, the Centers for Medicare and Medicaid Services reduced by 28 percent the rates at which Medicare would compensate hospitals and clinics for the costs of 340b drugs. Further reductions are being actively debated. In addition, specialty pharmacies are increasingly sending drugs to physicians but billing insurers directly after prior authorization. The potential for bundling payments by commercial insurers to private oncologists rather than using hospital owned clinics is also emerging as an alternative pathway.

Medicare Part D

Enacted in 2003, Part D went into effect on January 1, 2006, and now comprises about 85 percent of drug spending by Medicare. The Medicare Modernization Act includes specific language ("the noninterference clause") that prohibits the secretary of the Department of Health and Human Services (HHS) from negotiating directly with drug manufacturers on behalf of Medicare Part D beneficiaries. Instead, the legislation provides a mechanism for drug coverage through private plans that compete for business based on costs and coverage. That structure means that each plan separately negotiates drug prices with the pharmaceutical companies, usually through pharmacy benefit managers (figure 19.2), who can negotiate with drug companies as discussed earlier. To protect the health plans from financial risk and to promote their participation, Part D reinsurance was also included at the inception of Part D, which kicks in when patients reach their catastrophic coverage threshold ($5,000 in 2018). Both the noninterference and reinsurance provisions significantly impact pharmaceutical pricing.

Noninterference Clause

The goal of including an outpatient drug benefit for seniors is consistent with the intent of the original legislation. There were a number of unsuccessful legislative attempts to achieve that goal between 1965 and 2003.[20] While outpatient drug coverage was finally accomplished in the 2003 Medicare Modernization Act, however, it came at a steep price: the pharmaceutical lobby ensured that (1) the new drug benefit would be administered by private companies, (2) the federal government would not use its bargaining power to negotiate lower prices, and (3) reimportation of cheaper drugs from Canada would be banned.[21]

Insurers spent $32.2 million on federal lobbying in favor of this bill in 2003 and hired 222 individual lobbyists to work on its passage. Of the lobbyists hired by the pharmaceutical and health insurance firms, 45 percent previously worked for the federal government and 30 of these lobbyists were former US senators and representatives.[22] Despite the enormous lobbying and expense, the votes needed to pass the bill in the House of Representatives were not all in place until the final minutes of a vote at 3:00 a.m., steered by Congressman Billy Tauzin of Louisiana. A few months after the bill passed, Congressman Tauzin became the chief lobbyist for the pharmaceutical industry.[23] Combined with the use of patents and associated monopoly pricing, the provisions of the Medicare Modernization Act contribute significantly to the high and rising prices for pharmaceuticals in the United States.

Reinsurance

Recall that Parts B and D of Medicare (and the corresponding components of Part C) are not funded through the Medicare payroll tax, which is restricted to hospital services. Rather, the base outpatient drug benefit premium—whether administered in a doctor's office or at home—is funded by a combination of contributions from patients and their health plans. Under Part D, patients are responsible for 25 percent of drug costs through out-of-pocket premiums up to the catastrophic threshold, while Medicare subsidizes the remaining 75 percent (from general taxpayer revenues) with payments to the health plans. The health plans, in turn, typically funnel these funds through pharmacy benefit managers, who can obtain discounted prices from the drug companies. When drug costs exceed patients' catastrophic threshold, 80 percent of the additional cost is covered through reinsurance by Medicare (i.e., taxpayers), 15 percent by the health plan and 5 percent by the patient.

Part D premiums have been rising relatively slowly, but this apparent success in cost containment belies the fact that Medicare expenditures on reinsurance have been increasing rapidly because an increasing number of Medicare patients are exceeding their catastrophic thresholds due to high and increasing drug prices and a provision of the ACA in which enrollees are relieved of most of their cost-sharing through manufacturer discounts that count as enrollee out-of-pocket spending. Even though these discounts are not true out-of-pocket expenses, counting them as such means that Medicare beneficiaries reach their catastrophic threshold more quickly, transferring liability from themselves and their insurance plan to the reinsurance program (i.e., taxpayers). Based on data from the Medicare Board of Trustees, the increase in reinsurance cost has led to more than a doubling of total Medicare spending on Part D—from $47 billion in 2006 when the program commenced to $100 billion in 2017.[24] In 2017, 70 percent of total Part D expenditures by Medicare were for reinsurance, while only 30 percent was for base premium subsidies under the catastrophic threshold.

Economist Austin Frakt has cogently explained the unintended incentives that have been created by the reinsurance provision of Medicare modernization. Because reinsurance costs are outside the expenses of the Part D plans on which insurers bid, the resulting premiums "do not accurately reflect the 80 percent of reinsurance cost that is borne by taxpayers. . . . Therefore, insurers have a relatively weak incentive to minimize enrollee entry into and costs within the catastrophic range."[25] He summarizes the overall operation of the Part D reinsurance program by stating that it "is not functioning as reinsurance at all, which should mitigate against unpredictable risk. Instead, high drug spending exhibits considerable persistence. . . . Part D insurers can predict it to some degree and craft coverage and utilization management policies that shift liability from them to the reinsurance program."[26] Frakt further describes analyses by MedPAC that point to additional technical peculiarities in the way the program functions, leading to insurers being perversely incentivized to cover medications that are *more* expensive, not less expensive.

MedPAC has made several suggestions for reform of the reinsurance provision (chapter 22), and several legislative proposals have been put forward. This is an active area that may result in further modernizing the Medicare Modernization Act.

Patents

The US Patent and Trademark Office (USPTO), an agency of the US Department of Commerce, grants patents to protect inventions for a limited period of time. In the case of a drug, it becomes a property right of the inventor, issued by the USPTO, for 20 years from the date on which the patent was filed. The owner of the patent is, according to statute, granted "the right to exclude others from making, using, offering for sale, or selling" the invention in the United States.[27]

Historically, the idea of a patent was to grant exclusive use of a new innovation for a relatively brief period of time, after which the public would benefit in perpetuity. As such, the concept of a patent is to balance the benefits to the inventor with those of the nation and its citizens. There is a philosophical distinction, however, between patents for a digital communication technology or a manufacturing process, for example, and those for drugs that impact human life. A car powered by a patented electric motor may be preferred over one powered by a conventional gasoline engine because of considerations related to performance, maintenance, and carbon footprint, but market forces determine how many people will decide to pay more for the electric car. By contrast, cure of hepatitis C in a short period of time with a patented direct-acting antiviral (DAA) drug for $80,000 is, in principle, essentially taken out of the market; once approved by the FDA, it is (for the most part) covered under Medicare and by most Medicaid and commercial plans at its high (nonnegotiated) price with relatively little out-of-pocket cost to the patient. (That said, problems with access have developed: depending on a particular patient's clinical circumstances and the details of his or her insurer's health plan, one in three patients seeking insurance coverage for DAA medication through their health plans are denied.)[28]

Philosophically, patent protection was never intended to create monopoly pricing that would restrict the availability of life-saving medication; such an outcome would run counter to the balance between patent holder and public welfare. Indeed, it has been argued that this balance has been tipping more and more toward the inventor/owner and away from the public good. Elisabeth Rosenthal summarizes it: "By the mid-1990s, the basic rules of engagement, determined by the FDA and the US Patent and Trademark Office, had been settled to the lasting benefit of business: a strong patent system and no pricing restrictions."[29]

The tipped balance toward the pharmaceutical industry and away from consumers partly reflects powerful lobbying efforts: one estimate is that the pharmaceutical lobbying budget is 42 percent larger than the next highest-lobbying industry and equal to the combined lobbying budgets of the oil industry and defense contractors.[30] Beyond lobbying, there have evolved several contributory factors: monopoly pricing, oligopoly pricing, evergreening of patents, and the exploitation of off-patent, sole-source drugs. These will be considered in turn.

Monopoly Pricing

Given that about 10 years can elapse (give or take) between a patent application for a drug and its approval for commercial sale, there may be only 10 years left on the patent to generate revenues and obtain a return on investment. Such revenues also cover the costs of the patented drugs that didn't make it through the pipeline to commercialization. It is understood as a matter of public policy that being granted a monopoly will enable the drug manufacturer to set a higher price than if competitors were not excluded from the market.

In contrast to the price-taking producer in a competitive market, monopolists are in a position to be "price searchers," setting the highest price that each buyer (segment of the market) will bear. But, analogous to the situation with physicians and hospitals, there is a key difference between a typical monopolist whose customers pay full price for its products and the patent-holding monopolist of a drug in which the patient pays only a fraction of its price (or zero). If the manufacturer of a patented hepatitis C combination drug had to sell its drug directly to patients, it would have to reduce its price significantly along the path of a negatively sloping demand curve to sell it to most patients with the disease. At the full price, few would able to afford it; they would have to use less expensive (and less effective) treatments that would invariably lead to significant morbidity and premature mortality.

Prices for patented drugs can be set for Medicare patients at high levels because the Medicare Part D drug benefit program created under the 2003 Medicare Modernization Act included the "noninterference clause" discussed earlier, which stated that the HHS secretary "(1) may not interfere with the negotiations between drug manufacturers and pharmacies and PDP [Part D plan] sponsors; and (2) may not require a particular formulary or institute a price structure for the reimbursement of covered part D drugs."[31]

Concerns have been expressed about the influence of the pharmaceutical industry in the addition of this language to the bill. The noninterference that prevents Medicare from negotiating drug prices under Medicare Part D stands in contrast to the policy of other governments that directly negotiate drug pricing in their national health plans. But also of note in this regard is the fact that, among various US government programs, Medicare is unique in this prohibition as there is a statutory requirement for mandatory drug price rebates in Medicaid as well as a requirement that drug manufacturers charge the Department of Veterans Affairs no more than the lowest price paid by any private-sector purchaser.

In practice, once a drug is approved for safety and efficacy by the FDA and appears on Medicare formularies, commercial insurance coverage generally follows. In both cases, the setting of a list price for a drug by the manufacturer, and the subsequent distribution of discounts and rebates among the stakeholders, follow the scheme shown in figure 19.2 and described earlier, which incentivizes escalations in list prices over time. As continued increases in list prices have come under public and political scrutiny, drug companies have increasingly turned to ensuring that prices are high at the launch of a patented drug, taking advantage of their monopoly position.[32] These high list prices are backed by the prohibition of cross-border drug importation, despite the same drugs being available at a fraction of the US price in other countries. Many news reports document the quandary faced by patients who need life-sustaining drugs that are priced at an unaffordable level in the United States. A 2019 article in a Minnesota newspaper, for example, describes patients with diabetes driving to Canada to obtain their insulin at one-tenth the price, taking the legal risk against smuggling because they cannot otherwise afford it.[33]

Oligopoly Pricing

An oligopoly occurs when there are a small number of sellers of a similar product with significant barriers to entry. Under an oligopoly, prices can be as high as if there were a single monopolist if firms followed one another in pricing ("price leadership") or functioned as a cartel (i.e., acting as though there were only one firm). They can do this behaviorally without explicitly colluding on price.

There are many examples of this phenomenon in pharmaceutical pricing, especially specialty pricing. One prime example is the drug imatinib (brand name, Gleevec) in the treatment of chronic myelogenous leukemia (CML). The story of Gleevac was told in chapter 1 as an example of a breakthrough advance in medical science that translated into saving lives. Prior to Gleevac, patients with CML were treated with toxic chemotherapy or even bone marrow transplants, but they rarely lived more than three years. Recognizing that CML was due to a single genetic defect that resulted in a "fusion protein" that caused CML, Dr. Brian Drucker found, after great persistence in assessing the inhibitory actions of numerous molecules, that imatinib successfully inhibited the tyrosine kinase responsible for the activity of the fusion protein. Patients on imatinib (and the newer tyrosine kinase inhibitors, or TKIs) now have a 10-year survival rate of greater than 80 percent, as compared with less than 20 percent historically. According to a group of 100 experts in chronic myeloid leukemia who wrote an editorial commenting on the pricing of Gleevac and the newer TKIs, many people can now have normal lifespans so long as the TKI is continued.[34] In 2013, they wrote,

> Being one of the most successful cancer targeted therapies, imatinib may have set the pace for the rising cost of cancer drugs. Initially priced at nearly

$30,000 per year when it was released in 2001, its price has now increased to $92,000 in 2012, despite the fact that (1) all research costs were accounted for in the original proposed price, (2) new indications were developed and FDA approved, and (3) the prevalence of the CML population continuing to take imatinib was dramatically increasing. This resulted in numerous appeals by patients and advocates to lower the price of imatinib, to no avail so far.[35]

At the time of their writing, the $92,000 annual price for Gleevac in the United States was almost twice the next highest price (Germany) among 14 other nations, and about three times as high as most of them. The authors reported that all five of the other TKIs approved for use in the treatment of CML were higher-priced than Gleevac. Subsequently, Rosenthal points out that the makers of the various TKIs all increased their prices to meet the higher price point,[36] behavior consistent with the "leadership pricing" model of an oligopoly. Thus, by 2018, the price for *all* the TKIs was about $150,000 per year, and the list price for the first generic version of Gleevac was only slightly lower, at $140,000.[37]

Evergreening

The monopoly protection provided by a patent is sufficiently valuable that many different approaches have emerged to maintain and extend the patent on a drug. Rosenthal provides an insightful summary, with examples, from the perspective of an investigative journalist-physician.[38] One way is simply to increase the number of patents on a given drug. It's not just the molecular structure that can be patented, but many other features. To maximize the patent term, additional patent protection is now routinely sought for such features after launching the new drug, or even before its launch, including patents on manufacturing methods, modified dosing ranges and routes, drug delivery systems, additional methods of treatment, biological targets, and combination products with other drugs. AbbVie's Humira, for example, has a patent shield of more than 100 patents.[39]

Many of the techniques currently used to "evergreen" a patent resulted, ironically, from legislation that was designed to speed the availability of generics when patents expire. This legislation, the Drug Price Competition and Patent Term Restoration Act (usually referred to as the Hatch-Waxman Act), was passed by Congress in 1984,[40] at which time there were significant barriers to the development and commercialization of generics. This act, which was the first change in US patent terms since 1861,[41] simultaneously lowered the barriers to entry for generic drugs and provided various ways for pharmaceutical companies to extend their patents. Makers of generics no longer had to repeat clinical trials; they only had to demonstrate chemical identity and bioequivalence (similar metabolism in the body). To achieve "balance," however, manufacturers were allowed a three-year extension for certain types of changes in the drugs that were supported by clinical trials and a seven-year period of exclusivity for drugs to treat conditions affecting a small number of individuals (less than 200,000 in the United States), called "orphan drugs," and they received other benefits related to pediatric drugs and the extension of patents based on the recovery of time that was considered "lost" by regulatory review.[42]

Generics are now commonly used in the United States, so the legislation achieved a major part of its goal. However, it also led to a number of practices that were contrary to its intent. The Hatch-Waxman Act provided for an automatic 30-month stay of FDA approval (similar to a preliminary injunction) for patent holders that sue generics.[43] This provision has led to widespread patent litigation against attempted generic entrants that would have the greatest financial impact, delaying entry of generics for high-priced drugs into the market. Often, the patent-holding manufacturer settles these lawsuits by paying the generic competitor to hold its product off the market for a period of time. The arithmetic is straightforward: Suppose that a brand manufacturer has $1 billion in sales annually from a drug, and a generic manufacturer plans to offer a generic at an 80 percent discount at the time of patent expiration. The brand company can pay the generic manufacturer $200 million per year to delay bringing the generic to market, retaining $800 million in sales. This is a win-win for the two drug manufacturers, but a lose-lose for patients and national health care costs. These so-called "pay for delay" or "reverse payment" agreements are, thus far, considered legal. However, legal scholars have expressed the view that "given the Act's clear purpose to promote patent challenges, as well as the parties' aligned incentives and the severe anticompetitive potential of reverse payments, courts should treat such settlements as presumptively illegal."[44] The Federal Trade Commission has formally recommended that Congress pass legislation against these anticompetitive agreements, which they estimate cost consumers $3.5 billion per year.[45]

Other types of actions and legal settlements can also subvert the entry of generics into the market of a high-priced branded drug when its patent it due to expire. A generic manufacturer is granted a 180-day exclusivity period under the Hatch-Waxman Act when it brings its drug to market, but as interpreted by the courts thus far, the brand manufacturer is allowed to produce their own "authorized generic" drug. A study by the Federal Trade Commission found that although prices are reduced by about 5 percent due to this competition, revenues to the generic manufacturer are reduced by 40 to 52 percent during the exclusivity period, and by 53 to 62 percent in the subsequent 30 months.[46] This has led to several anticompetitive results: the generic manufacturer can increase its price to make up for the anticipated lost sales, decide not to enter the market entirely, or enter into a legal pay-to-delay agreement in which part of the payment is the brand manufacturer's promise not to introduce an authorized generic to compete with the true generic after the delay.

As already noted, brand manufacturers typically obtain additional patents on an already patented drug that modify the branded drug slightly. These reformulations typically have little or no therapeutic advantage but may be more convenient in one way or another. There may be a slightly different dose, a slow-release formulation, a change from a liquid to a tablet or a spray, or some other modification. Using a technique that the industry calls "product hopping," the new branded drug is marketed to physicians and patients near the old brand's patent expiration date to induce switching to the newer formulation, and the manufacturer may even withdraw the older branded drug from the market entirely before patent expiration. A generic based on the initial formulation cannot be substituted for the new brand formulation because such substitution is allowed only if the dosage strength, time-release characteristics, and other properties of the drug are the same. Under this type of scenario, when patients are forced to switch from a drug that has an about-to-expire patent to a new formulation, it has been reported that only 10 to 20 percent choose the generic version of the original drug once it becomes available.[47]

Another method of patent evergreening takes advantage of the 1983 US Orphan Drug Act. This legislation was intended to promote the investment by pharmaceutical companies in drug development for rare diseases affecting very small patient populations. Incentives included market exclusivity for seven years, extensions for pediatric indications, reduced regulatory fees, and subsidies for clinical trials. These incentives worked, but the interpretation of "rare diseases" was broadened. Soon drugs that were approved to treat a common condition (e.g., Humira for rheumatoid arthritis) was granted approvals for additional indications with orphan disease designation (e.g., juvenile rheumatoid arthritis and pediatric Crohn's disease). And drugs to treat prevalent conditions were divided into small, biomarker-defined, or genetics-defined categories that enabled orphan designation.[48] From 2009 to 2015, 229 new drugs were approved by the FDA, of which 84 were granted orphan designation. Of these, 13 were for biomarker-derived subsets of more prevalent diseases.[49] In 2017, the average price for the top 100 orphan drugs was $147,308 per year per patient.[50]

Trends on evergreening for the period 2005–2015 have been summarized by Robin Feldman.[51] Her key findings were as follows:

- 78 percent of new patents were issued for reformulations of old drugs, with only a relatively small minority issued for new drugs;
- Patent extensions were focused on high-priced "blockbuster" drugs, of which 80 percent had their patent extended at least once and 50 percent more than once; and
- this overall trend is becoming more pronounced over time.

Quite apart from its contribution to "evergreening" patents, the passage of the Orphan Drug Act, along with its subsidies for clinical trials, tax incentives, and additional monopoly protection, have led to the development of drugs to treat truly rare diseases. Although drug companies generally avoided a focus on rare diseases because of the small patient population that would constitute its market, this legislation along with scientific advancements have led to the development of drugs priced at $1 million or more for treatments such as enzyme replacement therapy for single-gene disorders and gene therapy for a variety of genetic conditions. The treatment of single patients, and potential children in the family who inherit the disorder, could jeopardize the financial viability of an entire health plan for unions or self-insured companies.[52]

Off-Patent, Sole-Source Drugs

Symptomatic of the market failure that can be exploited under current law are situations in which off-patent, sole-source drugs can be acquired by a company that could then exercise de facto monopoly power and raise prices by several thousand percent, literally overnight. A well-publicized example was that of Turing Pharmaceuticals, which raised the price of Daraprim, a

Table 19.2. Case studies of seven off-patent, single-source drugs

Drug	First developed	Therapeutic use	Price increase
Daraprim	1953	Toxoplasmosis	$13.50 to $100 per pill
Thiola	1988	Cystinurea	$1.50 to $30 per pill
Seromycin	1964	Drug-resistant tuberculosis	$500 to $10,800 for 30 pills
Cuprimine	1956	Wilson's disease	$445 to $26,189
Syprine	1969	Wilson's disease	$652 to $21,267
Isuprel	1956	Cardiac arrest, emergencies, and other cardiac abnormalities	$2,183 to $17,901 for 10 5ml vials
Nitropress	19th century	Congestive heart failure and life-threatening hypertension	$2,148 to $8,809 for 10 2ml vials

Source: Special Committee on Aging, *Sudden Price Spikes in Off-Patent Prescription Drugs.*[53]

65-year-old drug that effectively treats toxoplasmosis, by more than 5,000 percent to $360,000 per year.[53] Other examples are shown in table 19.2. This business model involves a drug company (or hedge fund as in the case of Turing) acquiring a gold-standard drug serving a small patient population for which there was only one manufacturer, and then controlling access to the drug through a specialty pharmacy or other closed distribution system. Prices could then be raised as much as possible as quickly as possible. During the course of their investigation, the Special Committee on Aging in the US Senate noted extraordinary price increases in other drugs that are used by much larger patient populations: "The mean price of insulin, a lifeline therapy for the 29 million Americans with diabetes, increased from $4.34 per milliliter in 2002 to $12.92 per milliliter in 2013, a 200 percent increase. . . . Naloxone, the antidote to prescription painkiller overdoses, increased by 1,000 percent amid an opioid health crisis . . . and a 500 percent price spike in the epinephrine auto-injector, EpiPen, which is used to save lives during allergic emergencies."[54]

The "fine balance" anticipated in the Hatch-Waxman Act has not materialized. The patent system in the United States, combined with prohibitions against price negotiation by Medicare and against cross-border importation of pharmaceuticals, has tipped the balance away from consumers and toward the pharmaceutical industry, causing higher prices. Higher drug costs, in turn, have increased overall health care costs and health insurance premiums. Suggestions for addressing some of these issues are provided in chapter 22.

Medical Devices

As defined by the Food, Drug & Cosmetic Act, a medical device is "an instrument, apparatus, implement, machine, contrivance, implant, in vitro reagent, or other similar or related article . . . which is . . . intended for use in the diagnosis of disease or other conditions, or in the cure, mitigation, treatment, or prevention of disease . . . and which does not achieve any of its primary intended purposes through chemical action."[55]

Progress in biomedical engineering has resulted in the development of medical devices that have extended and improved the quality of life. Among many examples, some of which were discussed in chapter 1, these innovations have included laparoscopic and robotic surgery; a variety of advanced imaging technologies; implantable defibrillators; endovascular surgery to treat heart disease, stroke, and other conditions; artificial joints and heart valves; radiosurgery; and left-ventricular assist devices. Procedures such as vascular surgery and joint replacement that were historically performed as inpatient surgery with lengthy postoperative recoveries are now done as same-day procedures with much faster recovery. For example, hip replacement surgery that used to involve cutting through muscles and tendons can now be done through an approach that separates these tissues without cutting across them, resulting in surgery that requires only an overnight stay, instead of a week in the hospital, and much quicker recovery at home.

These devices and procedures entail substantial cost. While there are far fewer data on the pricing of medical devices than of drugs, the medical device market is quite substantial globally—about half as large as pharmaceuticals ($370 billion vs. $740 billion, respectively, in 2015).[56] In the United States, about 6 percent of total health care expenditures were for medical devices.[57]

Some of the circumstances surrounding medical devices and their pricing have many parallels with drug pricing. Like pharmaceuticals, the FDA does not require evidence of cost effectiveness or of efficacy of a new device in comparison with an existing one. Unlike pharmaceuticals, however, medical devices often do not even have to show efficacy; generally all that is required is that they are "substantially equivalent" to other devices. This has impacted patient safety in a number of cases, many of which are now the subject of highly visible marketing to potentially affected patients by plaintiffs' attorneys. Class III devices require clinical studies of safety and efficacy, but few new products go through this process because Class III devices that arise from changes to previously approved devices are exempted from this requirement. Thus, in obtaining a patent on a medical device, there is less need to establish the efficacy of the device, build an actual prototype, or provide supporting data than is the case with patents on pharmaceutical products. This leads to high variability in efficacy and potential safety pitfalls.

With respect to pricing, in 2011 Medicare began a competitive bidding program (CBP) for some medical devices. Prior to the CBP, Medicare paid for nearly all medical devices on a fee-schedule basis, which was largely based on the manufacturer's list prices. In 2011, devices were divided into two groups—one group was subject to subsequent CBP, and the other group was not. Pricing for medical devices under Medicare has been studied by MedPAC. In 2011, Medicare spent $7.5 billion on devices subject to CBP and $3.3 billion on devices not subject to CBP. In 2015, four years after CBP implementation, expenditure for devices subject to CBP fell to $4.4 billion while those not subject to CBP increased to $4.0 billion. Devices not subject to CBP continue to be paid by Medicare based on fee schedules provided by manufacturers based on undiscounted list prices. Medicare's payment rates for medical devices not subject to CBP in 2015 were one-third higher than rates paid by commercial insurers.[58]

Also according to the MedPAC report, the top three non-CBP devices were continuous positive airway pressure (CPAP) masks for obstructive sleep apnea ($343 million), wearable automatic external defibrillators (AEDs) ($179 million), and "off-the-shelf" (i.e., not customized) lumbar-sacral support braces ($167 million). In the context of our conclusion in chapter 7 that health status is more influenced by behavioral factors than health care access, it is pertinent to note that the need for CPAP masks and back support braces are both related to obesity. One can also argue that obesity also increases the need for wearable AEDs because of obesity's etiologic link to heart disease.

MedPAC reported concerns about the pricing of each of these devices. Prices of CPAP masks are based on list prices from 30 years ago that have been updated over time for inflation. Many other non-CBP devices are also priced based on baselines that are decades old. Wearable AEDs are paid by Medicare as rental items with an implied purchase price of over $28,000 in

2018, as compared to direct purchase prices for nonwearable AEDs of $1,500–$2,000. And billing for off-the-shelf back braces increased by over 100 percent between 2014 and 2016 when rules were changed around quality requirements for custom-fitted braces.

In addition to issues around the pricing of medical devices that are not subject to the CBP, MedPAC also expressed concerns about physician-owned distributors (PODs), which allow physicians to benefit financially from sales of the medical products they prescribe and/or use in treatment. PODs are similar to specialist physicians taking ownership stakes in such entities as imaging centers and same-day surgery centers (chapters 5 and 15) but are more opaque in that physician ownership is often not disclosed. MedPAC called attention to physicians serving as an intermediary between the manufacturer and the hospital, taking profits as a "distributor" or as a "manufacturer/seller" of devices that another company manufactures on their behalf. PODs are mainly owned by spine surgeons and heart surgeons who sell devices to hospitals that are then used by the surgeons in their operative procedures. Referencing this behavior in relation to self-referral under the Anti-Kickback Statute and Stark law, the Office of the Inspector General released a Special Fraud Alert in 2013, in which PODs were described as "inherently suspect." In practice, however, government prosecutions have been limited. Despite the Special Fraud Alert, PODs continued to operate in 43 states as of December 2015.[59]

These practices have the potential to inflate prices and utilization. Although data on the prevalence of PODs are relatively limited, in 2011 the Office of the Inspector General found that PODs supplied spinal devices for about 20 percent of the spinal fusion operations billed to Medicare and sold about a third of such devices purchased by hospitals.

As previously discussed, drug companies have migrated from physician-directed marketing to a mix of physician- and consumer-directed advertising, with an increasing emphasis on the latter. Medical device manufacturers are navigating that same road somewhat differently because of the nature of their specific products and markets. Certain items are used exclusively within hospitals; for these, the device manufacturers target physician marketing since the ability of a vendor to create strong physician preferences for its particular product (i.e., pacemaker, artificial joint, stent, etc.) will greatly impact a hospital's purchasing decision. Other items, like back braces, devices to treat sleep apnea, and others, are increasingly being marketed directly and aggressively to consumers.

Pricing for medical devices is even more opaque than for pharmaceuticals, and large variations in purchasing discounts can occur across hospitals, depending on their market power. Sometimes a hospital negotiates directly with an imaging or device vendor, but often this is done through purchasing consortia (which themselves have administrative costs and profits). To explore variation in medical device pricing internationally, Wenzl and Mossialos studied cardiac implants as a test case.[60] They used 2006–2014 data from a commercial hospital panel survey and compared prices in the United States with four countries in the European Union. Data on hospital- and manufacturer-specific prices were available for coronary stents (both bare-metal and drug-eluting stents) and for six types of devices that manage cardiac rhythm (pacemakers, implantable defibrillators, and cardiac resynchronization devices). In a sample that comprised more than 30,000 unique hospital-manufacturer combinations, Wenzl and Mossialos found that prices were two to six times higher in the United States than in France, Italy, the United Kingdom, and Germany. Price variation among hospitals within a country was similar in magnitude.

The opacity and wide variation in the price of medical devices were highlighted by a study of pricing for hip replacement surgery using telephone interview survey data between May 2011 and June 2012.[61] A random sample of two hospitals from each state, as well as the 20 top-ranked hospitals for orthopedic services according to *US News and World Report* rankings, were contacted about the price of hip replacement surgery. Using a script that had been pilot tested and refined, one of the authors contacted each hospital and attempted to obtain the total price (bundled or not) for hip replacement surgery, indicating that she "would be comparing prices among several nearby hospitals under consideration for her [fictional] grandmother's upcoming surgery." Nine of 20 top-ranked hospitals provided a bundled price and an additional 3 provided a complete price by contacting the hospital and doctor separately (60 percent in total), as compared to 10 of the 102 non-top-ranked hospitals providing a bundled price and an additional 54 providing complete prices by contacting the hospital and doctor separately (63 percent in total). For hospitals in which a complete price could be obtained, prices in 2011–2012 ranged from $27,489 to $68,798 in top-ranked hospitals and from $36,923 to $46,409 in non-top-ranked hospitals.

Elisabeth Rosenthal tells the story of an architectural photographer and avid snowboarder who had hip replacement surgery performed in Belgium for $13,660, eloquently juxtaposing the contrast between surgical procedures involving medical devices in the United States and other countries.[62] The photographer had health insurance, but the medical condition that now required hip replacement was considered a "preexisting condition" due to an old sports injury and was not covered. In Belgium, the total price of $13,660 included all hospital and doctor charges, crutches, medicines, a week in rehab, and a round-trip ticket from the United States. A friend who worked for a medical device manufacturer arranged to provide the hip implant at a "no-markup" cost of $13,000 (essentially equal to the entire cost of the surgery in Belgium, including travel), but his hospital estimated that its charges would add another $65,000, not including the fees for the surgeon and anesthesiologist. Dr. Rosenthal reports that based on estimates of production costs for an artificial hip by the CEO of a company developing generic implants, the manufacturing cost is about $350. Like the pharmaceutical supply chain, there are many intermediaries, each of whom adds to the price along the way: based on interviews, Dr. Rosenthal reports that "there are as many as 13 layers of vendors between the physician and the patient for a hip replacement."[63]

As is the case with drug companies, the small number of medical device manufacturers, combined with pricing opacity, can lead to oligopolistic pricing in practice even if there is no overt cartel-like collusion. Facilitating such behavior may be physical proximity. Of the four major manufacturers of artificial joints in the United States, three are headquartered in the small town of Warsaw, Indiana. In 2011, all three generated sales of over $1 billion while spending only about 5 percent on research and development, a quarter of the percentage of revenues spent by pharmaceutical companies.[64]

Summary

Growth in the prices of both drugs and medical devices in the United States have contributed greatly to the overall rise in the price of health care services, which have in turn been primarily responsible for the growth in health care spending. There are a number of parallels between pharmaceuticals and medical devices with respect to FDA oversight, pricing opacity, numbers of intermediaries, direct-to-consumer advertising, and the potential for monopoly and oligopoly pricing.

FDA approval for both drugs and medical devices do not require demonstration of cost effectiveness relative to available drugs or devices.

Pharmaceuticals require the demonstration of safety and efficacy, but in most cases medical devices require only "substantial equivalence" to an existing approved device.

By statute, Medicare cannot negotiate price with drug manufacturers. With respect to medical devices, competitive bids are requested for only a subset of new products. A number of other statutes and policies have led to the potential for induced demand (chapter 17) and for monopoly or oligopoly pricing. These include methods for approvals and patents, price opacity, direct-to-consumer advertising, layers of intermediary vendors, buy-and-bill business models, and Part D reinsurance. Revisions in these statutes and policies will be necessary to control the growth in expenditures on drugs and devices in the United States.

20 INEQUALITY OF ACCESS

Since 1965, access to health care has been improved for older adults and poor children in the United States through Medicare and Medicaid. Now, more than 50 years later, remaining gaps in access are partly being filled through Medicaid expansion and the health care marketplace. Although the number of uninsured individuals has fallen significantly from almost 50 million in 2010 when the Affordable Care Act (ACA) was enacted, in 2017 there remained 28.5 million Americans under age 65 who did not have health insurance.[1]

In addition to those who have limited access to health care in the United States because of a lack of health insurance, others may have restricted access to health care if they are "underinsured" (i.e., have insurance with limited benefits and/or high deductibles and coinsurance rates).

Access to health care in the United States is out of balance relative to health care expenditures. Compared to other high-income countries, we have the highest per capita health care expenditures yet have the most inequitable access to care.[2] In this chapter, we review access from several different angles: overall trends in health insurance rates, demographic differences between the insured and uninsured, characteristics of those who remain uninsured and those who are underinsured, and the impact of Medicaid expansion on access and health status.

Overall Trends in Rates of Health Care Insurance

At this writing, the most recent data on rates of health care insurance pertain to 2017, as reported by the US Census Bureau in September 2018.[3] For comparison, the report also contains data for 2013, the year before the key

ACA provisions took effect. Data on insurance rates are drawn from the results of the Current Population Survey Annual Social and Economic Supplement (CPS ASEC). Insurance coverage is divided into two major categories:

- *Private health insurance*: a plan provided through an employer or purchased directly by an individual from an insurance company (including purchases through the ACA health care exchanges).
- *Government insurance*: programs such as Medicare, Medicaid, the Children's Health Insurance Program (CHIP), and "military health care," defined as civilian health insurance (TRICARE and CHAMPVA) as well as care provided by the Department of Veterans Affairs. As noted previously, federal and state programs are increasingly outsourced to private health insurance through Medicare Advantage and state Medicaid Managed Care programs. Thus, much of "government" insurance is really becoming a financing mechanism for private health insurance.

The fraction of the US population that was uninsured declined from 13.2 percent in 2013 to 8.8 percent in 2017 (table 20.1). This was partly due to a 1.0 percent change in the share of the population covered by employment-based health insurance or by military plans. Three contributors to the reduction in the uninsured rate were the following:

Table 20.1. Health insurance coverage by type of insurance, 2013 and 2017

	2013		2017	
Type of coverage	Number of people in millions	Percentage of total US population (%)	Number of people in millions	Percentage of total US population (%)
Employment-based	174,418	55.7	181,036	56.7
Direct purchase	35,755	11.4	51,821	16.0
Medicare	49,020	15.6	55,623	17.2
Medicaid	54,919	17.5	62,492	19.3
Military health care	14,016	4.5	15,532	4.8
Uninsured	41,795	13.3	28,543	8.8
Total US population	313,401[a]	N/A	323,156	N/A

Source: Berchick, Hood, and Barnett, *Health Insurance Coverage in the United States.*[1]

[a] Numbers and percents by type of coverage do not add to total US population because people can be covered by more than one type of insurance in the course of a year.

- Population aging: As the population shifted toward older ages, the fraction covered by Medicare increased by 1.6 percent, from 15.6 to 17.2 percent.
- Medicaid expansion: As a result of Medicaid expansion in some states, the fraction of the population covered by Medicaid increased by 1.8 percent, from 17.5 to 19.3 percent.
- Federally subsidized health care marketplace: Due to introduction of the health care exchanges, the direct purchase of private health insurance increased by 4.6 percent, from 11.4 to 16.0 percent.

Despite these improvements in the rate of uninsured individuals, there remained over 28.5 million individuals in the United States who did not have health insurance for any part of the year 2017.

Characteristics of Individuals According to Health Insurance Status

Age

Over half of those over 64 years of age in 2017 had some type of private health insurance (figure 20.1). Medicare ensures that virtually all (98.7 percent) Americans older than 64 have coverage. A combination of private health insurance and government programs also provides health insurance for a large fraction of children under age 19 (94.6 percent). Much

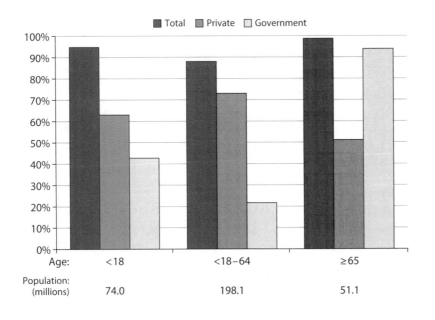

Figure 20.1. Percentage of people with health insurance, by age and type of insurance, 2017. Berchick, Hood, and Barnett, *Health Insurance Coverage in the United States*, 7.[1]

Figure 20.2.
Uninsured rate by
single year of age:
2013, 2016, and
2017. Berchick, Hood,
and Barnett, *Health
Insurance Coverage in
the United States*, 9.[1]

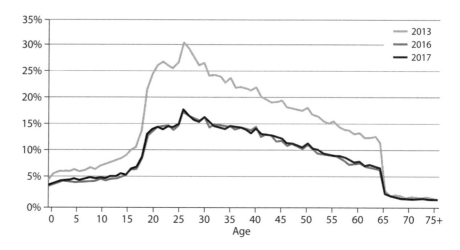

of this coverage (41.9 percent) is the result of government programs. The group with the largest fraction of uninsured individuals is adults between 19 and 64 years of age. In this age group, 12.1 percent overall did not have insurance for any part of 2017. Of the 87.9 percent who were insured (with some overlap), 72.8 percent had private insurance for some part of the year and 21.6 percent had some form of coverage by a government program.

In 2013, 2016, and 2017, there were markedly higher rates of uninsured among those aged 18 to 64 (figure 20.2). While the uninsured rate in this age group has clearly declined since 2013, it remains in the 10–15 percent range in 2017. Insuring Americans in the education/work years between childhood and retirement, and doing so without adding significantly to overall cost and while enhancing the quality of care, remains a critical health care conundrum facing our nation.

Education and Income

The percentage of people with health insurance is directly correlated with education, employment status, and income (figures 20.3, 20.4, and 20.5). Only 73.7 percent of those with no high school diploma had health insurance in 2017, increasing with higher levels of educational attainment and reaching 95.8 percent for those with graduate or professional degrees. About 90 percent of those who worked full-time, year-round were covered by health insurance. They mainly had private insurance (84.4 percent) but also some government insurance (10.9 percent), depending on income and with some overlap. Those who did not work for at least one week had

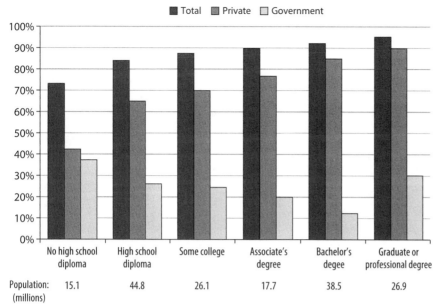

Figure 20.3.
Percentage of people with health insurance, by education and type of insurance, ages 26–64 (N = 164 million), 2017. Adapted from Berchick, Hood, and Barnett, *Health Insurance Coverage in the United States*, 10.[1]

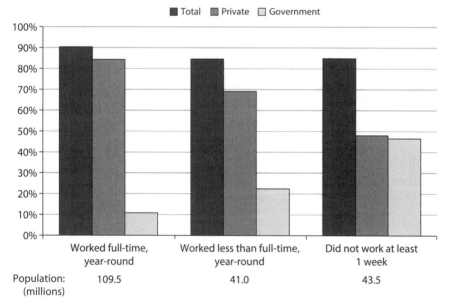

Figure 20.4.
Percentage of people with health insurance, by employment and type of insurance, ages 19–64 (N = 150.5 million), 2017. Adapted from Berchick, Hood, and Barnett, *Health Insurance Coverage in the United States*, 10.[1]

an 85 percent rate of health insurance, only 5 percent lower than that of individuals with full-time employment, but they had a much higher rate of government insurance (46.5 percent), as would be expected. People in this group also had a relatively high rate of private insurance (47.9 percent), which is mainly coverage through a spouse (or on their parents' policies through age 26).

Figure 20.5.
Percentage of people with health insurance, by household income and type of insurance, all ages, 2017. Adapted from Berchick, Hood, and Barnett, *Health Insurance Coverage in the United States*, 11.[1]

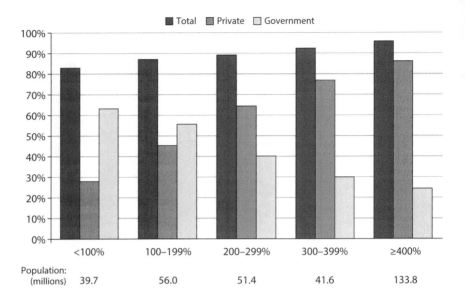

There is also a direct link between income and health insurance coverage, although the data in figure 20.5 do not show as strong a correlation as was evident with education, since all ages are considered. Thus, children and adults over 64 years of age have access to coverage independent of income through Medicaid, CHIP, and Medicare. The rate of health insurance coverage ranges from 83 percent for those below the federal poverty line (with 63 percent government insurance) to 96 percent for those whose household incomes are 400 percent of the federal poverty line or greater (with 24.2 percent government insurance). In dollar terms, those with household incomes of $100,000–$124,999 had a health insurance rate of 94.6 percent in 2017, while those with incomes of $125,000 or more had an insurance rate of 95.7 percent.

Race

Overall, 93 and 94 percent of Asians and Whites, respectively, had health insurance for at least part of 2017, as compared with lower percentages for Blacks (89.4 percent) and Hispanics (83.9 percent) (figure 20.6). Whites and Asians were also similar in the percentage of private health insurance (73 and 72 percent, respectively), while the percentage of private insurance among Blacks (56.5 percent) and Hispanics (53.5 percent) was lower.

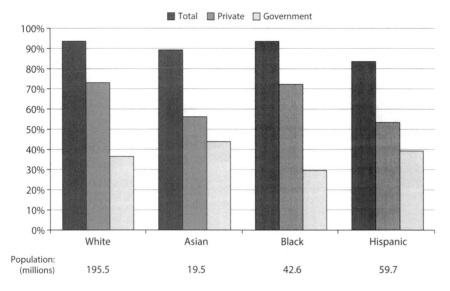

Total ■ Private □ Government

| Population: (millions) | White 195.5 | Asian 19.5 | Black 42.6 | Hispanic 59.7 |

Figure 20.6.
Percentage of people
with health insur-
ance, by race and
type of insurance, all
ages, 2017. Adapted
from Berchick, Hood,
and Barnett, *Health
Insurance Coverage in
the United States*, 16.[1]

Trends since Implementation of the Affordable Care Act

Data as summarized so far does not include trend information on insurance status across time by demographic characteristics. Those data have been
compiled by the Kaiser Family Foundation for the time period between implementation of the ACA in 2013 and 2016. Uninsured rates over that time
declined more in non-Whites, individuals with lower incomes, and adults
less than age 65 (figure 20.7). This is understandable, since these groups began with higher uninsurance rates before the ACA.

Characteristics of the Remaining Uninsured Population

As noted earlier, almost 100 percent of individuals over age 64 are covered
by Medicare and/or private insurance. Among individuals younger than 65,
however, 8.5 percent remained without health insurance during some part
of 2017 despite the improvements in coverage that occurred under the ACA.

It is illuminating to understand the characteristics of people who remain
uninsured and the degree to which they are eligible for Medicaid expansion
or premium tax credits under the health care marketplace exchange program. These data have been compiled by the Urban Institute, based on the
March 2017 CPS ASEC, which provides "snapshot" data at a point in time
(table 20.2). (Thus, this database is slightly different than that used earlier
comparing the insured vs. uninsured.) The share of uninsured for some

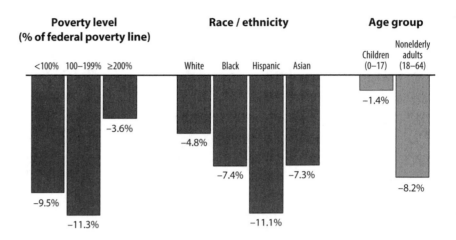

Poverty level **Race / ethnicity** **Age group**
(% of federal poverty line)

| <100% | 100–199% | ≥200% | White | Black | Hispanic | Asian | Children (0–17) | Nonelderly adults (18–64) |

−3.6%

−4.8%

−7.4% −7.3%

−9.5%

−11.3% −11.1%

−1.4%

−8.2%

Figure 20.7. Percentage change in uninsured rate among the nonelderly population by selected characteristics, 2013–2016. Jennifer Tolbert, Kendal Orgera, Natalie Singer, and Anthony Damico, "Key Facts about the Uninsured Population" (issue brief), Kaiser Family Foundation, December 7, 2018, http://files.kff.org/attachment//fact-sheet-key-facts-about-the-uninsured-population.

demographic groups is clearly out of proportion to their representation in the general population. For example, while Hispanics make up 12.5 percent of the US population,[4] they comprise 31.9 percent of those who remain without health insurance. Similarly, people without college degrees make up 55.6 percent of the population,[5] yet comprise 82.8 percent of the uninsured.

Overall, of the 30.1 million individuals who remained uninsured at the time of the March 2017 survey, it is remarkable that 7.5 million were eligible for coverage under Medicaid/CHIP and 3.1 million more were eligible for exchange products that would have included large premium tax credits (i.e., for those with household incomes at or below 200 percent of the federal poverty line). Thus, 35.2 percent of uninsured individuals in March 2017 were already eligible for coverage under current rules for Medicaid/CHIP eligibility or the health exchanges.

Individuals across demographic groups show significant potential for reductions in their uninsured rate if eligible individuals with each characteristic were enrolled in Medicaid/CHIP or the health exchanges. The potential for reduction in the uninsured is about 35 percent overall (7.5 million eligible for Medicaid/CHIP plus 3.1 million eligible for premium tax credits divided by 30.1 million total uninsured), and some groups can take more advantage of this opportunity than others. While those with family

Table 20.2. Selected characteristics of the remaining nonelderly uninsured, 2017

Characteristic	Number uninsured remaining, nonelderly	Share of uninsured in category (%)	Number uninsured eligible for Medicaid/CHIP	Number uninsured eligible for premium tax credits with incomes at or below 200% of federal poverty line
Total	30,089,000	100.0	7,522,000	3,122,000
Age				
0–17	4,602,000	15.3	2,800,000	4,000
18–34	11,413,000	37.9	2,426,000	1,457,000
35–49	8,012,000	26.6	1,302,000	872,000
50–64	6,062,000	20.1	993,000	790,000
Race/ethnicity				
White, single race, non-Hispanic	13,637,000	45.3	3,247,000	1,558,000
Black, single race, non-Hispanic	4,507,000	15.0	1,590,000	525,000
Hispanic	9,601,000	31.9	2,008,000	774,000
Other	2,344,000	7.8	677,000	264,000
Self-reported health status				
Excellent or very good	18,779,000	62.4	4,744,000	1,827,000
Good	8,541,000	28.4	1,997,000	961,000
Fair or poor	2,769,000	9.2	780,000	334,000
Citizenship status				
Citizen	24,004,000	79.8	N/R	2,754,000
Legal noncitizen resident	1,222,000	4.1	N/R	368,000
Undocumented immigrant	4,863,000	16.2	N/R[a]	N/A
Family income relative to federal poverty line				
At or below 200%	17,143,000	57.0	7,195,000	3,122,000
Greater than 200% but less than 400%	7,950,000	26.4	327,000	N/A
At or above 400%	4,996,000	16.6	N/R	N/A
Educational attainment (ages 18 and older)				
Less than high school	5,183,000	20.3	904,000	575,000
High school degree	9,143,000	35.9	1,889,000	1,236,000
Some college	6,785,000	26.6	1,378,000	899,000
College degree or more	3,173,000	17.2	550,000	408,000
Urban/rural				
Metropolitan Statistical Area (MSA)	25,479,000	84.7	6,311,000	2,553,000
Non-MSA	4,282,000	14.2	1,153,000	524,000

Table 20.2. *(continued)*

Characteristic	Number uninsured remaining, nonelderly	Share of uninsured in category (%)	Number uninsured eligible for Medicaid/CHIP	Number uninsured eligible for premium tax credits with incomes at or below 200% of federal poverty line
Employment status / usual weekly hours worked at main job at time of survey				
Full time (30 hrs/week or more)	13,323,000	44.3	1,231,000	1,595,000
Part time (less than 30 hrs/week or hours vary)	3,607,000	12.0	818,000	578,000
Unemployed	1,754,000	5.8	503,000	276,000
Not in labor force	7,660,000	25.5	2,673,000	669,000
Armed forces member or younger than 15	3,746,000	12.4	2,297,000	3,000

Source: Adapted from Linda J. Blumberg, John Holahan, Michael Karpman, and Caroline Elmendorf, *Characteristics of the Remaining Uninsured: An Update*, US Health Reform—Monitoring and Impact (Washington, DC: Urban Institute, July 2018), https://www.urban.org/research/publication/characteristics-remaining-uninsured-update.

[a] Not reported. Undocumented immigrants are not eligible for Medicaid, and legal noncitizen residents are eligible only in very restricted circumstances.

incomes less than 200 percent of the federal poverty line would have the most to gain from enrollment in Medicaid/CHIP or the exchanges, 60 percent were eligible but did not enroll. Among Blacks, 47 percent of uninsured individuals were eligible for Medicaid/CHIP or the health exchanges but did not enroll. Among individuals who did not reside in a metropolitan area, 39 percent were eligible but did not enroll. Facilitating enrollment by currently eligible individuals in Medicaid/CHIP or the health exchanges would appear to be a relatively uncomplicated way of improving access for those who remain uninsured.

The Underinsured

The concept of "underinsured" pertains to individuals who have some form of health insurance but experience significant financial strain because of high out-of-pocket costs due to limited coverage benefits, high deductibles, and/or high co-pays. To quantify this, the Commonwealth Fund has suggested that underinsurance occurs when there are

- out-of-pocket medical expenses of at least 10 percent of a family's total annual income,

- out-of-pocket medical expenses of at least 5 percent of annual income for households with income less than 200 percent of the federal poverty line, or
- health plan deductible expenses of at least 5 percent of annual income.[6]

The Commonwealth Fund conducts biennial health insurance surveys consisting of a 25-minute telephone interview with a random, nationally representative sample of adults age 19 and over.[7] The 2016 sample comprised data from telephone surveys of 6,005 individuals. An increasing underinsured rate is evident when the results related to the underinsured for 2016 are compared in a trend line that includes prior data since 2003 (figure 20.8). Using the criterion of out-of-pocket medical expenses of at least 10 percent of a family's total annual income, underinsurance among adults ages 19–64 has increased from 7 percent in 2003 to 17 percent in 2016. For households with annual income less than 200 percent of the federal poverty line and out-of-pocket medical expenses of at least 5 percent of that income, the underinsured rate has increased from 12 percent in 2003 to 28 percent in 2016. Extrapolating to the US population between the ages of 19 and 64, the estimated number of underinsured Americans increased from 16 million in 2003 to 41 million in 2016.

While the overall rate of underinsurance is 28 percent, the rate for those with individual coverage or coverage in the ACA health care marketplaces is much higher (44 percent) than for those covered under employer-sponsored health plans. Underinsurance has grown because of the growth in deductibles in private health plans (figure 20.9) and in other out-of-pocket

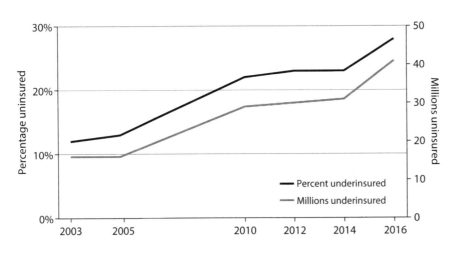

Figure 20.8. Underinsured among adults, ages 19–64, insured all year. Adapted from Collins, Gunja, and Doty, "How Well Does Insurance Coverage Protect Consumers from Health Care Costs."[6]

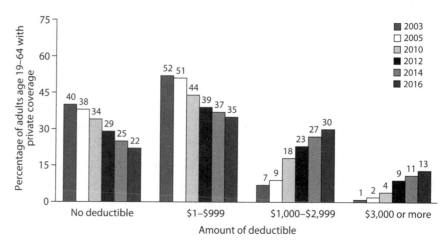

Figure 20.9.
Changes in the profile of deductibles in private insurance plans, 2003–2016. Collins, Gunja, and Doty, "How Well Does Insurance Coverage Protect Consumers from Health Care Costs," exhibit 4.[6]

costs. The underinsured rate is higher for those whose household incomes are less than 200 percent of the federal poverty line and for those in fair or poor health (figure 20.10).

In some respects, those who were underinsured in 2016 were similar to those who were uninsured: for example, over 50 percent of both groups had at least one medical bill problem or debt, in comparison with 25 percent of insured individuals (figure 20.11). In most respects, the underinsured were between the insured and uninsured. This was the case with respect to those who, because of medical bills, received a lower credit rating, had to declare bankruptcy, had a medical problem but did not go to a doctor or clinic, did not fill a prescription, and did not see a specialist when their doctor thought this was needed.

Even before the recent uptick in underinsurance, the financial strain of deductibles was evident, based on data from the Federal Reserve Board's 2013 Survey of Consumer Finances. A study from the Kaiser Family Foundation found that more than a third of adults less than age 65 did not have sufficient liquid assets to pay a deductible of $2,500 for single coverage or $5,000 for family coverage.[8]

A more recent report from a 2019 Kaiser Health Tracking Poll found that 34 percent of insured adults report difficulty affording their deductible.[9] About half of adults reported that they or a family member put off or skipped some sort of needed health care, and about a fifth have not filled a prescription for a medicine given to them by their physician.

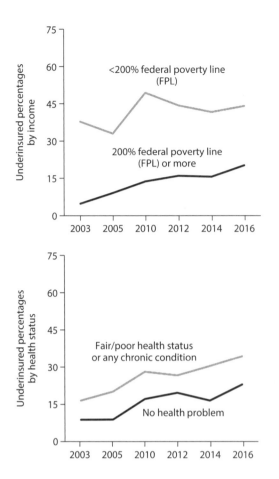

Figure 20.10. Underinsured rate trends by income and health status, ages 19–64. Adapted from Collins, Gunja, and Doty, "How Well Does Insurance Coverage Protect Consumers from Health Care Costs," exhibit 6.[6]

Figure 20.11. Percentages of underinsured, uninsured, and insured individuals, ages 19–64, in selected scenarios, 2016. Adapted from Collins, Gunja, and Doty, "How Well Does Insurance Coverage Protect Consumers from Health Care Costs."[6]

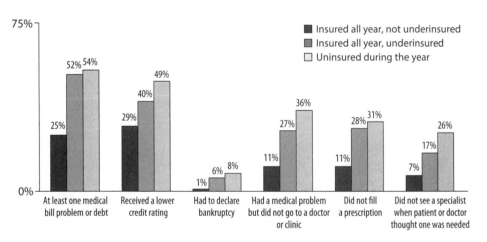

Impact of Medicaid Expansion on Access and Health Status

There are conflicting data on the relation between expanded coverage under Medicaid and improved access and health status. An early randomized trial of Medicaid eligibility in Oregon prior to the ACA showed improved access but mixed health benefits.[10] Longitudinal data before and after the 2006 health care reform in Massachusetts, however, indicate a significant reduction in all-cause mortality. More recent cross-sectional studies following implementation of the ACA suggest demonstrable benefits in both access and health status.

The Oregon Health Insurance Experiment

Occurring prior to the ACA, the Oregon Health Insurance Experiment was an important study regarding the impact of expanded Medicaid eligibility on enrollment and health status. At that time, Medicaid in Oregon consisted of two programs, collectively called the Oregon Health Plan (OHP). OHP Plus served the categorically eligible Medicaid population (children in low-income families, low-income pregnant women, etc.), and OHP Standard was designed to cover low-income adults who were not categorically eligible for OHP Plus. Individuals were eligible for OHP Standard if they were without insurance for at least six months, had income below the federal poverty line, and assets below $2,000.

Depending on state budget availability, OHP Standard covered a variable number of individuals over the years, reaching a peak of 110,000 in 2002 and declining to 19,000 by 2008. In 2008, state funds became available to add 10,000 eligible individuals and their first-degree family members to OHP Standard. A waiver was obtained from the Centers for Medicare and Medicaid Services to add these new members through a lottery. Almost 90,000 individuals asked to participate in the lottery. Ultimately, 35,169 individuals representing 29,664 households were selected by lottery, of whom about 30 percent successfully enrolled.[11] (About 40 percent never sent back applications and half of those who applied were deemed ineligible based on income, assets, or other criteria.)[12]

This scenario gave rise to a natural experiment (The Oregon Health Insurance Experiment), in which the outcomes of those who became eligible by lottery to enroll in Medicaid could be compared with those who were not selected by the lottery.[13] Two types of analyses were performed: (1) an intent-to-treat analysis provided estimates of the effect of winning the *ability to apply* for Medicaid (i.e., *access* to Medicaid) through the lottery, and (2) the effect of *actual* Medicaid coverage on outcomes.

In general, the effect of actually being enrolled in Medicaid was about four times greater than the effect of having been chosen by the lottery.[14] Other important results included the following:

- *Overall access to care*: As compared with controls, 68 percent more Medicaid enrollees had a usual source of clinic-based care, 57 percent more had a personal doctor, 35 percent more received all the care they needed in the past six months; and 25 percent more received all needed prescription medicines.[15]
- *Hospital utilization*: The probability of a hospital admission was 30 percent higher among those with Medicaid compared with controls; most admissions did not originate from the emergency room (e.g., planned admissions for surgery).[16]
- *Preventive care*: In the outpatient setting, preventive care was enhanced, including 15 percent higher testing for blood sugar among Medicaid enrollees than controls, 18 percent higher testing for blood cholesterol, and 62 percent higher mammography rates.[17]

All bulleted results were statistically significant at $p < .0001$, except for hospital admissions ($p = .004$), depression screen ($p = .001$), days of good physical health ($p = .019$), and days of good mental health ($p = .001$).

These findings are consistent with the conclusion that coverage through Medicaid indeed worked in promoting access to health care. They are also consistent with data that, across all types of medical services, including the emergency department, individuals who don't have health care coverage use less service. Thus, in 2013, uninsured adults in the United States who were less than 65 years old had 60 percent fewer doctor visits and 80 percent fewer hospital admissions than those with health insurance; although it may be counterintuitive, the uninsured also had 40 percent fewer emergency department visits, despite the Emergency Medical Treatment and Active Labor Act.[18] The uninsured use less health care, across the board.

Two years after the lottery, based on detailed personal interviews of 6,293 Medicaid enrollees and 5,746 controls, a significantly higher percentage of Medicaid enrollees had filled prescription medications for a variety of chronic illnesses, including cardiovascular disease, diabetes, and mental health conditions.[19] The number of prescription medications per person was also significantly higher among Medicaid enrollees (2.02) than controls (1.56). These findings complement the other results initially reported from the Oregon Health Study Group, showing greater use of primary and preventive care among Medicaid enrollees. Importantly, Medicaid coverage virtually eliminated the use of medications that were prescribed for someone else. Overall, the authors concluded that "Medicaid plays an important role in access to medicines for chronic conditions for low-income populations."[20]

In addition to improved access to physicians, hospitals, and pharmaceuticals as an outcome of the Oregon Health Insurance Experiment, preliminary data were analyzed on the survey results of self-reported health status: Compared with controls, 24 percent more Medicaid enrollees reported good or very good health (not fair or poor), 12 percent fewer Medicaid enrollees screened positive for depression (75 percent vs. 67 percent), and Medicaid enrollees had 1.3 more days of good physical health and 2.1 more days of good mental health in the month prior to the survey.[21]

To evaluate further the impact of Medicaid enrollment on clinical outcomes, investigators from the Oregon Health Study Group were able to conduct in-person interviews on 6,387 Medicaid enrollees and 5,842 control subjects in which a variety of health measures were obtained: blood pressure, cholesterol, glycated hemoglobin, screening for depression, self-reported health status, and out-of-pocket spending. Compared with controls two years after the lottery, there was no statistically significant difference between Medicaid enrollees and controls in the prevalence of hypertension, diabetes, or hypercholesterolemia or in the estimated risk for a cardiovascular event (table 20.3). There were statistically significant improvements in self-reported health status, depression, and avoidance of financial strain.

Much has been made of the fact that, despite greater use of primary care and prevention services by Medicaid enrollees as reported in the one-year results, there was no difference from controls in the prevalence of hypertension, hypercholesterolemia, or diabetes. (It was also found that new diagnoses of these conditions after the lottery were not different between enrollees and controls.) There are several possible explanations for this paradox:[22]

- First, there is evidence that behavioral factors are much more important in determining health status than access to medical services

Table 20.3. Selected effects of Medicaid clinical and financial outcomes from the Oregon Health Insurance Experiment

Variable	Percentage from control group (%)	Percentage change with Medicaid Coverage (%)	P value[b]
Hypertension prevalence	16.3	−1.3	0.65
Total cholesterol ≥ 240mg/dl	14.1	−2.4	0.37
HDL cholesterol < 40 mg/dl	28.0	−2.8	0.46
Glycated hemoglobin with diabetes	5.1	−0.9	0.61
High Framingham risk score[a]	8.2	−0.2	0.76
Positive screening for depression	30.0	−9.2	0.02
Health same or better vs. one year earlier	80.4	−7.8	0.02
Catastrophic expenditures	5.5	−4.5	0.02
Any medical debt	56.8	−13.3	0.002
Borrowed money to pay bills or skipped payment	24.4	−14.2	< 0.001

Source: Adapted from Baicker et al., "The Oregon Experiment."[14]
[a] A Framingham risk score predicts 10-year cardiovascular risk. These scores were calculated separately for men and women over 30 years of age and range from 0.99 percent to 30 percent.
[b] P values less than 0.05 are considered statistically significant.

(chapter 7). These behaviors begin in childhood and adolescence, and then accumulate through the life cycle.

- Second, one to two years of access to primary care and prevention services is probably not enough time to make a difference when it comes to hypertension, diabetes, and heart disease. Pertinent to this point is the finding that the prevalence of smoking and obesity was the same for Medicaid enrollees and controls.
- Third, all of the differences with Medicaid coverage were in the direction of improvement—less hypertension, high cholesterol, and diabetes—although not sufficiently so to be statistically significant. Thus, the sample size may not have been large enough to detect these differences, or the duration of follow may have been too short. For example, the estimated percent of Medicaid enrollees with high total cholesterol was 11.7 percent versus 14.1 percent in controls. Thus, high cholesterol was almost one fifth lower among enrollees than controls, but the small sample and relatively low prevalence created a wide variance around this difference, leading to a nonsignificant result.

- Fourth, it would appear that the controls had a relatively low baseline prevalence of hypertension (16.3 percent), hypercholesterolemia (14.1 percent), and diabetes (5.1 percent). From these low levels, it is more difficult to show a significant reduction in these diseases in one to two years.

On the flip side of these negative findings regarding hypertension, diabetes, and heart disease were the positive findings around less depression, better self-reported overall health status, and less financial strain.

Mortality Effects after Health Care Reform in Massachusetts in 2006

In 2006, the Massachusetts legislature passed comprehensive health care reform that expanded Medicaid, offered subsidized private insurance, and created an individual mandate. Indeed, this legislation was a model for the Affordable Care Act. As summarized by Sommers, Long, and Baicker, health insurance among adults aged 19 to 64 years increased by 3 to 8 percentage points following enactment of this reform bill, with an associated improvement in access, self-reported physical and mental health, use of preventive services, and functional status.[23]

To evaluate the impact of reform on mortality, Sommers and his collaborators compared death rates for adults aged 20 to 64 in Massachusetts between two periods: 2001 and 2005 (pre-reform) vs. 2007 to 2010 (post-reform). These differences were compared to a control group of similar counties in other states that did not experience health care reform. Adjusted for changes in the control group, the Massachusetts reforms were associated with a statistically significant decrease in all-cause mortality of 2.9 percent and a 4.5 percent reduction in deaths from causes amenable to health care.

Cross-Sectional Studies of Medicaid Expansion in Relation to Access and Health

Medicaid expansion under the ACA has moved forward nationally in a manner that is operationally different from the Oregon experiment. Finkelstein et al. pointed to a number of other considerations regarding the generalizability of their results from Oregon:

- They had limited time for follow-up.
- In contrast to their study of increased coverage of a relatively small number of people while "holding constant the rest of the health system," larger expansions might elicit supply-side responses from providers.
- Their population was different from the general low-income, uninsured population in a number of demographic characteristics.
- Selection bias was possible due to volunteering for the lottery.
- There is heterogeneity across states in the specifics of the Medicaid program.
- Oregon Medicaid was essentially free to enrollees.

Recognizing the methodologic advantages of the Oregon natural experiment over cross-sectional comparisons, but also these cautions about generalizing the results beyond Oregon and its unique system, there is a growing body of cross-state analyses indicative of a positive effect of Medicaid expansion under the ACA on access and a variety of health outcomes.

- Sommers et al. compared Texas, which has not expanded Medicaid, with two Medicaid expansion states—Kentucky and Arkansas.[24] Prior to ACA, the uninsured rates of low-income adults in all three states was in the range of 38–42 percent. Three years after ACA, however, the rate of individuals without health care coverage in Kentucky and Arkansas dropped to 10–15 percent, while the rate in Texas declined only to about 30 percent. In addition, people gaining coverage under Medicaid expansion experienced a 41 percentage point increase in having a usual source of care, a $337 reduction in annual out-of-pocket spending, significant increases in preventive health visits and glucose testing, and a 23 percentage point increase in "excellent" self-reported health.
- A cross-sectional study of 1.4 billion emergency room visits between 2006 and 2016, and 405 million hospital discharges between 2006 and 2016, compared clinical volumes before and after the 2014 ACA insurance expansions.[25] There was a decline in uninsured emergency room visits from 16 percent to 8 percent and in uninsured hospital stays from 6 percent to 4 percent. Among patients aged 18 to 64 years, declines in emergency room visits and hospital discharges were from 20 percent to 11 percent and 10 percent to 7 percent, respectively.

- Using a similar strategy of comparing a Medicaid expansion state (Michigan) with a nonexpansion state (Virginia), Charles et al.[26] reported improved outcomes from cardiac surgery in Medicaid populations. In Michigan, pre-operative risk measures declined after Medicaid expansion (attributed to better access to primary care and pre-operative evaluation), and there was a 31 percent reduction in the risk-adjusted rate of major postoperative morbidity from cardiac surgery in their Medicaid population. By contrast, in Virginia there was no difference between pre- and post-expansion eras in the pre-operative risk status of patients or in postoperative morbidity.
- Comparing expansion and nonexpansion states nationally, Bhatt and Beck-Sagué found that reductions in statewide infant mortality rates (for the entire population, not just Medicaid patients) were greater in expansion states, particularly among African-Americans.[27] Specifically, these investigators found that the decline in African American infant mortality in Medicaid expansion states (from 11.7 per 1,000 live births in 2010 to 10.0 per 1,000 live births in 2015), was more than twice the decline in nonexpansion states.
- Using data from the 2014 Behavioral Risk Factor Surveillance System survey conducted by the Centers for Disease Control and Prevention, Rogers and Zhang estimated the impact of Medicaid expansion on heart health.[28] Poor heart health was defined if there was a "yes" answer to any one of three questions on the survey that asked whether a physician or other health professional ever told the respondent that they had (1) a heart attack, (2) angina or coronary artery disease, or (3) stroke. Controlling for known contributors to poor heart health such as older age, diabetes, obesity, inactivity, and smoking, respondents in a Medicaid expansion state were 23 percent less likely to have poor heart health compared to low-income individuals in non–Medicaid expansion states.

Longitudinal Analysis of Medicaid Expansion in Relation to Financial Health

An important result of the Oregon Health Insurance Experiment was that uninsured individuals who won the Medicaid lottery and enrolled in the program had reduced financial strain. The impact of expanding access to health care through Medicaid expansion was studied in more detail by

Sarah Miller and her colleagues, drawing on Michigan's experience with Medicaid expansion under the Healthy Michigan Program (HMP). As reported in a National Bureau of Economic Research Working Paper, administrative data on HMP enrollees were matched against credit report data sets to study changes in the "financial health" of enrollees before and after HMP.[29] Up to twenty months of follow-up were available. HMP enrollment was associated with a significant decline in bill collections, amounts past due, bankruptcy, and number of months overdrawn on credit cards.

Impact of Health Insurance Marketplaces on Access

Limited data are available on the impact of the ACA exchanges on health care access. As noted in chapter 12, legal and policy decisions made and implemented since enactment of the ACA have led to a reduction in choice among exchange health plans in many counties, which may constrain the impact of ACA on access in the future. At this writing, there are only two analyses of the impact of the ACA on access. One study showed a favorable impact on the proportion of emergency department visits by uninsured patients. Using a national database that included both Medicaid expansion and nonexpansion states, the overall increased rate of insurance post-ACA was associated with a 2.1 percent per year decline in the proportion of uninsured emergency department patients between 2014 and 2016. For emergency department visits by patients between the ages of 18 and 64, there was a decline from 20 percent to 11 percent in the proportion uninsured.[30]

The other study focused on data when the ACA exchanges were in their "pure" form (i.e., prior to the potential effects on access of the mandate repeal, promotion of association health plans and short-term, limited duration plans, cancellation of payments to insurers for cost-sharing reductions, and other actions).[31] Data were obtained from the nationally representative Medical Expenditure Panel Survey conducted by the Agency for Healthcare Research and Quality, which is available in two-year, longitudinal data sets. Study data were analyzed across a two-year time period for both "intervention" and "control" groups:

- The intervention group consisted of adults ages 18–63 with 2013 family incomes of 138 to 400 percent of the federal poverty line who had been uninsured for at least six months. Data on this group were collected before (2013, "year 1") and after (2014, "year 2") the first open enrollment period for the ACA health insurance marketplace. Eighty-three percent of this group was employed.

- The control group consisted of two cohorts of individuals of the same age and income groups who had employer-sponsored health insurance in either 2011 or 2012. Data on this group were collected for 2011 or 2012 as "year 1" and compared with the following year as "year 2."

The intervention group had lower family income (mean = $35,272) than the control group (mean = $48,539) and was slightly younger (38.8 vs. 40.7 years), more likely male (57.2 vs. 46.1 percent), and more likely Hispanic (31.2 vs. 13.7 percent). Attempts were made to control for these and other potentially confounding variables in the statistical analyses.

Comparing year 2 to year 1, the control group showed a 4.4 percentage point increase in health insurance (from 93.3 to 97.7 percent) while the intervention group showed a 15.2 percentage point increase (from 27.6 percent to 42.8 percent). Adjusting for potentially confounding factors in multivariate analysis, the intervention group improved its insurance rate by 10.8 percentage points more than the control group, which was statistically significant at $p < 0.001$.

Summary

Access to health care in the United States is out of balance relative to expenditures. Compared to other high-income countries, we spend the most on health care per person yet have the most inequitable access to care. After implementation of the Affordable Care Act, there remains almost 30 million Americans without health care coverage. This represented a reduction from 13 percent uninsured in 2013, due to aging of the population and enrollment in Medicare, the introduction of Medicaid expansion in some states, and the availability of federally subsidized health care exchanges. Although the overall rate of uninsured in 2017 was 8.8 percent, the age group with the largest fraction of uninsured was among those aged 19–64, at 12.1 percent. Covering Americans in the education/work years between childhood and retirement remains the critical challenge in health care access facing our nation.

The percentage of people with health insurance is directly correlated with education, employment, and income and inversely associated with Black and Hispanic race and ethnicity. Consistent with these insured-versus-uninsured comparisons, those remaining uninsured are weighted heavily toward individuals who are less educated, have lower incomes, and are Black or Hispanic. It is potentially important that one third of individuals uninsured in 2017 were eligible for coverage through Medicaid/CHIP or the health exchanges but did not enroll.

The ranks of the underinsured are growing due to higher health plan deductibles and other changes in benefit design associated with higher out-of-pocket costs. It has been estimated that the number of underinsured Americans increased from 16 million in 2013 to 41 million (or 28 percent of those insured) in 2016. About half of the underinsured in 2016 had at least one medical bill problem or debt and received a lower credit rating, and about one third had a medical problem but did not go to a doctor or clinic.

Based on a pre-ACA randomized trial in Oregon, and post-ACA analyses comparing states that did and did not expand Medicaid, it is clear that Medicaid expansion improved access to care—doctor visits, hospitalization, pharmaceuticals—and reduced financial strain. Availability of the health insurance marketplace also improved access. Analyses of the impact of Medicaid expansion on health are early and somewhat mixed. The Oregon randomized trial showed a favorable effect on self-reported health status and depression but no difference between Medicaid enrollees and controls in objective assessments of hypertension, diabetes, or high cholesterol. Evidence from a quasi-experimental study of health care reform in Massachusetts indicates that expansion in access led to a 4.5 percent reduction in deaths from causes amenable to health care. Subsequent cross-sectional studies of expansion vs. nonexpansion states have confirmed a large (23 percent) difference in "excellent" self-reported health as well as significant improvement in a variety of specific health outcomes such as postoperative morbidity from heart surgery, infant mortality rates, and heart health (myocardial infarction, angina, coronary artery disease, and/or stroke).

PART IV

IMPROVING THE BALANCE OF CARE, COST, AND ACCESS

21 IMPROVING THE BALANCE I
MACRO CONSIDERATIONS

The twentieth century was a time of extraordinary breakthroughs in biomedical science. As these advances were translated into effective medical treatments, the duration and quality of our lives improved. The strong upward trajectory of biomedical science, technology, and medical innovation continues to this day.

As effective treatments for disease accelerated during the past century, so did the health care industry that now represents almost one fifth of our nation's economy. This industry evolved around a fee-for-service, claims-based backbone of health insurance, both private and public. Employer-sponsored health plans were stimulated by tax subsidies, and government-sponsored programs were enacted through legislation to cover older adults, children, and the poor. Due to price subsidies, individuals now pay out of pocket only a small fraction of the total cost of their health care, while the full price is paid by third parties to providers, hospitals, drug companies, and medical device manufacturers. In comparison with other high-income nations, we are first in health care spending but last in life expectancy, infant mortality, and other measures of health outcomes. Not all of us are destined to poor health, however; there is wide variability in our health status and longevity, with education and income profoundly influencing these outcomes. And although health care coverage through private health insurance and government programs is extensive in the United States, almost 30 million people remain uninsured and an additional 40 million are underinsured.

Thus, US health care is characterized by an imbalance of care, cost, and access. Having identified specific flaws in these three core and interrelated aspects of US health care, we will now consider ways in which the balance can be improved. The discussion on remedies can be framed by calling attention to broad, powerful forces that affect health and health care but which cannot be addressed with levers pertaining to the health care industry *per se*. These forces are social, behavioral, and environmental determinants of disease; biomedical and population health research; and the overall economy and federal budget.

Social, Behavioral, and Environmental Determinants of Disease
Social and Behavioral Determinants

Based on estimates of the impact of health care on mortality reduction in common diseases, a 1994 report concluded that about 40 percent of the improved life expectancy between 1950 and the early 1990s was due to medical interventions,[1] mainly because of a reduction in infant mortality and deaths from heart disease. This leaves 60 percent of the improvement being due to other factors, including environmental, social, and behavioral determinants of disease. In recent years, however, there has not been continuing improvement in United States life expectancy but rather a decline due to increased deaths from causes such as opioid overdose, alcohol abuse, and gun violence. Moreover, life expectancy in the United States lags behind other high-income countries due to social and behavioral determinants. Thus, countering the benefits of the extraordinary advances in biomedical science and medical treatments, environmental, social, and behavioral determinants of disease are a key macro consideration affecting population health.

These disease determinants vary inversely with income, so it is not surprising that life expectancy within the United States is higher for those with greater income:

- Men and women in the upper quartile of income can expect to live about 10.5 years and 6.0 years longer than men and women in the lowest quartile of income.
- The difference in life expectancy between high and low individuals is expanding across time in association with the widening difference in income.

Morover, since the United States trails other high-income nations in life expectancy, it is not surprising that it lags in most measures of health across the life cycle:

- A higher teen pregnancy rate leads to greater prematurity and, consequently, to greater neonatal and infant morbidity and mortality.
- Markers of poor health for adults between the ages of 20 and 50—obesity, inactivity, high cholesterol, and smoking—are associated with the development of diabetes, cardiovascular disease, and cancer.

With a high prevalence of these behaviorally based risk factors, Americans enter their later years in poorer health than their counterparts in other nations and are therefore more likely to develop a variety of diseases as they age.

According to a report from the National Research Council and National Academy of Medicine using 2010 data, 48 percent of all premature deaths in the United States are due to behavioral and other preventable factors.[2] The two greatest risk factors are tobacco and diet/activity, which are estimated to account for 15 and 18 percent, respectively, of all premature deaths. Using 2003–2006 data from the National Health and Nutrition Examination Survey to measure risk factors and mortality data from the National Center for Health Statistics, Danaei et al. estimated that smoking and hypertension were responsible for 467,000 deaths in the United States (i.e., about one in five to six deaths among US adults).[3] It was also estimated that obesity and physical inactivity were each responsible for nearly one in ten deaths.

The finding that variation in mortality within the United States depends strongly on behavioral factors (which are in turn associated with education, income, and racial/ethnic differences) is consistent with insights from international comparisons. In a National Academy of Medicine report, Michael McGinnis concludes that the low ranking of the United States among peer nations in life expectancy at age 50 is due mainly to our greater prevalence of smoking and obesity.[4] Along similar lines, the World Health Organization's Global Burden of Disease Study compared the United States and 34 Organisation for Economic Co-operation and Development countries with regards to 67 risk factors for 291 diseases and injuries, and it was found that years lost due to premature mortality plus years lived with disability were high in the United States mainly because of diet, obesity, smoking, high blood pressure, high fasting blood glucose, physical inactivity, and alcohol use[5]—all behavior-based risk factors.

In 2017, the three leading causes of mortality in the United States were heart disease (647,457 deaths), cancer (599,108 deaths), and "unintentional injuries" (169,936 deaths).[6] These three mortality threats are all linked to behavioral factors:

- Acquired heart disease is largely related to diet, activity, body weight, and weight distribution.
- Lung cancer is due mainly to smoking. (Although a decline in lung cancer mortality contributed to a 2.2 percent decline in overall cancer mortality rates between 2016 and 2017—the largest single-year decline ever—lung cancer still has the highest mortality rate, causing more deaths in 2017 than breast, prostate, colorectal, and brain cancers combined.)[7]
- Unintentional injuries reflect a variety of behavioral factors that include drug overdose, motor vehicle deaths due to intoxication, and violent deaths with firearms.

Greater health care utilization and cost follow from the occurrence of diseases that are behaviorally based. For example, the three medical devices for which taxpayers make the greatest Medicare expenditures are sleep apnea devices, wearable defibrillators, and back braces (chapter 19), all of which have etiologies strongly linked to obesity. A host of other medical, surgical, and pharmaceutical treatments are linked to diseases and injuries that have behavioral etiologies. When the higher rate of neonatal and infant mortality due to teen pregnancy is added to the picture, it is clear that behavioral factors across the life cycle—which are linked to income, education, and race/ethnicity—are responsible for a large share of morbidity and mortality in the United States.

How much benefit would be possible if interventions were effective in changing behavior? Using longitudinal data on risk factors and subsequent mortality from the Nurses' Health Study (1980–2014, N = 78,865) and the Health Professionals Follow-Up Study (1986–2014, N = 44,354), Yanping Li and a large group of national and international collaborators estimated the potential reduction in mortality risk associated with five lifestyle factors.[8] Low-risk lifestyle behaviors were not smoking, having a body mass index (BMI) less than overweight (18.5–24.9 kg/m^2), getting 30 minutes or more of moderate to vigorous exercise each day, moderate alcohol intake, and a high-quality diet. Comparing individuals having all five low-risk factors with those having none, and adjusting for potentially confounding variables, the low-risk group had an estimated risk reduction of about 75 percent for all-cause mortality, 65 percent for cancer mortality, and 80 percent for cardiovascular mortality. At age 50, comparing people with all five low-risk factors to those with none, the average life expectancy was projected to be 14.0 years longer for women and 12.2 years for men.

To what extent, however, are interventions actually effective in changing behavior? Can rates of smoking, obesity, and inactivity be altered by public health or individual interventions? Since publication of the first surgeon general's report on the health effects of smoking in 1964, tobacco control programs—including tobacco excise taxes, media campaigns, smoke-free policies, and restricted youth access—have markedly reduced smoking use and smoking-related morbidity and mortality in the United States.[9] This has been a success story. Nonetheless, as noted earlier, lung cancer remains the most common cause of cancer mortality, accounting for about one in four cancer deaths. Moreover, education, income, and geography have a tremendous influence on smoking; for instance, among adults whose highest degree is GED certification, tobacco use is eight times higher than those with a graduate degree; 25 percent of those below the poverty line smoke, as compared with 14 percent above the poverty line; and 9 to 12 percent of people living in California and Utah smoke, as compared with 22 to 25 percent of people who live in Kentucky and West Virginia.[10] Thus, social, cultural, and behavioral factors will continue to challenge tobacco control efforts, although the overall trend for smoking and lung cancer is going in a downward direction.

It has been challenging to impact behavioral risk factors for cardiovascular disease on a population basis, although widespread news coverage about the importance of reducing risk factors appears to have had some impact: it has been estimated that about half of the decline in US deaths from coronary heart disease from 1980 through 2000 was attributable to reductions in major risk factors, with evidence-based medical therapies accounting for the other half.[11] Promising results regarding diabetes were also obtained initially from research studies. Most prominent among these was the Diabetes Prevention Program (DPP), a major US study involving over 3,234 participants at risk for type 2 diabetes in 27 centers. The DPP was a randomized trial of intensive lifestyle intervention, metformin (an oral medication used to treat type 2 diabetes), and placebo to determine whether intensive lifestyle intervention or metformin (or both) would prevent or delay the onset of diabetes in comparison with placebo.[12] Participants receiving placebo or metformin pills did not know which of these two pills they were receiving. Providers were also blinded to treatment.

The lifestyle modification protocol consisted of 16 group sessions on dieting and exercise followed by monthly individualized sessions with the goals of decreasing weight by 7 percent and engaging in physical activity for at least 150 minutes per week. Participants were 51 years of age, on average, with a BMI of 34.0; 68 percent were women, and 45 percent were members of minority groups.

Based on data obtained through May 2001, the DPP trial was terminated one year early on the advice of the study's data monitoring board. By then, 65 percent of the planned person-years of observation had occurred. With an average follow-up of 2.8 years, the incidence of diabetes was 11.0 cases per 100 person-years in the placebo group, as compared with 7.8 in the metformin group, and 4.8 in the lifestyle group. Compared to placebo, the incidence of type 2 diabetes was reduced by 58 percent with the lifestyle intervention and by 31 percent with metformin, making lifestyle intervention significantly more effective than metformin. To prevent one case of diabetes during a period of three years, 6.9 persons would have to participate in the lifestyle-intervention program, and 13.9 would have to receive metformin.

Of the original participants, 2,766 enrolled in a longitudinal study; the median additional time of follow-up was 5.7 years. All three original groups were offered the group-implemented lifestyle intervention. Treatment with metformin was also continued in the original metformin group. After 10 years, as compared with the placebo group, the cumulative incidence of diabetes was 34 percent lower in the original lifestyle group and 18 percent lower in the metformin group. Importantly, in comparison with the baseline incidence rate of 11.0 new cases per 100 people for type 2 diabetes in the placebo group during the original DPP, the three groups in the follow-up trial (all of whom had access to lifestyle intervention) had similarly reduced incidence rates by year 10, in the range of 4.9 to 5.9 cases per 100 people. This occurred despite the fact that body weight in all three groups had returned close to baseline by 10 years.

In an effort to disseminate and implement the results of the DPP more widely, Congress authorized the Centers for Disease Control and Prevention (CDC) to establish the National Diabetes Prevention Program. Now an ongoing program, the National DPP is scaling the lifestyle intervention to achieve a population health impact for individuals at risk for type 2 diabetes. In collaboration with private-sector partners, the CDC developed a year-long curriculum, along with a training guide for lifestyle coaches. Organizations throughout the United States meeting CDC criteria have been implementing the program. In March 2016, the Centers for Medicare and Medicaid certified that the National DPP was both cost-saving and effective. Results from the first four years of implementation were reported in *Diabetes Care* in 2017.[13] Overall, participants reported a weekly average of 152 minutes of physical activity per week, and 35.5 percent achieved the goal of a 5 percent weight loss.

Unlike tobacco use, however, which has been declining in the United States, the prevalence of obesity has been rising, along with poor dietary habits and a sedentary lifestyle. Between 1999 and 2016, obesity rates increased from 30.5 to 39.6 percent among adults and from 13.9 to 18.5 percent among children 19 years of age or younger.[14] Thus, while the National DPP has been somewhat successful, the problem is like the situation described by the Red Queen in Lewis Carroll's *Through the Looking Glass*: "Now, here, you see, it takes all the running you can do, to keep in the same place. If you want to get somewhere else, you must run at least twice as fast!" Recent data show that the reduction in age-adjusted mortality rates from cardiometabolic disease has plateaued, being essentially constant for stroke and diabetes since 2011, and somewhat higher for hypertension.[15] Reductions in obesity from the DPP and similar programs, despite the extraordinary effort expended, have not kept up with the rise in obesity rates. Thus, obesity, diet, and exercise represent social and behavioral determinants of disease that must be addressed in the broader context of cultural and public health initiatives.

Environmental Determinants

In chapter 1, a "theory of epidemiologic transition" was described in which man-made diseases overtake infection pandemics as the principal cause of morbidity and mortality.[16] Indeed, this transition has played out in the United States and globally over the past century.

While some of these man-made diseases can be classified as behavioral, as just discussed, an increasing burden of disease can be attributed to environmental causes associated with industrialization. A longitudinal cohort study of air pollution involving 8,111 indivuduals across six US cities found a 26 percent higher risk of mortality attributable to particulate air pollution after adjusting for smoking and other potentially confounding factors.[17] Air pollution is thought to increase the risk of exacerbations of asthma symptoms and can contribute to new-onset asthma in both children and adults.[18] Prenatal exposure to pesticides, as measured in umbilical cord blood, has been found to have a substantial adverse impact on psychomotor development and IQ by three years of age.[19]

The health impact of exposure to asbestos, lead, secondhand smoke, and other environmental hazards, as well as the association between certain occupations (from coal miners to chimney sweeps) with cancer, lung disease, and premature mortality, are well known. It is also becoming apparent, however, that other diseases have an environmental etiology as part of their pathophysiology. For example, Parkinson's disease was rare in most of human history but has increased dramatically since the Industrial Revolution in association with exposure to specific solvents, pesticides, and heavy metals.[20] As well, the greatest increase in the incidence of Parkinson's disease has occurred across time in countries experiencing the most rapid industrialization.[21]

Research

Research is fundamentally important in improving health outcomes on an individual and population level. People with heart disease, cancer, and other diseases are now treated with drugs, surgery, and medical devices that extend the duration and quality of their lives. These treatments—evaluated for their efficacy through clinical trials (chapter 13)—are the result of fundamental scientific discoveries that have been translated into effective clinical practice, including a host of transformational biomedical discoveries (chapter 1).

Basic science and clinical research have been the mainstays of work supported by the National Institutes of Health (NIH). But for conditions that are preventable—including much of acquired heart disease, many cancers, and many causes of "unintentional injuries"—it is also important to conduct research that leads to a better understanding of social and behavioral determinants on a population basis under real-world conditions and of how public health programs and individual interventions can prevent their onset and development. Funding for this type of research has been less reliable than funding for biomedical science. So too has funding for research on how alternative policies regarding health care finance and delivery impact access to care as well as its cost and quality. We spend trillions of dollars on health care but only a tiny fraction of 1 percent to learn about which financing and delivery systems work best and should be enhanced and which are counterproductive and should be discontinued. Support for these types of research efforts has been part of the scientific portfolios of the Centers for Disease Control and Prevention, the Agency for Healthcare Improvement and Quality, and the Patient-Centered Outcomes Research Institute. Other agencies and foundations also provide funding for such studies, but overall this category of research has been supported in a less robust manner than NIH-funded investigations.

As an overarching matter, given that there has never been a time in the history of biomedical science when there is more promise for transformational discoveries that can lead to improved health, it will be essential for the United States to continue its historical trajectory of increasing support for the NIH. As well, greater amounts of steady, predictable support are needed for other types of research that focus on prevention, population science, real-world evidence, and systems of health care delivery and finance.

Biomedical Research and the Role of the National Institutes of Health

"If you think research is expensive, try disease." This phrase was coined by Mary Lasker, the philanthropist credited with leading the crusade for escalation in funding for the NIH, and specifically for the 1971 National Cancer Act.[22] In 1942, she and her husband, Albert, established the Lasker Awards, which have become regarded as "America's Nobels" for biomedical science.

NIH developed a funding model in which it distributed its research awards to a broad cross-section of universities and research institutes using a competitive, merit-based, peer-review process (chapter 9). This distributed model, combined with a dramatic increase in the federal funding of NIH that began in the 1940s, led to a surge in biomedical scientific discoveries and their subsequent translation into clinical practice. Federal support for NIH increased steadily between 1990 and 2010 and underwent a nominal doubling between 1998 and 2003 (figure 21.1). Between 2003 and 2015, however, the budget for NIH plateaued in nominal terms and declined

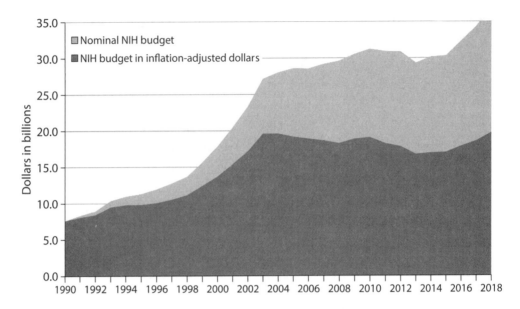

Figure 21.1. National Institutes of Health (NIH) budget trend in nominal dollars and inflation-adjusted dollars. "Spending History by Institute/Center, Mechanism, etc. (1983 to Present)," National Institutes of Health, Office of Budget, accessed January 30, 2019, https://officeofbudget.od.nih.gov/spending_hist.html.

in purchasing power. Since 2015, the NIH budget has increased from $30.3 billion to $37.3 billion, with a return in purchasing power to 2003 levels.

Jonathan Rothberg, the founder of a company that pioneered personal genome sequencing, opined, "The wealth of the nation comes from research and then innovation, which is the process of bringing research to market."[23] Taxpayer investment in NIH over the years has indeed created significant national wealth, while at the same time extending and improving lives and establishing the preeminence of American biomedical science in the world. A few examples among many can be counted:

- The NIH's Human Genome Project and its downstream ripple effects have resulted in nearly $1 trillion of economic growth. This represents a 178-fold return on investment.[24]
- Between 2010 and 2016, NIH-supported research was associated with every one of the 210 new drugs approved by the Food and Drug Administration (FDA) during that period.[25] Complementing industry research, the NIH-funded science focused on the biological targets for drug action rather than the drugs themselves.

- Private investment has been stimulated by NIH investment: on average, every $1.00 in NIH research funding stimulates an estimated $2.35 in additional industry clinical research over three years and $8.38 of additional industry basic research over eight years.[26]
- NIH-supported research was responsible for the first example of the class of protein kinase inhibitors that led to life-extending immunotherapy for patients with metastatic melanoma and other cancers (chapter 1).
- NIH-supported research was instrumental in developing the Hib vaccine, which immunizes young children against *Haemophilus influenzae* type b, a bacterium that causes the most common form of childhood bacterial meningitis. For the 2009 birth cohort alone, routine childhood immunization prevented an estimated 42,000 early deaths and 20 million cases of disease, with net savings of $13.5 billion in direct costs and $68.8 billion in total societal costs, respectively.[27]
- As discussed in chapter 13, the NIH-funded Women's Health Initiative fundamentally changed clinical practice regarding hormone replacement for menopausal women. It has been estimated that, as of 2014, the knowledge gained from this clinical trial led to financial and health outcomes worth an estimated $37.1 billion in net economic gain since the study was published in 2002, a return of approximately $140 per dollar invested in this research.[28]

Using a model of economic development maintained by the Bureau of Economic Analysis of the US Department of Commerce, it has been estimated that NIH research funding in 2016 directly and indirectly supported 379,471 jobs nationwide, which produced $64.8 billion in new economic activity, taking into account the income generated by these jobs as well as the purchase of research-related equipment, services, and materials cycling through the economy.[29]

Continued progress in fundamental biomedical science, and its translation into clinical practice, are critical building blocks for the future of health care and health in the United States and the world. Thus, it is disconcerting that national funding for NIH has plateaued. While the total investment in medical research funding from governmental and private sources continues to be greater in the United States than elsewhere in the world (e.g., $117.2 billion in the United States, with the next largest investments being $88.6 billion in Europe and $37.8 billion in Japan), the compound annual growth rate in research funding between 2004 and 2011 was 1.0 percent in the United States compared with 3.5 percent globally.[30] In some countries, much higher rates of growth in research investment have been occurring in recent years, such as China (16.9 per percent), Australia (9.3 percent), and Japan (6.8 percent).[31]

In 2013, after several years of flat funding that produced reduced purchasing power after accounting for inflation, Dr. Frances Collins, director of the NIH, commented in an interview at the Washington Ideas Forum that "we used to be the envy of the world" in making discoveries that led to cures and economic progress, but "we are starting to be the puzzle of the world as people look at our trajectory and wonder how we lost our way."[32] As chair of an international group of research funding directors, Dr. Collins asked the other directors about biomedical science funding in each of their countries. The answers reflected an increase in funding across all countries—from 5 percent to 15 percent. When Dr. Collins responded that, at a time of sequester funding in the United States, "we'll be lucky to go down by only 5 percent," the other national research leaders responded, "Are you guys crazy? We're reading your playbook from 10 years ago. Have you forgotten your own success story?"[33]

Among the many things in which the United States excels, biomedical research is high on the list. Why would we want to create deep, self-inflicted wounds in our biomedical research? Would France want to ravage its vineyards? In the years since the interview with Dr. Collins in 2013, the NIH budget has remained essentially flat (with the welcome exception of 2018). At a time when the prospects for scientific progress that can be directly translated to improved treatments and health outcomes have never been greater—in fields such as computational sciences, bioengineering, genomics, cellular reprogramming, and cell-based therapies, vaccine development, regenerative medicine, and others—it is a sad paradox that the growth in NIH funding has slowed over the past decade. Not only are the prospects for fundamental discoveries and new treatments threatened, but the attractiveness of biomedical research careers for those with the best scientific minds has been waning.

The uptick in 2018 funding for NIH is encouraging and hopefully represents a new inflection point. We return to Mary Lasker's insight: "If you think research is expensive, try disease." In addition to increased federal support of NIH, a number of other possibilities for supporting biomedical research have been advanced, including the creation of a national long-term strategy for research that would stabilize multiyear research budgets, enhanced coordination across public and private funding sources and research institutions, and improved operational efficiencies.[34]

John Porter, who served for 21 years as a Republican congressman from Illinois, and who is chair emeritus of Research!America, put it this way: "A nation's leadership must view research through the prism of future generations: our children and grandchildren, who will benefit from both a health and economic standpoint as a result of today's scientific discoveries. Imagine a world free of cancer, free of AIDS, free of Alzheimer's, free of heart disease. It's certainly possible if elected officials get beyond the rhetoric and take decisive action to strengthen our nation's investments in research."[35]

Outcomes and Policy Research

In clinical research, a distinction is drawn between a treatment's "efficacy" and its "effectiveness." The conceptual difference is that "efficacy" refers to whether a treatment produces a beneficial effect under ideal conditions, while "effectiveness" refers to a treatment's utility when deployed in communities under routine, "real-world" conditions. Efficacy addresses the question "Can it work?" Effectiveness addresses the question "Does it work in practice?"

The gold standard for evidence of efficacy is the double-blind, randomized clinical trial (RCT) (chapter 13). Such trials are funded by industry for pharmaceutical agents and by the NIH when there are important research questions regarding the outcome of major clinical practices involving medications, devices, or other technologies.

While the results of RCTs provide the most definitive evidence possible and have changed clinical practice in many fields, RCTs have a number of drawbacks. Principal among these is the enormous cost in time and money that it takes to complete a trial that has sufficient sample size. Among other, more specific, drawbacks and complexities are

- standardization across many practice sites;
- rigid inclusion and exclusion criteria that slow recruitment;
- many study obligations for participants (completing survey instruments, diagnostic testing, monitoring, etc.);

- multilayered governance structures with centralized data coordinating centers, data safety monitoring boards, cumbersome decision-making processes, and a multitude of oversight bodies and agencies;
- participant dropout rates, resulting in missing values that introduce potential bias and decrease statistical power;
- relatively short duration of follow-up to the initial end point, which may be too early to detect longer-term adverse events; and
- tightly controlled clinical/research settings that potentially limit the generalizability and applicability of the results.

In recent years, the advent of electronic medical records, combined with the ability to capture clinical data from these records in conjunction with medical and pharmaceutical claims from insurers, has led to research studies using "real-world data" to address questions that previously were addressed mainly through RCTs. These studies, sometimes called "pragmatic clinical trials," or more generally "real-world evidence" (RWE) research, can also complement RCTs. They collect data pertaining to effectiveness and safety once a treatment is approved for use and provide information on how factors such as clinical setting, provider, geography, race, education, income, and health system characteristics may modify the effectiveness of treatment in real-world practice.

In cases where a population registry can be linked to databases on medical and surgical diagnoses and treatments as well as filled prescriptions, longitudinal observation can lead to research designs that closely mimic a randomized trial. For example, Sweden's national civic registration system, combined with its national health program that includes electronic medical records, allows investigators to capture data from the entire population. In this circumstance, longitudinal observation of subsets of individuals with particular diagnoses who are treated, for example, with drug A or drug B can be monitored across time in large numbers, adjusting for potentially confounding variables and thus mimicing a prospective trial.[36] In the United States, a number of pragmatic clinical trials are underway in an NIH Collaboratory Demonstration Project,[37] funded by the NIH Common Fund in partnership with various US health care systems. Diverse and timely clinical questions, in areas such as colorectal cancer screening, self-management skills for chronic pain, hemodialysis care, reduction of hospital-acquired infections, suicide prevention, and post-traumatic stress disorder, are addressed with RWE studies.

While progress has been made in the area of RWE research, it is at an early stage. Its importance was recognized by passage of the 21st Century Cures Act in 2016, which requires the FDA to develop a framework and issue guidance regarding the use of RWE in relation to regulatory approval of drugs. In addition, the Prescription Drug User Fee Act reauthorization in November 2018 instructs the FDA to incorporate stakeholder input as it develops guidance for RWE research.

Key to the implementation of RWE research is the Patient-Centered Outcomes Research Institute (PCORI), which was first discussed in chapter 14 in connection with cost-effectiveness analysis. PCORI's focus is on comparative clinical effectiveness research; these studies compare different options for the prevention and treatment of disease. Its five national priorities are

- comparative assessment of prevention, diagnosis, and treatment options;
- improving health care systems;
- communication and dissemination of information to patients so that they can make informed health care decisions;
- addressing disparities; and
- accelerating patient-centered and methodologic research that can efficiently reach conclusions in a manner that includes patients and caregivers.

Since PCORI was founded in 2010, it has invested nearly $2.4 billion in more than 600 patient-centered comparative-effectiveness research studies and related projects that support comparative-effectiveness research. One of PCORI's key initiatives was the development of the National Patient-Centered Clinical Research Network (PCORnet), which is a national network for conducting comparative-effectiveness research, pragmatic clinical trials, and observational studies through partnerships with large clinical networks and patient organizations, making it highly representative of a diverse population of patients. As of December 2018, the PCORnet clinical network sites have health data for over 123 million patients in the United States.

PCORI's goal is to be self-sustaining and its value is highly regarded. A 2018 report issued by the Government Accountability Office noted, "PCORI research awards have increasingly focused on conditions that impose a substantial health or financial burden on patients and the healthcare system. . . . Officials from most stakeholder organizations we interviewed generally agreed that PCORnet offers value by improving the data available to conduct comparative effectiveness research."[38]

The clinical networks comprising PCORnet continue to work collaboratively toward a sustainable funding model that would reduce the infrastructure support currently provided through federal funding. Sustainability plans include continued development of industry partnerships and multisite studies funded through federal, foundation, and/or industry sponsors. Increasingly diverse funders are showing interest in research focused on patient engagement in health care decision-making, use of big data to examine health outcomes, and interventions to improve population health. Funders also have shown increasing interest in implementation science to promote the uptake of evidence-based best practices into diverse real-world settings. PCORnet and PCORI are uniquely positioned to continue to provide a national venue for these kinds of research efforts.

Policy Research

Virtually every page in Part III of this book pertains to health care policy or data that can inform health care policy. Sometimes these analyses may relate to the impact of policy decisions that have already been made. For example, what is the impact on health care exchanges of creating rules that facilitate the growth of high-deductible plans in the individual market? In other cases, the issue under consideration relates to the likely impact of a new policy that is being debated. For example, what would be the effect on drug development and innovation if Medicare negotiated lower prices for their products?

When changes in health policy occur at the national or state level, a natural experiment is created by default in which the benefits and risks affecting millions of Americans are poorly understood.[39] It makes sense that a deep dive into the myriad of implications that would result from a new health care policy—both positive and negative—should be done before it is enacted. Some examples currently exist, such as the pilot studies being undertaken to understand the effect of alternative payment models in affordable care organizations. It also makes sense that the numerous effects of a new policy on intended and unintended outcomes should be analyzed following its implementation, which could inform any changes that could improve its effectiveness. An analogy would be the extensive research that occurs around the safety and efficacy of a proposed new drug, and the follow-on tracking and analysis of data on adverse events. Of course, drug approvals do not have the associated political complexity of health policy. Nonetheless, information on the benefits and risks of implementing a new policy would seem to be an important part of the process. Yet, this type of research attracts the least amount of funding in comparison to laboratory studies, clinical trials, or outcomes research. From a macro perspective, it is important to support all of these categories of research, each of which make complementary contributions to improvements in health care and health.

Fiscal Propriety

The last macro consideration is that of fiscal propriety. All other high-income countries in the world provide universal coverage, while the United States spends almost twice as much per capita on health care but has 70 million residents who are uninsured or underinsured, and worse health outcomes overall. Using fiscal "propriety" in the sense of "appropriateness to the circumstances," "rightness," and "justness," it seems appropriate to state that the United States should be able to achieve enhanced access to health care and better health outcomes without spending *more* than twice as much as other countries.

Fiscal propriety is a matter of what's right, but it also reflects the realities of our national economy and governmental budgets. If the growth of national health care expenditure (HCE) exceeds the growth of gross domestic product (GDP), then it follows arithmetically that HCE will be an increasing share of GDP. Since GDP is equal to national population size times its productivity per capita, and since HCE is equal to national population times HCE per capita, in order for HCE *not* to increase as a percentage of GDP, it must grow at the same or slower rate than the rate of productivity in the overall economy. Productivity growth is expected to be in the range of 1.5–2.0 percent for the foreseeable future; thus, HCEs must slow to that rate on a sustained basis for it not to absorb an increasing fraction of the nation's economic output. From 2001 through 2017, HCE growth exceeded GDP growth for all but two years (figure 21.2). In the absence of significant reforms directed at reduced health care prices and utilization, however, the overall trajectories of GDP and HCE would suggest that the percentage of

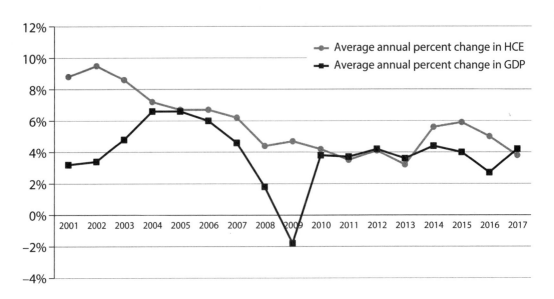

Figure 21.2. Annual percentage change in health consumption expenditures (HCE) versus gross domestic product (GDP). "National Health Expenditure Data: Historical," Centers for Medicare and Medicaid Services, https://www.cms.gov/Research -Statistics-Data-and-Systems/Statistics-Trends-and-Reports/NationalHealthExpendData /NationalHealthAccountsHistorical; "Gross Domestic Product (GDP)," FRED Economic Data, Federal Reserve Bank of St. Louis Economic Research, fred.stlouisfed.org/series/GDP.

GDP devoted to health care will increase across time. Legislation that would significantly increase access without also addressing price and per capita utilization will amplify this trend.

The realities of government budgets are also highly pertinent. The federal deficit from 2007 to 2018 included an increase that occurred in association with the Great Recession of 2008–2009, a decline that occurred with economic recovery, and another increase in recent years in association with increased government spending and reduced tax revenues from the Tax Cuts and Jobs Act of 2017 (figure 21.3). Any deficit in a given year adds to cumulative debt (figure 21.4). In 2018, the federal debt of $21.658 trillion was 5 percent greater than the GDP, which was $20.029 trillion. If state and local debt were considered, this would add $3.1 trillion to total debt.

Additionally, there are significant unfunded liabilities that are not included in the official, on-the-books federal debt.[40] As of 2019, both Social Security and the Hospital Insurance (HI) Trust Fund (Part A of Medicare) are in negative cash flow, which means that general revenues from the federal government have to make up the losses in order to pay the promised benefits. It is currently estimated that Social Security will run out of reserves

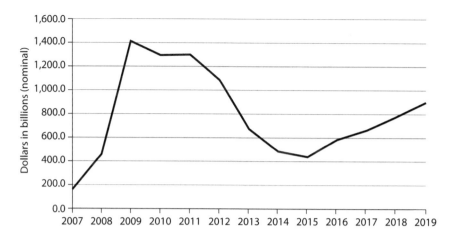

Figure 21.3. Federal deficit, 2007–2019 (estimated). "What Is the Deficit," USGovernmentSpending.com, accessed February 12, 2019, www.usgovernmentspending .com/us_deficit.

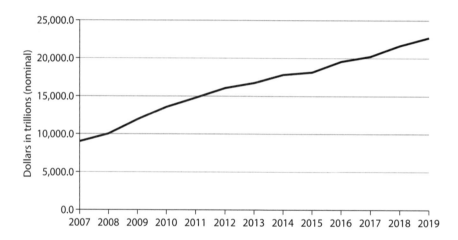

Figure 21.4. Federal debt, 2007–2019 (estimated). "Government Debt Chart Gallery: Federal Debt," USGovernmentSpending.com, accessed February 12, 2019, www .usgovernmentspending.com/debt_charts.

in 2034 and has a current unfunded liability of $13.2 trillion over the next 75 years. Solvency for Social Security would require raising the payroll tax rate and/or cutting benefits. An immediate increase in payroll taxes to 15.2 percent of taxable payroll (from today's combined employer-employee rate of 12.4 percent) would be needed, or a cut in benefits by about 17 percent.

Similarly, it is estimated that the Medicare HI trust fund will run out of reserves in 2026. Parts B and D of Medicare (i.e., physician and outpatient services and prescription drugs), and therefore Part C (Medicare Advantage), are considered "solvent" because they are 25 percent funded on a current basis from beneficiary premiums, but the other 75 percent comes from the US Treasury's general fund, so this too is an unfunded liability. Overall, Medicare's unfunded liability over 75 years is estimated to be more than $37 trillion.

It has been pointed out that the $50 trillion estimate for the combined unfunded liabilities of Social Security and Medicare is probably optimistic for two reasons:[41]

- On the cost side, the Medicare actuaries assume deep, permanent cuts in payment rates for physicians and hospitals that, although included in the Medicare Access and CHIP Reauthorization Act of 2015 and the Affordable Care Act (ACA) of 2010, have been repeatedly delayed and have not been implemented thus far. Indeed, the actuaries warn that such cuts might result in hospital closures and hinder access to physician services. Added to this is the planned reduction in disproportionate share payments to hospitals that was to occur under the ACA as Medicaid expansion took hold. As yet, these reductions have also been delayed. Substantial cost reductions are built into the projections, but the longer they do not occur, the more is added to unfunded liability.
- On the revenue side, births in the United States are now occurring at their lowest rate in 40 years. Compared to a population replacement rate of 2.1 births per 1,000 women of childbearing age, the birth rate in 2017 was 1.76. Since Social Security and Medicare depend on future growth of the taxpaying workforce to remain solvent, especially given the increasing percentage of the population 65 years of age or older in future decades, fewer workers who pay Social Security and Medicare payroll taxes means greater shortfalls for these programs. If the fertility rate remains at about 1.8, it is estimated that the unfunded liability for these programs will be about 25 percent greater than projected.

The presence of significant debt at the federal, state, and local levels will exert tremendous pressure to constrain government spending, especially new government spending. In August 2019, the nonpartisan Congressional Budget Office (CBO) released updated estimates of the federal deficit of

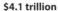
$4.1 trillion

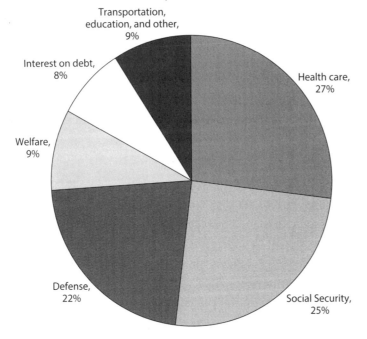

Transportation,
education, and other,
9%

Interest on debt,
8%

Welfare,
9%

Defense,
22%

Health care,
27%

Social Security,
25%

Figure 21.5. Breakdown of US federal budget, 2018. "Government Spending Chart Gallery," USGovernmentSpending.com, accessed February 12, 2019, www .usgovernmentspending.com/fed_chart_gallery.

$960 billion for 2019, which was $63 billion higher than the CBO estimate just three months earlier.[42] It was projected that the deficit would exceed $1 trillion in 2020 and average $1.2 trillion between 2020 and 2029.

Health care makes up 27 percent of current federal expenditures (divided about 55 percent to 45 percent between Medicare and Medicaid) (figure 21.5). For reasons already cited, expenditures on Social Security will inexorably rise and probably more than projected. The 8 percent of the federal budget absorbed by interest payments on the debt will also likely grow. This is partly because the total amount of debt is increasing as each new year of deficit is added and partly because the interest rates to be paid on this debt will likely rise over a moderate time horizon, given their historically low current levels and the upward pressure on interest rates caused by the sale of more and more government bonds.

Defense spending is potentially one area from which reallocation could occur to support other parts of the budget, including Social Security and Medicare. It is more in keeping with the historical record, however, to assume no reduction in defense spending given its sensitive political nature and the ever-present uncertainty of global events. One might argue that the problem could be solved by increasing income taxes, but a strong case could be made that increased tax revenues should be applied first to the deficit and promised Social Security payments before it is spent on new or incremental health care programs, especially given a baseline of high per capita spending. An increase in the Medicare payroll tax rate is another possible approach, but there are competing policy proposals that seek to *reduce* Medicare spending in a variety of ways; thus, it is not politically likely that a Medicare payroll tax increase can be enacted.

In view of these considerations, it is hard to escape the conclusion that the federal health care budget is squeezed on all sides and under pressure to remain at no more than 27 percent of the total federal budget, although the forces at work will naturally push it to a larger share. These forces, as described, include the Medicare shortfalls currently in place, the demographic and legislative factors that will increase these shortfalls, and the increase in the Medicaid part of the health care budget that will occur as more states opt for Medicaid expansion, whether by legislative action or ballot referendum.

The budgetary pressures outlined above make it unrealistic—from both fiscal and political perspectives—to conclude that there is much room for additional government funding of health care programs beyond what is already codified by statute and implemented in practice. Rather, to repeat the opening statement in this section, there is a justness and rightness in achieving enhanced access and better health outcomes without spending *more* than twice as much as other countries.

Summary

Before turning to specifics on how to improve the quality of health care in the United States, reduce cost, and enhance access, the concepts surrounding health care delivery and finance must be considered in the context of overarching forces and trends that will enhance or constrain their impact. Three of these "macro" forces are the social, behavioral, and environmental determinants of disease, research, and fiscal propriety.

The three leading causes of mortality in the United States—heart disease, cancer, and "unintentional injuries" (which includes opioid overdose, alcoholism, and violent deaths with firearms)—are all linked to behavioral factors, including obesity, activity levels, smoking, and drug dependency.

While there has been significant success in reducing smoking rates, lung cancer remains responsible for one in four cancer deaths. Lifestyle intervention to reduce obesity and diabetes has also had demonstrated success, but obesity rates continue to increase. Man-made, environomental causes of disease are well known, but in many cases, the political will to eliminate exposure to environmental toxins has not materialized. Population health status is determined to a greater extent by social, behavior, and environmental determinants than issues of health care, finance, delivery, and access. Thus, significant improvements in population health will depend importantly on favorably impacting these determinants.

Advances in biomedical research have been the basis for extraordinary progress in effective medical treatments in the United States and internationally. Historically, federal funding for this research, through a peer-reviewed, merit-based process at the National Institutes of Health and other federal agencies, has been a signature achievement that set the United States apart from other nations. Not only have there been important discoveries emanating from this research directly, but its impact has been multiplied by industry investment. In the past decade, however, funding for research in the United States has slowed relative to other nations. Moreover, critical work on social, behavioral, and environmental determinants of disease has been lagging, as has research on the effects of alternative policies on health care financing and delivery. From a macro perspective, it will be important to support biomedical, population, and health policy research to improve health outcomes while constraining cost.

Finally, a critical macro consideration is the need to achieve improvements in care, cost, and access while maintaining fiscal propriety. The federal debt and deficit are growing and seem hardwired for continued escalation. This will cause pressure on discretionary federal spending, including expenditures on government health care programs, which themselves are projected to be in deficit due to demographic changes, legislative factors, and continued increases in the prevalence of diseases that are behaviorally based. There is, therefore, a need to identify concepts that will improve the quality of care and enhance access while reducing costs. This is the subject of the next and final chapter.

IMPROVING THE BALANCE II
ENHANCING CARE, REDUCING COST,
AND IMPROVING ACCESS

Can the United States improve the balance of care, cost, and access in its health care industry without blowing it up? The answer is affirmative. For 90 percent of the population who have health care coverage, there are many ways to improve the quality of care while reducing cost. Moreover, to a large degree it should also be possible to enhance access for the uninsured 10 percent in an expenditure-neutral manner and bring better care to those individuals. The extent to which the United States will move from 10 percent uninsured toward 0 percent, however, will depend on the political process as well as individual choices by health care consumers.

While virtually all of the stakeholders in the health care industry acknowledge the imbalance in care, cost, and access and endorse the need to enhance access and improve the quality of care in a fiscally prudent manner, most will point to a need for change in some part of the industry *other* than their own. Any alteration of the current environment that adversely affects a given stakeholder—whether insurers, drug and device manufacturers, employers, patients, physicians, or hospitals—will be opposed by that stakeholder. Put differently, there are many examples of strategies to improve the balance of care, cost, and access that are clear and acceptable to everyone *except* the affected stakeholder.

Summary of the Key Drivers of Imbalance in Care, Cost, and Access

The first three parts of this book reviewed the economic underpinnings and historical roots of the US health care industry and analyzed its current functioning. Of the major themes that emerged, the following key drivers of the imbalance between care, cost, and access were identified:

1. Care
   a. Asymmetry of information between providers and patients
   b. Tension between provider autonomy and the need for standardized approaches to care that produce high reliability and quality
   c. Incomplete data on the comparative effectiveness of treatments, leading to medical overuse of low-value care and underuse of high-value care
   d. Limited data on the efficacy of public health initiatives to modify behavioral determinants of disease
   e. A paucity of data regarding the impact of alternative methods of financing and delivering health care on quality, cost, and outcomes
2. Cost: Expenditures = quantity × price. Imperfections in health care markets increase *both* utilization and price, resulting in multiplicatively higher expenditures.
   a. Quantity (utilization)
      i. Moral hazard: Producer subsidies paid by health plans and government translate to low out-of-pocket prices for patients that result in higher demand and utilization than if they faced the full price.
      ii. Provider-induced demand: Supply and demand are not independent in health care. Providers (and drug and device manufacturers) can induce demand due to a combination of information asymmetry, patient trust, lack of comparative-effectiveness data, and direct-to-consumer advertising.
      iii. Prevalence: Behavioral factors and the aging of the population increase the prevalence of disease and health care utilization.
   b. Price
      i. Negotiated prices: Instead of health care prices being determined at the intersection of supply and demand by large numbers of consumers and producers, they are primarily negotiated by a small number of large entities—government, health plans, pharmacy benefit managers, health systems, hospitals, and physician practices.
      ii. Opacity: There is a lack of price transparency throughout the industry.
      iii. Billing and insurance-related administrative costs: These expenses incurred by insurers and providers account for at least 20 to 25 percent of health insurance premiums.

iv. Restrictions in research: Prohibition against cost-effectiveness and cost-utility analysis in the evaluation of alternative treatments facilitates the utilization of higher-priced treatments that are no more effective than lower-priced treatments.

v. Government restrictions: Drug prices are pushed upward by the statutory prohibition against price negotiation with drug manufacturers and by limitations on the exclusion of drugs from national coverage decisions.

vi. Elements of monopoly/oligopoly: The market power of hospitals, providers, drug companies, device manufacturers, pharmacy benefit managers, and electronic medical records vendors lead to increased prices, a process amplified by consolidation and vertical integration.

vii. A paucity of data on the effect of alternative methods of health care delivery and finance on price.

3. Access

a. Constraints on further reductions in the percent of uninsured Americans under current law

i. Incomplete uptake of Medicaid expansion by states

ii. Potential impediments to the success of the Affordable Care Act (ACA) health care exchanges:

- individual mandate penalty repeal
- legal challenges as to whether the mandate penalty repeal invalidates the exchanges as a whole (and the ACA as a whole)
- facilitation of association health plans and short-term, limited duration plans
- barriers to enrollment such as reduced open enrollment periods and reduced resources devoted to navigators and marketing.

iii. Individuals who are eligible for Medicaid expansion or marketplace subsidies who choose not to enroll in these programs

iv. Social and geographic factors

b. Increasing numbers of underinsured Americans

i. More employer health plans with limited benefits and high deductibles

ii. Purchase of individual health plans with limited benefits and high deductibles

c. National financial constraints
   i. The need for fiscal propriety given the prospect of increasing federal deficits and debt and the demographically driven increases in government spending on health care
   ii. Cost inefficiencies due to medical overuse, monopoly pricing, and bloated billing and insurance-related administrative costs, which represent wasted resources that could otherwise be used to cover the uninsured and underinsured

Reform or Fundamental Change?

The key drivers of imbalance have produced specific shortcomings that, if addressed, could improve the quality of health care, constrain expenditures, and expand access to care for those who are uninsured. Indeed, addressing these shortcomings could improve the balance of quality and cost for the 90 percent of Americans who are insured, *independent* of any new national financing mechanism, which mainly addresses access.

Some observers champion fundamental change, arguing that the current health care industry is so intrinsically flawed that it can't be meaningfully reformed. Examples of a radical restructuring of US health care include a government-sponsored, single-payer system of universal coverage with generous benefits;[1] a system of means-tested tax credits providing health insurance premium support, with an expanded emphasis on high-deductible health plans and associated health savings accounts;[2] or implementation of a national health system of universal coverage (whether single-payer or insurance-based) modeled after another country. Others have offered specific ideas about how better to align incentives using the current industry chassis but with major restructuring of health insurance by eliminating the tax exemption for employer-based health insurance offset by a reduction in marginal tax rates.[3]

It is possible that the US political process will soon produce a radical restructuring of health care finance and delivery. A century of repeated failed experience with such efforts, however, combined with entrenchment of the key industry stakeholders, lead us to consider reforms *within* the existing industry structure that include both private and government actors while incorporating some of the concepts embedded in the proposals for more fundamental change. With the exception of proposed reforms on access, these ideas are not dependent on whether Medicaid expansion and the

ACA exchanges survive legal challenge. Instead, they are presented here with the full understanding that each of them would be strongly opposed by at least one stakeholder who is adversely affected and by a political environment that is highly influenced by lobbyists and mired in bunkered partisanship. For comparison with ideas for reform, then, two proposals for fundamental restructuring, at opposite ends of the political spectrum, are also analyzed.

Improving the Balance of Care, Cost, and Access through Reform: Big-Picture Concepts

The three core issues of care, cost, and access are intertwined such that a change in one invariably affects the other two in some way. Seven big-picture concepts for improving the balance of care, cost, and access flow directly from our foregoing analysis:

1. Create, disseminate, and utilize information on comparative effectiveness, cost effectiveness, and price.
2. Improve the quality and safety of health care through enhanced reliability.
3. Reduce provider-induced demand.
4. Reduce billing and insurance-related administrative costs.
5. Reduce expenditures on pharmaceuticals and medical devices.
6. Rationalize hospital pricing.
7. Improve access.

These big-picture reforms would build on the strengths of the current US health care industry and mitigate many of its weaknesses. Although perhaps viewed as "incremental," taken together these reforms would profoundly improve US health care by enhancing the quality of care, constraining cost, and improving access. Since care, cost, and access are intertwined, some proposals apply to more than one category of reform.

Create, Disseminate, and Utilize Information on Comparative Effectiveness, Cost Effectiveness, and Price

In my opinion, the single reform that would most substantially improve the balance of care, cost, and access in the US health care industry is the creation, dissemination, and utilization of information on the clinical efficacy, cost effectiveness, and price of health care services and products. High-quality information is a key assumption that underlies a well-functioning market economy. While the ideal of "perfect information" will never be achieved, a well-functioning market depends on accurate information about the product or service being sold, and its price.

Information about Price, Including Reference Pricing

The list prices of health care services are not typically known by consumers in advance, a drawback that especially affects those with high-deductible plans. Even more important, the contracted prices that hospitals and physician groups negotiate with health care plans are also hidden from view, allowing providers to exercise monopolistic pricing by charging different health plans different amounts. Layers of pricing among the various intermediaries of the pharmaceutical supply chain are similarly hidden, increasing the overall cost of drugs. The lack of transparency in all of these prices, coupled with low out-of-pocket expenses for patients that discourages shopping, are major drivers of the overall spiral in health care expenditures. Disclosure of the negotiated prices of health care products and services would reduce the impact of monopoly elements in the system and thereby constrain price growth.

During 2019, the House and Senate of the US Congress actively pursued legislation regarding price disclosure by hospitals and was resisted by the hospital industry. Additional legislation regarding the pricing of emergency and other out-of-network care ("surprise billing") was also in play. At year's end, however, not only was none of this legislation enacted but the health care industry won other gains through determined lobbying.[4]

Recently, a federal policy rule that would have required drug manufacturers to disclose prices in TV marketing was struck down in the courts. The US District Court for the District of Columbia held that the Department of Health and Human Services (HHS) exceeded its authority in attempting to create and enforce a rule requiring the disclosure of price in pharmaceutical advertising. The court found that neither the text of the Social Security Act, nor its structure or context, "evince an intent by Congress to empower HHS to issue a rule that compels drug manufacturers to disclose list prices. The Rule is therefore invalid."[5] This judiciary finding suggests that price transparency in health care may require legislative action.

Disclosure of contracted prices would be even more powerful if coupled with reference pricing to promote shopping.[6] Under reference pricing, reimbursement to providers for clinically equivalent treatments, devices, and pharmaceuticals are pegged to the lowest cost option.[7] For example, in 2011 the California Public Employees' Retirement System (Calpers) began to set a maximum dollar amount it would pay toward a hospital charge for knee and hip replacement surgery, arthroscopy, colonoscopy, cataract removal surgery, and several other elective procedures. The patient is responsible for any amount above this maximum contribution. Patients flocked to hospitals with prices at or below the maximum state contribution. Higher-priced hospitals reduced their prices. On average, the state saved 20 percent of costs for these procedures.[8] As another example, Whaley, Brown, and Robinson found that when Safeway offered a price transparency tool to employees there were no price-shopping effects, but when this tool was combined with reference pricing, there was a reduction in the prices paid for laboratory and imaging tests of 27 percent and 13 percent, respectively.[9] Since reference pricing has been used to a limited extent thus far, identification and quantitation of benefits and risks from health economics and health policy research would be informative before widespread adoption.

Information on Efficacy and Cost Effectiveness

While asymmetry in knowledge between a patient and physician or other health care professional will always be present, and while the natural and desired trust between patient and provider profoundly influences health care decisions, high quality and readily available information on the clinical and cost effectiveness of alternative treatments would help patients make a choice that is best for them, given their particular clinical, social, and financial circumstances.

In this age of digital information, it is becoming much more feasible to reduce the asymmetry of information between patient and provider (chapter 3) than it was when Professor Kenneth Arrow wrote his classic 1963 paper on the welfare economics of medical care and introduced the concept.[10] Moreover, with progress in the use of real-world information contained in large clinical and claims-based data sets, it is increasingly possible to generate estimates of efficacy and cost effectiveness on a wide variety of clinical questions about which there are gaps in knowledge.

Virtually all other high-income countries have created an entity in which experts in each medical field—along with epidemiologists, statisticians, patient representatives, and others—review the available evidence and make assessments about the clinical and cost effectiveness of alternative treatments for a given medical condition (chapter 14). A good example is the United Kingdom's National Institute for Health and Care Excellence (NICE). Three potential reforms for the United States along these lines are (1) the evaluation of existing knowledge, (2) research to fill any gaps in that knowledge, and (3) evidence-based coverage decisions.

Evaluation of Existing Knowledge

An ongoing independent review process focused on the efficacy and cost effectiveness of medical care could greatly improve the balance of care, cost, and access by improving the quality and dissemination of health care information. Technical summaries of the comparative and cost effectiveness of alternative drugs, devices, surgical procedures, and medical protocols could be prepared for clinicians, and lay summaries could be written for patients. This undertaking could be carried out under the auspices of a respected body such as the National Academy of Medicine. The compendium of analyses performed by NICE and similar entities in other countries could serve as a starting point while being complemented by the Cochrane Database of Systematic Reviews (chapter 13) and Choosing Wisely (recommendations by specialty societies).[11]

This idea, which is not new, would face staunch opposition. To understand how difficult it would be to implement this critically important reform, one has to look no further than the aftermath of the Independent Payment Advisory Board (IPAB), which was created under the Affordable Care Act to slow the growth in Medicare spending through an evidence-based process that would remove the political influence of stakeholders from Medicare payment decisions. Due to a backlash symbolized by referring to the IPAB as a "death panel," no members of IPAB were ever appointed. On February 9, 2018, Congress voted to repeal the Independent Payment Advisory Board as a part of the Bipartisan Budget Act of 2018.

Research to Fill Gaps in Knowledge

In addition to the evaluation of existing research data, when there are important gaps in knowledge it would also be important to fund research on comparative effectiveness and cost effectiveness. Recent reauthorization of the Patient-Centered Outcomes Research Institute (PCORI) through 2029 is an extraordinay step in this direction.[12] Additional research that focuses on comparative- or cost-effectivness comparisons that are outside of the strict purview of PCORI could potentially be conducted under the auspices of the National Insitutes of Health, the Centers for Disease Control and Prevention, the Agency for Healthcare Research and Quality, and/or a research arm of other entities (government or private). Requests for applications could be issued for specific comparative- and cost-effectiveness research questions as they arise and in which applicants would be funded according to merit based on a peer-review process. Such research alongside PCORI would produce a timely and relevant mix of analytic studies using real-world evidence and prospective, milestone-driven pilots and trials. Broad availability of these research results, and promotion of their use by social media and other marketing, should reduce the provision of services that are overused (chapter 17) and enhance services that are underused.

Evidence-Based Coverage Decisions

Once the infrastructure is in place to produce the best evidence on comparative and cost effectiveness, the next level of reform would be for the Centers for Medicare and Medicaid Services (CMS) to make decisions about the coverage of drugs and devices under Medicare and Medicaid based on this information. Such an approval process would imply the exclusion of some FDA-approved drugs from national coverage, based on lack of cost effectiveness in comparison with alternative treatments. This would require a change in current CMS practice that would be strongly opposed by drug and device manufacturers.

Although language in the 1965 Medicare legislation requires that medical services covered under Parts A and B be "necessary and reasonable," in practice CMS excludes very few FDA-approved drugs and devices from Medicare coverage. Moreover, while the "necessary and reasonable" language is silent on the issue of cost, there has been a longstanding tradition for Medicare administrators to make coverage approval decisions without considering cost. High-priced chemotherapy drugs and five other categories of drugs are defined as "protected classes" in which "all or substantially all drugs" are required by CMS to be covered under Part D plans without regard to cost. A revised set of criteria for Medicare approvals would be needed for Medicare to include cost-effectiveness data in coverage decisions. Commercial insurers would likely follow the CMS lead.

Implementation of coverage decisions based on comparative effectiveness and cost effectiveness would improve the quality of care by enhancing evidence-based practice and reduce cost. As Phelps and Parente have opined, "One cannot ask for cost control and at the same time deny the most powerful tools available to achieve that goal. . . . The time has come to remove the inconsistency and not only allow but specifically endorse the use of cost considerations in Medicare coverage determinations."[13]

Industry stakeholders are not consistently incentivized to support evidence-based practice and cost-effectiveness analysis. While greater use of these methods would benefit individual patients and the nation as a whole, reforms that utilize data on efficacy and cost effectiveness would financially harm drug companies, device manufacturers, and providers who induce demand. The insights conveyed by Patashnik, Gerber, and Dowling in *Unhealthy Politics*[14] suggest that political incentives, societal polarization, and the misuse of professional authority will undermine any effort to utilize evidence on comparative effectiveness and cost in coverage decisions. The instinct of the affected stakeholder is to cry foul, and the path of least resistance for the government is to stand on the sidelines. In the meantime, insurers are working with employers to leverage the best data available on efficacy and cost effectiveness and using increasingly detailed data on physician practice styles to design health plans with narrow networks of providers that exemplify high-value practice (chapter 17).

Improve the Quality and Safety of Health Care through Enhanced Reliability

In a 2008 lecture to the Royal College of General Practitioners titled "The Epitaph of Profession," Donald Berwick, MD (president and CEO of the Institute for Healthcare Improvement) spoke eloquently about the professional life of his father, one of two general practitioners in a rural Connecticut town.[15] Dr. Berwick's father was clearly a supremely dedicated physician who selflessly practiced medicine with great skill and autonomy, but who would no doubt be confused about physicians who, in Berwick's words, "traded prerogative for reliability." He goes on to say:

That's a subtle trade; surely the toughest one for my father, to be handled with caution. Overshoot, and patients lose the benefit of the poetry and art of individual expression from each caring doctor; but, undershoot, and patients play dice—gambling that this particular doctor knows that particular fact—up-to-date, accurate and precise. The aim is to promise every single patient the benefit of the best possible science, and that inevitably places the autonomy of the individual physician in some jeopardy. But, the new professional must make the choice: either treat the patient, your patient, according to your own store of knowledge and facts, or give up total self-reliance so as to promise the patient, your patient, treatment according to the entire world's store of knowledge and facts.[16]

Regardless of the industry—from manufacturing enterprises to airlines to hospitality—standardization ensures reliable, high-quality outcomes. Should it be any different in a hospital or ambulatory care environment? Promoting evidence-based, uniform protocols based on "the entire world's store of knowledge" in caring for patients regardless of their medical condition—from managing inpatients on ventilators to avoid pneumonia, to caring for outpatients with insulin-requiring diabetes so that they can live a full life free of complications, to providing counseling on wellness/prevention to those at risk for cardiovascular disease, and everything in between—represents the trade of prerogative for reliability; it reduces physician autonomy but produces better outcomes.

Recognizing that there will always be ambiguity in many aspects of the knowledge base that will benefit from the "art" of medicine, the writer's opinion is that transition from "experience" to "evidence" by all members of the health care team is a critical step in enhancing the reliability, and hence the quality, of health care.

Reduce Provider-Induced Demand

Health care providers function as the patient's agent. From the standpoint of ethical principles, acting as the patient's agent means that providers balance beneficence and nonmaleficence. In terms of economic modeling, providers act as the patient's agent by taking into account the nature of his or her medical condition, the perceived benefit of a potential treatment, and the patient's financial and social circumstances, but they do this while taking into account their own personal considerations.

In some circumstances, the provider will recommend diagnostic testing and/or treatments that are not indicated by current clinical guidelines. Overtesting leads to overdiagnosis and overtreatment (chapter 13). Given asymmetric information, trust, and low out-of-pocket cost, most patients will generally decide to go forward with their providers' recommendations. This phenomenon of induced demand (chapters 5 and 17) has the effect of shifting the demand curve outward and thus expanding health care expenditures.

Induced demand can be motivated by the provider's "belief" that the treatment will be of net benefit to a patient, notwithstanding the weight of the evidence. Recommendations like these fall under a category that has been referred to as "practice style." On the other hand, some induced demand is based largely on financial motivation. A natural experiment of "Medicare movers" (chapter 5) indicates that about half of the variation in medical spending between geographic areas can be attributed to these supply-side behaviors. In end-of-life care alone, data indicate that about one-third of expenditures could be saved if recommended clinical guidelines were followed.

There are potentially a number of ways to reduce provider-induced demand (based on the foregoing analyses in chapters 5, 10, 13, 15, 17, and 19), some of which will have a more realistic chance of making an important impact than others.

Counter Utilization-Driven Incentives with Fully Capitated, Risk-Bearing Organizations

A fully capitated entity is motivated to limit the overuse of health care services and products. Physicians in fully capitated, risk-bearing organizations are typically salaried and have no financial motivation to induce demand. In fact, their compensation usually depends in part on the extent to which they follow clinical guidelines. Such organizations are rare, however, and there are no major structural incentives for new ones to develop in the current US health care industry. Entities such as accountable care organizations (whether CMS or commercial), Medicare Advantage plans or Medicaid Managed Care plans, for example, are capitated at the health plan level, but these plans then usually subcontract services with physicians and hospitals on a fee-for-service basis. Thus, utilization-driven incentives remain. Moreover, physicians whose practice styles include services that go beyond recommended clinical guidelines, whether rooted in personal finance or beliefs, are unlikely to join a fully capitated organization where the incentives are in the reverse direction. In the absence of a movement toward an increase in the number of risk-bearing, fully capitated entities with owned hospitals and employed physicians, we must retreat to measures that can reduce supplier-induced demand under the claims-based system of payment.

Foster the Widespread Use of Best Evidence

One strategy that would reduce provider-induced demand without a fully capitated financing structure is broad dissemination of recommended clinical guidelines, reinforced by demonstrated knowledge of these guidelines for specialty recertification. Initiatives that encourage evidence-based practice by physicians and other providers are directed at the vast majority of providers who place a high value on evidence-based practice. These initiatives also pertain to the educational system for physicians and other providers, in which training environments are being created that will result in the embrace of evidence-based practice as a career-long imperative. Significant activity along these lines is underway, although the process will take time. It must be recognized, however, that such initiatives will not materially constrain induced demand by the subset of providers who remain motivated by financial gain and/or strongly held practice-style beliefs.

Redesign Insurance Benefits

Two innovations in insurance benefit design are increasingly being used to constrain utilization of "low-value" services that can be induced by providers or advertising. The first is high-deductible health plans (HDHPs) in association with employer-funded health savings accounts (HSAs). Since premiums are lower in HDHPs, some large employers are offering them to employees while simultaneously using the premium dollars saved to fund employee HSAs. HDHPs have increased from about 10 percent to 30 percent of employees over the past decade but with mixed results (chapter 17). A large number of studies indicate that HDHPs have indeed reduced utilization but that the reduction has been across the board, including both low-value and high-value care.

The second innovation is value-based insurance design (VBID). The concept behind VBID is to lower or eliminate co-payments for high-value services and increase co-payments for low-value services (chapter 17). Thus far, there has been more attention to the former and less to the latter. Employers appear to be hesitant to raise co-payments for low-value services, but modifications at both ends of the co-pay scale will be essential for VBID to work as an enduring strategy.

Conceptually, both HDHPs and VBID should reduce utilization of low-value health care services. The use of high deductibles is a relatively blunt instrument, in that both high-value and low-value services are reduced. VBID would appear to be a more fine-tuned approach, but outcome data are limited thus far. This is an area in which health policy research on accumulating real-world data will be informative.

Enact CMS Reforms

The Centers for Medicare and Medicaid has introduced several new approaches to the financing and delivery of Medicare and Medicaid services, including Medicare Advantage, accountable care organizations, the Merit-based Incentive Payment System (MIPS), and advanced alternative payment models (chapters 10 and 11). CMS has been innovative in piloting different versions of these programs and in refining them iteratively based on accumulating data on their strengths and weaknesses. While results have been mixed, recent encouraging data suggest that these programs will at least partly achieve the goal of improving quality while constraining cost.

Repeal or Change Policies or Laws That Incentivize Supplier-Induced Demand

Several actions can be taken to mitigate supplier-induced demand:

- Legislatively ban direct-to-consumer advertising for prescription drugs. If this is not possible, legislatively establish rules on disclosure regarding price, magnitude of benefit, comparative effectiveness, and cost effectiveness.
- Reform the process by which national coverage determinations are made, with the option of excluding drugs, including those in protected classes, based on comparative effectiveness and cost effectiveness.
- Revise the Stark law so that it can limit more effectively the use of physician-owned distributorships for medical devices (chapter 19). This can be done by closing loopholes in the language of the Stark law, as recommended by MedPAC,[17] that often allow physician-owned distributorships to skirt its intent and spirit.

- Consider revising the Stark law to reverse the safe harbor accorded to physicians who self-refer to an owned imaging center, ambulatory surgical facility, or other entity. This would reduce provider-induced demand but may not be cost-effective if the alternative is hospital-owned facilities in which prices are higher. This matter deserves study from legal, health economics, and health policy perspectives.
- Similarly, consolidation in the health care market involves benefits and risks that are deserving of study. Consolidation can produce efficiencies up to a point, but higher levels of consolidation will confer monopoly power that can result in higher prices and the potential for induced-demand lower quality. Legal, health economics, and health policy research can guide antitrust agencies on the right balance of antitrust enforcement.

Reduce Billing and Insurance-Related Administrative Costs

It has been estimated that 20 to 25 percent of private health insurance premiums are absorbed by billing and insurance-related (BIR) administrative costs, counting BIR costs for both insurers and providers and including both claims processing costs and profits for insurers (chapter 18). This estimate is for small-group and large-group plans. BIR administrative costs, including profits, can be far greater for association health plans and short-term, limited duration plans. These BIR administrative costs, which are much higher than those in other high-income countries, are due to the internationally unique US system of claims-based reimbursement for health care services. Here are several ways to reduce these costs.

Enforcement of Minimum Insurer Spending on Medical Care as a Fraction of Premiums

The Bureau of Labor Statistics defines retained earnings (i.e., what remains of collected premiums after medical costs are paid) as representing the insurer's contribution to the price of medical care. Overall, the price of medical care would decline if all health plans were required to pay out the ACA minimums for medical expenses: at least 80 percent of premiums in small-group and individual plans (including association health plans and short-term, limited duration plans) and at least 85 percent of premiums in the large group market.

Retained earnings of insurers represent the operating revenues of insurers. From these revenues, the costs of claims processing are paid, leaving the residual as profits. While limiting retained earnings has been criticized as being akin to treating health insurers as a regulated utility with constrained profitability, the capacity of insurers to earn profits with these thresholds remains considerable. In a standard large-group commercial health insurance plan, if the 85 percent threshold is reached for pass-through medical expenses, leaving 15 percent as operating revenues, and if 12 percent of premiums go to claims processing in all of its aspects (a typical estimate) leaving 3 percent as profit, the profit margin is 20 percent of operating revenues (i.e., 3 percent profit divided by 15 percent operating revenue). At an 80 percent threshold for medical care payments, profits would clearly be much higher if claims processing costs remained about the same.

Expansion of Self-Insurance

Large companies, major universities, and public entities increasingly utilize self-insurance programs to cover the costs of employee medical expenses. Insurers provide services as third-party administrators for these plans. Using a plan with 20,000 employees and 40,000 total members (including family members) as an example, the typical BIR cost for administering a plan of this size is about 4.6 percent; about 2.8 percent is paid to the third-party administrator and the remainder represents the employer cost of running the plan, including administrative costs and fees to the plan's pharmacy benefit manager and reinsurance carrier.[18] These are much lower BIR costs than the 15 to over 20 percent retained earnings under commercial health insurance plans. Expansion of self-insurance (and the consequent reduction of commercial insurance) is ongoing and will significantly reduce overall BIR administrative costs for US health care as a whole.

Direct Contracting

A higher-level step in this process is direct contracting between a local self-insured firm (which is already taking on risk and reinsurance costs) and a local health system, or between a nationwide employer and a network of hospitals and physicians who join together as providers. At scale, direct contracting would significantly lower BIR administrative costs in employer-sponsored plans nationally. While in its early stages currently, direct contracting is becoming more widely used by major firms such as General

Electric, General Motors, Boeing, Walmart and Lowe's, especially for targeted, high-cost treatments. In these cases, employees have the option to seek care for contracted conditions from a limited set of high-value providers, often using a bundled payment reimbursement model. Under these arrangements, employees typically receive lower deductibles and co-pays as an incentive for utilizing the contracted providers.

Direct Contracting with Capitation

Still more evolved would be a contract in which the self-insured employer pays the health system on a capitated basis (subject to specified expectations about coverage benefits, timeliness, outcome metrics, etc.), giving providers the incentive to shift from utilization-centric strategies for care to patient-centric strategies that emphasize a continuum of care. Global payment models better align the interests of patients and providers than do checkpoints in the claims-based process such as prior authorization, concurrence of chart documentation and billing codes, negotiation on claims denials, and so on.

Direct contracting with capitation, which harkens back to the "prepayment" contracts paid to the Permanente Health Plan by Kaiser Shipyards to cover its workers (chapter 9), achieves much more than the reduction of administrative complexity and cost; it establishes a payment system that, by its nature, encourages prevention and diminishes provider-induced demand.

Standardized Rules and Processes for Electronic Claims Processing

As Lee and Blanchfield have pointed out, the "US credit card system operates on one set of payment rules and processes that enable a plethora of bank credit cards to compete on interest rates, fees, loyalty programs, and more."[19] Additional examples of standardization to reduce administrative costs in other industries are the Federal Reserve's requirements for computer systems from different banks to communicate with one another and Walmart's rules regarding digital standards that must be met by suppliers of their retail products.[20]

HIPAA regulations require the use of common code sets, common identifiers, and common electronic claim formats, but these "requirements" have not been fully implemented. Insurers have lobbied successfully to retain customization of their own approaches, and each state has created its own rules for privacy, Medicaid, and Medicare. Moreover, while international standards are available for transfer of clinical and administrative data between software applications (e.g., Health Level Seven standards), vendors have added their own customized modifications, resulting in proprietary electronic health record (EHR) systems in the United States that each have their own way of handling BIR and patient-care data. Hospitals, physicians, and other providers must adapt to the particular EHR system of a particular vendor, which generally does not communicate efficiently and accurately with another vendor's EHR. Providers must also adapt their EHR to the numerous claims requirements of the various payers (e.g., commercial plans, health maintenence organizations, accountable care organizations, Medicare Advantage, fee-for-service Medicare, Medicaid Managed Care, etc.). Thus, the number of unique templates and rules for claims, given the number of EHR-payer-provider-patient combinations in the health care industry, is extraordinarily high, with proportionately high administrative and legal/compliance costs.

Universal adoption of standards for electronic records, claims processing, and data sharing would reduce BIR costs substantially. While it might seem like a pipe dream, imagine a world in which the following elements were standardized:

- A national unique patient identifier for each individual. It is recognized that this type of proposal has gained little traction in Congress thus far, despite attempts by a large number of professional organizations and health care systems.[21]
- Adoption of Medicare inpatient and outpatient diagnostic groupings by all health plans (public and private) in a standardized format. An analogous schedule for pediatrics could be developed.
- A national claims database that would require all insurers to submit data on the specific services they paid for, and the prices they paid, to a central repository.
- A uniform set of provider payment requirements across all payers.
- Common templates for step-therapy drug protocols, based on evidence-based guidelines and recorded in a uniform, streamlined manner across EHR platforms. Once that is successful, the next step would be to do the same regarding clinical protocols for common diagnoses.
- Real-time audits of claims by comparison with medical record documentation prior to claim submission (analogous to credit card

freezes and fraud alerts to cardholders when unusual transactions occur). This would become more realistic once streamlined and standardized diagnostic groupings were adopted, and medical necessity could be electronically verified against evidence-based practice guidelines.

- A clinical record summary in a uniform format that could be downloaded on a phone or USB drive for each patient.

Uniformity would be less of a pipe dream if there were a requirement for providers, insurers, and venders to participate or not get paid. The technology exists, recognizing that many details would require careful resolution (e.g., HIPPA protections for the national claims database); all that is needed is political will. Establishing uniformity would simplify the EHR and thereby reduce cost and allow the EHR to become the clinical support tool that was intended rather than something that, to most providers, seems mainly to enforce compliance with a myriad of tortured regulations while substantially increasing the level of frustration about the doctor-patient relationship and the costs of doing business.

Reduce Expenditures on Pharmaceuticals and Medical Devices

In 2016, $482 billion was spent on retail prescription drugs. Of this amount, $323 billion was retained by drug companies after rebates and discounts, $73 billion went to pharmacies, and the remaining $86 billion went to wholesalers, pharmacy benefit managers, providers, and insurers.[22] In 2013, spending on medical devices and in vitro diagnostics totaled about $172 billion.[23] Taken together, drugs and devices together absorb over 20 percent of national health consumption expenditures.

In the discussions of cost-benefit and cost-effectiveness analysis (chapter 14) and on pharmaceutical and medical device pricing (chapter 19), a number of opportunities were identified that, if addressed, could substantially reduce expenditures on pharmaceuticals and medical devices while enhancing quality. Some relate to utilization and some to price.

Implement Evidence-Based Practice

The best way to reduce expenditures on pharmaceuticals and medical devices while enhancing quality is to implement evidence-based practice (i.e., obtain and analyze data on comparative effectiveness and cost effectiveness, and then implement the findings). Collection and dissemination of this information would reduce the use of ineffective treatments, mitigate the impact of induced demand, and retard the acceptance of treatments that have comparable efficacy to standard of care but are more expensive. The balance of care and cost would improve by improving the efficacy of care at the same or lower cost.

Update the Medicare Modernization Act

Expenditure would decline and quality of care would improve if the Medicare Modernization Act (MMA) were updated so that

- Medicare could negotiate prices with pharmaceutical companies;
- the buy-bill difference under Part B was changed from a percentage of list price to a fixed amount;
- the reinsurance plan under Part D was restructured;
- more stringent requirements for the award and extension of exclusivity rights were established and enforced;
- policies that would ensure the timely availability of generics, including generic forms of biologic drugs, were developed and enforced (a first step could be legislation that would protect consumers from anticompetitive agreements such as "pay for delay" or "reverse payment" agreements); and
- safe reimportation of drugs from Canada and other countries were considered in certain circumstances (e.g., a drug company that holds a patent on a drug that has no substitute but refuses to sell the drug below an inflated list price).

In regards to negotiating prices with pharmaceutical companies, the United States is unique in its prohibition against government negotiation of drug prices. For example, despite Switzerland being home to Abbott, Alcon, Bayer, Hoffmann-La Roche, and Novartis, some of the largest drug companies in the world, the Swiss government negotiates drug prices.[24] Most countries negotiate drug prices using a reference price list that reflects an average of prices in other countries. The countries that should be used to compile such a list in the United States could be negotiated. Other considerations are that innovation and patent formation for pharmaceuticals do not appear to be hindered by lower prices. Adjusted for gross domestic product, the United States is in the middle of the pack in patent creation among other high-income countries in which drug prices are half that of the United States, net of rebates, discounts, and coupons (chapter 17).[25]

Some proposals are focused on limiting the rise in drug prices to a benchmark such as the consumer price index. This would moderate price growth but accept the current high price levels of specialty drugs as a floor. Moreover, such proposals would not mitigate the major reason for increased spending on prescription drugs in recent years, which is their high launch prices (chapter 17). Use of international reference pricing would provide a better standard.

In the argument against the government being involved in negotiating price, too, some legislators say price should be left to the "free market." The market for prescription drugs, however, is neither "free" nor a true "market." Rather, prices are protected by the issuance of patents, the evergreening of patents, and written statutory language prohibiting negotiation by Medicare. And in contrast to a true market in which buyers make decisions about drug purchases based on price, patients make decisions often without regard to price (due to low out-of-pocket cost), while the true buyers are health plans and government that pay the actual price using other people's money.

In regards to restructuring the reinsurance plan under Part D (an idea that has been advanced by MedPAC), this solution could

- reset the catastrophic cap to the 99th percentile (rather than the current 90th percentile) to mitigate against unpredictable risk and bring this percentile more in line with commercial health insurance plans,
- stop treating manufacturer co-pay coupons as "out-of-pocket" expenditures toward catastrophic thresholds (and a similar reform could apply to coupons in commercial plans being counted toward patient deductibles), and
- invert the cost of the reinsurance program from 80 percent Medicare to 20 percent Medicare, while relieving beneficiaries of financial responsibility once their catastrophic limit is reached.

Lastly, the results of health economics and health policy research on the benefits and risks of reimportation should guide such considerations of that potential MMA update. As opined by Califf and Slavitt, reimportation amounts to "a workaround born of desperation" and is the "least favored long-term approach."[26] The reality of underinsured diabetics taking legal risk by driving across the Canadian border to obtain needed insulin at one-tenth the price (chapter 19) is an example of an issue that can be resolved in the short term while we await the long-term solution.

Reduce Drug List Prices and Eliminate Rebates and Coupons

If CMS-negotiated prices become the new "list prices," pharmacy benefit manager rebates and co-pay patient coupons could be eliminated. It is important to note that list price reduction and the elimination of rebates and coupons go hand in hand; it won't work to do one without the other. If only rebates and coupons are eliminated, there is no guarantee that list prices will decline. Under that scenario, health insurance premiums and overall health care costs would likely go up, not down.

Deincentivize Orphan Drugs and Evergreening

The Orphan Drug Act (ODA) was enacted with the laudable intention of promoting the development of drugs to treat diseases of low prevalence that had been ignored because of small market potential (chapter 19). The ODA has been successful in achieving this goal, but the spirit of the act has been subverted in some areas. Biomarkers and molecular genetics have allowed the definition of an "orphan disease" (i.e., affecting less than 200,000 people) to become a subset of a common disease with a particular biomarker or genetic mutation. Defined in this way, the relative ease of obtaining approval for orphan drugs, the availability of other incentives, and the potential for high prices have led to a shift among pharmaceutical companies toward orphan drug development. It can be argued that since orphan drug sales in 2017 were $125 billion worldwide, and since the top 10 orphan therapies each generated more than $1 billion in sales in 2017, it is unclear that there is still a need to incentivize the development of such drugs.[27]

Repeal of ODA should be studied from a health economics and health policy standpoint. In the absence of a repeal, modifications in the definition of "orphan drug" and reduction in incentives should be considered so that societal resources are not directed at a process in which every new biomarker and genetic mutation defines a "new" disease with a low prevalence that becomes eligible for an orphan drug designation at stratospheric prices.

Restrictions against the evergreening of patents should also be considered, subject to health policy analysis of available real-world data. Awarding a patent for a temporary monopoly to reward innovation and account for development costs is a fair trade up to a point. The benefits of the trade are tipped toward the manufacturers and away from the public, however, when patent shields are created around manufacturing processes, dosing ranges, routes of administration, and so on. Industry is also favored by "authorized generics," product hopping, and other techniques of patent evergreening.

Enhance Value in Medical Devices

Several initiatives could reduce price and/or improve quality around medical devices:

- Expand the FDA's Competitive Bidding Program to a much larger number of devices, as appropriate after review of pertinent data.
- Disseminate information on comparative and cost effectiveness of alternative devices.
- Modernize the 1976 "substantial equivalence" criterion for new devices by creating a threshold for the duration of time from approval of a predicate device. (The FDA is considering a 10-year cutoff.)
- Modernize device approvals by implementing criteria based on efficacy metrics. These metrics would be in addition, or as alternative, to the substantial equivalence criterion.

Direct-to-Consumer Advertising for Prescription Drugs

Besides New Zealand, the United States is the only country that allows direct-to-consumer advertising (DTCA) of prescription drugs. Of note, no law in the United States was enacted to legalize DTCA nor was there any public or congressional debate on the matter. Rapid growth of the practice in the United States began in 1997 when the FDA relaxed its guidance on drug advertising. DTCA has induced demand for expensive medications, facilitated by the small fraction of the price that is borne by patients directly (chapter 19).

In 2015, the American Medical Association proposed a ban on DTCA that garnered widespread support. The ban was opposed by the pharmaceutical lobby, however, and never gained legislative traction. The political and judicial environment around First Amendment rights also dims the prospect for banning DTCA. That said, this is a worthwhile topic for public debate. Recognizing that DTCA for prescription drugs in the United States will likely be present for the foreseeable future, but also accepting that a well-functioning market requires that consumers have comprehensive and accurate information on all aspects of a good or service and that the courts have ruled against price disclosure in DTCA, any reforms in this area will likely require legislative action. Two suggestions for legislation that could improve the quality of information in an environment of continued DTCA are (1) wide dissemination of information readily available to patients on comparative and cost effectiveness of alternative medications, and (2) a requirement that drug ads include a listing of risks, the price of the advertised medication, and a statement of the magnitude of the expected benefit, on average.

Rationalize Hospital Pricing

Hospital prices have been escalating at a faster rate than other components of the medical care price index. Therefore, rationalizing hospital pricing is an important part of the puzzle. In doing so, one must be mindful that hospitals have the four-part structure of payment sources summarized in chapter 18: commercial insurance (highly profitable); Medicare (break-even at best); Medicaid (a major share of which is uncompensated); and uninsured (almost entirely uncompensated). Nationally, about 85 percent of the costs of uncompensated care are offset by government safety-net funding, but this is highly variable across states and municipalities. Inner city safety-net hospitals and rural hospitals are at a significant disadvantage.

Initiatives that reduce hospital prices, especially in safety-net hospitals, must be offset by other initiatives, such as those that improve publicly funded access to care among those currently uninsured. With that caveat, and the reminder that health economics and health policy research on the multi-faceted effects of these initiatives would be important before implementation, suggested measures that would rationalize hospital pricing include

- instituting a common diagnostic-related group (DRG) system for all claims, whether publicly funded or commercial, as suggested in the discussion of standardization of medical records;
- establishing a base price for each DRG, perhaps modeled after Medicare, and placing a cap on the DRG multiple that can be charged to any insurer;
- reducing the buy-bill difference in a manner that reduces supernormal profits but achieves the intent of the 340B program in relation to safety-net populations;[28]

- effectively addressing the "surprise bill" phenomenon,[29] due to the provision of out-of-network services, which is a conspicuous example of the absurdities of health care pricing and a cause of unnecessary hardship for affected patients;
- effectively addressing the differential prices for hospital vs. physician facility fees through bundled payment programs or other means; and
- establishing a cap on activation fees for trauma patients.

It bears repeating that these reforms, if they include concepts pertaining to disclosed multiple-of-Medicare prices for commercial payers with caps, must also include adequate payments for the care of uninsured and underinsured patients. Otherwise, safety-net hospitals would be at a distinct competitive disadvantage relative to for-profit hospitals and not-for-profit hospitals that are geographically located in areas with well-insured populations.

Improve Access

About 90 percent of Americans have some form of coverage for health care expenses. Most people are covered through employer-sponsored health insurance or government programs, who we will call "insured" for short. We have seen that the price of health care for insured individuals is high (chapter 18), and that the medical care provided, while the best in the world for some, is uneven in its quality for others (chapter 16). All of the reforms so far discussed represent ideas about how the quality and efficiency of care for the 90 percent of insured Americans can be improved and made more uniform within the existing structure of the US health care industry.

Much of the attention in the ongoing health care debate, however, is directed at the 10 percent of Americans *without* insured access to health care, who we will call "uninsured" for short. Proposals to improve access are largely financing mechanisms that are independent of the first six sets of reforms discussed thus far. Whether the current structure is retained, modified, or replaced by universal single-payer health care, any such reform could be done with or without utilization of comparative-effectiveness and cost-effectiveness data, negotiated pharmaceutical prices, changes in patent law, standardization of health care records, and so on. That said, what would it take to improve access to health care in the United States? Let's define the scope of the problem, consider how it can be addressed under current law, and then briefly analyze proposals for fundamental restructuring at the two ends of the political spectrum.

Defining the Scope of the Problem

What does "access to health care" mean and how much would it cost to establish universal access? The range of views about the meaning of access is quite broad, with correspondingly wide differences in cost. Those who do not view access to the full spectrum of health care as a fundamental right argue that the uninsured *already* have access to health care through hospital emergency rooms under the Emergency Medical Treatment and Active Labor Act (EMTALA) (chapter 15). From this viewpoint, there is already universal access and no added cost is needed. At the other extreme would be those who believe that uninsured members of the US population are entitled, as a fundamental right, to the same spectrum of health care services as those who are covered under employer-sponsored plans or Medicare. (In some proposals, the spectrum of covered health care benefits are expanded to include vision, dental, and other services.) Improving access under current law would lie somewhere in between. Let's consider the two extremes more carefully and then return to what can be done under current law.

Under EMTALA, hospitals must evaluate and stabilize anyone who presents to their emergency room, including the uninsured. Almost all bills sent to uninsured patients will not be paid. Through Disproportionate Share Hospital (DSH) funding and other safety-net support (chapter 11), hospitals are partly reimbursed for uncompensated care and offset remaining losses with profits from commercial-pay patients. Total DSH payments nationally in 2017 were $12.1 billion.[30]

While it is true that uninsured patients have access to health care through hospital emergency rooms under EMTALA, this care suffers from a number of limitations:

- Uninsured patients are understandably concerned about medical bills they can't afford. Consequently, they often allow an acute medical condition that could be readily addressed early in its course to become more serious before presenting to an emergency room, resulting in greater morbidity and more intensive treatment.
- Uninsured patients with chronic medical conditions (e.g., diabetes, epilepsy, asthma, heart disease, and many others), in the absence of

access to a provider who could help them achieve day-to-day control of their disease, instead have periodic flare-ups requiring emergency treatment. These patients become "regulars" in emergency rooms. Due to a lack of day-to-day control of their condition, the underlying disease process progresses in an accelerated manner, leading to greater morbidity and premature mortality.

- Many patients whose financial resources are so limited that they are *not* concerned about cost (because they know their bills will be written off as charity care) use emergency rooms as primary care clinics for routine problems that could be readily addressed in an outpatient setting. These emergency room visits, which are highly prevalent, represent an extreme mismatch of resources.

- The emergency room bills of patients with incomes above a defined threshold (usually 200–300 percent of the federal poverty line) are not written off as charity care and are pursued by hospital-contracted collection agencies. These bills will be extremely high because of the nature of hospital pricing, especially if there is an associated hospital admission. For low- and moderate-income individuals, these bills will cause financial hardship. Patients who do not pay their bills will see their credit scores adversely impacted; many will end up declaring bankruptcy.

- If uninsured patients have a medical condition requiring highly specialized and expensive treatments, such as organ transplants or chemotherapy, they will often have difficulty accessing such treatment.

Now let's consider the other extreme. Figure 4.1 (chapter 4) shows a line representing a continuum of medical need. At the top are treatments for serious medical conditions and accidents and at the bottom are elective treatments like aesthetic plastic surgery and testimonial-style therapies for which there is no scientific evidence. Where should the threshold lie in this continuum for defining universal access to treatment? Let's assume a threshold in which the currently uninsured accessed the same spectrum of health care in the same way as the currently insured. Translated into 2018 dollars, this would add 10 percent to the current $3.5 trillion spent on personal health care, or $350 billion. Expressed as a percent of gross domestic product, health care would increase from about 18 percent (where it has plateaued for now) to almost 20 percent. And since the incremental expense to pay for care of the uninsured would be drawn from public funds, the goal of fiscal propriety in terms of government deficit and debt (chapter 21) would be shattered.

The limitations of EMTALA at one extreme, and the fiscal impropriety of universal access to the full spectrum of health care under the current industry structure at the other, leads to the need for either reforms under the current structure or a fundamental restructuring of the industry.

Reforms to Enhance Access within Existing Industry Structure

Mechanisms for enhanced access through Medicaid expansion and health care exchanges are already in the ACA law, and their budgetary implications (both costs and revenues) are included in Congressional Budget Office projections (chapter 11), although future projections will have to be revised to account for the reduction in ACA revenues resulting from congressional repeal of the major tax revenue in the original bill. While Medicaid expansion and the ACA exchanges have been incompletely implemented, they have been successful in reducing the number of uninsured individuals by about 45 percent from the pre-ACA baseline. Further reductions in uninsured rates, however, face significant challenges. These challenges partly reflect barriers erected in recent years by the executive branch and legislators at the federal and state levels but also by the nature of the population comprising the remaining uninsured (table 22.1). Of the 27.5 million uninsured in 2016,

- 10.5 million are ineligible for financial assistance (3.9 million due to immigration status, 3.7 million because they declined an offer of employer-sponsored insurance, and 2.9 million because their income is too high for subsidies or tax credits under the health care exchanges);
- 6.8 million are individuals who are eligible for Medicaid coverage in expansion states, but have not enrolled (4.1 million adults and 2.7 million children);
- 7.8 million are eligible for subsidies under the exchanges but chose not to purchase insurance; and
- 2.2 million fall into the "coverage gap" of Medicaid eligibility in nonexpansion states, which is the difference between the eligibility threshold set by the state and the federal povertly line (above which uninsured individuals would have access to exchange products with

Table 22.1. Distribution of uninsured by Affordable Care Act eligibility categories, 2016

Category	Number of people in millions
Ineligible due to	
Income over 400% of federal poverty line	2.9
Immigration status	3.9
Decline of employer-sponsored insurance offered	3.7
In the coverage gap, residing in a nonexpansion state	2.2
Eligible but chose not to enroll	
Tax credit eligible	7.8
Medicaid, adult	4.1
Medicaid, child	2.7
Total	27.5

Source: Rachel Garfield, Anthony Damico, Kenal Orgera, Gary Claxton, and Larry Levitt, "Estimates of Eligibility for ACA Coverage among the Uninsured in 2016" (data note), Kaiser Family Foundation, June 2018, http://files.kff .org/attachment/Data-Note-Estimates-of-Eligibility-for-ACA-Coverage-among-the-Uninsured-in-2016.

Medicaid	No coverage (Coverage gap)	Marketplace subsidies

0% federal poverty line (FPL)	43% FPL	100% FPL	400% FPL
Single adult, 2018	$8,935	$12,140	$48,560

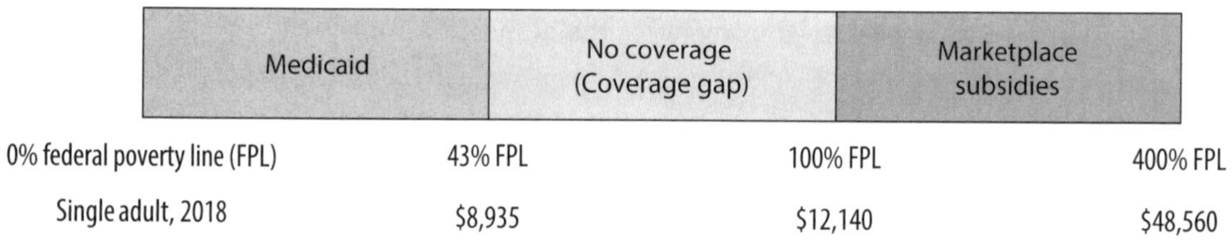

Figure 22.1. Gap in health insurance coverage among adults who live in states that have not expanded Medicaid under the Affordable Care Act. Adapted from Rachel Garfield, Anthony Damico, and Kendel Orgera, "The Coverage Gap: Uninsured Poor Adults in States that Do Not Expand Medicaid" (issue brief), Kaiser Family Foundation, March 2019, http://files.kff.org/attachment/Issue-The-Coverage-Gap-Uninsured -Poor-Adults-in-States-that-Do-Not-Expand-Medicaid.

subsidies) (figure 22.1). On average, in nonexpansion states the threshold for Medicaid eligibility is income less than 43 percent of the federal poverty line.

Much attention has been directed toward closing the coverage gap by extending Medicaid expansion to the remaining nonexpansion states. In the 2018 election cycle, voters in Idaho, Nebraska, and Utah approved ballot initiatives to include in their Medicaid programs adults with incomes up to 138 percent of the federal poverty line. (These voter-approved Medicaid expansions have not yet been implemented by state legislatures.) Ballot referendums in a number of other nonexpansion states are being developed.

Of those in the coverage gap across all of the remaining nonexpansion states, 29 percent reside in Texas, which has both a large uninsured population and strict limitations on Medicaid eligibility. Adding Florida, Georgia, and North Carolina, which share the same characteristics, accounts for two-thirds of all individuals in the coverage gap nationally. While these states currently have legislative bodies that are politically opposed to Medicaid expansion, there are several reasons to believe that some of these states, and others, may expand Medicaid through ballot referendums or legislative action across time. These reasons include favorable experience in other states, growing recognition of the financial benefits to citizens of the state by leveraging 10 percent of the cost with state general revenue to draw 90 percent of the cost from the federal government, the multiplier effects on economic development from these extra dollars coming into the state, and shifts in the political winds that occur in cycles over time.

But here's the conundrum. Even if Medicaid expansion were extended to all 14 states that have not yet participated, this would only add eligibility to 2.2 million additional adults in the coverage gap and an additional 1.5 million who would become eligible for Medicaid between 100 and 138 percent of the federal poverty line. Moreover, as previously noted, and as shown in the Oregon natural experiment (chapter 20), a significant fraction of Medicaid-eligible individuals don't enroll. Thus, even if Medicaid expansion is complete, there would still remain about 25 million uninsured people in the United States.

The fact that so many individuals do not have health insurance is the Achilles' heel of US health care; while many shortcomings are relatively tractable by implementing some of the reforms described already (and/or others), the conundrum of uninsurance has thus far been relatively intractable. This problem is multifaceted, given the different categories of the uninsured:

- The 7 million people who are eligible for Medicaid, but who have not enrolled, are living in the shadows of society and/or lack trust in the "system." When they become acutely ill, they tend to present to emergency rooms.
- The almost 4 million employed individuals who decline employer-sponsored health insurance are making a statement about what they perceive as the unaffordability of the employee cost of premiums relative to their wages.

- The 3 million who are above 400 percent of the federal poverty line, but who choose not to purchase health insurance on the individual market, are making a similar statement.
- The 8 million who are eligible for subsidized health insurance on the ACA marketplace exchanges but decline to do so are also making a financial decision knowing there is a chance of an unpredictable major illness or accident. It's not that they don't want coverage *per se*—that applies to only 2 percent of the uninsured based on survey data. Rather, survey results indicate that people make the decision to remain uninsured mainly because of ongoing concerns about cost or a lack of awareness about affordable options.

Perhaps the greatest opportunity for reductions in the uninsured population is in this last group of individuals whose incomes make them eligible for ACA marketplace subsidies. Enrollment of this group would be facilitated by stabilizing the exchanges, devoting more resources to providing information about exchange products, and removing barriers to enrollment.[31]

Among the many ways that have been proposed to stabilize the exchange markets, some key initiatives are as follows:

- For markets (counties) that have no insurer, or only one or two insurers, consider a "public option," perhaps using the model of the Federal Employees Health Benefits Plan, which is operated by large private insurers, or enacting one of the public options being advanced in Congress such as a "Medicare buy-in" or "Medicaid buy-in."
- As in Medicare Advantage, provide regulatory relief by lowering the initial barriers to market entry. This could be done, for example, by offering insurers a longer-term path to meeting network adequacy requirements.
- Reconsider changes in federal rules that have been made to risk adjustment, reinsurance, and risk corridors. All of these methods guard against insurer risk when a new product is launched with no underwriting history. They were written into the ACA law following the approach used in the Medicare Part D program. However, the ACA risk corridor program was subsequently disabled by Congress, leading to significant insurer losses and uncertainty. Study of the benefits and risks of alternative approaches to managing insurer risk

is warranted, with the goal of producing an outcome that at once stabilizes the exchange markets and produces efficient premium pricing for patients. A study by Avalere found that a reinsurance programs started in seven states, for example, reduced average exchange premiums by 20 percent.[32]

- Reconsider the policy on allowing association health plans and short-term, limited duration plans to circumvent consumer protections built into the ACA. These products create adverse selection by drawing away healthy patients from exchange products, thereby leaving sicker patients in the exchanges and increasing premiums.

Initiatives to improve enrollment could include

- extending the period of open enrollment with widespread announcements of start and end dates;
- investing in both broad and targeted outreach campaigns, as CMS did with the launch of Part D of Medicare;
- restoring funding for in-person assisters or "navigators," as with Part D;
- conveying to potential low-income enrollees (whether with navigators, social media, or other marketing) that they may be eligible for zero premium (albeit high-deductible) plans, which at least would provide catastrophic coverage; and
- quieting the political polarization, misinformation, and other headwinds in the public sphere and focusing instead on how to help potential enrollees choose an exchange plan that can work in their particular circumstance.

Four final points can be made about reforms to enhance health care access:

1. The ACA has been successful in reducing the number of uninsured Americans by almost half, a noteworthy accomplishment.
2. Just as care can be improved while reducing cost for the insured 90 percent, the reforms listed here to achieve this goal (i.e., evidence-based practice, highly reliable clinical protocols, streamlined administrative processes, reduced pharmacy cost, value-based insurance design, more capitation and less fee-for-service, diminished induced

demand, and rationalized hospital pricing) can also be applied to the uninsured 10 percent as they gain access.

3. If the number of uninsured were reduced by enrolling those eligible for the exchanges by half—from 8 million to 4 million—this would be considered a home run even if the various strategies for exchange stabilization and enrollee marketing are highly successful. But this would still leave over 20 million uninsured.

4. Therefore, even if Medicaid expansion is complete across all states and the exchange markets are stabilized, under the present industry structure we are still left with a hybrid: insured access to health care for perhaps as many as 92 to 94 percent of the population (albeit with many underinsured) and suboptimal access to health care through emergency rooms under EMTALA for the remaining 6 to 8 percent.

As the noted health economist Victor Fuchs has commented, universal health care insurance coverage can be achieved by reforms less comprehensive than single-payer, but "universal coverage requires (1) subsidies for individuals who are too poor or too sick to acquire insurance at actuarial correct premiums, and (2) compulsion (i.e., a mandate) for everyone else to participate and implicitly contribute to the subsidies. No country achieves universal coverage without subsidies and compulsion."[33]

Regarding Fuchs's requirements for universal access, restoring a mandate for health insurance seems extremely unlikely, as is an increased level of subsidy for Medicaid and marketplace exchanges, given macroeconomic considerations (chapter 20). We are left with two broad choices: reform the current health care industry as discussed so far or completely replace the current structure with a new one that entails fundamental restructuring.

Alternatives to Reform: Fundamental Restructuring

For reasons cited at many junctures in this book, none of the plans that will radically restructure the century-old health care industry in the United States is politically likely. For completeness and context, however, it's important to summarize two proposals at opposite ends of the political spectrum. One sees private health insurance as the fundamental flaw in US health care, makes it illegal, and establishes the federal government as the single payer; the other sees government as being the primary culprit and converts everything to private insurance.

Universal Tax Credit Plan

The Universal Tax Credit Plan (UTCP) was developed by Avik Roy, a physician who became an investment analyst early after medical training and then a hedge fund manager focused on health care. Over the past decade, Roy has been recognized as a thoughtful conservative commentator on matters related to health policy. He founded the Foundation for Research on Equal Opportunity, which "conducts original research on expanding economic opportunity to those who least have it."[34]

A central idea of the UTCP is a means-tested, universal tax credit that would be used to purchase private health insurance. This is often referred to as "premium support," which Roy points out dates back to a 1978 proposal by the economist Alain Einthoven for a "consumer-choice health plan," with later variants carried forward by both liberal and conservative policy analysts and legislators. The UTCP reflects serious thought about the US health care industry. Roy's monograph *Transcending Obamacare* and a more recent update entitled "Bringing Private Health Insurance into the 21st Century" contain projected fiscal and coverage outcomes as well as considerable discussion about how it would operate with respect to employer-sponsored health insurance, Medicaid, Medicare, care for veterans, and pharmacy costs.[35]

The concept of a federal set of essential health benefits is included, as is protection against adverse selection by requiring identical premiums for men and women and for those of varying health statuses. To expand access and encourage consumer involvement in health care decisions, a combination of high-deductible plans and health savings accounts would be emphasized. On a sliding scale, to defray the cost of deductibles and co-pays, the UTCP would provide a version of HSAs that are referred to as "health reimbursement accounts" in the update.[36] These would average $1,800 for eligible individuals. Projected deductibles for the benchmark plan, however, are $7,000 for individuals and $14,000 for families. For the marketplace exchanges, the actuarial values of the different insurance tiers (bronze, silver, gold, and platinum) would be reduced, which means there would be more out-of-pocket medical cost for the consumer and less cost for the plan. One critique of an early version of the plan put it this way: The UTCP "would create essentially doughnut hole plans for individuals, where routine costs could be covered out of the HSA, catastrophic costs would be insured, but everything in between would be the responsibility of the individual."[37] This appears to be intended: the utilization-constraining "consumer driven" part of the plan relies on patients making more direct choices about their consumption of medical care with out-of-pocket cash.

There is no compulsion (i.e., mandate), but enrollment would be encouraged by establishing a penalty (defined in terms of foregoing a potential benefit, modeled after Germany): states would have the flexibility "to conduct open enrollment less frequently, up to once every five years."[38] Thus, although there would not be a financial penalty as under the initial design of the individual mandate, people who don't enroll when eligible must wait up to five years. There is also a provision in which states have the option of auto-enrolling their residents in a state-assigned default health insurance plan and HSA. Across time, the intent is for the system of UTCP health insurance plans and HSAs to create an umbrella that would encompass Medicaid, Medicare, and veterans health care. In the case of Medicaid, the UTCP would gradually migrate acute-care enrollees into the benchmark insurance plan in their state, leaving responsibility for long-term care to the state. Fees to doctors and hospitals under the UTCP's benchmark plans would be higher than is currently the case under Medicaid, thereby increasing costs. Provisions to constrain drug prices under the UTCP include the ability for insurance plans to exclude drugs from its formularies and price negotiation with pharmaceutical companies by private insurers in each state.

Roy's description of the UTCP contains numerous important insights about the US health care industry, and the plan itself presents a vision that would comprehensively change health care delivery in a fundamental way by transitioning publicly funded programs to private health insurance. In terms of framing the balance between care, cost, and access, however, the overarching emphasis on private health insurance that largely retains the fee-for-service payment mechanism creates clear challenges for improving the balance of care, cost, and access:

- Since expenditures equal price multiplied by quantity, any constraint on expenditures due to reduced utilization associated with high deductibles would still face the dual headwinds of incentivized provider-induced demand in a fee-for-service system and monopolistic pricing by providers and pharmaceutical companies.
- Reduction in utilization associated with high-deductible plans tends to be across the board; that is, both high-value and low-value care are reduced.

- Based on public pushback against high-deductible plans that are currently in use, there is likely to be widespread dissatisfaction with a national plan that imposes high deductibles and co-pays throughout the health care industry.
- High billing and insurance-related administrative costs, associated with retained earnings by insurers and claims-based billing by providers, would remain unless reforms around standardization are enacted as discussed.
- Insurer-negotiated drug discounts would not be as effective as government negotiation (US drug prices after rebates and discounts, as negotiated by pharmacy benefit managers, are still twice as high as the prices negotiated by other governments).
- The costs of caring for patients currently in Medicaid would increase due to higher fee schedules.
- The extent of reduction in the uninsured rate, if any, is unclear. Individuals currently eligible for Medicaid who choose not to enroll would not necessarily be drawn to the UTCP plans. This will depend on their level of awareness and trust and the specific manner in which the HSA funds and out-of-pocket "doughnut hole" expenses play out. The same is true for currently uninsured individuals who are eligible for marketplace exchange subsidies but choose not to enroll as well as for individuals currently uninsured whose incomes exceed the subsidy threshold but who choose not to enroll.

If such a plan were seriously considered, health economics and health policy research on these issues would be critical before implementation.

Medicare for All

While many versions of a single-payer system have been implemented in other countries or proposed for the United States, we will use as our example the Medicare for All Act of 2019 sponsored by Senator Bernie Sanders of Vermont and others.[39] The key provisions of this act are as follows:

- It applies to all US residents.
- Auto-enrollment occurs at birth, with transitional enrollment for all others over four years.

- Benefits include "medically necessary" services in 13 categories, including dental, hearing, and vision.
- There are no premiums and no cost sharing, except a small amount for prescription drugs to encourage use of generics and none for low-income individuals.
- Fee schedules for providers are established by the Secretary of Health and Human Services using a process like that under Medicare.
- Drug prices are negotiated by the HHS Secretary.
- A global national health budget is established, which specifies total spending for covered services, capital expenditures, health professions education, reserves, and other categories.
- A beneficiary ombudsman is available to assist consumers, including filing and resolving appeals.
- It replaces the current Medicare program and private health insurance (employer, marketplace exchanges, Federal Employees Health Benefits, and TriCare), and it prohibits employers from providing duplicative health benefits.
- It replaces the Medicaid acute care program but retains state administration of long-term care.
- It establishes the Universal Medicare Trust Fund, with appropriations from current federal health spending offsets (e.g., marketplace subsidies, tax exclusion for employer-sponsored health plans, Medicaid, and Medicare). Additional financing would be needed, though not specified in the bill but discussed in a white paper[40] and elsewhere. Suggested options include income-based premiums paid by employers and/or households, a wealth tax on billionaires, and general revenues raised by increasing income taxes on individuals in the upper percentiles of income.

There are clear strengths to Medicare for All (which we shall call "M4A"). The problem of access—uninsurance and underinsurance—is essentially solved, as Fuchs's two requirements of subsidy and compulsion are met. Administrative costs associated with claims processing would be reduced, because the billing expenses of the large single payer would be much lower than the retained earnings of insurers, and because claims processing for providers would be streamlined by having only one set of rules. Pharmacy prices would be reduced and rebates and coupons could be eliminated. Cost-effectiveness analysis could be implemented in a straightforward manner because the results would be applied uniformly across all populations. And evidence-based practice that promotes highly reliable medical care could be more readily promulgated because of a uniform set of diagnostic groups for which care could be tracked.

While the strengths of M4A are clear, so are its weaknesses. Chief among these is placing the entire health care enterprise under the executive branch of the federal government. What happens when political considerations, a recession, and/or rising levels of deficit and debt (chapter 21) cause the executive branch and/or Congress to implement austerity measures around government spending, including health care? Freezing or reducing global health care budgets is a blunt mechanism that will constrain the amount and quality of care. The government and/or providers may have to decide which procedures or drug therapy can no longer be offered unless some threshold of clinical severity is reached, and hospitals may cut corners on the quality and safety protocols that had been so carefully honed. Queues for various treatments might develop. Moreover, and perhaps even more fundamental, health care may receive more priority in some administrations and less in others depending on the priorities of the executive branch at any point in time. Given the experience in recent years of relatively unchecked rules, revisions, and rollbacks in virtually all executive branch agencies, the prospect of new rules governing all of health care being unilaterally implemented by a Department of Health and Human Services secretary reporting directly to the president will be unsettling for many on both sides of the political aisle.

A second major problem with M4A is its financial feasibility and sustainability. No doubt, there would be substantial savings to national health care expenditures from reduction in drug prices and administrative expenses. Additional savings would occur because of lower payments to hospitals, doctors, and other providers (since the Medicare fee schedule is less than that of commercial plans), but any reductions will be hard fought by providers, and the subset of savings that are successfully achieved won't flow back directly to the federal government to offset costs. Against these savings, the aggregate incremental costs of the plan's universal coverage, combined with more generous benefits and the zero premium/zero deductible/zero co-pay provision, means the plan comes up significantly short financially. At least as it is presently written, one experienced and sympathetic analyst has concluded that "even with generous assumptions about potential revenue and savings, there would still be a substantial gap between the additional spending and the new revenue."[41] Estimates from the Commonwealth Fund using detailed microsimulations of large national data sets indicate a shortfall of $32 trillion over a decade.[42]

The degree to which M4A produces a funding gap depends on the extent to which its outcomes would be in line with its assumptions: for example, the amount of savings in administrative and drug costs; the amount of health care spending that would remain out-of-pocket; the increase in utilization that would result from universal coverage and zero premiums, deductibles, and co-pays; the increase in costs from assuming responsibility for the state share of Medicaid and the insurance costs of state employees; and the amount of revenues from provisions like eliminating employer-sponsored insurance (which would raise wages and tax revenues but by an unknown amount), among others. Better information on the impact of each of these assumptions would help refine the plan so that it can be modified to become more financially feasible. Political feasibility is quite another matter.

Related to the issue of financial feasibility and sustainability is the fundamental single-payer principle of M4A, in which the federal government budget for health care grows from about $1.2 trillion currently to encompass the entire cost of US health care—$4.2 trillion in the first year based on the Commonwealth Fund estimate. Payments currently being made by states (for state employee health plans and its share of Medicaid), employers, and individuals would now be made by the federal government, requiring substantially higher federal revenues. The $4.2 trillion expenditure in the first year would represent a $3 trillion increase in the federal budget for health care, almost doubling the entire current federal budget of $3.5 trillion. Moreover, accepting the likelihood that highly optimistic incremental revenues will be insufficient to cover incremental costs, M4A would add to the current $1 trillion of annual federal overspending.

All of this will occur in a macroeconomic environment in which the consequences of eliminating private health insurance will be quite disruptive, with no precedent in US history.[43] Substantial impact on employment, financial markets, and the national money supply and its turnover would be unavoidable.

Partly in response to these concerns, alternative proposals retain the major components of the current structure (private employer health plans, Medicare, and Medicaid), but add Medicare or Medicaid buy-ins for different population groups. These are, essentially, proposals to reform access to the current health care industry. A nonmandated "buy-in" option would re-duce the uninsured rate to some extent but would probably not have a large impact. This is because, as noted in the discussion earlier, a large per-centage of the people who are currently eligible for Medicaid in an expan-sion state simply choose not to enroll. Similarly, many who are eligible for a subsidized plan in the ACA marketplace exchanges choose not to enroll. Individuals in both groups would likely also decide not to buy a similar "public option" plan. Moreover, even if one of the buy-in plans were enacted, the need for the other reforms would still be needed to improve care and reduce cost.

Summary and Final Assessment

Health and health care in the United States are uniquely paradoxical:

- Truly extraordinary breakthroughs in biomedical science and biomed-ical engineering have been translated into treatments that are extend-ing the length and quality of many lives—yet life expectancy in the United States has recently declined for the third straight year because of diseases of despair (opioid abuse, alcoholism, and suicide).
- The behavioral etiologies of common diseases are now widely understood—yet the behaviors responsible for the major causes of morbidity and mortality continue.
- There has never been more wealth in the United States than today—yet inequality in wealth is reaching historic levels and is widening, as is inequality in health.

The evolution of the US health care industry reflects these paradoxes, which are embedded in the core values of its citizens. For the most part, people believe that health care is a right (up to a point), but they also be-lieve in the fundamental strengths of a market economy while accepting that this economic system will mean that some people will be able to pur-chase more goods and services than others, including health care goods and services. As biomedical science took hold in the twentieth century and gave rise to treatments that cured disease, an industry arose that reflected these values but also exploited—as will occur in a capitalist system—the inher-ent imperfections in the markets for medical goods and services. These mar-ket imperfections, fundamentally arising from the distinctive features of health care, have led to an imbalance of care, cost, and access. Thus, 90 percent of the US population has access to health care through private insurance or government programs, but the quality of care is variable and the cost is high.

Key drivers of the imbalance in care, cost, and access can be identified, and concepts can be advanced that would materially improve the balance. Working within the industry structure, the opportunity for improving the balance through incremental reform is very substantial but every action that would make things better overall will be staunchly opposed by at least one powerfully entrenched stakeholder.

Some believe that the current balance of care, cost, and access cannot be materially improved through reform and that radical restructuring is needed. One type of restructuring would create a system of private health insurance with means-based government subsidies; this might help with expenditures, but the market imperfecions associated with claims-based, subsidized health insurance would remain, the impact on access might not be any better than with reform, and improvements in care would depend on the same concepts (evidence-based practice, high reliability, and reduction in medical overuse) that are needed under reform. At the opposite extreme, another type of restructuring would create universal access to health care with a single government payer, eliminating private health insurance and employer-sponsored plans, eliminating out-of-pocket cost sharing (with minor exceptions), and expanding benefits. This would improve access but would place the entire health care system under the executive branch of the federal government, potentially without effective checks and balances, and produce almost a doubling of the federal government's need for tax revenue in an economy that is already facing rapidly growing government deficits and debt.

The final assessment is that incremental reform of the current health care industry is possible—entrenched stakeholders aside—in a manner that will greatly improve care while constraining cost and also expanding access to many, but not all, Americans who are currently uninsured or underinsured. There is no silver bullet that cuts through the complexity of the US health care industry and comprehensively achieves a perfect solution.

REFERENCES

Preface

1. Irene Papanicolas, Liana R. Woskie, and Ashish K. Jha, "Health Care Spending in the United States and Other High-Income Countries," *JAMA* 319, no. 10 (2018): 1024–39, doi:10.1001/jama.2018.1150.

2. Raj Chetty, Michael Stepner, Sarah Abraham, Shelby Lin, Benjamin Scuderi, Nicholas Turner, Augustin Bergeron, and David Cutler, "The Association between Income and Life Expectancy in the United States, 2001–2014," *JAMA* 315, no. 16 (2016): 1750–66, doi:10.1001/jama.2016.4226.

3. Uwe Reinhardt, "Is Health Care Special?," *Economix* (blog), *New York Times*, August 6, 2010, https://economix.blogs.nytimes.com/2010/08/06/is-health-care -special.

1. Setting the Stage

1. Elizabeth Arias, Melonie Heron, and Jiaquan Xu, "United States Life Tables, 2014," *National Vital Statistics Reports* 66, no. 4 (August 2017): 1–64, https://www .cdc.gov/nchs/data/nvsr/nvsr66/nvsr66_04.pdf.

2. Sherry L. Murphy, Jiaquan Xu, Kenneth D. Kochanek, and Elizabeth Arias, *Mortality in the United States, 2017*, NCHS Data Brief No. 328 (Hyattsville, MD: National Center for Health Statistics, 2018), https://www.cdc.gov/nchs/data /databriefs/db328-h.pdf.

3. Arias, Heron, and Xu, "United States Life Tables, 2014."

4. Centers for Disease Control and Prevention, "Achievements in Public Health, 1900–1999: Control of Infectious Diseases," *MMWR Weekly* 48, no. 29 (1999): 621–29, https://www.cdc.gov/mmwr/preview/mmwrhtml/mm4829a1.htm.

5. Abdel R. Omran, "The Epidemiologic Transition: A Theory of the Epidemiology of Population Change," *Milbank Quarterly* 83, no. 4 (December 2005): 731–57, doi:10.1111/j.1468-0009.2005.00398.x.

6. Steven H. Woolf and Heidi Schoomaker, "Life Expectancy and Mortality Rates in the United States, 1959–2017," *JAMA* 322, no. 20 (2019): 1996–2016, doi:10.1001 /jama.2019.16932.

7. Dorothy P. Rice and Barbara S. Cooper, "National Health Expenditures, 1950–67," *Social Security Bulletin* 32, no. 1 (January 1969): 3–20, https://www.ssa.gov/policy/docs/ssb/v32n1/v32n1p3.pdf.

8. Rice and Cooper, "National Health Expenditures, 1950–67."

9. "All Items in US City Average, All Urban Consumers," BLS Data Viewer, Bureau of Labor Statistics, accessed January 21, 2020, https://beta.bls.gov/dataViewer/view/timeseries/CUUR0000SA0; "Medical Care in US City Average, All Urban Consumers," BLS Data Viewer, Bureau of Labor Statistics, accessed January 21, 2020, https://beta.bls.gov/dataViewer/view/timeseries/CUUR0000SAM.

10. Henri Hartman, *Gynecological Operation including Non-Operative Treatment and Minor Gynecology* (Philadelphia: P. Blakiston's Son,1913), 460.

11. Laurence A. Cole, Jaime M. Sutton-Riley, Sarah A. Khanlian, Marianna Borkovskaya, Brittany B. Rayburn, and William F. Rayburn, "Sensitivity of Over-the-Counter Pregnancy Tests: Comparison of Utility and Marketing Messages," *Journal of the American Pharmacists Association* 45, no. 5 (2005): 608–15, doi:10.1331/1544345055001391.

12. Howard Wilbur Jones, *In Vitro Fertilization Comes to America: Memoir of a Medical Breakthrough* (Williamsburg, VA: Jamestown Bookworks, 2014).

13. Gina Kolata, "Edwards Dies at 87; Changed Rules of Conception with First 'Test Tube Baby,'" *New York Times*, April 10, 2013, https://www.nytimes.com/2013/04/11/us/robert-g-edwards-nobel-winner-for-in-vitro-fertilization-dies-at-87.html.

14. "Assisted Reproductive Technology (ART)," Centers for Disease Control and Prevention, accessed April 21, 2019, https://www.cdc.gov/art/artdata/index.html.

15. Debbie Saslow, Diane Solomon, Herschel W. Lawson, Maureen Killackey, Shalini L. Kulasingam, Joanna Cain, Francisco A. R. Garcia, et al., "American Cancer Society, American Society for Colposcopy and Cervical Pathology, and American Society for Clinical Pathology Screening Guidelines for the Prevention and Early Detection of Cervical Cancer," *CA: A Cancer Journal for Clinicians* 62, no. 3 (May/June 2012): 147–72, doi:10.3322/caac.21139.

16. Fangjian Guo, Leslie E. Cofie, and Abbey B. Berenson, "Cervical Cancer Incidence in Young US Females after Human Papillomavirus Vaccine Introduction," *American Journal of Preventive Medicine* 55, no. 2 (August 2018): 197–204, doi:10.1016/j.amepre.2018.03.013.

17. Hannah C. Glass, Andrew T. Costarino, Stephen A. Stayer, Claire M. Brett, Franklyn Cladis, and Peter J. Davis, "Outcomes for Extremely Premature Infants," *Anesthesia & Analgesia* 120, no. 6 (June 2015): 1337–51, doi:10.1213/ane.0000000000000705.

18. "Preterm Birth," Reproductive Health, Centers for Disease Control and Prevention, accessed July 9, 2018, https://www.cdc.gov/reproductivehealth/maternalinfanthealth/pretermbirth.htm.

19. Glass et al., "Outcomes for Extremely Premature Infants."

20. Bernard Fisher, Joseph P. Costantino, D. Lawrence Wickerham, Carol K. Redmond, Maureen Kavanah, Walter M. Cronin, Victor Vogel, et al., "Tamoxifen for Prevention of Breast Cancer: Report of the National Surgical Adjuvant Breast and

Bowel Project P-1 Study," *JNCI: Journal of the National Cancer Institute* 90, no. 18 (September 1998): 1371–88, doi:10.1093/jnci/90.18.1371.

21. Dennis J. Slamon, Brian Leyland-Jones, Steven Shak, Hank Fuchs, Virginia Paton, Alex Bajamonde, Thomas Fleming, et al., "Use of Chemotherapy plus a Monoclonal Antibody against HER2 for Metastatic Breast Cancer that Overexpresses HER2," *New England Journal of Medicine* 344, no. 11 (2001): 783–92, doi:10.1056 /nejm200103153441101.

22. Edward H. Romond, Edith A. Perez, John Bryant, Vera J. Suman, Charles E. Geyer, Nancy E. Davidson, Elizabeth Tan-Chiu, et al., "Trastuzumab plus Adjuvant Chemotherapy for Operable HER2-Positive Breast Cancer," *New England Journal of Medicine* 353, no. 16 (2005): 1673–84, doi:10.1056/nejmoa052122; Martine J. Piccart-Gebhart, Marion Procter, Brian Leyland-Jones, Aron Goldhirsch, Michael Untch, Ian Smith, Luca Gianni, et al., "Trastuzumab after Adjuvant Chemotherapy in HER2-Positive Breast Cancer," *New England Journal of Medicine* 353, no. 16 (2005): 1659–72, doi:10.1056/nejmoa052306.

23. Brian J. Druker, Moshe Talpaz, Debra J. Resta, Bin Peng, Elisabeth Buch-dunger, John M. Ford, Nicholas B. Lydon, et al., "Efficacy and Safety of a Specific Inhibitor of the BCR-ABL Tyrosine Kinase in Chronic Myeloid Leukemia," *New England Journal of Medicine* 344, no. 14 (2001): 1031–37, doi:10.1056/nejm 200104053441401.

24. George D. Demetri, Margaret von Mehren, Charles D. Blanke, Annick D. Van den Abbeele, Burton Eisenberg, Peter J. Roberts, Michael C. Heinrich, et al., "Efficacy and Safety of Imatinib Mesylate in Advanced Gastrointestinal Stromal Tumors," *New England Journal of Medicine* 347, no. 7 (2002): 472–80, doi:10.1056 /nejmoa020461.

25. Jedd D. Wolchok, Vanna Chiarion-Sileni, Rene Gonzalez, Piotr Rutkowski, Jean-Jacques Grob, C. Lance Cowey, Christopher D. Lao, et al., "Overall Survival with Combined Nivolumab and Ipilimumab in Advanced Melanoma," *New England Journal of Medicine* 377, no. 14 (2017): 1345–56, doi:10.1056/nejmoa1709684.

26. Charles Daniel, "Worldwide Hepatitis Statistics: Incidence and Prevalence of the Five Types of Hepatitis," *Verywell Health*, updated September 7, 2019, https:// www.verywellhealth.com/how-many-people-have-hepatitis-1760012.

27. Poonam Mishra, Jeffry Florian, Joy Peter, Monika Vainorius, Michael W. Fried, David R. Nelson, and Debra Birnkrant, "Public-Private Partnership: Targeting Real-World Data for Hepatitis C Direct-Acting Antivirals," *Gastroenterology* 153, no. 3 (September 2017): 626–31, doi:10.1053/j.gastro.2017.07.025.

28. Daniel P. Webster, Paul Klenerman, and Geoffrey M. Dusheiko, "Hepatitis C," *The Lancet* 385, no. 9973 (2015): 1124–35, doi:10.1016/s0140-6736(14)62401-6.

29. Lisa I. Backus, Pamela S. Belperio, Troy A. Shahoumian, and Larry A. Mole, "Direct-Acting Antiviral Sustained Virologic Response: Impact on Mortality in Patients Without Advanced Liver Disease," *Hepatology* 68, no. 3 (2018): 827–38, doi:10.1002/hep.29811.

30. Jeffrey V. Lazarus, Stefan Wiktor, Massimo Colombo, and Mark Thursz, "Micro-Elimination—A Path to Global Elimination of Hepatitis C," *Journal of Hepatology* 67, no. 4 (2017): 665–66, doi:10.1016/j.jhep.2017.06.033.

31. Vincenza Calvaruso, Salvatore Petta, and Antonio Craxì, "Is Global Elimination of HCV Realistic?," *Liver International* 38, suppl. 1 (2018): 40–46, doi:10.1111/liv.13668.

32. Elizabeth G. Nabel and Eugene Braunwald, "A Tale of Coronary Artery Disease and Myocardial Infarction," *New England Journal of Medicine* 366, no. 1 (2012): 54–63, doi:10.1056/nejmra1112570.

33. William B. Kannel, Thomas R. Dawber, Abraham Kagan, Nicholas Revotskie, and Joseph Stokes, "Factors of Risk in the Development of Coronary Heart Disease—Six-Year Follow-Up Experience: The Framingham Study," *Annals of Internal Medicine* 55, no. 1 (1961): 33–50, doi:10.7326/0003-4819-55-1-33.

34. Nabel and Braunwald, "A Tale of Coronary Artery Disease and Myocardial Infarction," 55–56.

35. Daniel B. Mark, Kevin J. Anstrom, Shubin Sheng, Jonathan P. Piccini, Khaula N. Baloch, Kristi H. Monahan, Melanie R. Daniels, et al., "Effect of Catheter Ablation vs Medical Therapy on Quality of Life among Patients with Atrial Fibrillation," *JAMA* 321, no. 13 (2019): 1275–85, doi:10.1001/jama.2019.0692.

36. "Stroke Facts," Centers for Disease Control and Prevention, last modified September 6, 2017, accessed July 12, 2018, https://www.cdc.gov/stroke/facts.htm.

37. National Institute of Neurological Disorders and Stroke rt-PA Stroke Study Group, "Tissue Plasminogen Activator for Acute Ischemic Stroke," *New England Journal of Medicine* 333, no. 24 (1995): 1581–88, doi:10.1056/nejm199512143332401.

38. Substance Abuse and Mental Health Services Administration, *Key Substance Use and Mental Health Indicators in the United States: Results from the 2017 National Survey on Drug Use and Health*, HHS Publication No. SMA 18-5068, NSDUH Series H-53 (Rockville, MD: Center for Behavioral Health Statistics and Quality, Substance Abuse and Mental Health Services Administration, 2018), retrieved from https://www. samhsa.gov/data.

39. "Disability Weights, Discounting and Age Weighting of DALYs," Health Statistics and Information Systems, World Health Organization, accessed April 7, 2019, https://www.who.int/healthinfo/global_burden_disease/daly_disability_weight/en.

40. Thomas R. Insel, "Assessing the Economic Costs of Serious Mental Illness," *American Journal of Psychiatry* 165, no. 6 (June 2008): 663–65, doi:10.1176/appi.ajp.2008.08030366.

41. Joel T. Braslow and Stephen R. Marder, "History of Psychopharmacology," *Annual Review of Clinical Psychology* 15, no. 1 (2019): 25–50, doi:10.1146/annurev-clinpsy-050718-095514.

42. Stefan Leucht, Sandra Hierl, Werner Kissling, Markus Dold, and John M. Davis, "Putting the Efficacy of Psychiatric and General Medicine Medication into Perspective: Review of Meta-Analyses," *British Journal of Psychiatry* 200, no. 2 (February 2012): 97–106, doi:10.1192/bjp.bp.111.096594.

43. Lars Leksell, "The Stereotaxic Method and Radiosurgery of the Brain," *Acta Chirurgica Scandinavica* 102, no. 4 (1951): 316–19.

44. William A. Friedman, Frank J. Bova, and William M. Mendenhall, "Linear Accelerator Radiosurgery for Arteriovenous Malformations: The Relationship of Size

to Outcome," *Journal of Neurosurgery* 82, no. 2 (1995): 180–89, doi:10.3171/jns.1995 .82.2.0180.

2. Perfect Competition and Its Applicability to Health Care Services

1. Vilfredo Pareto, *Manual of Political Economy*, ed. Aldo Montesano, Alberto Zanni, Luigino Bruni, John S. Chipman, and Michael McLure M., Critical and Variorum Edition (Oxford: Oxford University Press, 2014). First published 1906.

2. Adam Smith, *The Wealth of Nations* (Hollywood, FL: Simon & Brown, 2011). First published in 1776 as *An Inquiry into the Nature and Causes of the Wealth of Nations*.

3. Alfred Marshall, *Principles of Economics*, 8th ed. (London: MacMillan, 1946). First published in 1890.

4. Adam Smith, *The Theory of Moral Sentiments* (Los Angeles: Enhanced Media, 2016). First published in 1759.

5. Smith, *Theory of Moral Sentiments*, part 4, chap. 1, 162.

6. Smith, *Wealth of Nations*, book 1, chap. 2, 15.

7. Smith, *Wealth of Nations*, book 4, chap. 2, 279.

8. Smith, *Wealth of Nations*, book 1, chap. 7, 45.

9. Antoine Cournot, *Researches on the Mathematical Principles of the Theory of Wealth*, trans. Natanial T. Bacon (New York: MacMillan, 1897; Whitefish, MT: Kessinger Legacy Reprints, 2010). First published in 1839.

10. Marshall, *Principles of Economics*, book 5, chap. 3, 348.

11. Marshall, *Principles of Economics*, book 5, chap. 3, 345.

12. Marshall, *Principles of Economics*, appendix H.

13. Marshall, *Principles of Economics*, book 5, chap. 3, 345–46.

3. Imperfections in the Market for Health Care Services

1. "Health Status: Maternal and Infant Mortality," OECD.Stat, Organisation for Economics Co-operation and Development, accessed December 12, 2018, https://stats .oecd.org/index.aspx.

2. "Health Status: Life Expectancy," OECD.Stat, Organisation for Economics Co-operation and Development, accessed December 12, 2018, https://stats.oecd.org /index.aspx.

3. Committee on Quality of Health Care in America, Institute of Medicine, *To Err Is Human: Building a Safer Health System* (Washington, DC: National Academies Press, 2000); Committee on Quality of Health Care in America, Institute of Medicine, *Crossing the Quality Chasm: A New Health System for the 21st Century* (Washington, DC: National Academies Press, 2001); Pierre Yong, Robert S. Saunders, and LeighAnne Olsen, eds., *The Healthcare Imperative: Lowering Costs and Improving Outcomes—Workshop Series Summary*, Institute of Medicine (US) Roundtable on Value & Science-Driven Health Care (Washington, DC: National Academies Press, 2010).

4. Irene Papanicolas, Liana R. Woskie, and Ashish K. Jha, "Health Care Spending in the United States and Other High-Income Countries," *JAMA* 319, no. 10 (2018): 1024–39. doi:10.1001/jama.2018.1150.

5. Edward Chamberlain, *The Theory of Monopolistic Competition*, 8th ed. (Cambridge, MA: Harvard University Press, 1962). First published 1933.

6. Sunita Desai, Laura A. Hatfield, Andrew L. Hicks, Michael E. Chernew, and Ateev Mehrotra, 2016. "Association between Availability of a Price Transparency Tool and Outpatient Spending," *JAMA* 315, no. 17 (2016): 1874, doi:10.1001/jama.2016.4288.

7. Michael Chernew, Zack Cooper, Eugene Larsen-Hallock, and Fiona Scott Morton, "Are Health Care Services Shoppable? Evidence from the Consumption of Lower-Limb MRI Scans," National Bureau of Economic Research, Working Paper No. 24869, July 2018.

8. Kenneth Arrow, "Uncertainty and the Welfare Economics of Medical Care," *American Economic Review* 53 (1963), 951.

9. "Infertility Coverage by State," Resolve: The National Infertility Association, accessed July 18, 2018, https://resolve.org/what-are-my-options/insurance-coverage/infertility-coverage-state.

10. Tarun Jain, Bernard L. Harlow, and Mark D. Hornstein, "Insurance Coverage and Outcomes of In Vitro Fertilization," *New England Journal of Medicine* 347, no. 9 (2002): 661–66, doi:10.1056/nejmsa013491.

4. Implications of an Imperfect Market I

1. David Card, Carlos Dobkin, and Nicole Maestas, "The Impact of Nearly Universal Insurance Coverage on Health Care Utilization and Health: Evidence from Medicare," *American Economic Review* 98, no. 5 (December 2008): 2242–58, doi:10.3386/w10365.

2. Willard G. Manning, Joseph P. Newhouse, Naihua Duan, Emmett B. Keiler, Arleen Leibowitz, and Susan Marquis, "Health Insurance and the Demand for Medical Care: Evidence from a Randomized Experiment," *American Economic Review* 77, no. 3 (1987): 251–77.

3. Jeanne S. Ringel, Susan D. Hosek, Ben A. Volaard, and Sergej Mahnovski, *The Elasticity of Demand for Health Care: A Review of the Literature and its Application to the Military Health System*," RAND Monograph Report (Santa Monica, CA: RAND Corporation, 2002), https://www.rand.org/pubs/monograph_reports/MR1355.html.

4. Jeffrey R. J. Richardson and Stuart J. Peacock, "Supplier-Induced Demand: Reconsidering the Theories and New Australian Evidence," *Applied Health Economics and Health Policy* 5, no. 2 (June 2006): 87–98, doi:10.2165/00148365-200605020-00003.

5. Yasushi Iwanmoto and Kensaku Kishida, "An Estimation of Price Elasticity of Medical Care Demand: Evidence from Japanese Policy Reforms During 40 Years" (preliminary paper), Kyoto University, May 2001, http://www.ier.hit-u.ac.jp/~iwaisako/mmws/papers/Iwamoto_0510.pdf.

6. "Out-of-Pocket Expenditure Per Capita (Current US$)," World Health Organization Global Health Expenditure Database, The World Bank, accessed August 2, 2018, https://data.worldbank.org/indicator/SH.XPD.OOPC.PC.CD.

7. Irene Papanicolas, Liana R. Woskie, and Ashish K. Jha, "Health Care Spending in the United States and Other High-Income Countries," *JAMA* 319, no. 10 (2018): 1024–39, doi:10.1001/jama.2018.1150.

8. Michael E. Martinez, Emily P. Zammitti, and Robin A. Cohen, *Health Insurance Coverage: Early Release of Estimates from the National Health Interview Survey, January–June 2018* (Hyattsville, MD: National Center for Health Statistics, November 2018), https://www.cdc.gov/nchs/data/nhis/earlyrelease/insur201811.pdf.

9. Sara R. Collins, Munira Z. Gunja, Michelle M. Doty, and Herman K. Bhupal, "Americans' Views on Health Insurance at the End of a Turbulent Year" (survey brief), Commonwealth Fund, March 2018, https://www.commonwealthfund.org/sites/default/files/documents/___media_files_publications_issue_brief_2018_mar_collins_views_hlt_insurance_turbulent_year_aca_tracking_survey.pdf.

10. Ricardo Alonso-Zaldivar and Laurie Kellman, "AP-NORC Poll: Shift to Political Left Seen on Health Care," *Associated Press*, July 20, 2017, http://www.apnorc.org/news-media/Pages/AP-NORC-Poll-Shift-to-political-left-seen-on-health-care.aspx.

5. Implications of an Imperfect Market II

1. Glen S. Hazlewood, Cheryl Barnabe, George Tomlinson, Deborah Marshall, Daniel JA Devoe, and Claire Bombardier, "Methotrexate Monotherapy and Methotrexate Combination Therapy with Traditional and Biologic Disease Modifying Anti-Rheumatic Drugs for Rheumatoid Arthritis: A Network Meta-Analysis," *Cochrane Database of Systematic Reviews*, no. 8 (2016): CD010227, doi:10.1002/14651858.cd010227.pub2.

2. Jack Hadley, John Holahan, and William Scanlon, "Can Fee-for-Service Reimbursement Coexist with Demand Creation?," *Inquiry* 16, no. 3 (1979), 249.

3. Cam Donaldson and Karen Gerard, *Economics of Health Care Financing: The Visible Hand* (Basingstoke, England: Macmillan, 1994): 116–17.

4. Erin M. Johnson, "Physician-Induced Demand," in *Encyclopedia of Health Economics*, ed. Anthony J. Culyer (Oxford: Elsevier, 2014): 78.

5. Jonathan Skinner, "Causes and Consequences of Regional Variations in Health Care," in *Handbook of Health Economics*, ed. Mark V. Pauly, Thomas G. Msguire, and Pedro P. Barros (Oxford: Elsevier, 2011), 50.

6. Skinner, "Causes and Consequences."

7. Victor R. Fuchs, "The Supply of Surgeons and the Demand for Operations," *Journal of Human Resources* 13 (1978): 35, doi:10.2307/145247.

8. Amitabh Chandra and Jonathan Skinner, "Technology Growth and Expenditure Growth in Health Care," *Journal of Economic Literature* 50, no. 3 (2012): 645–80, doi:10.1257/jel.50.3.645.

9. John Wennberg and Alan Gittelsohn, "Small Area Variations in Health Care Delivery," *Science* 182, no. 4117 (1973): 1102–8, doi:10.1126/science.182.4117.1102.

10. Skinner, "Causes and Consequences," 54–56.

11. Gary Schwartz, "Hippocrates Revisited," *Einstein Journal of Biology and Medicine* 21 (2004): 33–34.

12. Bruce J.Hillman and Jeff Goldsmith, "Imaging: The Self-Referral Boom and the Ongoing Search for Effective Policies to Contain It," *Health Affairs* 29, no. 12 (2010): 2231–36, doi:10.1377/hlthaff.2010.1019.

13. J. Alison Glover, "The Incidence of Tonsillectomy in School Children," *Proceedings of the Royal Society of Medicine* 31, no. 10 (1938): 1219–36.

14. Glover, "The Incidence of Tonsillectomy," 1226.

15. Glover, "The Incidence of Tonsillectomy," 1232.

16. Wennberg and Gittelsohn, "Small Area Variations in Health Care Delivery."

17. Emily F. Boss, Jill A. Marsteller, and Alan E. Simon, "Outpatient Tonsillectomy in Children: Demographic and Geographic Variation in the United States, 2006," *Journal of Pediatrics* 160, no. 5 (2012): 814–19, doi:10.1016/j.jpeds.2011.11.041.

18. Martin J. Burton, Paul P. Glasziou, Lee Yee Chong, and Roderick P. Venekamp, "Tonsillectomy or Adenotonsillectomy versus Non-Surgical Treatment for Chronic/Recurrent Acute Tonsillitis," *Cochrane Database of Systematic Reviews*, no. 11 (2014): CD001802, doi:10.1002/14651858.cd001802.pub3.

19. David C. Goodman and Greg J. Challener, "Tonsillectomy: A Procedure in Search of Evidence," *Journal of Pediatrics* 160, no. 5 (2012): 716–18, doi:10.1016/j.jpeds.2012.01.033.

20. Max Shain and Milton I. Roemer, "Hospital Costs Relate to the Supply of Beds," *Modern Hospital* 92, no. 4 (1959): 71–73.

21. Milton I. Roemer, "Bed Supply and Hospital Utilization: A Natural Experiment," *Hospitals* 35 (1961): 36–42.

22. Martin S. Feldstein, "Hospital Cost Inflation: A Study of Nonprofit Price Dynamics," *American Economic Review* 61, no. 5 (1971): 853–72.

23. Paul B. Ginsburg and Daniel M. Koretz, "Bed Availability and Hospital Utilization: Estimates of the 'Roemer Effect,'" *Health Care Finance Review* 5, no. 1 (1983): 87–92.

24. "Understanding Geographic Variation in Health Care," Dartmouth Atlas Project, www.dartmouthatlas.org; Institute of Medicine, *Variation in Health Care Spending: Target Decision Making, Not Geography* (Washingon, DC: National Academies Press, 2013).

25. Stephen Zuckerman, Timothy Waidmann, Robert Berenson, and Jack Hadley, "Clarifying Sources of Geographic Differences in Medicare Spending," *New England Journal of Medicine* 363, no. 1 (2010): 54–62, doi:10.1056/nejmsa0909253.

26. Institute of Medicine, *Variation in Health Care Spending*, xxiv.

27. Louise Sheiner, "Why the Geographic Variation in Health Care Spending Cannot Tell Us Much about the Efficiency or Quality of Our Health Care System," *Brookings Papers on Economic Activity*, no. 2 (Fall 2014): 1–72, doi:10.1353/eca.2014.0012.

28. Sheiner, "Why the Geographic Variation in Health Care Spending Cannot Tell Us Much," 3.

29. Yunjie Song, Jonathan Skinner, Julie Bynum, Jason Sutherland, John E. Wennberg, and Elliott S. Fisher, "Regional Variations in Diagnostic Practices," *New England Journal of Medicine* 363, no. 1 (2010): 45–53, doi:10.1056/nejmsa0910881.

30. James D. Reschovsky, Jack Hadley, and Patrick S. Romano, "Geographic Variation in Fee-for-Service Medicare Beneficiaries' Medical Costs Is Largely Explained by Disease Burden," *Medical Care Research and Review* 70, no. 5 (2013): 542–63, doi:10.1177/1077558713487771.

31. Zuckerman et al., "*Clarifying Sources.*"

32. Amy Finkelstein, Matthew Gentzkow, and Heidi Williams, "Sources of Geographic Variation in Health Care: Evidence from Patient Migration," NBER Working Paper No. 20789, National Bureau of Economic Research, Cambridge, MA, December 2014, https://www.nber.org/papers/w20789.pdf.

33. David J. Ciesla, Etienne E. Pracht, Pablo T. Leitz, David A. Spain, Kristan L. Staudenmayer, and Joseph J. Tepas, "The Trauma Ecosystem," *Journal of Trauma and Acute Care Surgery* 82, no. 6 (2017): 1014–22, doi:10.1097/ta.0000000000001442.

34. Kristan L. Staudenmayer, Renee Y. Hsia, N. Clay Mann, David A. Spain, and Craig D. Newgard, "Triage of Elderly Trauma Patients: A Population-Based Perspective," *Journal of the American College of Surgeons* 217, no. 4 (2013): 569–76, doi:10.1016/j.jamcollsurg.2013.06.017.

35. Atul Gawande, "The Cost Conundrum: What a Texas Town Can Teach Us about Health Care," *New Yorker*, June 1, 2009, https://www.newyorker.com/magazine/2009/06/01/the-cost-conundrum.

36. David Cutler, Jonathan S. Skinner, Ariel Dora Stern, and David Wennberg, "Physician Beliefs and Patient Preferences: A New Look at Regional Variation in Health Care Spending," *American Economic Journal: Economic Policy* 11, no. 1 (2019): 192–221, doi:10.1257/pol.20150421.

37. Austin Frakt, "Painkiller Abuse, a Cyclical Challenge," *New York Times*, December 14, 2014, https://www.nytimes.com/2014/12/23/upshot/painkiller-abuse-a-cyclical-challenge.html.

6. The Role of Price in Health Care Spending Growth

1. Gerard F. Anderson, Uwe E. Reinhardt, Peter S. Hussey, and Varduhi Petrosyan, "It's the Prices, Stupid: Why the United States Is So Different from Other Countries," *Health Affairs* 22, no. 3 (2003), 103, doi:10.1377/hlthaff.22.3.89.

2. Gerard F. Anderson, Peter Hussey, and Varduhi Petrosyan, "It's Still the Prices, Stupid: Why the US Spends So Much on Health Care, and a Tribute to Uwe Reinhardt," *Health Affairs* 38, no. 1 (2019), 87, doi:10.1377/hlthaff.2018.05144.

3. Irene Papanicolas, Liana R. Woskie, and Ashish K. Jha, "Health Care Spending in the United States and Other High-Income Countries," *JAMA* 319, no. 10 (2018): 1024–39, doi:10.1001/jama.2018.1150.

4. Papanicolas, Woskie, and Jha, "Health Care Spending," 1031.

5. Papanicolas, Woskie, and Jha, "Health Care Spending," 1035.

6. Papanicolas, Woskie, and Jha, "Health Care Spending," Supplement 1, eTable 1.

7. Ezekiel J. Emanuel, "The Real Cost of the US Health Care System," *JAMA* 319, no. 10 (2018): 983, doi:10.1001/jama.2018.1151.

8. David U. Himmelstein, Miraya Jun, Reinhard Busse, Karine Chevreul, Alexander Geissler, Patrick Jeurissen, Sarah Thomson, Marie-Amelie Vinet, and Steffie Woolhandler, "A Comparison of Hospital Administrative Costs in Eight Nations: US Costs Exceed All Others by Far," *Health Affairs* 33, no. 9 (2014): 1586–94, doi:10.1377/hlthaff.2013.1327.

9. Phillip Tseng, Robert S. Kaplan, Barak D. Richman, Mahek A. Shah, and Kevin A. Schulman, "Administrative Costs Associated with Physician Billing and Insurance-Related Activities at an Academic Health Care System," *JAMA* 319, no. 7 (2018): 691–97, doi:10.1001/jama.2017.19148.

10. Centers for Medicare and Medicaid Sevices, "Table 02: National Health Expenditures, Aggregate and Per Capita Amounts, by Type of Expenditure" (data file), National Health Expenditure Data: NHE Tables, accessed January 22, 2020. https://www.cms.gov/Research-Statistics-Data-and-Systems/Statistics-Trends-and -Reports/NationalHealthExpendData/NationalHealthAccountsHistorical.

11. Charles S. Roehrig and David M. Rousseau, "The Growth in Cost Per Case Explains Far More of US Health Spending Increases than Rising Disease Prevalence," *Health Affairs* 30, no. 9 (2011): 1657–63, doi:10.1377/hlthaff.2010.0644.

12. A. Dunn, Eli Liebman, and Adam Hale Shapiro, "Decomposing Medical-Care Expenditure Growth," Federal Reserve Bank of San Francisco, Working Paper 2012-26, November 2012, https://www.frbsf.org/economic-research/files/wp12-26bk .pdf.

13. Joseph L. Dieleman, Ellen Squires, Anthony L. Bui, Madeline Campbell, Abigail Chapin, Hannah Hamavid, Cody Horst, et al. "Factors Associated with Increases in US Health Care Spending, 1996–2013," *JAMA* 318, no. 17 (2017): 1668–78, doi:10.1001/jama.2017.15927.

7. Inequality of Wealth, Health, and Access to Care

1. Barack Obama, "United States Health Care Reform: Progress to Date and Next Steps," *JAMA* 316, no. 5 (2016): 525, doi:10.1001/jama.2016.9797.

2. Irene Papanicolas, Liana R. Woskie, and Ashish K. Jha, "Health Care Spending in the United States and Other High-Income Countries," *JAMA* 319, no. 10 (2018): 1024–39, doi:10.1001/jama.2018.1150.

3. Papanicolas, Woskie, and Jha, "Health Care Spending," 1037.

4. US Department of Health and Human Services, Office of Disease Prevention and Health Promotion, "Healthy People 2020 Framework" [fact sheet], accessed November 12, 2018, https://www.healthypeople.gov/sites/default/files/HP 2020Framework.pdf.

5. Michael I. Norton and Dan Ariely, "Building a Better America—One Wealth Quintile at a Time," *Perspectives on Psychological Science* 6, no. 1 (2011): 9–12, doi:10.1177/1745691610393524.

6. Angus Deaton, "On Death and Money," *JAMA* 315, no. 16 (2016): 1703, doi:10.1001/jama.2016.4072.

7. Raj Chetty, Michael Stepner, Sarah Abraham, Shelby Lin, Benjamin Scuderi, Nicholas Turner, Augustin Bergeron, and David Cutler, "The Association between Income and Life Expectancy in the United States, 2001–2014," *JAMA* 315, no. 16 (2016): 1750–66, doi:10.1001/jama.2016.4226.

8. Jonas Minet Kinge, Jørgen Heibø Modalsli, Simon Øverland, Håkon Kristian Gjessing, Mette Christophersen Tollånes, Ann Kristin Knudsen, Vegard Skirbekk, Bjørn Heine Strand, Siri Eldevik Håberg, and Stein Emil Vollset, "Association of Household Income with Life Expectancy and Cause-Specific Mortality in Norway, 2005–2015," *JAMA* 321, no. 19 (2019): 1916, doi:10.1001/jama.2019.4329.

9. Laura Dwyer-Lindgren, Amelia Bertozzi-Villa, Rebecca W. Stubbs, Chloe Morozoff, Johan P. Mackenbach, Frank J. van Lenthe, Ali H. Mokdad, and Christopher J. L. Murray, "Inequalities in Life Expectancy among US Counties, 1980 to 2014," *JAMA Internal Medicine* 177, no. 7 (2017): 1003, doi:10.1001/jamainternmed.2017.0918.

10. National Research Council and Institute of Medicine, *US Health in International Perspective: Shorter Lives, Poorer Health,* edited by Steven H. Woolf and Laudan Y. Aron (Washington, DC: National Academies Press, 2013).

11. Uwe Reinhardt, "Is Health Care Special?," *Economix* (blog), *New York Times*, August 6, 2010, https://economix.blogs.nytimes.com/2010/08/06/is-health-care-special.

12. Rachel Garfield, Kendal Orgera, and Anthony Damico, *The Unisured and the ACA: A Primer* (San Francisco: Kaiser Family Foundation, January 2019), 13, http://files.kff.org/attachment/The-Uninsured-and-the-ACA-A-Primer-Key-Facts-about-Health-Insurance-and-the-Uninsured-amidst-Changes-to-the-Affordable-Care-Act.

13. Karen Davis and Jeromie Ballreich, "Equitable Access to Care—How the United States Ranks Internationally," *New England Journal of Medicine* 371, no. 17 (2014): 1567–70, doi:10.1056/nejmp1406707.

14. Gary Claxton, Larry Levitt, and Michelle Long, "Payments for Cost Sharing Increasing Rapidly over Time," *Peterson-KFF Health System Tracker*, April 12, 2016, https://www.healthsystemtracker.org/brief/payments-for-cost-sharing-increasing-rapidly-over-time/#item-start.

15. Zarek C. Brot-Goldberg, Amitabh Chandra, Benjamin R. Handel, and Jonathan T. Kolstad, "What Does a Deductible Do? The Impact of Cost-Sharing on Health Care Prices, Quantities, and Spending Dynamics," *Quarterly Journal of Economics* 132, no. 3 (2017): 1261–1318, doi:10.1093/qje/qjx013.

16. National Research Council and Institute of Medicine, *US Health in International Perspective,* 46–51.

17. John S. Santelli, Laura Duberstein Lindberg, Lawrence B. Finer, and Susheela Singh, "Explaining Recent Declines in Adolescent Pregnancy in the United States: The Contribution of Abstinence and Improved Contraceptive Use," *American Journal of Public Health* 97, no. 1 (2007): 150–56, doi:10.2105/ajph.2006.089169.

18. Melissa S. Kearney and Phillip B. Levine, "Why the Teen Birth Rate in the United States Is So High and Why Does It Matter?," NBER Working Paper No. 17965, National Bureau of Economic Research, Cambridge, MA, March 2012, https://www.nber.org/papers/w17965.pdf.

19. Cynthia Ferré, William Callaghan, Christine Olson, Andrea Sharma, and Wanda Barfield, "Effects of Maternal Age and Age-Specific Preterm Birth Rates on Overall Preterm Birth Rates—United States, 2007 and 2014," *Morbidity and Mortality Weekly Report* 65, no. 43 (2016): 1181–84, doi:10.15585/mmwr.mm6543a1.

20. Ali S. Khashan, Philip N. Baker, and Louise C. Kenny, "Preterm Birth and Reduced Birthweight in First and Second Teenage Pregnancies: A Register-Based Cohort Study," *BMC Pregnancy and Childbirth* 10, no. 1 (2010): 36, doi:10.1186/1471-2393-10-36.

21. Brian M. D'Onofrio, Quetzal A. Class, Martin E. Rickert, Henrik Larsson, Niklas Långström, and Paul Lichtenstein, "Preterm Birth and Mortality and Morbidity," *JAMA Psychiatry* 70, no. 11 (2013): 1231, doi:10.1001/jamapsychiatry.2013.2107.

22. James A. Levine, "Poverty and Obesity in the US," *Diabetes* 60, no. 11 (2011): 2667–68, doi:10.2337/db11-1118.

23. Peter Franks, Paul C. Winters, Daniel J. Tancredi, and Kevin A. Fiscella, "Do Changes in Traditional Coronary Heart Disease Risk Factors over Time Explain the Association between Socio-Economic Status and Coronary Heart Disease?," *BMC Cardiovascular Disorders* 11, no. 1 (2011): 28, doi:10.1186/1471-2261-11-28.

24. Mark Lemstra, Marla Rogers, and John Moraros, "Income and Heart Disease," *Canadian Family Physician* 61, no. 8 (2015): 698–704, PMID:26836056.

25. Chetty et al., "Association between Income and Life Expectancy."

26. Chetty et al., "Association between Income and Life Expectancy," 1763.

27. Dwyer-Lindgren et al., "Inequalities in Life Expectancy," 1008.

8. Origins and Structural Underpinnings of the US Health Care Industry

1. Kenneth J. Arrow, "Uncertainty and the Welfare Economics of Medical Care," *American Economic Review* 53, no. 5 (1963): 941–73, http://www.jstor.org/stable/1812044.

2. Sources for the following historical account are mainly Odin W. Anderson, *The Uneasy Equilibrium: Private and Public Financing of Health Services in the United States 1875–1965* (New Haven, CT: College & University Press, 1968); Paul Starr, *The Social Transformation of American Medicine* (New York: Basic Books, 1986); Institute of Medicine Committee on Employment-Based Health Benefits, *Employment and Health Benefits: A Connection at Risk,* edited by Marilyn J. Field and Harold T. Shapiro (Washington, DC: National Academies Press, 1993); William Bynum, *The History of Medicine: A Very Short Introduction* (Oxford: Oxford University Press, 2008); Michael A. Morrisey, *Health Insurance* (Chicago: Health Administration Press, 2008); and Christy Ford Chapin, *Ensuring America's Health: The Public Creation of the Corporate Health Care System* (Cambridge: Cambridge University Press, 2015). Specific references are given for quotations or other detailed information, and additional sources are cited when appropriate.

3. US Bureau of Labor Statistics, "100 Years of US Consumer Spending," released May 2006 with revisions on June 2 and August 3, 2006, data from Table 5, https://www.bls.gov/opub/100-years-of-u-s-consumer-spending.pdf.

4. Abraham Flexner, *Medical Education in the United States and Canada: A Report to the Carnegie Foundation for the Advancement of Teaching, with an Introduction by Henry S. Pritchett* (New York: Carnegie Foundation, 1910; reproduced by Merrymount Press in 1960), http://archive.carnegiefoundation.org/pdfs/elibrary/Carnegie_Flexner_Report.pdf.

5. Lu Wang Adams, Carol A. Aschenbrenner, Timothy T. Houle, and Raymond C. Roy, "Uncovering the History of Operating Room Attire through Photographs," *Anesthesiology* 124, no. 1 (2016): 19–24, doi:10.1097/aln.0000000000000932.

6. Starr, *Social Transformation*, 209.

7. Starr, *Social Transformation*, 116–17.

8. Institute of Medicine Committee, *Employment and Health Benefits*, chapter 2, "Origins and Evolution of Employment-Based Health Benefits."

9. Anderson, *Uneasy Equilibrium*, 75.

10. Starr, *Social Transformation*, 237–39.

11. Institute of Medicine Committee, *Employment and Health Benefits*, chapter 2.

12. Institute of Medicine Committee, *Employment and Health Benefits*, chapter 2.

13. Starr, *Social Transformation*, 265.

14. Anderson, *Uneasy Equilibrium*, 101.

15. Chapin, *Ensuring America's Health*, 23.

16. Anderson, *Uneasy Equilibrium*, 98.

17. Starr, *Social Transformation*, 295.

18. Michael M. Davis and C. Rufas Rorem, *The Crisis in Hospital Finance and Other Studies in Hospital Economics* (Chicago: University of Chicago Press, 1932).

19. Starr, *Social Transformation*, 296.

20. "About Us: The Blue Cross Blue Shield System," Blue Cross Blue Shield, accessed September 3, 2018. https://www.bcbs.com/about-us/the-blue-cross-blue-shield-system.

21. Starr, *Social Transformation*, 298.

22. Anderson, *Uneasy Equilibrium*, 196.

23. Starr, *Social Transformation*, 297–98.

24. Chapin, *Ensuring America's Health*, 122–23.

25. Chapin, *Ensuring America's Health*, 122.

26. Chapin, *Ensuring America's Health*, 25–26.

27. Sylvia A. Law, *Blue Cross: What Went Wrong?* (New Haven, CT: Yale University Press, 1974).

9. The US Health Care Industry Takes Shape

1. Paul Starr, *The Social Transformation of American Medicine* (New York: Basic Books, 1982), 340.

2. National Institutes of Health Office of Budget, "Appropriation History by Institute/Center (1938 to Present)," accessed September 16, 2018, https://officeofbudget.od.nih.gov/approp_hist.html.

3. Richard Carter, *Breakthrough: The Saga of Jonas Salk* (New York: Trident Press, 1965), 268.

4. Starr, *Social Transformation*, 350.

5. Pierre de Vise, *Misused and Misplaced Hospitals and Doctors: A Locational Analysis of the Urban Health Care Crisis* (Washington, DC: Association of American Geographers, 1973), 76.

6. Louis S. Reed, "Private Health Insurance Coverage and Financial Experience, 1940–66," *Social Security Bulletin* (November 1967): 3–19, https://www.ssa.gov/policy/docs/ssb/v30n11/v30n11p3.pdf.

7. Herman M. Somers and Anne R. Somers, *Doctors, Patients, and Health Insurance* (Washington, DC: Brookings Institution, 1961), 261.

8. Health Insurance Institute, *Source Book of Health Insurance Data, 1965* (New York: Health Insurance Institute, 1966).

9. Michael Morrisey, *Health Insurance* (Chicago: Health Administration Press, 2008), 12.

10. Marie Gottchalk, *The Shadow Welfare State: Labor, Business, and the Politics of Health Care in the United States* (Ithica: Cornell University Press, 2000), 48.

11. Christy Ford Chapin, *Ensuring America's Health: The Public Creation of the Corporate Health Care System* (Cambridge: Cambridge University Press, 2015), 61.

12. Chapin, *Ensuring America's Health*, 62.

13. "How It All Started," Our Story: Our history, Kaiser Permanente, accessed September 17, 2018, https://share.kaiserpermanente.org/about-us/history.

14. "Fast Facts," Who We Are, Kaiser Permanente, accessed September 17, 2018, https://share.kaiserpermanente.org/about-us/fast-facts.

15. Starr, *Social Transformation*, 321.

16. Starr, *Social Transformation*, 324–27.

17. Gottchalk, *Shadow Welfare State*, 48.

18. Starr, *Social Transformation*, 313.

19. Bureau of Labor Statistics, "94 Percent of Union Workers Had Access to Medical Care Benefits in March 2017," *TED: The Economics Daily*, October 6, 2017, https://www.bls.gov/opub/ted/2017/94-percent-of-union-workers-had-access-to-medical-care-benefits-in-march-2017.htm.

10. Medicare

1. Ronald Anderson, Joanna Lion, and Odin W. Anderson, *Two Decades of Health Services: Social Survey Trends in Use and Expenditure* (Cambridge, MA: Ballinger, 1976).

2. The historical summary presented here is based on the excellent accounts by Richard Harris, *A Sacred Trust* (New York: New American Library, 1966); Theodore R. Marmor, *The Politics of Medicare*, 2nd ed. (New York: Routledge, 2017); Jonathan Oberlander, *The Political Life of Medicare* (Chicago: University of Chicago Press, 2003); Paul Starr, *The Social Transformation of American Medicine* (New York:

Basic Books, 1982); and Julian E. Zelizer, "How Medicare Was Made," *New Yorker*, February 15, 2015, https://www.newyorker.com/news/news-desk/medicare-made.

3. Stephen M. Weiner, "'Reasonable Cost' Reimbursement for Inpatient Hospital Services Under Medicare and Medicaid: The Emergence of Public Control," *American Journal of Law & Medicine* 3, no. 1 (1977): 1–47.

4. Brian M. Kinkead, "Medicare Payment and Hospital Capital: The Evolution of Policy," *Health Affairs* 3, no. 3 (1984): 49–74, doi:10.1377/hlthaff.3.3.49.

5. Kinkead, "Medicare Payment and Hospital Capital."

6. *2018 Annual Report of the Boards of Trustees of the Federal Hospital Insurance and Federal Supplementary Medical Insurance Trust Funds* (Washington, DC: Boards of Trustees, Federal Hospital Insurance and Federal Supplementary Medical Insurance Trust Funds, 2018), https://www.cms.gov/Research-Statistics-Data-and -Systems/Statistics-Trends-and-Reports/ReportsTrustFunds/downloads/tr2018.pdf.

7. Gretchen Jacobson, Matthew Rae, Tricia Neuman, Kendal Orgera, and Cristina Boccuti, *Medicare Advantage: How Robust Are Plans' Physician Networks?* (Menlo Park, CA: Kaiser Family Foundation, 2017), https://www.kff.org/medicare /report/medicare-advantage-how-robust-are-plans-physician-networks.

8. Thomas G. McGuire, Joseph P. Newhouse, and Anna D. Sinaiko, "An Economic History of Medicare Part C," *Milbank Quarterly* 89, no. 2 (2011): 289–332, doi:10.1111/j.1468-0009.2011.00629.x.

9. Bob Blancato and Meredith P. Whitmire, "The Good News for Medicare Beneficiaries," *Forbes*, April 17, 2018, https://www.forbes.com/sites/nextave nue/2018/04/17/the-good-news-for-medicare-beneficiaries.

10. Medicare Payment Advisory Commission (MEDPAC), *Report to the Congress: Medicare Payment Policy* (Washington, DC: MEDPAC, 2009), 258, http://www .medpac.gov/docs/default-source/reports/march-2009-report-to-congress-medicare -payment-policy.pdf.

11. Stephen Zuckerman, Laura Skopec, and Stuart Guterman, "Do Medicare Advantage Plans Minimize Costs? Investigating the Relationship between Benchmarks, Costs, and Rebates" (issue brief), Commonwealth Fund, December 2017, https://www .commonwealthfund.org/sites/default/files/documents/___media_files_publications _issue_brief_2017_dec_zuckerman_medicare_advantage_benchmarks_ib.pdf.

12. Zuckerman, Skopec, and Guterman, "Do Medicare Advantage Plans Minimize Costs?," 4.

13. Zuckerman, Skopec, and Guterman, "Do Medicare Advantage Plans Minimize Costs?," 5.

14. Zuckerman, Skopec, and Guterman, "Do Medicare Advantage Plans Minimize Costs?," 3.

15. Christina Farr, "Devoted Health, a Start-Up Selling Health Insurance to Seniors, Is Worth $1.8 Billion," *CNBC*, October 17, 2018, https://www.cnbc.com /2018/10/17/devoted-health-is-valued-at-1point8-billion-in-funding-led-by-andreessen .html.

16. Bruce Japsen, "Google Bets $375M on Medicare Advantage with Oscar Health Stake," *Forbes*, August 14, 2018, https://www.forbes.com/sites/brucejapsen/2018/08/14 /google-bets-375m-on-medicare-advantage-with-oscar-health-investment.

17. *Medicare Advantage: CMS Should Use Data on Disenrollment and Beneficiary Health Status to Strengthen Oversight*, GAO-17-393 (Washington, DC: US Government Accountability Office, April 2017).

18. *Medicare Advantage*, GAO-17-393, GAO Highlights page.

19. John Z. Ayanian, Bruce E. Landon, Alan M. Zaslavsky, Robert C. Saunders, L. Gregory Pawlson, and Joseph P. Newhouse, "Medicare Beneficiaries More Likely to Receive Appropriate Ambulatory Services in HMOs than in Traditional Medicare," *Health Affairs* 32, no. 7 (2013): 1228–35, doi:10.1377/hlthaff.2012.0773.

20. Ayanian et al., "Medicare Beneficiaries," 1228.

21. Marsha Gold and Giselle Casillas, *What Do We Know about Health Care Access and Quality in Medicare Advantage Versus the Traditional Medicare Program?* (Menlo Park, CA: Kaiser Family Foundation, 2014), https://www.kff.org/medicare /report/what-do-we-know-about-health-care-access-and-quality-in-medicare -advantage-versus-the-traditional-medicare-program.

22. Dan Mendelson, Christie Teigland, and Sean Creighton, *Medicare Advantage Achieves Cost-Effective Care and Better Outcomes for Beneficiaries with Chronic Conditions Relative to Fee-for-Service Medicare* (Washington, DC: Avalere Health, 2018), http://img04.en25.com/Web/AvalereHealth/%7B914072d2-41c3-4645-84e0 -2ac8f761be2e%7D_BMA_Report.pdf.

23. Susan Morse, "CMS Touts Medicare Advantage Plans Ahead of October 15 Open Enrollment," *Healthcare Finance*, September 28, 2018, https://www.healthcare-financenews.com/news/cms-touts-medicare-advantage-plans-ahead-october-15 -open-enrollment; Tricia Neuman, "Traditional Medicare . . . Disadvantaged?," Kaiser Family Foundation, March 31, 2016, https://www.kff.org/medicare/perspective /traditional-medicare-disadvantaged.

24. Centers for Medicare and Medicaid Services, "Medicare Physician Group Practice Demonstration: Physicians Groups Continue to Improve Quality and Generate Savings under Medicare Physician Pay-for-Performance Demonstration" (fact sheet), July 2011, https://innovation.cms.gov/Files/fact-sheet/PGP-Fact-Sheet.pdf.

25. Elliott S. Fisher, Mark B. McClellan, John Bertko, Steven M. Lieberman, Julie J. Lee, Julie L. Lewis, and Jonathan S. Skinner, "Fostering Accountable Health Care: Moving Forward in Medicare," *Health Affairs* 28, no. 2 (2009): w219-w231, doi:10.1377/hlthaff.28.2.w219.

26. Donald M. Berwick, Thomas W. Nolan, and John Whittington, "The Triple Aim: Care, Health, and Cost," *Health Affairs* 27, no. 3 (2008): 759–69, doi:10.1377 /hlthaff.27.3.759.

27. Centers for Medicare and Medicaid Services, "Medicare Program; Medicare Shared Savings Program; Accountable Care Organizations—Pathways to Success and Extreme and Uncontrollable Circumstances Policies for Performance Year 2017," *Federal Register* 83, no. 249 (2018): 67816–68082, https://www.govinfo.gov/content /pkg/FR-2018-12-31/pdf/2018-27981.pdf.

28. Tianna Tu, David Muhlestein, S. Lawrence Kocot, and Ross White, "The Impact of Accountable Care: Origins and Future of Accountable Care Organizations" (issue brief), Leavitt Partners, May 2015, https://leavittpartners.com/the-impact-of -accountable-care.

29. David Peiris, Madeleine C. Phipps-Taylor, Courtney A. Stachowski, Lee-Sien Kao, Stephen M. Shortell, Valerie A. Lewis, Meredith B. Rosenthal, and Carrie H. Colla, "ACOs Holding Commercial Contracts Are Larger and More Efficient than Noncommercial ACOs," *Health Affairs* 35, no. 10 (2016): 1849–56, doi:10.1377/hlthaff .2016.0387.

30. Jacqueline LaPointe, "MSSP ACOs Improve Care Quality, Struggle to Realize Savings," *RevCycle Intelligence*, November 27, 2017, https://revcycleintelligence.com /news/mssp-acos-improve-care-quality-struggle-to-realize-savings.

31. Adam A. Markovitz, John M. Hollingsworth, John Z. Ayanian, Edward C. Norton, Phyllis L. Yan, and Andrew M. Ryan, "Performance in the Medicare Shared Savings Program After Accounting for Nonrandom Exit," *Annals of Internal Medicine* 171, no. 1 (2019): 27–36, doi:10.7326/m18-2539.

32. Jacqueline LaPointe, "71% of MSSP ACOs Likely to Quit Rather than Assume Downside Risk," *RevCycle Intelligence*, May 4, 2018, https://revcycleintelligence.com /news/71-of-mssp-acos-likely-to-quit-rather-than-assume-downside-risk.

33. Francis J. Crosson, Kate Bloniarz, David Glass, and James Mathews, "MedPAC's Urgent Recommendation: Eliminate MIPS, Take a Different Direction," *Health Affairs* blog, March 16, 2018, https://www.healthaffairs.org/do/10.1377/hblog 20180309.302220/full.

34. *2018 Annual Report of the Boards of Trustees of the Federal Hospital Insurance and Federal Supplementary Medical Insurance Trust Funds*, 7.

11. Medicaid

1. Wilbur J. Cohen and Robert J. Myers, "Social Security Act Amendments of 1950: A Summary and Legislative History," In-Depth Research, Social Security Administration, accessed December 16, 2018, https://www.ssa.gov/history/1950 amend.html.

2. Judith D. Moore and David G. Smith, "Legislating Medicaid: Considering Medicaid and Its Origins," *Health Care Financing Review* 27, no. 2 (2005): 45–52.

3. "HHS Poverty Guidelines for 2018," Office of the Assistant Secretary for Planning and Evaluation, US Department of Health and Human Services, accessed October 23, 2018, https://aspe.hhs.gov/poverty-guidelines.

4. "Medicaid Waiver Tracker: Approved and Pending Section 1115 Waivers by State," Kaiser Family Foundation, March 1, 2019, accessed March 5, 2019, https:// www.kff.org/medicaid/issue-brief/medicaid-waiver-tracker-approved-and-pending -section-1115-waivers-by-state/#Table2.

5. Sandhya Raman, "States Grapple with Medicaid Work Requirments," *Roll Call*, July 9, 2019, https://www.rollcall.com/news/congress/states-grapple-medicaid -work-requirements.

6. Robin Rudowitz and Rachel Garfield, "10 Things to Know about Medicaid: Setting the Facts Straight" (issue brief), Kaiser Family Foundation, published April 12, 2018, updated March 2019, accessed December 12, 2018, https://www.kff.org /medicaid/issue-brief/10-things-to-know-about-medicaid-setting-the-facts -straight.

7. "Federal Medicaid Assistance Percentage (FMAP) for Medicaid and Multiplier," Kaiser Family Foundation, accessed April 7, 2019, https://www.kff.org/medicaid/state-indicator/federal-matching-rate-and-multiplier.

8. "Federal Medicaid Assistance Percentage (FMAP) for Medicaid and Multiplier," Kaiser Family Foundation.

9. MACPAC, *Medicaid Base and Supplemental Payments to Hospitals* (Washington, DC: Medicaid and CHIP Payment and Access Commission, March 2019), https://www.macpac.gov/wp-content/uploads/2018/06/Medicaid-Base-and-Supplemental-Payments-to-Hospitals.pdf.

10. MACPAC, *Medicaid Base and Supplemental Payments to Hospitals*, 4.

11. MACPAC, *Medicaid Base and Supplemental Payments to Hospitals*, 5.

12. MACPAC, *Medicaid Base and Supplemental Payments to Hospitals*, Appendix A.

13. Robert Nelb, James Teisl, Allen Dobson, Joan E. DaVanzo, and Lane Koenig, "For Disproportionate-Share Hospitals, Taxes and Fees Curtail Medicaid Payments," *Health Affairs* 35, no. 12 (2016): 2277–81, doi:10.1377/hlthaff.2016.0602.

14. Nelb et al., "For Disproportionate-Share Hospitals," Appendix B, https://www.healthaffairs.org/doi/suppl/10.1377/hlthaff.2016.0602/suppl_file/2016-0602_nelb_appendix.pdf.

15. "Medicaid-to-Medicare Fee Index, 2016," State Health Facts, Kaiser Family Foundation, https://www.kff.org/medicaid/state-indicator/medicaid-to-medicare-fee-index.

16. Peter Ubel, "Why Many Physicians Are Reluctant to See Medicaid Patients," *Forbes*, November 7, 2013, https://www.forbes.com/sites/peterubel/2013/11/07/why-many-physicians-are-reluctant-to-see-medicaid-patients/#7518863d1045.

17. Sandra L. Decker, "In 2011 Nearly One-Third of Physicians Said They Would Not Accept New Medicaid Patients, but Rising Fees May Help," *Health Affairs* 31, no. 8 (2012): 1673–79, doi:10.1377/hlthaff.2012.0294.

18. John Holahan, Teresa Coughlin, Leighton Ku, Debra J. Lipson, and Shruti Rajan, "Insuring the Poor Through Section 1115 Medicaid Waivers," *Health Affairs* 14, no. 1 (1995): 199–216, doi:10.1377/hlthaff.14.1.199.

19. Robert E. Hurley and Stephen A. Somers, "Medicaid and Managed Care: A Lasting Relationship?," *Health Affairs* 22, no. 1 (2003): 77–88, doi:10.1377/hlthaff.22.1.77.

20. Mathematica Policy Research, *Medicaid Managed Care Enrollment and Program Characteristics, 2016* (Washington, DC: Centers for Medicare and Medicaid Services, 2018), https://www.medicaid.gov/medicaid/managed-care/downloads/enrollment/2016-medicaid-managed-care-enrollment-report.pdf.

21. Jeff Goldsmith, David Mosley, and Anne Jacobs, "Medicaid Managed Care: Lots of Unanswered Questions (Part 1)," *Health Affairs* blog, May 3, 2018, https://www.healthaffairs.org/do/10.1377/hblog20180430.387981/full.

12. The Affordable Care Act

1. Carmen DeNavas-Walt, Bernadette D. Proctor, and Jessica C. Smith, *Income, Poverty, and Health Insurance Coverage in the United States: 2010*, US Census Bureau Current Population Reports (Washington, DC: US Government Printing Office, 2011), 60–239, https://www.census.gov/prod/2011pubs/p60-239.pdf.

2. Steven Brill, *America's Bitter Pill: Money, Politics, Backroom Deals, and the Fight to Fix Our Broken Healthcare System* (New York: Random House, 2015).

3. "Summary of the Affordable Care Act," Kaiser Family Foundation, April 15, 2013, https://www.kff.org/health-reform/fact-sheet/summary-of-the-affordable-care-act.

4. Barack Obama, "United States Health Care Reform: Progress to Date and Next Steps," *JAMA* 316, no. 5 (2016): 525–32.

5. Edward R. Berchick, Jessica C. Barnett, and Rachel D. Upton, *Health Insurance Coverage in the United States: 2018*, US Census Bureau Current Population Reports (Washington, DC: US Government Printing Office, 2019), 2, https://www.census.gov/content/dam/Census/library/publications/2019/demo/p60-267.pdf.

6. Carmen DeNavas-Walt, Bernadette D. Proctor, and Jessica C. Smith, *Income, Poverty, and Health Insurance Coverage in the United States: 2011*, US Census Bureau Current Population Reports (Washington, DC: US Government Printing Office, 2012), 60–243, http://sfes.info/IMG/pdf/income_poverty_and_health_insurance_coverage_in_usa_2011.pdf.

7. "Selected Characteristics of the Uninsured in the United States: 2017 American Community Survey 1-Year Estimates," American Fact Finder, US Census Bureau, accessed Oct. 27, 2018, https://factfinder.census.gov/faces/tableservices/jsf/pages/productview.xhtml?pid=ACS_17_1YR_S2702&prodType=table.

8. "Women and the Health Care Law in the United States" (fact sheet), National Women's Law Center, May 16, 2013, https://nwlc.org/resources/women-and-health-care-law-united-states.

9. Institute of Medicine, *Essential Health Benefits: Balancing Coverage and Cost* (Washington, DC: National Academies Press, 2012), xi.

10. Sabrina Corlette, Kevin W. Lucia, and Max Levin, "Implementing the Affordable Care Act: Choosing an Essential Health Benefits Benchmark Plan," *Realizing Health Reform's Potential*, Commonwealth Fund pub. 1677, vol. 15 (March 2013), https://www.commonwealthfund.org/sites/default/files/documents/___media_files_publications_issue_brief_2013_mar_1677_corlette_implementing_aca_choosing_essential_hlt_benefits_reform_brief.pdf.

11. Justin Giovannelli, Kevin W. Lucia, and Sabrina Corlette, "Implementing the Affordable Care Act: Revisiting the ACA's Essential Health Benefits," *Realizing Health Reform's Potential*, Commonwealth Fund pub. 1783, vol. 28 (October 2014), https://www.commonwealthfund.org/sites/default/files/documents/___media_files_publications_issue_brief_2014_oct_1783_giovannelli_implementing_aca_essential_hlt_benefits_rb.pdf.

12. "Health Insurance Exchanges 2018 Open Enrollment Period Final Report" (fact sheet), Centers for Medicare and Medicaid Services, April 3, 2018, https://www

.cms.gov/newsroom/fact-sheets/health-insurance-exchanges-2018-open-enrollment
-period-final-report.

13. Stuart M. Butler, *Assuring Affordable Health Care for All Americans*, The
Heritage Lectures, no. 218 (Washington, DC: Heritage Foundation, 1989), 6, https://
healthcarereform.procon.org/sourcefiles/1989_assuring_affordable_health_care_for
_all_americans.pdf.

14. Stuart M. Butler, ed., *A Heritage Foundation Conference: Is Tax Reform the
Key to Health Care Reform?*, The Heritage Lectures, no. 298 (Washington, DC:
Heritage Foundation, 1991), 16, https://www.heritage.org/health-care-reform/report
/tax-reform-the-key-health-care-reform.

15. Stuart M. Butler, "Don't Blame Heritage for Obamacare Mandate," Heritage
Foundation, February 6, 2012, https://www.heritage.org/health-care-reform/commen
tary/dont-blame-heritage-obamacare-mandate.

16. James Taranto, "Heritage Rewrites History," *WSJ Opinion*, February 8, 2012,
https://www.wsj.com/articles/heritage-rewrites-history-1383157826.

17. Christine Eibner and Sarah Nowak, *The Effect of Eliminating the Individual
Mandate Penalty and the Role of Behavioral Factors* (New York: Commonwealth
Fund, July 2018), https://www.commonwealthfund.org/publications/fund-reports/2018
/jul/eliminating-individual-mandate-penalty-behavioral-factors.

18. K.K. Rebecca Lai and Alicia Parlapiano, "Millions Pay the Obamacare Penalty
Instead of Buying Insurance. Who Are They?," *New York Times*, November 28, 2017,
https://www.nytimes.com/interactive/2017/11/28/us/politics/obamacare-individual
-mandate-penalty-maps.html.

19. Sarah Kliff, "This Princeton Health Economist Thinks Obamacare's Marketplaces Are Doomed," *Vox*, August 25, 2016, https://www.vox.com/2016/8/25
/12630214/obamacare-marketplaces-death-spiral.

20. "Poll: Survey of the Non-Group Market Finds Most Say the Individual
Mandate Was Not a Major Reason They Got Coverage in 2018, and Most Plan to
Continue Buying Insurance Despite Recent Repeal of the Mandate Penalty," Kaiser
Family Foundation, April 3, 2018, https://www.kff.org/health-reform/press-release
/poll-most-non-group-enrollees-plan-to-buy-insurance-despite-repeal-of-individual
-mandate-penalty.

21. State of Texas et al. v. United States et al. No. 19-10011 (5th Cir. 2019),
http://www.ca5.uscourts.gov/opinions/pub/19/19-10011-CV0.pdf.

22. Department of Labor, Employee Benefits Security Administration, "Definition of 'Employer' under Section 3(5) of ERISA—Association Health Plans," *Federal
Register* 83, no. 120 (2018): 28912–64, https://www.gpo.gov/fdsys/pkg/FR-2018-06
-21/pdf/2018-12992.pdf.

23. Departments of Treasury, Labor, and Health and Human Services, "Short-
Term, Limited-Duration Insurance," *Federal Register* 83, no. 150 (2018): 38212–43,
https://www.gpo.gov/fdsys/pkg/FR-2018-08-03/pdf/2018-16568.pdf.

24. Department of Labor, "Definition of 'Employer,'" 28912.

25. Rabah Kamal, Cynthia Cox, Rachel Fehr, Marco Ramirez, Katherine
Horstman, and Larry Levitt, "How Repeal of the Individual Mandate and Expansion
of Loosely Regulated Plans Are Affecting 2019 Premiums" (issue brief), Kaiser Family

Foundation, October 26, 2018, https://www.kff.org/health-costs/issue-brief
/how-repeal-of-the-individual-mandate-and-expansion-of-loosely-regulated-plans-are
-affecting-2019-premiums.

26. National Association of Insurance Commissioners, *2017 Accident and Health
Policy Experience Report* (Washington, DC: NAIC, 2018), https://www.naic.org
/prod_serv/AHP-LR-18.pdf.

27. Mark Hall, *Stabilizing and Strengthening the Individual Health Insurance
Market: A View from Ten States*, USC-Brookings Schaeffer Initiative for Health Policy
(Washington, DC: Brookings Institution, 2018), https://www.brookings.edu/wp
-content/uploads/2018/07/Stabilizing-and-Strenghtening-the-Individual-Health
-Insurance-Market2.pdf.

28. Congressional Budget Office, *Repealing the Individual Health Insurance
Mandate: An Updated Estimate* (Washington, DC: Congressional Budget Office,
2017), 3, https://www.cbo.gov/system/files/115th-congress-2017-2018/reports/53300
-individualmandate.pdf.

29. Ashley Kirzinger, Bianca DiJulio, Cailey Munana, and Mollyann Brodie,
"Kaiser Health Tracking Poll—November 2017: The Role of Health Care in the Republican Tax Plan," Kaiser Family Foundation, November 15, 2017, https://www.kff.org
/health-reform/poll-finding/kaiser-health-tracking-poll-november-2017-the-role-of
-health-care-in-the-republican-tax-plan.

30. Fritz Busch and Paul R. Houchens, "The Individual Mandate Repeal: Will It
Matter?" (white paper), Milliman, March 1, 2018, http://www.milliman.com
/uploadedFiles/insight/2018/will-individual-mandate-repeal-matter.pdf.

31. Eibner and Nowak, *The Effect of Eliminating the Individual Mandate Penalty.*

32. Hall, *Stabilizing and Strengthening the Individual Health Insurance Market.*

33. Cynthia Cox, Rachel Fehr, and Larry Levitt, "Individual Insurance Market
Performance in 2018," Kaiser Family Foundation, May 7, 2019, https://www.kff.org
/private-insurance/issue-brief/individual-insurance-market-performance-in-2018.

34. Samantha Liss, "ACA Market Continues to Lose Those Who Don't Qualify for
Financial Help," *HealthCareDive*, August 13, 2019, https://www.healthcaredive.com
/news/aca-market-continues-to-lose-those-who-dont-qualify-for-financial-help/560755.

35. Kevin Griffith, David K. Jones, and Benjamin D. Sommers, "Diminishing
Insurance Choices in the Affordable Care Act Marketplaces: A County-Based
Analysis," *Health Affairs* 37, no. 10 (2018): 1678–84, doi:10.1377/hlthaff.2018.0701.

36. Griffith, Jones, and Sommers, "Diminishing Insurance Choices."

37. Robin Rudowitz and Larisa Antonisse, "Implications of the ACA Medicaid
Expansion: A Look at the Data and Evidence" (issue brief), Kaiser Family Foundation, May 23, 2018, https://www.kff.org/medicaid/issue-brief/implications-of-the
-aca-medicaid-expansion-a-look-at-the-data-and-evidence.

38. Obama, "United States Health Care Reform."

39. Elizabeth Hinton, MaryBeth Musumeci, Robin Rudowitz, Larisa Antonisse,
and Cornelia Hall, "Section 1115 Medicaid Demonstration Waivers: The Current
Landscape of Approved and Pending Waivers" (issue brief), Kaiser Family Foundation,
February 12, 2019, https://www.kff.org/medicaid/issue-brief/section-1115-medicaid
-demonstration-waivers-the-current-landscape-of-approved-and-pending-waivers.

40. "Medicaid Waiver Tracker: Approved and Pending Section 1115 Waivers by State," Kaiser Family Foundation, updated December 4, 2019, https://www.kff.org /medicaid/issue-brief/medicaid-waiver-tracker-approved-and-pending-section-1115-wai vers-by-state/#Table2.

41. Jennifer Wagner, "New Arkansas Data Contradict Claims that Most Who Lost Medicaid Found Jobs," *Off the Charts* (blog), Center on Budget and Policy Priorities, March 19, 2019, https://www.cbpp.org/blog/new-arkansas-data-contradict-claims -that-most-who-lost-medicaid-found-jobs.

42. Douglas W. Elmendorf, "Estimating the Budgetary Effects of the Affordable Care Act," Congressional Budget Office blog, June 17, 2014, https://www.cbo.gov /publication/45447

43. Elmendorf, "Estimating the Budgetary Effects."

44. Congressional Budget Office, *CBO's Record of Projecting Subsidies for Health Insurance under the Affordable Care Act: 2014 to 2016* (Washington, DC: Congressional Budget Office, 2017), https://www.cbo.gov/system/files/115th-congress-2017-2018 /reports/53094-acaprojections.pdf.

13. Evidence-Based Practice

1. Quentin W. Smith, Richard L. Street, Robert J. Volk, and Michael Fordis, "Differing Levels of Clinical Evidence," *Medical Care Research and Review* 70, no. 1 Suppl (2012): 3S–13S. doi:10.1177/1077558712468491.

2. Tammy C. Hoffmann and Chris Del Mar, "Clinicians' Expectations of the Benefits and Harms of Treatments, Screening, and Tests," *JAMA Internal Medicine* 177, no. 3 (2017): 407–19, doi:10.1001/jamainternmed.2016.8254.

3. Eric Patashnik, Alan S. Gerber, and Conor M. Dowling, *Unhealthy Politics* (Princeton: Princeton University Press, 2017).

4. Elizabeth Barrett-Connor and Deborah Grady, "Hormone Replacement Therapy, Heart Disease and Other Considerations," *Annual Review of Public Health* 19, no. 1 (1998): 55–72, doi:10.1146/annurev.publhealth.19.1.55.

5. Adam L. Hersh, Marcia L. Stefanick, and Randall S. Stafford, "National Use of Postmenopausal Hormone Therapy: Annual Trends and Response to Recent Evidence," *JAMA* 291, no. 1 (2004): 47–53, doi:10.1001/jama.291.1.47.

6. David H. Kreling, David A. Mott, Joseph B. Wiederholt, Janet Lundy, and Larry Levitt, *Prescription Drug Trends: A Chartbook Update* (Menlo Park, CA: Kaiser Family Foundation, 2001), http://files.kff.org/attachment/report-prescription-drug -trends-a-chartbook-update.

7. Collaborative Group on Hormonal Factors in Breast Cancer, "Breast Cancer and Hormone Replacement Therapy: Collaborative Reanalysis of Data from 51 Epidemiological Studies of 52,705 Women with Breast Cancer and 108,411 Women without Breast Cancer," *The Lancet* 350, no. 9084 (1997): 1047–59, doi:10.1016 /s0140-6736(97)08233-0.

8. Stephen Hulley, Deborah Grady, Trudy Bush, Curt Furberg, David Herrington, Betty Riggs, and Eric Vittinghoff for the Heart and Estrogen/progestin Replacement Study (HERS) Research Group, "Randomized Trial of Estro-

gen Plus Progestin for Secondary Prevention of Coronary Heart Disease in Postmenopausal Women," *JAMA* 280, no. 7 (1998): 605–13, doi:10.1001/jama .280.7.605.

9. Writing Group for the Women's Health Initiative Investigators, "Risks and Benefits of Estrogen Plus Progestin in Healthy Postmenopausal Women: Principal Results from the Women's Health Initiative Randomized Controlled Trial," *JAMA* 288, no. 3 (2002): 321–33, doi:10.1001/jama.288.3.321.

10. Hersh, Stefanick, and Stafford, "National Use of Postmenopausal Hormone Therapy."

11. Rowan T. Chlebowski, Lewis H. Kuller, Ross L. Prentice, Marcia L. Stefanick, JoAnn E. Manson, Margery Gass, Aaron K. Aragaki et al., "Breast Cancer after Use of Estrogen Plus Progestin in Postmenopausal Women," *New England Journal of Medicine* 360, no. 6 (2009): 573–87, doi:10.1056/nejmoa0807684.

12. Graham A. Colditz, "Decline in Breast Cancer Incidence Due to Removal of Promoter: Combination Estrogen Plus Progestin," *Breast Cancer Research* 9, no. 4 (2007): article number 108, doi:10.1186/bcr1736.

13. Rowan T. Chlebowski, Thomas E. Rohan, JoAnn E. Manson, Aaron K. Aragaki, Andrew Kaunitz, Marcia L. Stefanick, Michael S. Simon et al., "Breast Cancer after Use of Estrogen Plus Progestin and Estrogen Alone," *JAMA Oncology* 1, no. 3 (2015): 296–305, doi:10.1001/jamaoncol.2015.0494.

14. JoAnn E. Manson, Aaron K. Aragaki, Jacques E. Rossouw, Garnet L. Anderson, Ross L. Prentice, Andrea Z. LaCroix, Rowan T. Chlebowski et al., "Menopausal Hormone Therapy and Long-Term All-Cause and Cause-Specific Mortality," *JAMA* 318, no. 10 (2017): 927–38, doi:10.1001/jama.2017.11217.

15. "The Experts Do Agree about Hormone Therapy," North American Menopause Society, accessed November 13, 2018, https://www.menopause.org/for-women /menopauseflashes/menopause-symptoms-and-treatments/the-experts-do-agree -about-hormone-therapy.

16. C. Anthony Blau, "E. Donnall Thomas, MD (1920–2012)," *Stem Cells* 31, no. 2 (2013): 221–22, doi:10.1002/stem.1311.

17. Michelle M. Mello and Troyen A. Brennan, "The Controversy over High-Dose Chemotherapy with Autologous Bone Marrow Transplant for Breast Cancer," *Health Affairs* 20, no. 5 (2001): 101–17, doi:10.1377/hlthaff.20.5.101.

18. Edward A. Stadtmauer, Anne O'Neill, Lori J. Goldstein, Pamela A. Crilley, Kenneth F. Mangan, James N. Ingle, Isadore Brodsky et al., "Conventional-Dose Chemotherapy Compared with High-Dose Chemotherapy Plus Autologous Hematopoietic Stem-Cell Transplantation for Metastatic Breast Cancer," *New England Journal of Medicine* 342, no. 15 (2000): 1069–76, doi:10.1056/nejm200004133421501.

19. Mello and Brennan, "The Controversy over High-Dose Chemotherapy."

20. David H. Howard, Carolyn Kenline, Hillard M. Lazarus, Charles F. LeMaistre, Richard T. Maziarz, Philip L. McCarthy Jr., Susan K. Parsons, David Szwajcer, James Douglas Rizzo, and Navneet S. Majhail, "Abandonment of High-Dose Chemotherapy / Hematopoietic Cell Transplants for Breast Cancer Following Negative Trial Results," *Health Services Research* 46, no. 6 Pt 1 (2011): 1762–77, doi:10.1111/j.1475-6773.2011.01296.x.

21. Marc E. Lippman, "High-Dose Chemotherapy Plus Autologous Bone Marrow Transplantation for Metastatic Breast Cancer," *New England Journal of Medicine* 342, no. 15 (2000): 1119–20, doi:10.1056/nejm200004133421508.

22. Howard et al., "Abandonment of High-Dose Chemotherapy."

23. Mello and Brennan, "The Controversy over High-Dose Chemotharapy."

24. Richard A. Rettig, Peter D. Jacobson, Cynthia M. Farquhar, and Wade M. Aubry, *False Hope: Bone Marrow Transplantation for Breast Cancer* (New York: Oxford University Press, 2007).

25. Sunny Kim, Jose Bosque, John P. Meehan, Amir Jamali, and Richard Marder, "Increase in Outpatient Knee Arthroscopy in the United States: A Comparison of National Surveys of Ambulatory Surgery, 1996 and 2006," *Journal of Bone and Joint Surgery-American Volume* 93, no. 11 (2011): 994–1000, doi:10.2106/jbjs.i.01618.

26. Nirav H. Amin, Waqas Hussain, John Ryan, Shannon Morrison, Anthony Miniaci, and Morgan H. Jones, "Changes within Clinical Practice after a Randomized Controlled Trial of Knee Arthroscopy for Osteoarthritis," *Orthopaedic Journal of Sports Medicine* 5, no. 4 (2017), doi:10.1177/2325967117698439.

27. J. Bruce Moseley, Kimberly O'Malley, Nancy J. Petersen, Terri J. Menke, Baruch A. Brody, David H. Kuykendall, John C. Hollingsworth, Carol M. Ashton, and Nelda P. Wray, "A Controlled Trial of Arthroscopic Surgery for Osteoarthritis of the Knee," *New England Journal of Medicine* 347, no. 2 (2002): 81–88, doi:10.1056/nejmoa013259.

28. Amin et al., "Changes within Clincal Pratice."

29. Ville M. Mattila, Raine Sihvonen, Juha Paloneva, and Li Felländer-Tsai, "Changes in Rates of Arthroscopy Due to Degenerative Knee Disease and Traumatic Meniscal Tears in Finland and Sweden," *Acta Orthopaedica* 87, no. 1 (2015): 5–11, doi:10.3109/17453674.2015.1066209.

30. Ian A. Harris, Navdeep S. Madan, Justine M. Naylor, Shanley Chong, Rajat Mittal, and Bin B. Jalaludin, "Trends in Knee Arthroscopy and Subsequent Arthroplasty in an Australian Population: A Retrospective Cohort Study," *BMC Musculoskeletal Disorders* 14, no. 1 (2013): 143–48, doi:10.1186/1471-2474-14-143.

31. Alexandra Kirkley, Trevor B. Birmingham, Robert B. Litchfield, J. Robert Giffin, Kevin R. Willits, Cindy J. Wong, Brian G. Feagan et al., "A Randomized Trial of Arthroscopic Surgery for Osteoarthritis of the Knee," *New England Journal of Medicine* 359, no. 11 (2008): 1097–107, doi:10.1056/nejmoa0708333.

32. Mattila et al., "Changes in Rates of Arthoscopy."

33. David H. Howard, "Trends in the Use of Knee Arthroscopy in Adults," *JAMA Internal Medicine* 178, no. 11 (2018): 1557–58, doi:10.1001/jamainternmed.2018.4175.

34. Aaron Potts, John J. Harrast, Christopher D. Harner, Anthony Miniaci, and Morgan H. Jones, "Practice Patterns for Arthroscopy of Osteoarthritis of the Knee in the United States," *American Journal of Sports Medicine* 40, no. 6 (2012): 1247–51, doi:10.1177/0363546512443946.

35. "Total/unicompartment knee arthroscopy per 1,000 Medicare beneficiaries with osteoarthritis/joint pain in the lower leg" (raw data file), Custom Atlas Rate Generator Rates, Dartmouth Atlas Data, accessed June 18, 2019, https://atlasdata.dartmouth.edu/static/custom_arg_rates.

36. David T. Felson, "Arthroscopy as a Treatment for Knee Osteoarthritis," *Best Practice & Research: Clinical Rheumatology* 24, no. 1 (2010): 47–50, doi:10.1016/j .berh.2009.08.002.

37. L. Stefan Lohmander, Jonas B. Thorlund, and Ewa M. Roos, "Routine Knee Arthroscopic Surgery for the Painful Knee in Middle-Aged and Old Patients—Time to Abandon Ship," *Acta Orthopaedica* 87, no. 1 (2015): 2–4, doi:10.3109/17453674.2015.11 24316.

38. Nina Jullum Kise, May Arna Risberg, Silje Stensrud, Jonas Ranstam, Lars Engebretsen, and Ewa M Roos, "Exercise Therapy versus Arthroscopic Partial Meniscectomy for Degenerative Meniscal Tear in Middle Aged Patients: Randomised Controlled Trial with Two Year Follow-Up," *BMJ* 354 (2016): i3740, doi:10.1136/bmj.i3740.

39. Reed A. C. Siemieniuk, Ian A. Harris, Thomas Agoritsas, Rudolf W. Poolman, Romina Brignardello-Petersen, Stijn Van de Velde, Rachelle Buchbinder, et al., "Arthroscopic Surgery for Degenerative Knee Arthritis and Meniscal Tears: A Clinical Practice Guideline," *BMJ* 357 (2017): j1982, doi:10.1136/bmj.j1982.

40. Ellen C. Keeley, Judith A. Boura, and Cindy L. Grines, "Primary Angioplasty versus Intravenous Thrombolytic Therapy for Acute Myocardial Infarction: A Quantitative Review of 23 Randomised Trials," *The Lancet* 361, no. 9351 (2003): 13–20, doi:10.1016/s0140-6736(03)12113-7.

41. Rita F. Redberg, "Informed Strategies for Treating Coronary Disease," *Archives of Internal Medicine* 172, no. 4 (2012): 321, doi:10.1001/archinternmed .2011.2313.

42. Eric J. Topol and Steven E. Nissen, "Our Preoccupation with Coronary Luminology," *Circulation* 92, no. 8 (1995): 2333–42, doi:10.1161/01.cir.92.8.2333.

43. William E. Boden, Robert A. O'Rourke, Koon K. Teo, Pamela M. Hartigan, David J. Maron, William J. Kostuk, Merril Knudtson, et al., "Optimal Medical Therapy with or without PCI for Stable Coronary Disease," *New England Journal of Medicine* 356, no. 15 (2007): 1503–16, doi:10.1056/nejmoa070829.

44. Kathleen Stergiopoulos and David Brown, "Initial Coronary Stent Implantation with Medical Therapy vs Medical Therapy Alone for Stable Coronary Artery Disease," *Archives of Internal Medicine* 172, no. 4 (2012): 312–19, doi:10.1001 /archinternmed.2011.1484.

45. Nicholas Bakalar, "No Extra Benefits Are Seen in Stents for Coronary Artery Disease, *New York Times*, February 27, 2002, https://www.nytimes.com/2012/02/28 /health/stents-show-no-extra-benefits-for-coronary-artery-disease.html.

46. David H. Howard and Yu-Chu Shen, "Trends in PCI Volume after Negative Results from the COURAGE Trial," *Health Services Research* 49, no. 1 (2013): 153–70, doi:10.1111/1475-6773.12082.

47. Frederick A. Masoudi, Angelo Ponirakis, James A. de Lemos, James G. Jollis, Mark Kremers, John C. Messenger, John W.M. Moore, et al., "Trends in US Cardiovascular Care: 2016 Report from 4 ACC National Cardiovascular Data Registries," *Journal of the American College of Cardiology* 69, no. 11 (2017): 1427–50, doi:10.1016 /j.jacc.2016.12.005.

48. Elizabeth A., McGlynn, Steven M. Asch, John Adams, Joan Keesey, Jennifer Hicks, Alison DeCristofaro, and Eve A. Kerr, "The Quality of Health Care Delivered

to Adults in the United States," *New England Journal of Medicine* 348, no. 26 (2003): 2635–45, doi:10.1056/nejmsa022615.

49. "Less Is More," *JAMA Internal Medicine* article series, accessed November 18, 2018, https://jamanetwork.com/collections/44045/less-is-more.

50. For example: Shannon Brownlee, *Overtreated: Why Too Much Medicine Is Making Us Sicker and Poorer* (New York: Bloomsbury USA, 2008); John Abramson, *Overdosed America: The Broken Promise of American Medicine* (New York: HarperCollins, 2008); H. Gilbert Welch, *Less Medicine, More Health* (Boston: Beacon Press, 2015).

51. Atul Gawande, "Overkill," *New Yorker*, May 11, 2015, https://www.newyorker.com/magazine/2015/05/11/overkill-atul-gawande.

52. Roger Chou, Rongwei Fu, John A. Carrino, and Richard A. Deyo, "Imaging Strategies for Low-Back Pain: Systematic Review and Meta-Analysis," *The Lancet* 373, no. 9662 (2009): 463–72, doi:10.1016/s0140-6736(09)60172-0.

53. Stephanie G. Wheeler, Joyce E. Wipf, Thomas O. Staiger, Richard A. Deyo, and Jeffrey G. Jarvik, "Evaluation of Low Back Pain in Adults," *UpToDate*, July 12, 2018, https://www.uptodate.com/contents/evaluation-of-low-back-pain-in-adults.

54. Daniel C. Cherkin, Richard A. Deyo, John D. Loeser, Terry Bush, and Gordon Waddell, "An International Comparison of Back Surgery Rates," *Spine* 19, no. 11 (1994): 1201–6, doi:10.1097/00007632-199405310-00001.

55. James N. Weinstein, Jon D. Lurie, Patrick R. Olson, Kristen K. Bronner, and Elliott S. Fisher, "United States' Trends and Regional Variations in Lumbar Spine Surgery: 1992–2003," *Spine* 31, no. 23 (2006): 2707–14, doi:10.1097/01.brs.0000248132.15231.fe.

14. Cost-Benefit, Cost-Effectiveness, and Cost-Utility Analysis

1. D. Pearce, "Cost Benefit Analysis and Environmental Policy," *Oxford Review of Economic Policy* 14, no. 4 (1998): 84–100, doi:10.1093/oxrep/14.4.84.

2. Burton A. Weisbrod, *Economics of Public Health* (Philadelphia: University of Pennsylvania Press, 1961).

3. David M. Cutler and Ellen Meara, "The Technology of Birth: Is It Worth It?," in *Frontiers in Health Policy Research 3,* National Bureau of Economic Research Series, ed. Alan M. Garber (Cambridge: MIT Press, 2000), 33–68.

4. David Cutler, *Your Money or Your Life: Strong Medicine for America's Health Care System* (New York: Oxford University Press, 2004).

5. Richard H. Morrow and John H. Bryant, "Health Policy Approaches to Measuring and Valuing Human Life: Conceptual and Ethical Issues," *American Journal of Public Health* 85, no. 10 (1995): 1356–60, doi:10.2105/ajph.85.10.1356.

6. Richard A. Hirth, Michael E. Chernew, Edward Miller, A. Mark Fendrick, and William G. Weissert, "Willingness to Pay for a Quality-Adjusted Life Year," *Medical Decision Making* 20, no. 3 (2000): 332–42, doi:10.1177/0272989x0002000310.

7. "Executive Order 12866," Regulatory Resource Center, Center for Effective Government, accessed November 20, 2018, https://www.foreffectivegov.org/node/2560.

8. "Guidelines and Discount Rates for Benefit-Cost Analysis of Federal Programs," Circular No. A-94, White House Office of Management and Budget, accessed November 20, 2018, https://www.whitehouse.gov/sites/whitehouse.gov/files/omb/circulars/A94/a094.pdf.

9. Molly J. Moran, "Guidance on Treatment of the Economic Value of a Statistical Live (VSL) in US Department of Transportation Analyses—2016 Adjustment" (memorandum), US Department of Transportation, Office of the Secretary of Transportation, accessed November 18, 2018, https://www.transportation.gov/office-policy/transportation-policy/revised-departmental-guidance-on-valuation-of-a-statistical-life-in-economic-analysis.

10. "Mortality Risk Valuation," Environmental Protection Agency, accessed November 18, 2018, https://www.epa.gov/environmental-economics/mortality-risk-valuation#means.

11. Richard Thaler and Sherwin Rosen, "The Value of Saving a Life: Evidence from the Labor Market," in *Household Production and Consumption*, Studies in Income and Wealth, ed. Nestor E. Terleckyj (New York: National Bureau of Economic Research, 1976), 265–302, https://www.nber.org/chapters/c3964.pdf.

12. CPI Inflation Calculator, US Bureau of Labor Statistics, accessed November 22, 2018, https://www.bls.gov/data/inflation_calculator.htm.

13. Peter J. Neumann, Theodore G. Ganiats, Louise B. Russell, Gillian D. Sanders, and Joanna E. Siegel, *Cost-Effectiveness in Health and Medicine*, 2nd ed. (New York: Oxford University Press, 2017).

14. Herbert E. Klarman, John Francis, and Gerald D. Rosenthal, "Cost Effectiveness Analysis Applied to the Treatment of Chronic Renal Disease," *Medical Care* 6, no. 1 (1968): 48–54, doi:10.1097/00005650-196801000-00005.

15. David A. Pettitt, S. Raza, B. Naughton, A. Roscoe, A. Ramakrishnan, A. Ali, B. Davies, et al., "The Limitations of QALY: A Literature Review," *Journal of Stem Cell Research & Therapy* 6, no. 4 (2016): 334, doi:10.4172/2157-7633.1000334.

16. Gerard Duru, Jean Paul Auray, Ariel Bresniak, Michel Lamure, Abby Paine, and Nicolas Nicoloyannis, "Limitations of the Methods Used for Calculating Quality-Adjusted Life-Year Values," *Pharmacoeconomics* 20, no. 7 (2002): 463–73, doi:10.2165/00019053-200220070-00004.

17. Wolfgang C. Winkelmayer, Milton C. Weinstein, Murray A. Mittleman, Robert J. Glynn, and Joseph S. Pliskin, "Health Economic Evaluations: The Special Case of End-Stage Renal Disease Treatment," *Medical Decision Making* 22, no. 5 (2002): 417–30, doi:10.1177/027298902236927.

18. Chris P. Lee, Glenn M. Chertow, and Stefanos A. Zenios, "An Empiric Estimate of the Value of Life: Updating the Renal Dialysis Cost-Effectiveness Standard," *Value in Health* 12, no. 1 (2009): 80–87, doi:10.1111/j.1524-4733.2008.00401.x.

19. Raymond Hutubessy, Dan Chisholm, Tessa Tan-Torres Edejer, and WHO-CHOICE, "Generalized Cost-Effectiveness Analysis for National-Level Priority-Setting in the Health Sector," *Cost Effectiveness and Resource Allocation* 1 (2003): article no. 8, doi:10.1186/1478-7547-1-8.

20. "Guide to the Methods of Technology Appraisal 2013," National Institute for Health and Care Excellence, published April 2013, https://www.nice.org.uk/process/pmg9/chapter/the-appraisal-of-the-evidence-and-structured-decision-making.

21. "Technology Appraisal Data: Appraisal Recommendations," National Institute for Health and Care Excellence, accessed January 19, 2020, https://www.nice.org.uk/about/what-we-do/our-programmes/nice-guidance/nice-technology-appraisal-guidance/data/appraisal-recommendations.

22. "Technology Appraisal Data: Appraisal Recommendations," Excel document file, Recommendation No. 840.

23. "Technology Appraisal Data: Appraisal Recommendations," Excel document file, Recommendation No. 842.

24. Mike Paulden, "Recent Amendments to NICE's Value-Based Assessment of Health Technologies: Implicitly Inequitable?," *Expert Review of Pharmacoeconomics & Outcomes Research* 17, no. 3 (2017): 239–42, doi:10.1080/14737167.2017.1330152.

25. Karl Claxton, Steve Martin, Marta Soares, Nigel Rice, Eldon Spackman, Sebastian Hinde, Nancy Devlin, Peter C. Smith, and Mark Sculpher, "Methods for the Estimation of the National Institute for Health and Care Excellence Cost-Effectiveness Threshold," *Health Technology Assessment* 19, no. 14 (2015): 1–504, doi:10.3310/hta19140.

26. Sir Andrew Dillon, "Carrying NICE over the Threshold," National Institute for Health and Care Excellence blog, February 19, 2015, https://www.nice.org.uk/news/blog/carrying-nice-over-the-threshold.

27. Institute for Clinical and Economic Review, "ICER Value Framework: Overview of Conceptual Elements and Procedures Related to Value Assessment Reports and Appraisal Committee Voting at Public Meetings" (presentation slides), January 2018, http://icer-review.org/wp-content/uploads/2018/05/ICER-value-framework-v1-21-18.pdf.

28. Caroline Humer, "CVS Drug Coverage Plan Based on Outside Pricing Review Is Off to a Slow Start," *Reuters Health News*, October 3, 2019, https://www.reuters.com/article/us-cvs-health-drugpricing-focus/cvs-drug-coverage-plan-based-on-outside-pricing-review-is-off-to-a-slow-start-idUSKBN1WI2IO.

29. Congressional Budget Office, *Research on the Comparative Effectiveness of Medical Treatments: Issues and Options for an Expanded Federal Role*, report prepared by Philip Ellis with contributions from Colin Baker and Morgan Hanger (Washington, DC: CBO, December 2007), 3, https://www.cbo.gov/sites/default/files/110th-congress-2007-2008/reports/12-18-comparativeeffectiveness.pdf.

30. Congressional Budget Office, *Research on the Comparative Effectiveness of Medical Treatments*, iii.

31. Health Care Financing Administration, "Medicare Program; Criteria for Making Coverage Decisions," *Federal Register* 65, no. 95 (2000): 31124–29, https://www.govinfo.gov/content/pkg/FR-2000-05-16/pdf/00-12237.pdf.

32. Patient Protection and Affordable Care Act, H.R. 3590, 111th Cong. (2010), 623, https://www.gpo.gov/fdsys/pkg/BILLS-111hr3590enr/pdf/BILLS-111hr3590enr.pdf#page=623.

33. Joseph Selby, "PCORI: History, Goals, Challenges, Potential Impact on Treatment Development," presented February 19, 2013, at the International Society for CNS Trials and Methodology (ISCTM) Annual Scientific Meeting, https://isctm .org/public_access/Feb_2013/presentations/19Feb2013_1045_Selby.pdf.

34. Tom Allen, "A Policymaker's Perspective on Comparative Effectiveness Research: History and Prospects," *Health Affairs* blog, October 11, 2018, https://www .healthaffairs.org/do/10.1377/hblog20181003.112848/full/.

35. Eric M. Patashnik, Alan S. Gerber, and Conor M. Dowling, *Unhealthy Politics: The Battle over Evidence-Based Medicine* (Princeton, NJ: Princeton University Press, 2017), 3.

36. Patashnik, Gerber, and Dowling, *Unhealthy Politics*, 9.

37. Patashnik, Gerber, and Dowling, *Unhealthy Politics*, 10–18.

15. Health Care Law

1. Malcolm Sparrow, *License to Steal: How Fraud Bleeds America's Health Care System* (Boulder: Westview Press, 2000), 39.

2. LexisNexis Health Care, "Bending the Cost Curve: Analytics-Driven Enterprise Fraud Control" (white paper), accessed February 27, 2019, http://lexisnexis.com /risk/downloads/idm/bending-the-cost-curve-analytic-driven-enterprise-fraud -control.pdf.

3. Margit Sommersguter-Reichmann, Claudia Wild, Adolf Stepan, Gerhard Reichmann, and Andrea Fried "Individual and Institutional Corruption in European and US Healthcare: Overview and Link of Various Corruption Typologies," *Applied Health Economics and Health Policy* 16, no. 3 (2018): 289–302.

4. 31 U.S.C. § 3739(d)(2) (1988).

5. 31 U.S.C. § 3729(a), 28 C.F.R. 85.3(a)(9).

6. Sheppard Mullin, "The 2017 Department of Justice False Claims Act Recovery Statistics," *Healthcare Law Blog*, January 22, 2018, https://www.sheppardhealthlaw .com/2018/01/articles/false-claims-act/the-2017-department-of-justice-false-claims -act-recovery-statistics.

7. 31 U.S.C. § 3729(a).

8. 42 U.S.C. § 1320a–7b.

9. *United States v. Greber*, 760 F.2d 68 (3rd Cir. 1985).

10. Section 1128B of the Social Security Act (42 USC 1320a–7b).

11. American Hospital Association, *Regulatory Overload: Assessing the Regulatory Burden on Health Systems, Hospitals, and Post-Acute Care Providers* (Chicago; Washington, DC: American Hospital Association, October 2017), https://www.aha .org/guidesreports/2017-11-03-regulatory-overload-report.

12. Sally Quinlan Yates, "Individual Accountability for Corporate Wrongdoing" (memorandum), US Department of Justice, Office of the Assistant Attorney General, September 9, 2015, https://www.justice.gov/archives/dag/file/769036/download.

13. "Hospital Chain Will Pay Over $513 Million for Defrauding the United States and Making Illegal Payments in Exchange for Patient Referrals" (press release), Justice

News, Office of Public Affairs, US Department of Justice, October 3, 2016, https://www.justice.gov/opa/pr/hospital-chain-will-pay-over-513-million-defrauding-united-states-and-making-illegal-payments.

14. "Medical Equipment Company Will Pay $646 Million for Making Illegal Payments to Doctors and Hospitals" (press release), Justice News, Office of Public Affairs, US Department of Justice, March 1, 2016, https://www.justice.gov/opa/pr/medical-equipment-company-will-pay-646-million-making-illegal-payments-doctors-and-hospitals.

15. Office of the Inspector General, US Department of Health and Human Services, "Medicare and State Health Care Programs: Fraud and Abuse; Request for Information Regarding the Anti-Kickback Statute and Beneficiary Inducements CMP," *Federal Register* 83, no. 166 (2018): 43607–11, https://www.federalregister.gov/documents/2018/08/27/2018-18519/medicare-and-state-health-care-programs-fraud-and-abuse-request-for-information-regarding-the.

16. Martin A. Makary, William E. Bruhn, and Elizabeth A. Fracica, "Group Purchasing Organizations, Health Care Costs, and Drug Shortages," *JAMA* 320, no. 18 (2018): 1859, doi:10.1001/jama.2018.13604.

17. Joe Carlson, "Pete Stark: Repeal the Stark Law," *Modern Healthcare*, August 2, 2013, https://www.modernhealthcare.com/article/20130802/BLOG/308029995/pete-stark-repeal-the-stark-law.

18. Carlson, "Pete Stark."

19. American Medical Association, *The Stark Law Rules of the Road* (Chicago: American Medical Association, 2011), https://coa.org/docs/LibraryofWebinars/AMAStarkLawRulesoftheRoad.pdf.

20. American Physical Therapy Association, comments to the Health Subcommittee of the House Committee on Ways and Means for a hearing titled "Modernizing Stark Law to Ensure the Successful Transition from Volume to Value in the Medicare Program, July 17, 2018, https://www.apta.org/uploadedFiles/APTAorg/Advocacy/Federal/Legislative_Issues/Self_Referral/Comments/APTAComments_StarkLaw.pdf.

21. American Health Lawyers Association (AHLA) Public Interest Committee, *A Public Policy Discussion: Taking the Measure of the Stark Law* (Washington, DC: AHLA), 2–3, accessed February 27, 2019, https://www.healthlawyers.org/hlresources/PI/ConvenerSessions/Documents/Stark%20White%20Paper.pdf.

22. AHLA Public Interest Committee, *A Public Policy Discussion*, 3.

23. "Fraud and Abuse Waivers," Centers for Medicare and Medicaid Services, last modified November 11, 2019, accessed February 27, 2019, https://www.cms.gov/medicare/fraud-and-abuse/physicianselfreferral/fraud-and-abuse-waivers.html.

24. David A. Ansell and Robert L. Schiff, "Patient Dumping: Status, Implications, and Policy Recommendations," *JAMA* 257, no. 11 (1987): 1500–1502, doi:10.1001/jama.1987.03390110076030.

25. Robert L. Schiff, David A. Ansell, James E. Schlosser, Ahamed H. Idris, Ann Morrison, and Steven Whitman, "Transfers to a Public Hospital: A Prospective Study of 467 Patients," *New England Journal of Medicine* 314, no. 9 (1986): 552–57, doi:10.1056/NEJM198602273140905.

26. Section 1867 of the Social Security Act [42 U.S.C. 1395dd].

27. 42 U.S.C. 1395dd(e).

28. 42 U.S.C. 1395dd(a)–(c).

29. 42 U.S.C. 1395dd(d).

30. 42 U.S.C. 1395dd(d)(2).

31. Nadia Zuabi, Larry Weiss, and Mark Langdorf, "Emergency Medical Treatment and Labor Act (EMTALA) 2002–15: Review of Office of Inspector General Patient Dumping Settlements," *Western Journal of Emergency Medicine* 17, no. 3 (2016): 245–51, doi:10.5811/westjem.2016.3.29705.

32. "The HIPAA Privacy Rule," Health Information Privacy, US Department of Health and Human Services, accessed March 1, 2019, https://www.hhs.gov/hipaa/for-professionals/privacy/index.html.

33. 45 C.F.R. § 160.103—Definitions.

34. 45 C.F.R. § 160.103—Definitions.

35. 45 C.F.R. 164.512(f)(2).

36. Institute of Medicine Committee on Health Research and the Privacy of Health Information, *Beyond the HIPAA Privacy Rule: Enhancing Privacy, Improving Health through Research*, ed. Sharyl J. Nass, Laura A. Levit, and Lawrence O. Gostin (Washington, DC: National Academies Press, 2009), 2.

37. Institute of Medicine, *Beyond the HIPAA Privacy Rule*.

38. "Summary of 2018 HIPAA Fines and Settlements," *HIPAA Journal*, accessed March 1, 2019, https://www.hipaajournal.com/summary-2018-hipaa-fines-and-settlements.

39. Office of the Secretary, US Department of Health and Human Services, "Standards for Privacy of Individually Identifiable Health Information; Final Rule," *Federal Register* 65, no. 250 (2000): 82761.

40. Federico Girosi, Robin Meili, and Richard Scoville, *Extrapolating Evidence of Health Information Technology Savings and Costs* (Santa Monica, CA: RAND Corporation, 2005), http://www.rand.org/pubs/monographs/MG410.html.

41. "Reform of EU Data Protection Rules," European Commission, accessed March 1, 2019, https://ec.europa.eu/info/law/law-topic/data-protection/reform_en.

16. The Safety and Quality of Patient Care

1. David Cutler, *The Quality Cure* (Berkeley and Los Angeles: University of California Press, 2014), 1.

2. Donald A. Barr, *Introduction to Health Policy: The Organization, Financing, and Delivery of Health Care in America* (Baltimore, MD: Johns Hopkins University Press, 2016).

3. Barr, *Introduction to Health Policy*, 364.

4. David Leonhardt, "Making Health Care Better," *New York Times Magazine*, November 3, 2009, https://www.nytimes.com/2009/11/08/magazine/08Healthcare-t.html.

5. Emanuel Rivers, Bryant Nguyen, Suzanne Havstad, Julie Ressler, Alexandria Muzzin, Bernhard Knoblich, Edward Peterson, and Michael Tomlanovich, "Early

Goal-Directed Therapy in the Treatment of Severe Sepsis and Septic Shock," *New England Journal of Medicine* 345, no. 19 (2001): 1368–77, doi:10.1056/nejmoa010307.

6. R. P. Dellinger, Mitchell M. Levy, Andrew Rhodes, Djillali Annane, Herwig Gerlach, Steven M. Opal, Jonathan E. Sevransky, et al., "Surviving Sepsis Campaign: International Guidelines for Management of Severe Sepsis and Septic Shock, 2012," *Intensive Care Medicine* 39, no. 2 (2013): 165–228, doi:10.1007/s00134-012 -2769-8.

7. Committee on Quality of Health Care in America, *To Err Is Human: Building a Safer Health System* (Washington, DC: National Academies Press, 2000), xi.

8. Committee on Quality of Health Care in America, *To Err Is Human*, 3–5.

9. Committee on Quality of Health Care in America, *To Err Is Human*, 1.

10. Committee on Quality of Health Care in America, *To Err Is Human*, 1.

11. Rodney A. Hayward and Timothy P. Hofer, "Estimating Hospital Deaths Due to Medical Errors: Preventability Is in the Eye of the Reviewer," *JAMA* 286, no. 4 (2001): 415–20, doi:10:10.1001/jama.286.4.485

12. Clement J. McDonald, Michael Weiner, and Siu L. Hui, "Deaths Due to Medical Errors Are Exaggerated in Institute of Medicine Report," *JAMA* 284, no. 1 (2000): 93–95, doi:10.1001/jama.284.1.93.

13. "Initiatives Overview: 5 Million Lives Campaign," Institute for Healthcare Improvement. accessed December 13, 2018, http://www.ihi.org/Engage/Initiatives /Completed/5MillionLivesCampaign/Pages/default.aspx.

14. "HCUP Fast Stats: Trends in Inpatient Stays," Healthcare Cost and Utilization Project, Agency for Healthcare Research and Quality, accessed January 24, 2019, https://hcup-us.ahrq.gov/faststats/NationalTrendsServlet?measure1 =01&characteristic1=01&time1=10&measure2=05&characteristic2=01&time2 =20&expansionInfoState=hide&dataTablesState=hide&definitionsState =hide&exportState=hide.

15. Emily Le Coz, Josh Salmon J, and Lucille Sherman, "Failure to Deliver: Burgeoning Industry Fails to Hold Midwives Accountable," *Columbus Dispatch*, November 25, 2018, https://www.dispatch.com/news/20181125/failure-to-deliver-bur geoning-industry-fails-to-hold-midwives-accountable/1.

16. Elisabeth Rosenthal, *An American Sickness: How Healthcare Became Big Business and How You Can Take It Back* (New York: Penguin Press, 2017).

17. Peter B. Hutt, "The Regulation of Drug Products by the United States Food and Drug Administration," in *The Textbook of Pharmaceutical Medicine*, ed. Griffin J. O'Grady (London: Blackwell BMJ Books, 1992).

18. Atira H. Kaplan, "Fifty Years of Drug Amendments Revisited: In Easy-to-Swallow Capsule Form," *Food Drug Law Journal* 50 Spec (1995): 179–96.

19. Committee on the Assessment of the US Drug Safety System and the Board on Population Health and Public Health Practice, *The Future of Drug Safety: Promoting and Protecting the Health of the Public*, ed. Alina Baciu, Kathleen Stratton, and Sheila P. Burke (Washington, DC: National Academies Press, 2007), 152, https://www.nap.edu/read/11750/chapter/7#152.

20. "FDA Has Taken Steps to Strengthen the 510(k) Program," US Food and Drug Administration, November 2018, https://www.fda.gov/media/118500/download.

21. Rosenthal, *An American Sickness*, 132.

22. Rosenthal, *An American Sickness*, 133.

23. Rosenthal, *An American Sickness*, 134.

24. "510(k) Devices Cleared in 2017," US Food and Drug Administration, accessed December 14, 2018, https://www.fda.gov/MedicalDevices/ProductsandMed icalProcedures/DeviceApprovalsandClearances/510kClearances/ucm540522.htm.

25. "Novel Drug Approvals for 2017," US Food and Drug Administration, accessed December 14, 2018, https://www.fda.gov/drugs/developmentapprovalprocess /druginnovation/ucm537040.htm.

26. Rosenthal, *An American Sickness*, 133.

27. "2019 Medical Device Recalls," US Food and Drug Administration, accessed January 5, 2020, https://www.fda.gov/medical-devices/medical-device-recalls/2019 -medical-device-recalls.

28. "Medical Device Lawsuits," ClassAction.com, accessed January 5, 2020, https://www.classaction.com/lawsuits/medical-devices.

29. "Statement from FDA Commissioner Scott Gottlieb, MD, and Jeff Shuren, MD, Director of the Center for Devices and Radiological Health, on Transformative New Steps to Modernize FDA's 510(k) Program to Advance the Review of the Safety and Effectiveness of Medical Devices" (press release), US Food and Drug Administration, November 26, 2018, https://www.fda.gov/NewsEvents/Newsroom/PressAnnounce ments/ucm626572.htm.

30. Committee on Quality of Health Care in America, *Crossing the Quality Chasm: A New Health System for the 21st Century* (Washington, DC: National Academies Press, 2001).

31. Committee on Quality of Health Care in America, *Crossing the Quality Chasm*, 4.

32. Committee on Quality of Health Care in America, *Crossing the Quality Chasm*, 5.

33. Committee on Quality of Health Care in America, *Crossing the Quality Chasm*, 5–6.

34. Health Services Advisory Group and Mathematica Policy Research, *Project Evaluation Activity in Support of Partnership for Patients: Interim Evaluation Report, Final* (Woodlawn, MD: Center for Medicare and Medicaid Innovation, 2015), https://downloads.cms.gov/files/cmmi/pfp-interimevalrpt.pdf.

17. The Cost Conundrum I

1. "Measuring Price Change in the CPI: Medical Care," Consumer Price Index, US Bureau of Labor Statistics, last modified April 24, 2019, accessed February 1, 2019, https://www.bls.gov/cpi/factsheets/medical-care.htm.

2. "National Health Expenditure Data: Historical," Centers for Medicare and Medicaid Services, accessed December 19, 2018, https://www.cms.gov/Research -Statistics-Data-and-Systems/Statistics-Trends-and-Reports/NationalHealthExpend Data/NationalHealthAccountsHistorical.html.

3. Joseph L. Dieleman, Ellen Squires, Anthony L. Bui, Madeline Campbell, Abigail Chapin, Hannah Hamavid, Cody Horst, et al, "Factors Associated with

Increases in US Health Care Spending, 1996–2013," *JAMA* 318, no. 17 (2017): 1668–78, doi:10.1001/jama.2017.15927.

4. Ezekiel J. Emanuel, "The Real Cost of the US Health Care System," *JAMA* 319, no. 10 (2018): 983, doi:10.1001/jama.2018.1151.

5. Irene Papanicolas, Liana R. Woskie, and Ashish K. Jha, "Health Care Spending in the United States and Other High-Income Countries," *JAMA* 319, no. 10 (2018): 1024–39, doi:10.1001/jama.2018.1150.

6. "Current Health Care Expenditure Per Capita," World Health Organization Health Expenditure Database, The World Bank, accessed December 17, 2018, https://data.worldbank.org/indicator/SH.XPD.CHEX.PC.CD.

7. Papanicolas, Woskie, and Jha, "Health Care Spending in the United States."

8. Papanicolas, Woskie, and Jha, "Health Care Spending in the United States."

9. Michael E. Porter, "What Is Value in Health Care?," *New England Journal of Medicine* 363, no. 26 (2010): 2477–81, doi:10.1056/nejmp1011024.

10. Sari Harrar, "Insulin Prices Still High," OnTrack Diabetes, accessed April 21, 2017, https://www.ontrackdiabetes.com/type-1-diabetes/insulin-prices-still-high.

11. Jean Fuglesten Biniek and William Johnson, *Spending by Individuals with Type 1 Diabetes and the Role of Rapidly Increasing Insulin Prices* (Washington, DC: Health Care Cost Institute, 2019), https://www.healthcostinstitute.org/research/publications/entry/spending-on-individuals-with-type-1-diabetes-and-the-role-of-rapidly-increasing-insulin-prices.

12. Board of Governors of the Federal Reserve System, *Report on the Economic Well-Being of US Households in 2017* (Washington, DC: Federal Reserve Board, May 2018), https://www.federalreserve.gov/publications/files/2017-report-economic-well-being-us-households-201805.pdf.

13. J. Frank Wharam, Christine Y. Lu, Fang Zhang, Matthew Callahan, Xin Xu, Jamie Wallace, Stephen Soumerai, Dennis Ross-Degnan, and Joseph P. Newhouse, "High-Deductible Insurance and Delay in Care for the Macrovascular Complications of Diabetes," *Annals of Internal Medicine* 169, no. 12 (2018): 845, doi:10.7326/m17-3365.

14. Wharam et al., "High-Deductible Insurance and Delay in Care."

15. Gary Claxton, Matthew Rae, Michelle Long, Anthony Damico, and Heidi Whitmore, "Health Benefits in 2018: Modest Growth in Premiums, Higher Worker Contributions at Firms with More Low-Wage Workers," *Health Affairs* 37, no. 11 (2018): 1892–1900, doi:10.1377/hlthaff.2018.1001.

16. Zarek C. Brot-Goldberg, Amitabh Chandra, Benjamin R. Handel, and Jonathan T. Kolstad, "What Does a Deductible Do? The Impact of Cost-Sharing on Health Care Prices, Quantities, and Spending Dynamics," *Quarterly Journal of Economics* 132, no. 3 (2017): 1261–1318, doi:10.1093/qje/qjx013.

17. Brot-Goldberg et al., "What Does a Deductible Do?"

18. Rajender Agarwal, Olena Mazurenko, and Nir Menachemi, "High-Deductible Health Plans Reduce Health Care Cost and Utilization, Including Use of Needed Preventive Services," *Health Affairs* 36, no. 10 (2017): 1762–68, doi:10.1377/hlthaff.2017.0610.

19. Rachel Reid, Brendan Rabideau, and Neeraj Good, "Impact of Consumer-Directed Health Plans on Low-Value Healthcare," *American Journal of Managed Care* 23, no. 12 (2017): 741.

20. John Tozzi and Zachary Tracer, "Sky-High Deductibles Broke the US Health Insurance System," *Bloomberg*, June 26, 2018, https://www.bloomberg.com/news/features/2018-06-26/sky-high-deductibles-broke-the-u-s-health-insurance-system.

21. Tozzi and Tracer, "Sky-High Deductibles."

22. Tozzi and Tracer, "Sky-High Deductibles."

23. A. Mark Fendrick and Michael E. Chernew, "Precision Benefit Design—Using 'Smarter' Deductibles to Better Engage Consumers and Mitigate Cost-Related Non adherence," *JAMA Internal Medicine* 177, no. 3 (2017): 368, doi:10.1001/jamainternmed.2016.8747.

24. "Value-Based Insurance Design," National Converence of State Legislatures, accessed April 2, 2019, http://www.ncsl.org/research/health/value-based-insurance-design.aspx.

25. Kai Yeung, Anirban Basu, Ryan N. Hansen, John B. Watkins, and Sean D. Sullivan, "Impact of a Value-Based Formulary on Medication Utilization, Health Services Utilization, and Expenditures," *Medical Care* 55, no. 2 (2017): 191–98, doi:10.1097/mlr.0000000000000630.

26. "Less Is More," JAMA Network, accessed December 24, 2018, https://jamanetwork.com/collections/44045/less-is-more.

27. Deborah Grady and Rita Redberg, "Less Is More: How Less Health Care Can Result in Better Health," *Archives of Internal Medicine* 170, no. 9 (2010): 749, doi:10.1001/archinternmed.2010.90.

28. Allison Lipitz-Snyderman and Peter B. Bach, "Overuse: When Less is More . . . More or Less," *JAMA Internal Medicine* 173, no. 14 (2013): 1277–78, doi:10.1001/jamainternmed.2013.6181.

29. Timothy Sullivan, "Antibiotic Overuse and *Clostridium Difficile*: A Teachable Moment," *JAMA Internal Medicine* 174, no. 8 (2014): 1219, doi:10.1001/jamainternmed.2014.2299.

30. Nancy E. Epstein and Donald C. Hood, "'Unnecessary' Spinal Surgery: A Prospective 1-Year Study of One Surgeon's Experience," *Surgical Neurology International* 2, no. 1 (2011): 83, doi:10.4103/2152-7806.82249.

31. Bruce E. Lehnert and Robert L. Bree, "Analysis of Appropriateness of Outpatient CT and MRI Referred from Primary Care Clinics at an Academic Medical Center: How Critical Is the Need for Improved Decision Support?," *Journal of the American College of Radiology* 7, no. 3 (2010): 192–97, doi:10.1016/j.jacr.2009.11.010.

32. Paul S. Chan, Manesh R. Patel, Lloyd W. Klein, Ronald J. Krone, Gregory J. Dehmer, Kevin Kennedy, Brahmajee K. Nallamothu, et al., "Appropriateness of Percutaneous Coronary Intervention," *JAMA* 306, no. 1 (2011), doi:10.1001/jama.2011.916.

33. Wade Nicholson Harrison, John F. Dick, and Thom Walsh, "Patient Preferences and End-of-Life Care: A Teachable Moment," *JAMA Internal Medicine* 175, no. 7 (2015): 1087–88, doi:10.1001/jamainternmed.2015.1283.

34. Daniel J. Morgan, Sanket S. Dhruva, Eric R. Coon, Scott M. Wright, and Deborah Korenstein, "2017 Update on Medical Overuse," *JAMA Internal Medicine* 178, no. 1 (2018): 110–15, doi:10.1001/jamainternmed.2017.4361.

35. Daniel J. Morgan, Sanket S. Dhruva, Eric R. Coon, Scott M. Wright, and Deborah Korenstein, "2018 Update on Medical Overuse," *JAMA Internal Medicine* 179, no. 2 (2019): 240–46, doi:10.1001/jamainternmed.2018.5748.

36. Morgan et al., "2017 Update on Medical Overuse," 112.

37. Morgan et al., "2018 Update on Medical Overuse," 242.

38. Morgan et al., "2018 Update on Medical Overuse," 242–43.

39. Morgan et al., "2017 Update on Medical Overuse," 113.

40. H. Gilbert Welch, *Should I Be Tested for Cancer? Maybe Not and Here's Why* (University of California Press, 2006); H. Gilbert Welch, Lisa M. Schwartz, and Steven Woloshin, *Overdiagnosed: Making People Sick in the Pursuit of Health* (Boston: Beacon Press, 2011); H. Gilbert Welch, *Less Medicine, More Health: 7 Assumptions that Drive Too Much Medical Care* (Boston: Beacon Press, 2015).

41. Jane E. Brody, "Healthy in a Falling Apart Sort of Way," *New York Times*, May 2, 2015, https://well.blogs.nytimes.com/2015/03/02/healthy-in-a-falling-apart -sort-of-way/.

42. Heather Lyu, Tim Xu, Daniel Brotman, Brandan Mayer-Blackwell, Michol Cooper, Michael Daniel, Elizabeth C. Wick, Vikas Saini, Shannon Brownlee, and Martin A. Makary, "Overtreatment in the United States," *PLoS One* 12, no. 9 (2017): e0181970, doi:10.1371/journal.pone.0181970.

43. Lisa Rosenbaum, "The Less-Is-More Crusade—Are We Overmedicalizing or Oversimplifying?," *New England Journal of Medicine* 377, no. 24 (2017): 2392–97, doi:10.1056/nejmms1713248.

44. Rosenbaum, "The Less-Is-More Crusade," 2396.

45. John Mandrola, "In Defense of Less Is More," *Medscape*, January 9, 2018, https://www.medscape.com/viewarticle/891091.

46. Steven Woloshin and Lisa M Schwartz, "Overcoming Overuse: The Way Forward Is Not Standing Still," *BMJ* 361 (2018): k2035, doi:10.1136/bmj.k2035.

47. Rosenbaum, "The Less-Is-More Crusade," 2393.

48. Marta Wosinska, "Just What the Patient Ordered? Direct-to-Consumer Advertising and the Demand for Pharmaceutical Product," Harvard Business School Marketing Research Paper No. 02-04, October 2002, http://ssrn.com/abstract_id=347005.

49. Frank Celia, "Pharma Ups the Ante on DTC Advertising," *Pharmaceutical Commerce*, April 4, 2017, http://pharmaceuticalcommerce.com/brand-marketing -communications/pharma-ups-ante-dtc-advertising.

50. Food and Drug Administration, "Guidance for Industry: Consumer-Directed Broadcast Advertisements," August 1999, http://www.fda.gov/downloads/Regula toryInformation/Guidances/ucm125064.pdf.

51. Joseph A. DiMasi, Henry G. Grabowski, and Ronald W. Hansen, "Innovation in the Pharmaceutical Industry: New Estimates of R&D Costs," *Journal of Health Economics* 47 (2016): 20–33, doi:10.1016/j.jhealeco.2016.01.012.

52. Vinay Prasad and Sham Mailankody, "Research and Development Spending to Bring a Single Cancer Drug to Market and Revenues after Approval," *JAMA Internal Medicine* 177, no. 11 (2017): 1569, doi:10.1001/jamainternmed.2017.3601.

53. Jerry Avorn, "The $2.6 Billion Pill—Methodologic and Policy Considerations," *New England Journal of Medicine* 372, no. 20 (2015): 1877–79, doi:10.1056/nejm

p1500848; Matthew Herper, "The Cost of Developing Drugs Is Insane. That Paper that Says Otherwise Is Insanely Bad," *Forbes*, October 16, 2017, https://www.forbes.com /sites/matthewherper/2017/10/16/the-cost-of-developing-drugs-is-insane-a-paper -that-argued-otherwise-was-insanely-bad.

54. DiMasi, Grabowski, and Hansen, "Innovation in the Pharmaceutical Industry."

55. Jonathan D. Rockoff, "Big Pharma, Short on Blockbusters, Outsources the Science," *Wall Street Journal,* Decmber 6, 2016, https://www.wsj.com/articles/big -pharma-short-on-blockbusters-outsources-the-science-1481042583.

56. Salomeh Keyhani, Steven Wang, Paul Hebert, Daniel Carpenter, and Gerard Anderson, "US Pharmaceutical Innovation in an International Context," *American Journal of Public Health* 100, no. 6 (2010): 1075–80, doi:10.2105/ajph.2009.178491.

57. Barbara Mintzes, Morris L. Barer, Richard L. Kravitz, Ken Bassett, Joel Lexchin, Arminée Kazanjian, Robert G. Evans, Richard Pan, and Stephen A. Marion, "How Does Direct-to-Consumer Advertising (DTCA) Affect Prescribing? A Survey in Primary Care Environments with and without Legal DTCA," *CMAJ* 169, no. 5 (2003): 405–12.

58. Anthony Crupi, "Big Pharma Is Spending Lots of Money on Your Favorite Sitcoms," *AdAge*, November 12, 2018, https://adage.com/article/media/why-pharma -ads-are-so-prevalent-on-tv-sitcoms/315575.

59. Richard L. Kravitz, Ronald M. Epstein, Mitchell D. Feldman, Carol E. Franz, Rahman Azari, Michael S. Wilkes, Ladson Hinton, and Peter Franks, "Influence of Patients' Requests for Direct-to-Consumer Advertised Antidepressants," *JAMA* 163, no. 14 (2005): 1673–81, doi:10.1001/jama.293.16.1995.

60. John B. McKinlay, Felicia Trachtenberg, Lisa D. Marceau, Jeffrey N. Katz, and Michael A. Fischer, "Effects of Patient Medication Requests on Physician Prescribing Behavior," *Medical Care* 52, no. 4 (2014): 294–99, doi:10.1097 /mlr.0000000000000096.

61. Eric G. Campbell, Genevieve Pham-Kanter, Christine Vogeli, and Lisa I. Iezzoni, "Physician Acquiescence to Patient Demands for Brand-Name Drugs: Results of a National Survey of Physicians," *JAMA Internal Medicine* 173, no. 3 (2013): 237–39, doi:10.1001/jamainternmed.2013.1539.

62. Wosinska, "Just What the Patient Ordered?"

63. Hsien-Yen Chang, Irene Murimi, Matthew Daubresse, Dima M. Qato, Sherry L. Emery, and G. Caleb Alexander, "Effect of Direct-to-Consumer Advertising on Statin Use in the United States," *Medical Care* 55, no. 8 (2017): 759–64, doi:10.1097/mlr.0000000000000752.

64. Jalpa A. Doshi, Amy R Pettit, and Pengziang Li, "Addressing Out-of-Pocket Specialty Drug Costs in Medicare Part D: The Good, the Bad, the Ugly, and the Ignored," *Health Affairs* blog, July 25, 2018, https://www.healthaffairs.org/do/10 .1377/hblog20180724.734269/full.

65. Doshi, Pettit, and Li, "Addressing Out-of-Pocket Specialty Drug Costs."

66. "Conditions and Diseases," National Institute for Health and Care Excellence, accessed December 26, 2018, https://www.nice.org.uk/guidance/conditions -and-diseases.

18. The Cost Conundrum II

1. Elaine M. Cardenas, "Revision of the CPI Hospital Services Component," *Monthly Labor Review*, December 1996, https://www.bls.gov/opub/mlr/1996/12/art6full.pdf.

2. "Measuring Price Change in the CPI: Medical Care," US Bureau of Labor Statistics, last modified April 24, 2019, accessed February 1, 2019, https://www.bls.gov/cpi/factsheets/medical-care.htm.

3. Irene Papanicolas, Liana R. Woskie, and Ashish K. Jha, "Health Care Spending in the United States and Other High-Income Countries," *JAMA* 319, no. 10 (2018): 1024, doi:10.1001/jama.2018.1150.

4. *Delivering Better Health Care Value to Consumers: The First Three Years of the Medical Loss Ratio, Hearing before the Committee on Commerce, Science, and Transportation*, 113th Cong., 2nd Sess. (2014).

5. *Delivering Better Health Care Value to Consumers.*

6. Phillip Tseng, Robert S. Kaplan, Barak D. Richman, Mahek A. Shah, and Kevin A. Schulman, "Administrative Costs Associated with Physician Billing and Insurance-Related Activities at an Academic Health Care System," *JAMA* 319, no. 7 (2018): supplementary online content, eFigure, doi:10.1001/jama.2017.19148.

7. Tseng et al., "Administrative Costs."

8. Steffie Woolhandler, Terry Campbell, and David U. Himmelstein, "Costs of Health Care Administration in the United States and Canada," *New England Journal of Medicine* 349, no. 8 (2003): 768–75, doi:10.1056/nejmsa022033.

9. James G. Kahn, Richard Kronick, Mary Kreger, and David N. Gans, "The Cost of Health Insurance Administration in California: Estimates for Insurers, Physicians, and Hospitals," *Health Affairs* 24, no. 6 (2005): 1629–39, doi:10.1377/hlthaff.24.6.1629.

10. Julie Ann Sakowski, James G. Kahn, Richard G. Kronick, Jeffrey M. Newman, and Harold S. Luft, "Peering into the Black Box: Billing and Insurance Activities in a Medical Group," *Health Affairs* 28, no. 4 (2009): w544–54. doi:10.1377/hlthaff.28.4.w544; Lawrence P. Casalino, Sean Nicholson, David N. Gans, Terry Hammons, Dante Morra, Theodore Karrison, and Wendy Levinson, "What Does It Cost Physician Practices to Interact with Health Insurance Plans?," *Health Affairs* 28, no. 4 (2009): w533–43, doi:10.1377/hlthaff.28.4.w533.

11. Aliya Jiwani, David Himmelstein, Steffie Woolhandler, and James G. Kahn, "Billing and Insurance-Related Administrative Costs in United States' Health Care: Synthesis of Micro-Costing Evidence," *BMC Health Services Research* 14, 556 (2014), doi:10.1186/s12913-014-0556-7.

12. Tseng et al., "Administrative Costs."

13. Vivian S. Lee and Bonnie B. Blanchfield, "Disentangling Health Care Billing," *JAMA* 319, no. 7 (2018): 661, doi:10.1001/jama.2017.19966.

14. "Where Does Your Health Care Dollar Go?," AHIP, May 22, 2018, https://www.ahip.org/health-care-dollar/.

15. National Association of Insurance Commissioners (NAIC), *2017 Accident and Health Policy Experience Report* (Washington, DC: NAIC, 2018), https://www.naic.org/prod_serv/AHP-LR-18.pdf.

16. Jared Lane K. Maeda and Lyle Nelson, "How Do the Hospital Prices Paid by Medicare Advantage Plans and Commercial Plans Compare with Medicare Fee-For-Service Prices?," *INQUIRY: The Journal of Health Care Organization, Provision, and Financing* 55 (2018), doi:10.1177/0046958018779654.

17. Chapin White and Christopher Whaley, *Prices Paid to Hospitals by Private Health Plans Are High Relative to Medicare and Vary Widely: Findings from an Employer-Led Transparency Initiative* (Santa Monica, CA: RAND Corporation, 2019), https://www.rand.org/pubs/research_reports/RR3033.html

18. Ge Bai and Gerard F. Anderson, "Market Power: Price Variation among Commercial Insurers for Hospital Services," *Health Affairs* 37, no. 10 (2018): 1615–22, doi:10.1377/hlthaff.2018.0567.

19. Bai and Anderson, "Market Power."

20. Elsa Pearson and Austin Frakt, "Our Turn: Elsa Pearson and Austin Frakt: Hospital Mergers Don't Cut Prices," *Providence Journal*, August 4, 2019, https://www.providencejournal.com/opinion/20190804/our-turn-elsa-pearson-and-austin-frakt-hospital-mergers-dont-cut-prices.

21. Zack Cooper, Stuart Craig, Martin Gaynor, Nir J. Harish, Harlan M. Krumholz, and John Van Reenen, "Hospital Prices Grew Substantially Faster Than Physician Prices for Hospital-Based Care in 2007–14, *Health Affairs* 38, no. 2 (2019): 184–89, doi:10.1377/hlthaff.2018.05424.

22. Daria Pelech, *An Analysis of Private-Sector Prices for Physician Services*, Working Paper 2018-01 (Washington, DC: Congressional Budget Office, 2018), https://www.cbo.gov/publication/53441.

23. Eli Y. Adashi, Barak D. Richman, and Reuben C. Baker, "The New State Medical Board: Life in the Antitrust Shadow," *Health Affairs* blog, January 6, 2020, https://www.healthaffairs.org/do/10.1377/hblog20191226.86148/full.

24. IHS Markit Ltd., *The Complexities of Physician Supply and Demand: Projections from 2017 to 2030* (Washington, DC: Association of American Medical Colleges, 2019), https://aamc-black.global.ssl.fastly.net/production/media/filer_public/31/13/3113ee5c-a038-4c16-89af-294a69826650/2019_update_-_the_complexities_of_physician_supply_and_demand_-_projections_from_2017-2032.pdf.

25. "Survey of Over 17,000 Physicians Finds Shifting Practice Patterns Limit Patient Access to Care," *Business Wire*, September 21, 2016, https://www.businesswire.com/news/home/20160921005410/en/Survey-17000-Physicians-Finds-Shifting-Practice-Patterns.

26. Emily Gudbranson, Aaron Glickman, and Ezekiel J. Emanuel, "Reassessing the Data on Whether a Physician Shortage Exists," *JAMA* 317, no. 19 (2017): 1945–46, doi:10.1001/jama.2017.2609.

27. Leslie Kane, "Medscape Physician Compensation Report 2018," *Medscape*, April 11, 2018, https://www.medscape.com/slideshow/2018-compensation-overview-6009667.

28. "Employment Cost Index (NAICS)," Databases, Tables & Calculators by Subject, US Bureau of Labor Statistics, accessed February 2, 2019, https://data.bls.gov/timeseries/CIU1010000000000A.

29. Hannah T. Neprash, Michael E. Chernew, Andrew L. Hicks, Teresa Gibson, and J. Michael McWilliams, "Association of Financial Integration between Physicians and Hospitals with Commercial Health Care Prices," *JAMA Internal Medicine* 175, no. 12 (2015): 1932–39, doi:10.1001/jamainternmed.2015.4610.

30. Physician Advocay Institute, "Updated Physician Practice Acquisition Study: National and Regional Changes in Physician Employment 2012–2016" (presentation slides), March 2018, http://www.physiciansadvocacyinstitute.org/Portals/0/assets /docs/2016-PAI-Physician-Employment-Study-Final.pdf.

31. Joshua M. Sharfstein and Jamar Slocum, "Private Equity and Dermatology— First, Do No Harm," *JAMA Dermatology* 155, no. 9 (2019): 1007–8, doi:10.1001/jama dermatol.2019.1322.

32. Shriji N. Patel, Sylvia Groth, and Paul Sternberg, "The Emergence of Private Equity in Ophthalmology," *JAMA Ophthalmology* 137, no. 6 (2019): 601–2, doi:10.1001/jamaophthalmol.2019.0964.

33. Angie Stewart,."Private Equity Investments in Orthopedics Expected to Surge in 2019," *Becker's ASC Review*, January 9, 2019, https://www.beckersasc.com /asc-transactions-and-valuation-issues/private-equity-investments-in-orthopedics -expected-to-surge-in-2019-avoid-these-risks.html.

19. The Cost Conundrum III

1. Magellan Rx Management, *Medical Pharmacy Trend Report 2017*, 8th ed. (Orlando, FL: Magellan Rx Management, 2018), https://www1.magellanrx.com /documents/2019/03/medical-pharmacy-trend-report_2017.pdf.

2. Magellan Rx Management. *Medical Pharmacy Trend Report 2017*, 6.

3. Magellan Rx Management. *Medical Pharmacy Trend Report 2017*, 6.

4. Xinyang Hua, Natalie Carvalho, Michelle Tew, Elbert S. Huang, William H. Herman, and Philip Clarke, "Expenditures and Prices of Antihyperglycemic Medications in the United States: 2002–2013," *JAMA* 315, no. 13 (2016): 1400, doi:10.1001 /jama.2016.0126.

5. Adam J. Fein, "2018 MDM Market Leaders: Top Pharmaceutical Providers," Modern Distribution Management, accessed June 28, 2019, https://www.mdm.com /2017-top-pharmaceuticals-distributors.

6. Robert Langreth, David Ingold, and Jackie Gu, "The Secret Drug Pricing System Middlemen Use to Rake in Millions," *Bloomberg*, September 11, 2018, https://www.bloomberg.com/graphics/2018-drug-spread-pricing.

7. MedPAC Staff, "Factors Increasing Part D Spending for Catastrophic Benefits," *MedPAC Blog*, June 8, 2017, http://www.medpac.gov/-blog-/factors-increasing-part-d -spending-for-catastrophic-benefits/2017/06/08/factors-increasing-part-d-spending -for-catastrophic-benefits.

8. Bob Herman, "The Data Showing Drug Pricing Games," *Axios*, August 1, 2018, https://www.axios.com/data-showing-pbm-medicaid-drug-price-manipulation-15330 59892-c2a97bcd-8874-42c2-a161-503e89666678.html.

9. Herman, "Data Showing Drug Pricing Games."

10. US Government Accountability Office (GAO), *Drug Industry: Profits, Research and Development Spending, and Merger and Acquisition Deals*, Report to Congressional Requesters GAO-18-40 (Washington, DC: GAO, November 2017), https://www.gao.gov/assets/690/688472.pdf.

11. Leemore Dafny, Christopher Ody, and Matt Schmitt, "When Discounts Raise Costs: The Effect of Copay Coupons on Generic Utilization," *American Economic Journal: Economic Policy* 9, no. 2 (2017): 91–123, doi:10.1257/pol.20150588.

12. William G. Schiffbauer, "Let's Talk about Prescription Drug Copay Coupons: Do They Operate as Unregulated Secondary Insurance?," *Bloomberg Law*, April 18, 2018, https://news.bloomberglaw.com/health-law-and-business/lets-talk-about -prescription-drug-copay-coupons-do-they-operate-as-unregulated-secondary -insurance.

13. Schiffbauer, "Let's Talk about Prescription Drug Copay Coupons."

14. Sarah Karlin-Smith, "Co-Pay Support Orgs Rank High among Largest US Charities," *Politico*, May 15, 2017, https://www.politico.com/tipsheets/prescrip tion-pulse/2017/05/co-pay-support-orgs-rank-high-among-largest-us-charities -220316.

15. Brett Friedman, Alison Fethke, and Jamie Darch, "Emerging Enforcement Trends for Patient Support Programs," *Law 360*, May 15, 2018, https://www.ropesgray .com/en/newsroom/alerts/2018/05/Emerging-Enforcement-Trends-For-Patient-Sup port-Programs.

16. Blase N. Polite, Jeffery C. Ward, John V. Cox, Roscoe F. Morton, John Hennessy, Ray D. Page, and Rena M. Conti, "Payment for Oncolytics in the United States: A History of Buy and Bill and Proposals for Reform," *Journal of Oncology Practice* 10, no. 6 (2014): 357–62, doi:10.1200/jop.2014.001958.

17. "For Oncologists, It Is Bye to Buy-and-Bill and Hello to Value-Based Care," *Managed Care*, July 13, 2015, https://www.managedcaremag.com/archives/2015/7 /oncologists-it-bye-buy-and-bill-and-hello-value-based-care.

18. Medicare Payment Advisory Commission (MedPAC), *A Data Book: Health Care Spending and the Medicare Program* (Washington, DC: MedPAC, June 2018), http://medpac.gov/docs/default-source/data-book/jun18_databookentirereport_sec .pdf.

19. "For Oncologists, It Is Bye to Buy-and-Bill," *Managed Care*.

20. Thomas R. Oliver, Philip R. Lee, and Helene L. Lipton, "A Political History of Medicare and Prescription Drug Coverage," *Milbank Quarterly* 82, no. 2 (2004): 283–354, doi:10.1111/j.0887-378x.2004.00311.x.

21. "Drug Industry and HMOs Deployed an Army of Nearly 1,000 Lobbyists to Push Medicare Bill, Report Finds," Public Citizen, June 23, 2004, https://www.citizen. org/media/press-releases/drug-industry-and-hmos-deployed-army-nearly-1000-lobby ists-push-medicare-bill.

22. "Drug Industry and HMOs Deployed an Army," Public Citizen.

23. Michelle Singer, "Under the Influence: Steve Kroft Reports on Drug Lobby- ists' Role in Passing Bill the Keeps Drug Prices High," *CBS News*, March 29, 2007, https://www.cbsnews.com/news/under-the-influence.

24. *2018 Annual Report of the Boards of Trustees of the Federal Hospital Insurance and Federal Supplementary Medical Insurance Trust Funds* (Washington, DC: Boards of Trustees, Federal Hospital Insurance and Federal Supplementary Medical Insurance Trust Funds, 2018), https://www.cms.gov/Research-Statistics-Data-and-Systems/Statistics-Trends-and-Reports/ReportsTrustFunds/downloads/tr2018.pdf.

25. Austin Frakt and Mark Miller, "The Case for Restructuring the Medicare Prescription Drug Benefit," *Health Services Research* 53, no. 6 (2018): 4133, doi:10.1111/1475-6773.13019.

26. Frakt and Miller, "Case for Restructuring the Medicare Prescription Drug Benefit," 4134.

27. "General Information Concerning Patents," United States Patent and Trademark Office, October 2015, https://www.uspto.gov/patents-getting-started/general-information-concerning-patents.

28. Benjamin Ryan, "One in Three People Seeking Insurance Coverage for Hepatitis C Drugs Are Denied," *HEP*, June 8, 2018, https://www.hepmag.com/article/one-three-people-seeking-insurance-coverage-hep-c-drugs-denied.

29. Elisabeth Rosenthal, *An American Sickness: How Healthcare Became Big Business and How You Can Take It Back* (New York: Penguin Press, 2017), 96.

30. Gregory H. Jones, Michael A. Carrier, Richard T. Silver, and Hagop Kantarjian, "Strategies that Delay or Prevent the Timely Availability of Affordable Generic Drugs in the United States," *Blood* 127, no. 11 (2016): 1398–1402, doi:10.1182/blood-2015-11-680058.

31. "Subpart 2—Prescription Drug Plan; PDP Sponsors; Financing," Compilation of the Social Security Laws, Social Security Administration, accessed January 8, 2019, https://www.ssa.gov/OP_Home/ssact/title18/1860D-11.htm.

32. "Drug Price Increases Have Slowed, but New Analysis Shows Launch Prices Pushing Costs into Orbit," 46brooklyn Research, October 15, 2019, https://www.46brooklyn.com/research/2019/10/11/three-two-one-launch-rfmyr.

33. Glenn Howett, "Insulin Outlaws: High Cost of Medication Drives Minnesotans across the Border to Canada, *Star Tribune*, May 12, 2019, http://www.startribune.com/insulin-outlaws-high-cost-of-medication-drives-minnesotans-across-the-border/509802712.

34. Experts in Chronic Myeloid Leukemia, "The Price of Drugs for Chronic Myeloid Leukemia (CML) Is a Reflection of the Unsustainable Prices of Cancer Drugs: From the Perspective of a Large Group of CML Experts," *Blood* 121, no. 22 (2013): 4439–42, doi:10.1182/blood-2013-03-490003.

35. Experts in Chronic Myeloid Leukemia, "The Price of Drugs," 4440.

36. Elisabeth Rosenthal, "Why Competition Won't Bring Down Drug Prices," *New York Times*, June 21, 2018, https://www.nytimes.com/2018/06/21/opinion/competition-drug-prices.html.

37. Rosenthal, "Why Competition Won't Bring Down Drug Prices."

38. Rosenthal, *An American Sickness*, chapter 4.

39. Eric Saganowsky, "Pharma's Pervasive 'Evergreening' Is Driving Prices Up, Study Says," *FiercePharma*, November 3, 2017, https://www.fiercepharma.com/pharma/pharma-s-pervasive-evergreening-driving-prices-up-study-says.

40. Drug Price Competition and Patent Term Restoration Act of 1984 (Hatch-Waxman Act), Pub. L. No. 98-417, 98 Stat. 1585, codified as amended at 21 U.S.C. § 355 (2006).

41. Henry G. Grabowski and John M. Vernon, "Longer Patents for Increased Generic Competition: The Waxman-Hatch Act after One Decade," Duke Economics Working Paper #95-11, November 26, 1997, http://dx.doi.org/10.2139/ssrn .40940.

42. Drug Price Competition and Patent Term Restoration Act of 1984.

43. Michael A. Carrier, "Unsettling Drug Patent Settlements: A Framework for Presumptive Illegality," *Michigan Law Review* 108, no. 1 (2009): 37–80.

44. Carrier, "Unsettling Drug Patent Settlements," 38.

45. Federal Trade Commission, *Pay-for-Delay: How Drug Company Pay-Offs Cost Consumers Billions*, (Washington, DC: Federal Trade Commission, January 2010), https://www.ftc.gov/sites/default/files/documents/reports/pay-delay-how -drug-company-pay-offs-cost-consumers-billions-federal-trade-commission-staff-study /100112payfordelayrpt.pdf.

46. Federal Trade Commission, *Authorized Generic Drugs: Short-Term Effects and Long-Term Impact* (Washington, DC: Federal Trade Commission, August 2011), https://www.ftc.gov/sites/default/files/documents/reports/authorized-generic-drugs -short-term-effects-and-long-term-impact-report-federal-trade-commission/author ized-generic-drugs-short-term-effects-and-long-term-impact-report-federal-trade -commission.pdf.

47. Jonathan Lapook, "Forced Switch? Drug Cos. Develop Maneuvers to Hinder Generic Competition," *CBS News*, August 28, 2014, https://www.cbsnews.com/news /drug-companies-develop-maneuvers-to-hinder-generic-competition.

48. Aaron S. Kesselheim, Carolyn L. Treasure, and Steven Joffe, "Biomarker-Defined Subsets of Common Diseases: Policy and Economic Implications of Orphan Drug Act Coverage," *PLoS Medicine* 14, no. 1 (2017): e1002190, doi:10.1371/journal.pmed .1002190.

49. Kesselheim, Treasure, and Joffe, "Biomarker-Defined Subsets of Common Diseases."

50. Nicholas Bagley, Armitabh Chandra, Craig Garthwaite, and Ariel Stern, "It's Time to Reform the Orphan Drug Act," *NEJM Catalyst*, December 19, 2018, https:// catalyst.nejm.org/time-reform-orphan-drug-act.

51. Robin Feldman, "May Your Drug Price Be Evergreen," *Journal of Law and the Biosciences* 5, no. 3 (2018): 590–647, doi:10.1093/jlb/lsy022.

52. Katie Thomas and Reed Abelson, "The $6 Million Drug Claim," *New York Times*, August 26, 2019, https://www.nytimes.com/2019/08/25/health/drug-prices -rare-diseases.html.

53. Special Committee on Aging, *Sudden Price Spikes in Off-Patent Prescription Drugs: The Monopoly Business Model that Harms Patients, Taxpayers, and the US Health Care System* (Washington, DC: United States Senate, December 2016), https://www.aging.senate.gov/imo/media/doc/Drug%20Pricing%20 Report.pdf.

54. Special Committee on Aging, *Sudden Price Spikes*, 11.

55. "How to Determine if Your Product Is a Medical Device," US Food and Drug Administration, accessed January 23, 2019, https://www.fda.gov/MedicalDevices/Device RegulationandGuidance/Overview/ClassifyYourDevice/ucm051512.htm.

56. Martin Wenzl and Elias Mossialos, "Prices for Cardiac Implant Devices May Be Up to Six Times Higher in the US than in Some European Countries," *Health Affairs* 37, no. 10 (2018): 1570–77, doi:10.1377/hlthaff.2017.1367.

57. Wenzl and Mossialos, "Prices for Cardiac Implant Devices."

58. Medicare Payment Advisory Commission (MedPAC), *Medicare and the Health Care Delivery System: Report to the Congress* (Washington, DC: MedPAC, June 2018), http://medpac.gov/docs/default-source/reports/jun18_medpacreportto congress_sec.pdf.

59. MedPAC, *Medicare and the Health Care Delivery System*.

60. Wenzl and Mossialos, "Prices for Cardiac Implant Devices."

61. Jaime A. Rosenthal, Xin Lu, and Peter Cram, "Availability of Consumer Prices from US Hospitals for a Common Surgical Procedure," *JAMA Internal Medicine* 173, no. 6 (2013): 427–32, doi:10.1001/jamainternmed.2013.460.

62. Elisabeth Rosenthal, "In Need of a New Hip, but Priced Out of the US," *New York Times*, August 3, 2013, https://archive.nytimes.com/www.nytimes.com/2013/08 /04/health/for-medical-tourists-simple-math.html.

63. Rosenthal, "In Need of a New Hip."

64. Rosenthal, "In Need of a New Hip."

20. Inequality of Access

1. Edward R. Berchick, Emily Hood, and Jessica C. Barnett, *Health Insurance Coverage in the United States: 2017*, Current Population Reports P60-264 (Washington, DC: US Government Printing Office, September 2018), https://www.census.gov /content/dam/Census/library/publications/2018/demo/p60-264.pdf.

2. Irene Papanicolas, Liana R. Woskie, and Ashish K. Jha, "Health Care Spending in the United States and Other High-Income Countries," *JAMA* 319, no. 10 (2018): 1024–39, doi:10.1001/jama.2018.1150.

3. Berchick, Hood, and Barnett, *Health Insurance Coverage in the United States*.

4. "Population and Housing Unit Estimates," United States Census Bureau, accessed January 16, 2019, https://www.census.gov/programs-surveys/popest.html.

5. "Population and Housing Unit Estimates," United States Census Bureau.

6. Sara R. Collins, Munira Z. Gunja, and Michelle M. Doty, "How Well Does Insurance Coverage Protect Consumers from Health Care Costs" (issue brief), Commonwealth Fund, October 18, 2017, https://www.commonwealthfund.org/publica tions/issue-briefs/2017/oct/how-well-does-insurance-coverage-protect-consumers -health-care.

7. Collins, Gunja, and Doty, "How Well Does Insurance Coverage Protect Consumers from Health Care Costs."

8. Gary Claxton, Matthew Rae, and Nirmita Panchal, "Consumer Assets and Patient Cost Sharing" (issue brief), Kaiser Family Foundation, March 2015,

https://www.kff.org/health-costs/issue-brief/consumer-assets-and-patient-cost
-sharing.

9. Ashley Kirzinger, Cailey Muñana, Bryan Wu, and Mollyann Brodie, "Data Note: Americans' Challenges with Health Care Costs," Kaiser Family Foundation, June 11, 2019, https://www.kff.org/health-costs/poll-finding/data-note-americans-challenges -with-health-care-costs.

10. Amy Finkelstein, Sarah Taubman, Bill Wright, Mira Bernstein, Jonathan Gruber, Joseph P. Newhouse, Heidi Allen, and Katherine Baicker, "The Oregon Health Insurance Experiment: Evidence from the First Year," *Quarterly Journal of Economics* 127, no. 3 (2012): 1057–1106, doi:10.1093/qje/qjs020.

11. Finkelstein et al., "The Oregon Health Insurance Experiment."

12. Heidi Allen, Katherine Baicker, Amy Finkelstein, Sarah Taubman, and Bill J. Wright, "What the Oregon Health Study Can Tell Us about Expanding Medic-aid," *Health Affairs* 29, no. 8 (2010): 1498–1506, doi:10.1377/hlthaff.2010.0191.

13. Finkelstein et al., "The Oregon Health Insurance Experiment."

14. Katherine Baicker, Sarah L. Taubman, Heidi L. Allen, Mira Bernstein, Jonathan H. Gruber, Joseph P. Newhouse, Eric C. Schneider, Bill J. Wright, Alan M. Zaslavsky, and Amy N. Finkelstein, "The Oregon Experiment—Effects of Medicaid on Clinical Outcomes," *New England Journal of Medicine* 368, no. 18 (2013): 1713–22, doi:10.1056/nejmsa1212321.

15. Baicker et al., "The Oregon Experiment," table 10 (percentages derived from regression results).

16. Baicker et al., "The Oregon Experiment," table 4 (percentages derived from regression results).

17. Baicker et al., "The Oregon Experiment," table 6 (percentages derived from regression results).

18. Ruohua Annetta Zhou, Katherine Baicker, Sarah Taubman, and Amy N. Finkelstein, "The Uninsured Do Not Use the Emergency Department More—They Use Other Care Less," *Health Affairs* 36, no. 12 (2017): 2115–22, doi:10.1377 /hlthaff.2017.0218.

19. Katherine Baicker, Heidi L. Allen, Bill J. Wright, and Amy N. Finkelstein, "The Effect of Medicaid on Medication Use among Poor Adults: Evidence from Oregon," *Health Affairs* 36, no. 12 (2017): 2110–14, doi:10.1377/hlthaff.2017.0925.

20. Baicker et al., "The Effect of Medicaid on Medication Use," 2114.

21. Finkelstein et al., "The Oregon Health Insurance Experiment," table 9 (percentages derived from regression results).

22. Baicker et al., "The Oregon Experiment."

23. Benjamin D. Sommers, Sharon K. Long, and Katherine Baicker, "Changes in Mortality after Massachusetts Health Care Reform," *Annals of Internal Medicine* 160, no. 9 (2014): 585, doi:10.7326/m13-2275.

24. Benjamin D. Sommers, Bethany Maylone, Robert J. Blendon, E. John Orav, and Arnold M. Epstein, "Three-Year Impacts of the Affordable Care Act: Improved Medical Care and Health Among Low-Income Adults," *Health Affairs* 36, no. 6 (2017): 1119–28, doi:10.1377/hlthaff.2017.0293.

25. Adam J. Singer, Henry C. Thode, and Jesse M. Pines, "US Emergency Department Visits and Hospital Discharges among Uninsured Patients before and after Implementation of the Affordable Care Act," *JAMA Network Open* 2, no. 4 (2019): e192662, doi:10.1001/jamanetworkopen.2019.2662.

26. Eric J. Charles, Lily E. Johnston, Morley A. Herbert, J. Hunter Mehaffey, Kenan W. Yount, Donald S. Likosky, Patricia F. Theurer, et al., "Impact of Medicaid Expansion on Cardiac Surgery Volume and Outcomes," *Annals of Thoracic Surgery* 104, no. 4 (2017): 1251–58, doi:10.1016/j.athoracsur.2017.03.079.

27. Chintan B. Bhatt and Consuelo M. Beck-Sagué, "Medicaid Expansion and Infant Mortality in the United States," *American Journal of Public Health* 108, no. 4 (2018): 565–67, doi:10.2105/ajph.2017.304218.

28. Christopher K. Rogers and Ning Jackie Zhang, "An Early Look at the Association between State Medicaid Expansion and Disparities in Cardiovascular Diseases: A Comprehensive Population Health Management Approach," *Population Health Management* 20, no. 5 (2017): 348–56, doi:10.1089/pop.2016.0113.

29. Sarah Miller, Luojia Hu, Robert Kaestner, Bhashkar Mazumder, and Ashley Wong, "The ACA Medicaid Expansion in Michigan and Financial Health," National Bureau of Economic Research Working Paper No. 25053, published September 2018, accessed January 18, 2019, revised September 2019, https://www.nber.org/papers/w25053.

30. Singer, Thode, and Pines, "US Emergency Department Visits."

31. Anna L. Goldman, Danny McCormick, Jennifer S. Haas, and Benjamin D. Sommers, "Effects of the ACA's Health Insurance Marketplaces on the Previously Uninsured: A Quasi-Experimental Analysis," *Health Affairs* 37, no. 4 (2018): 591–99, doi:10.1377/hlthaff.2017.1390.

21. Improving the Balance I

1. John P. Bunker, Howard S. Frazier, and Frederick Mosteller, "Improving Health: Measuring Effects of Medical Care," *Milbank Quarterly* 72, no. 2 (1994): 225, doi:10.2307/3350295.

2. J. Michael McGinnis, "Actual Causes of Death, 1990–2010," presentation at Workshop on Determinants of Premature Mortality, September 18, 2013, National Research Council, Washington, DC.

3. Goodarz Danaei, Eric L. Ding, Dariush Mozaffarian, Ben Taylor, Jürgen Rehm, Christopher J. L. Murray, and Majid Ezzati, "The Preventable Causes of Death in the United States: Comparative Risk Assessment of Dietary, Lifestyle, and Metabolic Risk Factors," *PloS Medicine* 6, no. 4 (2009): e1000058, doi:10.1371/journal.pmed.1000058.

4. Committee on Population, National Research Council and Institute of Medicine, *Measuring the Risks and Causes of Premature Death: Summary of Workshops* (Washington, DC: National Academies Press, 2015), https://www.ncbi.nlm.nih.gov/books/NBK279981/#sec_000046.

5. US Burden of Disease Collaborators, "The State of US Health, 1990–2010: Burden of Diseases, Injuries, and Risk Factors," *Journal of the American Medical Association* 310, no. 6 (2013): 591–608, doi: 10.1001/jama.2013.13805.

6. Melonie Heron, "Deaths: Leading Causes for 2017," *National Vital Statistics Reports* 68, no. 6 (June 2019), https://www.cdc.gov/nchs/data/nvsr/nvsr68/nvsr68_06-508.pdf.

7. Rebecca L. Siegel, Kimberly D. Miller, and Ahmedin Jemal, "Cancer Statistics, 2020," *CA: A Cancer Journal for Clinicians* 70, no. 1 (2020): 7–30, doi:10.3322/caac.21590.

8. Yanping Li, An Pan, Dong D. Wang, Xiaoran Liu, Klodian Dhana, Oscar H. Franco, Stephen Kaptoge, et al., "Impact of Healthy Lifestyle Factors on Life Expectancies in the US Population," *Circulation* 138, no. 4 (2018): 345–55, doi:10.1161/circulationaha.117.032047.

9. Theodore R. Holford, Rafael Meza, Kenneth E. Warner, Clare Meernik, Jihyoun Jeon, Suresh H. Moolgavkar, and David T. Levy, "Tobacco Control and the Reduction in Smoking-Related Premature Deaths in the United States, 1964–2012," *JAMA* 311, no. 2 (2014): 164, doi:10.1001/jama.2013.285112.

10. Holford et al., "Tobacco Control."

11. Earl S. Ford, Umed A. Ajani, Janet B. Croft, Julia A. Critchley, Darwin R. Labarthe, Thomas E. Kottke, Wayne H. Giles, and Simon Capewell, "Explaining the Decrease in US Deaths from Coronary Disease, 1980–2000," *New England Journal of Medicine* 356, no. 23 (2007): 2388–98, doi:10.1056/nejmsa053935.

12. Diabetes Prevention Program Research Group, "Reduction in the Incidence of Type 2 Diabetes with Lifestyle Intervention or Metformin," *New England Journal of Medicine* 346, no. 6 (2002): 393–403, doi:10.1056/nejmoa012512.

13. Elizabeth K. Ely, Stephanie M. Gruss, Elizabeth T. Luman, Edward W. Gregg, Mohammed K. Ali, Kunthea Nhim, Deborah B. Rolka, and Ann L. Albright, "A National Effort to Prevent Type 2 Diabetes: Participant-Level Evaluation of CDC's National Diabetes Prevention Program," *Diabetes Care* 40, no. 10 (2017): 1331–41, doi:10.2337/dc16-2099.

14. "Obesity Rates & Trend Data," State of Childhood Obesity, accessed January 30, 2019, https://www.stateofobesity.org/data.

15. Nilay S. Shah, Donald M. Lloyd-Jones, Martin O'Flaherty, Simon Capewell, Kiarri Kershaw, Mercedes Carnethon, and Sadiya S. Khan, "Trends in Cardiometabolic Mortality in the United States, 1999–2017," *JAMA* 322, no. 8 (2019): 780, doi:10.1001/jama.2019.9161.

16. Abdel R. Omran, "The Epidemiologic Transition: A Theory of the Epidemiology of Population Change," *Milbank Quarterly* 83, no. 4 (2005): 731–57, doi:10.1111/j.1468-0009.2005.00398.x.

17. Douglas W. Dockery, C. Arden Pope, Xiping Xu, John D. Spengler, James H. Ware, Martha E. Fay, Benjamin G. Ferris, and Frank E. Speizer, "An Association between Air Pollution and Mortality in Six US Cities," *New England Journal of Medicine* 329, no. 24 (1993): 1753–59, doi:10.1056/nejm199312093292401.

18. Michael Guarnieri and John R. Balmes, "Outdoor Air Pollution and Asthma," *The Lancet* 383, no. 9928 (2014): 1581–92, doi:10.1016/s0140-6736(14)60617-6.

19. Virginia A. Rauh, Robin Garfinkel, Frederica P. Perera, Howard F. Andrews, Lori Hoepner, Dana B. Barr, Ralph Whitehead, Deliang Tang, and Robin W. Whyatt, "Impact of Prenatal Chlorpyrifos Exposure on Neurodevelopment in the First 3 Years of Life among Inner-City Children," *Pediatrics* 118, no. 6 (2006): e1845–59, doi:10.1542/peds.2006-0338.

20. E. Ray Dorsey, Todd Sherer, Michael S. Okun, and Bastiaan R. Bloem, "The Emerging Evidence of the Parkinson Pandemic," *Journal of Parkinson's Disease* 8, no. s1 (2018): S3–S8, doi:10.3233/jpd-181474.

21. Dorsey et al., "The Emerging Evidence of the Parkinson Pandemic."

22. Claire Pomeroy, "'Empress of All Maladies': Mary Lasker," *The Hill*, March 20, 2015, https://thehill.com/blogs/congress-blog/healthcare/236121-empress -of-all-maladies-mary-lasker.

23. United for Medical Research and Eric Wolff, *Profiles of Prosperity: How NIH-Supported Research Is Fueling Private Sector Growth and Innovation* (United for Medical Research, 2013), 3, http://www.unitedformedicalresearch.com/wp -content/uploads/2013/07/UMR_ProsperityReport_071913a.pdf.

24. Batelle Technology Partnership Practice, *The Impact of Genomics on the US Economy* (Columbus, OH: Battelle Memorial Institute, 2013), https://web.ornl.gov/sci /techresources/Human_Genome/publicat/2013BattelleReportImpact-of-Genomics -on-the-US-Economy.pdf.

25. Ekaterina Galkina Cleary, Jennifer M. Beierlein, Navleen Surjit Khanuja, Laura M. McNamee, and Fred D. Ledley, "Contribution of NIH Funding to New Drug Approvals 2010–2016," *Proceedings of the National Academy of Sciences* 115, no. 10 (2018): 2329–34, doi:10.1073/pnas.1715368115.

26. Andrew A. Toole, "Does Public Scientific Research Complement Private Investment in Research and Development in the Pharmaceutical Industry?," *Journal of Law and Economics* 50, no. 1 (2007): 81–104, doi:10.1086/508314.

27. Fangjun Zhou, Abigail Shefer, Jay Wenger, Mark Messonnier, Li Yan Wang, Adriana Lopez, Matthew Moore, Trudy V. Murphy, Margaret Cortese, and Lance Rodewald, "Economic Evaluation of the Routine Childhood Immunization Program in the United States, 2009," *Pediatrics* 133, no. 4 (2014): 577–85, doi:10.1542 /peds.2013-0698.

28. Joshua A. Roth, Ruth Etzioni, Teresa M. Waters, Mary Pettinger, Jacques E. Rossouw, Garnet L. Anderson, Rowan T. Chlebowski, et al., "Economic Return from the Women's Health Initiative Estrogen Plus Progestin Clinical Trial," *Annals of Internal Medicine* 160, no. 9 (2014): 594–602, doi:10.7326/m13-2348.

29. United for Medical Research, *NIH's Role in Sustaining the US Economy: 2017 Update* (United for Medical Research, 2017), http://www.unitedformedicalresearch .com/wp-content/uploads/2017/03/NIH-Role-in-the-Economy-FY2016.pdf.

30. Hamilton Moses, David H. M. Matheson, Sarah Cairns-Smith, Benjamin P. George, Chase Palisch, and E. Ray Dorsey, "The Anatomy of Medical Research: US and International Comparisons," *JAMA* 313, no. 2 (2015): 174, doi:10.1001/jama .2014.15939.

31. Moses et al., "Anatomy of Medical Research."

32. "Frances Collins at the Washington Ideas Forum" (video), *C-SPAN*, November 13, 2013, https://www.c-span.org/video/?316217-13/francis-collins-washington -ideas-forum.

33. "Frances Collins," *C-SPAN*.

34. Bruce Alberts, Marc W. Kirschner, Shirley Tilghman, and Harold Varmus, "Rescuing US Biomedical Research from Its Systemic Flaws," *Proceedings of the*

National Academy of Sciences 111, no. 16 (2014): 5773–77, doi:10.1073/pnas.14044 02111; Victor J. Dzau and Harvey V. Fineberg, "Restore the US Lead in Biomedical Research," *JAMA* 313, no. 2 (2015): 143, doi:10.1001/jama.2014.17660.

35. John Porter, "A Do-Nothing Congress Isn't Healthy," *CNN*, August 16, 2013, https://www.cnn.com/2013/08/16/opinion/porter-health-research-congress/index .html.

36. Thomas Cars, Lars Lindhagen, and Johan Sundström, "A Framework for Monitoring of New Drugs in Sweden," *Upsala Journal of Medical Sciences* 124, no. 1 (2019): 46–50, doi:10.1080/03009734.2018.1550454.

37. Leah Tuzzio, Eric B. Larson, David A. Chambers, Gloria D. Coronado, Lesley H. Curtis, Wendy J. Weber, Douglas F. Zatzick, and Catherine M. Meyers, "Pragmatic Clinical Trials Offer Unique Opportunities for Disseminating, Implementing, and Sustaining Evidence-Based Practices into Clinical Care: Proceedings of a Workshop," *Healthcare* 7, no. 1 (2019): 51–57, doi:10.1016/j.hjdsi.2018.12.003.

38. US Government Accountability Office (GAO), *Comparative Effectiveness Research: Activities Funded by the Patient-Centered Outcomes Research Trust Fund*, GAO-18-311 (Washington, DC: GAO, March 2018), 16, https://www.gao.gov/assets /700/690835.pdf.

39. Sumit R. Majumdar and Stephen B. Soumerai, "The Unhealthy State of Health Policy Research," *Health Affairs* 28, no. 5 (2009): w900–908, doi:10.1377/hlth aff.28.5.w900.

40. James C. Capretta, "Opinion: The Financial Hole for Social Security and Medicare Is Even Deeper Than the Experts Say," *MarketWatch*, June 16, 2018, https://www.marketwatch.com/story/the-financial-hole-for-social-security-and-medi care-is-even-deeper-than-the-experts-say-2018-06-15.

41. Capretta, "Opinion."

42. Phill Swagel, "Director's Statement on an Update to the Budget and Economic Outlook, 2019–2029," *CBO Blog*, Congressional Budget Office, August 21, 2019, https://www.cbo.gov/publication/55565.

22. Improving the Balance II

1. "Medicare for All Act of 2019," Bernie Sanders (website), accessed April 17, 2019, https://www.sanders.senate.gov/download/medicare-for-all-act-of-2019.

2. Avik S. A. Roy, *Transcending Obamacare: A Patient-Centered Plan for Near-Universal Coverage and Permanent Fiscal Solvency*, 2nd ed. (Austin, TX: Foundation for Research on Equal Opportunity, 2016), https://freopp.docsend.com/view/utmr2i6.

3. Charles E. Phelps and Stephen T. Parente, *The Economics of US Health Care Policy* (New York: Routledge, 2018).

4. Jeff Stein and Yasmeen Abutaleb, "Congress Showers Health Care Industry with a Multibillion-Dollar Victory after Wagging Finger at It for Much of 2019," *Washington Post*, December 20, 2019, https://www.washingtonpost.com/business /economy/congress-showers-health-care-industry-with-multi-billion-victory-after -wagging-finger-at-it-for-much-of-2019/2019/12/19/9422aa6a-2028-11ea-9146-6c3a3 ab1be6c_story.html.

5. Valerie C. Brannon, "Drug Price Disclosures and the First Amendment" (legal sidebar), Congressional Research Service, updated July 9, 2019, 1, https://fas.org/sgp /crs/misc/LSB10298.pdf.

6. Christopher Whaley, Timothy Brown, and James Robinson, "Consumer Responses to Price Transparency Alone versus Price Transparency Combined with Reference Pricing," *American Journal of Health Economics* 5, no. 2 (2019): 227–49, doi:10.1162/ajhe_a_00118.

7. Uwe E. Reinhardt, "The Disruptive Innovation of Price Transparency in Health Care," *JAMA* 310, no. 18 (2013): 1927, doi:10.1001/jama.2013.281854.

8. Austin Frakt, "How Common Procedures Became 20 Percent Cheaper for Many Californians," *New York Times*, August 8, 2016, https://www.nytimes.com/2016 /08/09/upshot/how-common-procedures-got-20-percent-cheaper-for-many-califor nians.html.

9. Whaley, Brown, and Robinson, "Consumer Responses to Price Transparency."

10. Kenneth Arrow, "Uncertainty and the Welfare Economics of Medical Care," *American Economic Review* 53 (1963): 941–73.

11. Choosing Wisely (website), American Board of Internal Medicine Foundation, accessed March 5, 2019, https://www.choosingwisely.org.

12. Further Consolidated Appropriations Act, 2020. H.R. 1865, 116th Cong. (2019), https://www.congress.gov/116/bills/hr1865/BILLS-116hr1865enr.pdf.

13. Phelps and Parente, *Economics of US Health Care Policy*, 137.

14. Eric A. Patashnik, Alan S. Gerber, and Conor M. Dowling, *Unhealthy Politics* (Princeton: Princeton University Press, 2017).

15. Donald M. Berwick, "The Epitaph of Profession," *British Journal of General Practice* 59, no. 559 (2009): 128–31, doi:10.3399/bjgp08x376438.

16. Berwick, "The Epitaph of Profession," 131.

17. Medicare Payment Advisory Commission (MedPAC), *Medicare and the Health Care Delivery System: Report to the Congress* (Washington, DC: MedPAC, June 2018), http://medpac.gov/docs/default-source/reports/jun18_medpacreporttocongress_sec .pdf.

18. These figures are based on data from GatorCare, the self insurance plan for University of Florida Health in Gainesville, Florida.

19. Vivian S. Lee and Bonnie B. Blanchfield, "Disentangling Health Care Billing," *JAMA* 319, no. 7 (2018): 661, doi:10.1001/jama.2017.19966.

20. David Cutler, Elizabeth Wikler, and Peter Basch, "Reducing Administrative Costs and Improving the Health Care System," *New England Journal of Medicine* 367, no. 20 (2012): 1875–78, doi:10.1056/nejmp1209711.

21. Letter to Senate committees on national unique patient identifier, August 27, 2019, https://strategichealthcare.net/wp-content/uploads/2019/09/Letter-On -National-Patient-ID.pdf.

22. Nancy L. Yu, Preston Atteberry, and Peter B. Bach, "Spending on Prescription Drugs in the US: Where Does All the Money Go?," *Considering Health Spending* (blog), *Health Affairs*, July 31, 2018, https://www.healthaffairs.org/do/10.1377 /hblog20180726.670593/full/.

23. Gerald Donahoe and Guy King, *Estimates of Medical Device Spending in the United States* (Washington, DC: Advance Medical Technology Association [AdvaMed], June 2015), https://www.advamed.org/sites/default/files/resource/994 _100515_guy_king_report_2015_final.pdf.

24. Ezekiel J. Emanuel, "Democrats Are Having the Wrong Health Care Debate," *New York Times*, August 2, 2019, https://www.nytimes.com/2019/08/02/opinion/demo crats-health-care.html.

25. Salomeh Keyhani, Steven Wang, Paul Hebert, Daniel Carpenter, and Gerard Anderson, "US Pharmaceutical Innovation in an International Context," *American Journal of Public Health* 100, no. 6 (2010): 1075–80, doi:10.2105/ajph.2009.178491.

26. Robert M. Califf and Andrew Slavitt, "Lowering Cost and Increasing Access to Drugs without Jeopardizing Innovation," *JAMA* 321, no. 16 (2019): 1571, doi:10.1001/jama.2019.3846.

27. Shailin Thomas and Arthur Caplan, "The Orphan Drug Act Revisited," *JAMA* 321, no. 9 (2019): 833–34, doi:10.1001/jama.2019.0290.

28. Rena M. Conti, Sayeh Nikpay, Gabriela Gracia, and Melinda J. Beeuwkes Buntin, "Proposed Reforms to the 340B Drug Discount Program," *Drugs and Medical Innovation* (blog), *Health Affairs*, March 7, 2019, https://www.healthaffairs.org/do/10 .1377/hblog20180306.70004/full/.

29. Loren Adler, Matthew Fiedler, Paul B. Ginsburg, Mark Hall, Erin Trish, Christen Linke Young, and Erin L. Duffy, *State Approaches to Mitigating Surprise Out-of-Network Billing*, white paper for USC-Brookings Schaeffer Initiative for Health Policy (Washington, DC: Brookings Institution, 2018), https://www.brookings. edu/wp-content/uploads/2019/02/Adler_et-al_State-Approaches-to-Mitigating-Sur prise-Billing-2019.pdf.

30. Medicaid and CHIP Payment and Access Commission (MACPAC), "Ex-hibit 24. Medicaid Supplemental Payments to Hospital Providers by State, FY2017" (data file), accessed March 11, 2019, https://www.macpac.gov/publication/medicaid -supplemental-payments-to-hospital-providers-by-state.

31. Sabrina Corlette and Jack Hoadley, *Strategies to Stabilize the Affordable Care Act Marketplaces: Lessons from Medicare* (Washington, DC: Georgetown University Health Policy Institute, August 2016), https://www.rwjf.org/en/library/research/2016 /08/strategies-to-stabilize-the-affordable-care-act-marketplaces.html.

32. Chris Sloan, Neil Rosacker, and Elizabeth Carpenter, "State-Run Reinsur-ance Programs Reduce ACA Premiums by 19.9% on Average" (press release), Avalere, March 13, 2019, https://avalere.com/press-releases/state-run-reinsurance-programs -reduce-aca-premiums-by-19-9-on-average.

33. Victor R. Fuchs, "Is Single Payer the Answer for the US Health Care System?," *JAMA* 319, no. 1 (2018): 15, doi:10.1001/jama.2017.18739.

34. Roy, *Transcending Obamacare*, 4.

35. Roy, *Transcending Obamacare*; Avik Roy, "Bringing Private Health Insurance into the 21st Century," FREEOP.org, April 21, 2019, https://freopp.org/bringing -private-health-insurance-into-the-21st-century-d1df138f1f0c.

36. Roy, "Bringing Private Health Insurance into the 21st Century."

37. Timothy Jost, "Transcending Obamacare? Analyzing Avik Roy's ACA Replacement Plan," *Following the ACA* (blog), *Health Affairs*, September 2, 2014, https://www.healthaffairs.org/do/10.1377/hblog20140902.041142/full.

38. Roy, "Bringing Private Health Insurance into the 21st Century."

39. "Medicare for All Act of 2019," Bernie Sanders (website).

40. "Financing Medicare for All" (white paper), Bernie Sanders (website), accessed April 17, 2019, https://www.sanders.senate.gov/download/medicare-for-all-2019-financing.

41. Dean Baker, "Can We Pay for Single Payer?," *Democracy Journal*, September 14, 2017, https://democracyjournal.org/arguments/can-we-pay-for-single-payer.

42. Linda J. Blumberg, John Holahan, Matthew Buettgen, Anuj Gangopadhyaya, Bowen Garrett, Adele Shartzer, Michael Simpson, Robin Wang, Melissa M. Favreault, and Diane Arnos, *From Incremental to Comprehensive Health Care Insurance Reform: How Various Reform Options Compare on Coverage and Costs* (Washington, DC: Urban Institute, October 2019), https://www.urban.org/sites/default/files/2019/10/15/from_incremental_to_comprehensive_health_insurance_reform-how_various_reform_options_compare_on_coverage_and_costs.pdf.

43. Reed Abelson and Margot Sanger-Katz, "Medicare for All Would Abolish Private Insusrance: 'There's No Precedent in American History,'" *New York Times*, March 23, 2019. https://www.nytimes.com/2019/03/23/health/private-health-insurance-medicare-for-all-bernie-sanders.html.

INDEX

asymmetric information, 284, 285, 459; induced demand and, 53, 59, 73, 77–78, 179, 253; reduction in, 464–67

Atherosclerosis Risk in Communities, 128

authority, of physicians, 284, 285

autonomy, of physicians, 135–36, 137, 284, 285, 313–15, 459; reliability *vs.*, 313–17, 459, 467–68

back braces, 404–5, 438

back pain, surgical treatment, 179, 180–82, 263–64

Balanced Budget Act, 176

bankruptcy, 130, 420, 421, 429, 484

Baruch, Bernard, 164

behavioral determinants, of disease/health status, 10, 125, 127–28, 424–25, 436–38, 457, 459, 497; interventions, 438–41; life expectancy and, 128–30

benchmarking, 184; value-based, 348

beneficence, 79

benefit-to-cost ratio, 265

Berwick, Donald, 190, 467–68

best-practice treatment, 260–61, 311, 313

Better Medicare Alliance, 188

billing: administrative costs, 105–6, 360–69, 459, 461, 472–74; diagnostic codes, 362–65; integrated system, 363, 365. *See also* claims processing

biological response modifiers, 72–73

biomedical research, 156–57, 444–45, 457; on comparative or cost effectiveness of care, 465–66; funding, 442–43; HIPAA Privacy rule effects, 306–7; pragmatic clinical trials, 242, 447–51; translational, 9–10. *See also* randomized controlled trials

biomedicine, advances in, 3, 173, 403, 435, 436, 442, 443, 457, 497; cancer treatment, 12–16; cardiovascular disease treatment, 19–21; childhood leukemia, 12–13; gynecology and reproductive endocrinology, 5–11; heart valve malfunction treatment,

22–24; hepatitis prevention and treatment, 16–18; historical overview, 138–39, 143, 153, 155–57, 166–67; mental health, 24–25; premature infant care, 11–12; prescription drugs, 349, 350–52, 356–57; radiosurgery, 25–26; stroke treatment, 21–22; transformative, 246–47, 442, 443

Bipartisan Budget Act, 192, 465

birth rate, 454

Blue Cross and Blue Shield, 147, 148, 149–50, 153, 159–61, 169, 220, 343

Blumberg, Baruch, 17

bone marrow transplant therapy, 155, 251–54, 255

Bradley, Daniel, 18

Brandeis, Louis, 140–41

Braunwald, Eugene, 20

breast cancer, 248, 249, 250, 438; prevention and treatment, 13–15, 251–54, 255

Bundled Payments for Care Improvement Initiative, 300

bundled payment systems, 214, 300, 474, 482

Bureau of Labor Statistics (BLS), 137–38, 164–65, 333, 359, 369, 472

Butler, Stuart, 219

California Public Employees' Retirement System (Calpers), 464

cancer, 1, 2, 5, 22, 336–37, 437–38; treatment, 12–16, 33–36, 37

capitalism, 38–40, 497

capitation payment systems, 162, 309, 378, 474; fully capitated, risk-bearing, 469–70; Medicaid, 203–4, 209; Medicare, 176, 183–86, 187, 189

cardiovascular disease, 22–24, 122, 125, 246, 336–37, 425, 426, 428; hormone replacement therapy and, 247–51; as mortality cause, 1, 2, 19–21, 122, 436, 437–38; risk factors, 19, 20–21, 125, 128, 437, 438, 439

Carr, Elizabeth Jordan, 8

case-control studies, 240–42

case series, 240

Center for Medicare and Medicaid Innovation, 327

Centers for Disease Control and Prevention (CDC), 17, 18, 58, 256, 428, 440–41, 443, 466

Centers for Medicare and Medicaid Services (CMS), 176, 275, 277, 303, 348, 366, 466–67, 471; Anti-Kickback Statute and, 296; Medicaid oversight role, 197, 199, 229; Medicare Advantage expenditures, 183–85; Medicare Physician Group Practice Demonstration, 190; value-based programs, 348

Certificate of Need statutes, 36, 49, 50, 54, 83, 95

certification/recertification requirements, 36, 49–50, 53–54, 140, 258, 321, 322

cervical cancer, 5, 8–11, 13

Chamberlin, Edward, 51

CHAMPVA, 410

chemotherapy, 12–16, 138, 246, 390–91, 445

Child Health and Medical Assistance Act, 196

children, 12–13; health insurance coverage, 168, 197, 198–99, 209, 214–16, 411, 414; mortality causes and rates, 121, 122; obesity in, 122, 123

Children's Health Insurance Program (CHIP), 112, 197, 198, 199–201, 207, 410, 414, 418; eligibility, 416

Choo, Qui-Lim, 18

Choosing Wisely, 465

chronic diseases, 4, 5, 125, 173, 187–89, 336–37; social and behavioral determinants, 436–41; in uninsured patients, 483–84; US/international comparison, 122–23, 125

claims processing, 362–65, 371; audits, 288, 291, 309, 475–76; denial of claims, 364, 365; electronic, 106, 242, 289, 363–65, 474–76; fraudu-

lent claims, 287, 288–91, 309; health care price effects, 371

clinical guidelines, 469–70

Clinical Outcomes Utilizing Revascularization and Aggressive Drug Evaluation (COURAGE) trial, 258–59

clinical practice, individual styles, 314–17

clinical trials, 324, 399; cooperative, 12; funding and subsidies, 248, 400, 401; pragmatic, 242, 447–51. *See also* randomized controlled trials

Cochrane Database of Systematic Reviews, 244–45, 465

cognitive behavioral therapy, 25

cohort studies, longitudinal, 241–42

coinsurance (co-pays), 54, 214, 363; health care utilization relationship, 61–64, 338; for low-value services, 470–71; Medicare, 177, 179–80; out-of-pocket costs and, 61, 64–65; for prescription drugs, 385–86, 388–89; price elasticity of demand and, 61–66; value-based, 338–39, 347–48

Collins, Frances, 446

colorectal cancer, 15, 438, 448

commercial health insurance, 478; 1920s through 1930s, 144, 148, 149, 150, 153; 1940s through 1965, 159–61; cost sharing, 126; hospital payments, 373–74, 375, 379–80, 481, 483, 495; pharmacy ad medical device payments, 381–81, 388, 394–95, 396, 406, 467; physician payments, 376, 379–80, 390–91, 495; retained earnings, 361, 473; spending per beneficiary, 88–90, 100. *See also* employer-sponsored health insurance; private health insurance

Committee on Quality of Health Care in America, *Crossing the Quality Chasm: A New Health System for the 21st Century*, 326–30

Committee on the Costs of Medical Care (CCMC), 144–47, 148, 149, 153

Committee to Coordinate Health and Welfare Activities, 148–49, 150 commodities, value of, 40–41

Commonwealth Fund, 419

comparative-effectiveness research, 283–84, 462–63, 464–67; patient-centered, 449–50

competition: monopolistic, 51, 52. *See also* perfect competition, assumptions of

Comprehensive Care for Joint Replacement, 300

conflict of interest, 80, 287. *See also* Anti-Kickback Statute; Stark law

confounding variables, 241

congestive heart failure, 321, 322

Congressional Budget Office (CBO), 190, 225, 227, 230–31, 281–82, 283, 454–55

Consolidated Omnibus Reconciliation Act, 301

consolidation, in health care market, 472

Consumer Price Index (CPI), 106, 176, 333, 358–60, 375, 376, 378, 381–82, 478

consumer-producer interactions, 31–32

consumers: as health care industry stakeholders, 136, 137; perfect knowledge of, 36–37; rationality, 36–37, 48, 50

consumption, in perfect competition, 37

continuous positive airway pressure (CPAP) masks, 404, 438

contraceptives, 5, 57, 127, 338

Copeland Act, 292

coronary artery disease, coronary stents for, 257–60

cost, of health care. *See* health care costs

cost-benefit analysis, 235–37, 265–72; classification of benefits, 268–69; constraints, 279–85, 460; valuation of life component, 269–72

cost-benefit ratio, 253

cost-effectiveness analysis, 266, 273–74, 287; constraints, 279–85, 459, 460; as health care reform component, 462–67

cost-plus reimbursement system, 151–52, 153, 171, 176–77, 236

cost sharing, 126, 202, 209, 212, 224, 226, 294, 343, 356

cost-to-charge ratio, 373–74

cost-utility analysis, 266, 273–79, 460

Cournot, Antoine, 39–40

CPAP masks (sleep apnea devices), 404, 438

credentialing, 140

Crossing the Quality Chasm: A New Health System for the 21st Century, 326–30

cross-sectional studies, 240–41

CT (computerized tomography) scans, 21, 26, 65, 338, 345

Current Procedural Terminology (CPT) codes, 171–72, 362

CVS-Caremark, 281

CVS Pharmacy, 342

Dartmouth Atlas, 84, 93

Davis, Michael, 147

"death panels," 280, 465

deaths, medical errors–related, 318–21, 322

decision-making: evidence-based, 245–46; with imperfect information, 261–64; marginal cost–marginal benefit model, 74–77, 99

deductibles, 177, 338, 363, 370; as underinsurance cause, 419–20, 431. *See also* high-deductible health insurance; out-of-pocket costs

defibrillators, wearable, 403, 404–5, 438

demand, health care expenditures and, 54–58. *See also* supply and demand

demand curves, 74–77

demand-side factors, in health care expenditures, 85, 94, 100

demand theory, of revealed preference strategy, 272

dentists/dental care, 62, 64, 109, 144, 155, 157, 196, 197, 359, 483, 494

designated health services (DHS), 297–99

diabetes, 90–91, 122, 125, 129, 336–37, 437, 441, 457; health care utilization

Freud, Sigmund, 25
Frost, Robert, 7
Fuchs, Victor, 76, 490, 494
fusion protein inhibitors, 15–16,
397–98

gainsharing, 300–301
gap payments, 63–64
Gardasil, 10–11
Garfield, Sidney, 162
gastric cancer, 15, 16
general equilibrium theory, 36–37
generic drugs, 337, 398–400, 477, 480
genetic disorders, 2
geographic variation, in health care
expenditures, 81–96, 336; cross-
sectional studies, 84–92; historical
studies, 81–84; natural experiments,
92–94, 100, 469; physician beliefs
and practice styles and, 96–98, 336
germ theory, 138–39
Gini coefficient, 114–17
government health insurance, 410
Great Depression, 117, 143, 147, 148–49,
162
Great Recession (2008–2009), 214, 452
Gross Domestic Product (GDP), 46, 107,
116, 214, 335, 353, 451–52, 477–78
Group Health Association of New York,
163
Group Health Cooperative of Puget
Sound, 163
Group Health Incorporated (GHI), 163
Group Health Incorporated (GHI)
Health Maintenance Organization,
163
group practice: Medicare Physician
Group Practice Demonstration,
190; prepaid health insurance plans,
146, 150–51, 162–64, 167, 474
group purchasing organizations (GPOs),
296–97
guaranteed issue, 213, 216–17, 218, 219,
220–21, 223
gun violence, 436, 438
gynecology and reproductive endocrinology, advances in, 5–11

Hatch-Waxman Act. *See* Drug Price
Competition and Patent Term
Restoration Act
health care: differentiation of services,
47–48, 51; as right, 66–71, 483, 497
health care access, 27; constraints, 460;
health outcomes effects, 426, 427–28;
imbalance with cost and quality, 312,
329, 435–36, 456–57, 497–98; in
perfect market, 60–61; strategies for
improvement, 482–90. *See also*
insured population; Medicaid;
Medicare; uninsured population
health care access inequalities, 47,
112–30, 312, 409–31, 482; income
and wealth inequalities and, 113–18;
strategies for improvement, 482–90
Health Care Cost Institute, 337
health care costs, 3–4, 8; of behaviorally
based disease, 438; as deterrent to
health care utilization, 47, 125–26; as
health care expenditures component,
459; health insurance contributions,
379; hospitals' contributions, 373–76,
379; imbalance with access, 435–36,
456–57; of ineffective treatment, 311;
major drivers, 336; of medical
devices, 403; of mental health
treatment, 24
health care exchanges, 211, 411, 416, 418,
429–30; challenges to, 223–25,
226–27, 231; enrollment, 224–25,
226, 488–89; stabilization, 488–89,
490; subsidies and tax credits,
217–18, 224–25, 485, 488
health care expenditures, 137–38, 455;
1940s through 1965, 165–66;
administrative costs component,
105–6, 361, 365–66; under Affordable Care Act, 213–14; federal deficit/
debt and, 452–55; fraud-based, 289,
291, 309; health care costs and, 459;
health outcomes and, 331; health
status and, 88–89, 90–92; per illness
episodes, 107, 108, 109; in imperfect
market, 54–58; induced demand
and, 331–32; longitudinal analyses,

design, 338–39, 342–43, 347–49,
470–71. *See also* coinsurance;
deductibles; Medicaid; Medicare;
premiums
health insurance, history of, 133–53;
1920s through 1930s, 143–52, 153;
1940s through 1965, 159–64;
hospital care coverage, 147–49
health insurance benefits, 265
health insurance companies, 136, 142;
administrative costs, 360–62,
365–69; consolidation with pharmacy chains, 387; health care price
effects, 369–71; medical loss ratio,
224, 361–62, 366–67, 369; retained
earnings (profits), 360, 361–62, 367,
369, 370–71, 472–73
health insurance industry, 435; 1920s
through 1930s, 143–52, 153; 1940s
through 1965, 159–64; stakeholders'
special interests, 134–37
Health Insurance Plan (HIP), 163
Health Insurance Portability and
Accountability Act (HIPAA), 304–9,
310; Privacy Rule, 304, 306–7, 474,
476
health maintenance organizations
(HMOs), 176, 187, 190, 374
health outcomes: causal link with
treatment, 238; cost-benefit analysis,
265–72; health policy research and,
447–51; heterogeneity, 47–48; of
Medicaid enrollees, 424–26, 427–28,
431; US/international comparison, 4,
46, 435
Health Professionals Follow-Up Study,
438
health reimbursement accounts, 491
health savings accounts, 470, 491–92,
493; combined with high-deductible
health insurance, 341, 342
health status: behavioral factors, 404,
424–25; health care expenditures
and, 88–89, 90–92; health care
utilization and, 86–87, 88–89, 90–92,
94; health insurance coverage and,
417, 420, 421; measures, 118–25; of

Medicaid enrollees, 424–26; US/
international comparison, 46
Healthy Michigan, 428–29
Healthy People 2020, 13, 14, 113
Healy, Bernadine, 248
Heart and Estrogen/progestin Replacement Study (HERS), 249
heart surgery, in Medicaid enrollees, 428
heart valve disease, 22–24, 156
hemodialysis, 273–74, 276–77, 280
hepatitis, 16–18
hepatitis vaccine, 17
heterogeneous health care products and
services, 51
high-deductible health insurance, 214,
339, 360, 370, 463, 470, 471, 491;
combined with health savings
accounts, 341, 342; health utilization
effects, 340–41
high-value health plans, 342
Hill-Burton Act, 158–59, 171
HIPAA. *See* Health Insurance Portability
and Accountability Act
Hippocrates, 79
hip replacement surgery, 403, 406–7
Hispanics, 414, 415, 416, 417, 430–31
HIV/AIDS, 122, 123, 126, 127, 246
Holmes, King, 10
homicide, 122, 126, 127
homogeneous health care products and
services, 36, 47–48, 51
hormone replacement therapy, 247–51,
255
hospital(s): Certificate of Need, 36, 49,
50, 54, 83, 95; commercial insurance
payments to, 481; cost-plus reimbursement system, 151–52; disproportionate share payments, 197,
203–5, 209, 214, 454, 483; expenditures on, 144; as health care industry
stakeholders, 136, 137; Medicaid
enrollees' utilization rate, 423, 427;
Medicare and Medicaid payments to,
171, 177–79, 203–5, 209, 481; mergers
and acquisitions, 375; operating
margins, 375; physicians employed
by, 377–79, 380, 391; post-WWII

insured population, 66, 160, 482, 490

Internal Revenue Act, 166

International Classification of Diseases, Version 10 (ICD-10), 362

International Federation of Health Plans (IFHP), 103–5

"invisible hand" theorem, 38–40, 42–43, 235

in vitro fertilization (IVF), 7–8; economic efficiency *vs.* societal values of, 32–33, 37; insurance coverage-utilization relationship, 54–58, 61; supply and demand curves, 41–42, 43–44

In Vitro Fertilization Comes to America (Jones Jr.), 7

Johnson, Lyndon B., 170

Jones, Georgeanna Segar, 8

Jones, Howard W., Jr., 7, 8

Kaiser Permanente (KP), 162, 163, 474

Kassebaum, Nancy, 304

Kennedy, Edward M., 68, 304

Kennedy, Jacqueline Bouvier, 11

Kennedy, John F., 11–12, 169, 170

Kennedy, Patrick Bouvier, 11

Kerr-Mills Act, 195–96, 208–9

Keynes, John Maynard, 40

Kimball, Justin Ford, 147

King, Cecil, 169, 170

knee osteoarthritis, arthroscopic treatment, 91, 254–57

Koch, Robert, 138

Kuo, George, 18

labor unions, 142, 144, 161, 164, 165–66

LaGuardia, Fiorello, 163

Lasker, Mary, 443, 446

Leksell, Lars, 26

Less Medicine, More Health (Welch), 346

Leucht, Stefan, 25

leukemia, 12–13, 15–16, 246, 397–98

License to Steal (Sparrow), 289

licensing requirements, 36, 49–50, 53–54, 140, 321, 322

life, valuation of, 269–72, 286

life expectancy, 1–3, 435; behavioral factors, 128–30, 436, 438–39, 497; chronic disease prevalence and, 336–37; income inequality and, 119–21; metabolic factors, 128–29; as population health status measure, 118–21; US/international comparison, 46, 119, 126–27

lifestyle interventions, for disease prevention, 438–41

limited liability, 148, 150

Lincoln Act. *See* False Claims Act

lobbying, 135, 142, 145, 392–93, 463

long-term care, 196–97, 209

lung cancer, 143, 156, 438, 439, 457

lung disease, chronic, 123

magnetic resonance imaging (MRI), 65, 263–64, 338

managed care: Medicaid plans, 203–4, 206, 207–8, 209. *See also* Medicare Advantage

Mandrola, John, 347

man-made diseases, 2–3, 441–42, 457

Manual of Political Economy (Pareto), 32

marginal behavior, 41

marginal cost, 41; perfect competition and, 31–32

marginal cost–marginal benefit model, of patient decision-making, 74–77, 99

market competition, 31. *See also* perfect competition, assumptions of

market imperfections, in health care, 46–59, 236, 497–98; health care expenditures and, 54–58; utilization–price subsidies relationship, 60–71

Marshall, Alfred, 38, 39–44, 45, 74–75

Massachusetts, health care reforms, 426

maternal-fetal medicine, 11–12

maternity care insurance coverage, 215, 223 224

McNary, William, 161

Medicaid, 1, 112, 195–209; administrative costs, 361; anti-kickback laws and, 297; coverage rates, 410; drug coverage, 355, 391; eligibility rules,

National Health Expenditure Accounts, 106, 107, 108–9
National Health Expenditure Data tables, 333–34
National Heart Institute, 157
National Institute for Health and Care Excellence (NICE) (UK), 279–80, 465
National Institute of Dental Research, 157
National Institute of Mental Health, 157
National Institutes of Health (NIH), 10; Collaboratory Demonstration Project, 448; funding, 157, 443–44, 445–47; research role, 155, 157, 442, 443–47, 457, 466; Women's Health Initiative clinical trial, 248–51, 445
National Labor Relations Act, 149
National Labor Relations Board, 165
National Patient-Centered Clinical Research Network (PCORnet), 449, 450
National Research Council, 122–23, 126, 318
National Survey of Ambulatory Surgery, 256
National War Labor Board, 166
neonatal medicine, 11–12, 246
neurologic disorders, 2
neurosurgery, 25–26
neurotransmitters, 24–25
new molecular entities, 353
Nixon, Richard M., 169
nonmaleficence, 79
not-for-profit hospitals/organizations, 49, 136, 171, 375
Nurses' Health Study, 438

Obama, Barack, 190
obesity, 122, 127–28, 129, 404, 425, 437, 438, 441, 457
observational studies, 87, 242–43, 253
Office of Civil Rights, 305, 307
Office of Management and Budget (OMB), 270
Office of the Inspector General (OIG), 289, 291, 293, 295, 296, 405
oligopolistic prices, 397–98, 407, 408, 460

Omnibus Budget Reconciliation Acts, 297–98
opioid abuse, 99, 436, 497
Oregon Health Insurance Experiment, 422–23, 424, 426–27, 428, 487
Organisation for Economic Co-operation and Development (OECD), 46, 101–2, 437
Orphan Drug Act, 400–401, 479
out-of-network services, 463, 482
out-of-pocket costs, 236, 253, 371, 435, 463; co-pays and, 61, 64–65; "doughnut hole," 356, 491, 493; drugs, 355–56; health care utilization effect, 126, 338, 339–43; in high-deductible insurance, 176, 340–42; under Medicare and Medicaid, 173, 174–76, 179, 183, 427; price subsidies and, 435, 459; for underinsured individuals, 418–20; US/international comparison, 65, 338; in value-based insurance design, 342–43
ovarian cancer, genetic factors, 15, 16
overuse, of health care. *See* medical overuse

pandemics, 2–3, 441
Pap smear, 8, 9, 143
Pareto efficiency, 37, 42–43, 44, 45, 66, 112; social welfare and, 32–36
Parkinson's disease, 442
Partnership for Patients (PfP) campaign, 327–28
Pasteur, Louis, 10, 138
patents: for medical devices, 404; for prescription drugs, 350, 394–97, 398–401, 477–78, 479–80
patient assistance programs, 389–90
patient-centered care, 327, 329
Patient-Centered Outcomes Research Institute (PCORI), 287, 443, 449–50, 466
"patient comes first" value, 313, 314
"patient dumping," 301–3
Patient Protection and Affordable Care Act (ACA), 209, 210–32; accountable

physician(s) (*cont.*)
321, 322; opposition to health
insurance, 141–42; patients' trust in,
52–53, 59, 285; prescription drug
profits, 387, 390–91; pricing by,
376–379, 371, 375
physician office consultations, 65, 71
physician-owned distributors (PODs),
405
physician-patient relationship, 52–54,
285, 313, 464. *See also* provider-
induced demand
pictorial displays, of levels of evidence,
243–45
Pigou, Arthur, 40
pneumonia, 1, 2–4, 65, 321, 322
poliomyelitis vaccine, 1–2, 155, 157
population growth, 106, 109, 111, 335
population health status, 457
population registries, 448
Porter, John, 447
preexisting conditions, 37, 215, 216–17,
220–21, 223–24, 232, 407; guaranteed issue provision, 213, 216–17, 218,
219, 220–21, 223
preferred provider organizations (PPOs),
374
pregnancy: adolescent, 122, 123–24, 126,
127, 437, 438; Medicaid coverage,
198–99, 209; probability rate, 57;
tubal ectopic, 5–7. *See also* in vitro
fertilization
premature infants, 11–12, 127
premiums, 360; administrative cost
component, 106, 369–70, 379; under
Affordable Care Act, 212, 216–17, 218,
219–20; association health plans,
223–24; under community rating,
159–60, 213, 219–20, 221–22, 223;
under experience rating, 159–61,
220–21; in fee-for-service payment
systems, 288; health care price
effects, 370; medical loss ratio, 224,
361–62, 366–67, 369; under
Medicare, 177; per capita
community-based, 152; percentage
spent on medical care, 369, 370,

472–73; preexisting conditions
coverage (guaranteed access), 213,
216–17, 218, 219, 220–21, 223;
risk-averse, 33, 134; short-term
limited duration, 223–24; tax credits
for, 416
prepaid group health insurance plans,
147, 150–51, 153, 162–64, 167, 474
prescription drugs: adverse effects, 319;
approval process, 324, 325, 329,
356–57, 407–8; cost-utility analysis,
275–76, 279, 280; development costs,
350–52, 351–53; evergreening
techniques for, 398–400, 478,
479–80; generic, 337, 398–400, 477,
480; importation, 397, 402, 477,
478–79; induced demand for,
343–44, 471–72; market, 403;
Medicaid enrollees' use of, 423–24;
Medicare coverage, 176, 183, 466;
off-label use, 282; off-patent,
sole-source, 401–3; "orphan drugs,"
400–401, 479–80; patented, 350,
394–97, 398–401, 477–78, 479–80;
prices, 282; reduction in expenditures on, 476–81; safety, 323–24;
standards of efficacy, 282; unaffordability, 397; underinsurance for, 420;
unequal access, 385; unnecessary
use, 347; utilization rate, 109, 110;
wholesale distributors, 384–85, 386,
476. *See also* direct-to-consumer
advertising; pharmaceutical prices
Prescription Drug User Fee Act, 449
prevention and wellness behaviors, 3
preventive care, 187, 189, 260, 261,
423, 425
price, of health care services: disclosure,
463–64; drivers, 369, 459; health
care expenditures and, 52, 101–11,
331–39; health insurers' contribution
to, 151–52, 369–71; information
about, 462–64; monopolistic, 39, 51,
52, 151, 371–80, 408, 460, 463;
negotiated, 51–52, 69, 371, 374, 459,
463; oligopolistic, 397–98, 407, 408,
460; paid by consumers *vs.* providers,

50, 54, 55, 59; in perfect competition market, 135; perfect knowledge of, 48, 52–53; predetermined, 236; reference pricing, 464; sliding scale, 151; supply and demand effects, 40–44, 50, 51–52; transparency, 463, 464. *See also* pharmaceutical prices

price discrimination, 151, 373–77

price shopping, 464

price subsidies. *See* subsidies, for health care

Principle of Economics (Marshall), 42

private health insurance, 285; coverage rates, 410–11; elimination under Medicare for All, 494, 496; establishment and growth, 164, 166–67; Universal Tax Credit Plan, 491–93, 498

profit: dynamic efficiency and, 44, 350; maximization, 36, 48–49; monopolistic, 39

prospective payment systems, 177–79

prostate cancer, 438

protected health information (PHI), 304–9

protein kinase inhibitors, 445

provider-induced demand, 71–100, 459; agency relationship and, 77–80, 236, 238, 343, 468–69; cross-sectional studies, 84–92; empirical data regarding, 80–98; health care utilization and, 54–59, 65, 331–32, 338, 343–49, 371; historical studies, 81–84; natural experiments–based data, 92–94, 95–96; provider's beliefs and, 80, 96–98, 99, 100, 343, 469; provider's clinical practice styles and, 96–98, 99, 100, 343, 469; provider's financial interests and, 73–74, 78, 80, 99, 343, 469; strategies for reduction, 468–72; warranted or unwarranted, 78–80

psychoactive drugs, 24–25

public health, 1–2

Public Health Service Act, 158

Pure Food and Drug Act, 323

quality, 140, 311–30; guidelines for improvement, 326–30; perfect knowledge of, 48, 52–53; professional autonomy *vs.* reliability issue, 313–17; regulatory safeguards, 321–26, 329

quality adjusted life-years (QALYSs), 265–66, 273–80; threshold value, 275–78, 283; utility value, 273

quantity, in health care. *See* health care utilization

racial and ethnic factors: in behaviorally related disease, 438; in health insurance coverage, 414–15, 416, 430–31; in life expectancy, 128–29; in premature births, 11

radiosurgery, 25–26, 403

RAND Health Insurance Experiment (RAND-HIE), 62–63

randomized controlled trials (RCTs), 242–44, 264; clinical practice effects, 247–53; clinical process effects, 246–47; drawbacks, 447–48; ineffective treatment discontinuation and, 247–53; lack of, 261–62; placebo effect, 25, 73, 157, 238, 240, 243, 275, 323, 324; of sepsis treatment, 316

rare diseases, drug therapy development for, 400–401, 479

rationing, of health care, 280

real value, 48

referrals, as conflict of interest. *See* Anti-Kickback Statute

regulation, cost considerations in, 279–85

Reichman, Richard, 10

Reinhardt, Uwe, 102

reliability, professional autonomy *vs.*, 313–17, 467–68

resource-based relative value scale, 171–72

resource redistribution, in health care, 112–13

respiratory distress syndrome (RDS), 11–12

rheumatoid arthritis, treatment cost, 72–73

right, health care as, 66–71, 483, 497

risk aversion, 133–34

risk factors, for disease, 436–41; lifestyle interventions for reduction of, 438–41

risk pools, 216–17, 220

Rockefeller Institute for Medical Research, 155–56

Roemer's law, 83–84, 95

Roosevelt, Franklin D., 148–49, 166

Rorem, C. Rufus, 147

Rose, Robert, 10

Rosen, Sherwin, 272

Rosenbaum, Lisa, 347

Rosenthal, Elisabeth, 325, 406–7

RowdMap, 348

Roy, Avik, 491

safe harbor laws, 293, 296–97, 309, 389, 472

Salk, Jonas, 157

Sanders, Bernie, 493

Self-Determination Act, 10

self-insurance plans, 473–74

self-interest, 38–39

self-referrals, 80, 309, 405, 472. *See also* Anti-Kickback Statute

Semmelweis, Ignaz, 138–39

sepsis, evaluation and treatment, 315–17, 320–21

sexually transmitted diseases, 122, 126

shared savings payment systems, 300

Shatner, William, 125

short-term limited duration (STLD) plans, 223–25, 226, 227, 460, 489

single-payer systems, 461, 490. *See also* universal health care insurance coverage: Medicare for All

smallpox vaccine, 1–2

Smith, Adam, 38–40, 235

smoking, 128, 129, 143, 156, 425, 437, 438, 439, 441, 457

social determinants, of disease, 436–41

socialized medicine, 164, 169

Social Security, 164, 452–53

Social Security Act, 148–49, 168, 178, 463; 1950 amendments, 195, 208–9;

Section 1115, 229; Title XVIII, 170, 171, 172, 300; Title XIX, 170, 196

specialist care, gatekeepers for, 183

specialists: board certification, 49–50, 53, 258, 321, 322; income, 378; Medicaid patients' access to, 126; Medicare reimbursement, 172; monetization of practices, 379; oversupply, 83; recommended standards of care, 260–61; self-referrals, 80; standard of care, 313; supply and utilization correlation, 86–87

spine surgery, hospital expenditures, 179, 180–82

stakeholders, in health care industry, 27, 46, 164, 167, 168, 210, 312–13, 467

standard patient technique, 353–54

standards of care, recommended, 260–61

Stark, Fortney "Pete," 297, 300

Stark law, 291, 297–301, 405; in-office ancillary services (IOAS) exception, 299, 309; proposed revisions, 471, 472; safe-harbor provision, 293, 296–97, 389, 472

stents, coronary, 257–60

Steptoe, Patrick, 7–8

stroke (cerebrovascular accident / "brain attack"), 21–22, 246, 321, 322, 336–37, 441

subsidies, for health care, 212, 331–32, 435; in health care exchanges, 217–18, 224–25, 488; health care utilization and, 54–58, 59, 61–66, 174, 337, 339, 459; for ineffective treatment, 338; of Medicare, 179; for prescription drugs, 356; societal acceptability, 66–71

substance abuse disorder, 25

suicide, 3, 123, 497

sulfanilamide, 323

supply and demand, 50, 459; commodity values, 40–41; information asymmetry and, 53; for physicians, 376, 377–79; price effects, 40–44, 50, 51–52 supply and demand curves, 40; classic economic analysis, 41–44; for in vitro fertilization, 55–58; shifts in, 43–44

supply chains, 407; pharmaceutical, 384–88

supply-side factors, in health care expenditures, 85–90, 94, 98, 100, 336, 469

surgery: advances in, 155, 403; development, 138–39; geographic variation in rates, 81–84; induced demand for, 65

surplus, consumer and producer, 42–43, 372

tamoxifen, 13–14

targeted chemotherapy, 15–16, 246, 397–98

Tauzin, Billy, 392

taxation, 37, 145, 146, 148–49, 153

tax credits: health exchanges–related, 415, 416, 417, 418, 485; means-tested universal, 461, 491–93; Medicaid/CHIP-related, 416, 417, 418; universal coverage system–related, 461

Tax Cuts and Jobs Act, 222, 452

tax-exempt status, of health insurance premiums, 112; in employer-paid health insurance, 37, 46, 77, 136, 161, 164, 166, 167, 168, 174, 363, 435, 481, 494

tax subsidies, for health insurance, 435

Tenet Healthcare Corporation, 295

testimonials, 239

Thaler, Richard, 272

thalidomide, 323

Thomas, E. Donnall, 251

tissue plasminogen activator (t-PA), 21

To Err Is Human: Building A Safer Health System (National Academy of Medicine), 318–21, 327, 328

tonsillectomy rates, 81–83

transcatheter aortic valve replacement (TAVR), 23

trastuzumab, 15

trauma centers, 95–96

treatment: advances in, 1, 3–4; alternative, 266, 460; new, 265

treatment overuse. See medical overuse

treatment rates, geographic variation in, 81–84

TRICARE, 410

Trudeau, Edward Livingstone, 138

Truman, Harry S., 158, 164

Trump, Donald, 191

tuberculosis, 1, 155

Tufts Center for the Study of Drug Development, 351–52

typhoid, immunization against, 1–2

tyrosine kinase inhibitors, 397–98

ultrasound, high-resolution transvaginal, 6–7

uncertainty, clinical decision-making effects, 261–64

underinsured population, 35, 47, 137, 418–21, 435, 451

underwriting, 216–17

Unhealthy Politics (Patashnik et al.), 467

uninsured population, 66, 199, 209, 410–11, 435, 451, 460, 482; under Affordable Care Act, 112–13, 213, 215, 217, 225, 227–29, 409, 415, 485, 489; characteristics, 199, 412, 415–18, 485–86, 487–88; emergency room care, 66–67, 112, 301–3, 309–10, 311, 423, 483–85, 487, 490; health care access, 47, 137, 287, 483–90; health care–related debt, 420, 421, 431, 484; health care utilization rate, 65, 77, 423; insurance eligibility, 415; low-income, 210, 211; under Medicaid and Medicare, 112–13, 213, 231; Medicaid/CHIP eligibility, 416, 418, 485–86; Medicaid coverage gap of, 485–87; Medicaid expansion and, 427–28, 430, 485–87; "patient dumping" problem, 301–3; prior to Affordable Care Act, 210

United Healthcare, 391

United Kingdom, National Institute for Health and Care Excellence (NICE), 279–80, 465